Progress
in the
Management
of the
Menopause

Progress
in the
Management
of the
Menopause

Edited by
Barry G. Wren
MD, BS, MHPEd, FRACOG, FRCOG

Director, Sydney Menopause Centre
Chairman, Scientific Committee of
the 8th International Menopause Society Congress

The Proceedings of the 8th International Congress on the Menopause,
Sydney, Australia, November 1996

The Parthenon Publishing Group
International Publishers in Medicine, Science & Technology

NEW YORK   LONDON

Published in the USA by
The Parthenon Publishing Group Inc.
One Blue Hill Plaza
PO Box 1564, Pearl River,
New York 10965, USA

Published in the UK and Europe by
The Parthenon Publishing Group Limited
Casterton Hall, Carnforth,
Lancs. LA6 2LA, UK

Library of Congress Cataloging-in-Publication Data

International Congress on the Menopause (8th : 1996 : Sydney, N.S.W.)
    Progress in the management of the menopause : proceedings of the
8th International Congress on the Menopause, Sydney, Australia, 3–7
November 1996 / edited by Barry Wren.
      p. cm.
    Includes bibliographical references and index.
    ISBN 1-85070-799-5 (hardcover)
    1. Menopause—Congresses.   I. Wren, Barry G.   II. Title.
    [DNLM: 1. Menopause—congresses.   2. Estrogen Replacement Therapy-
-congresses.   3. Estrogens—therapeutic use—congresses.   WP 580
I61p 1997]
RG186.I57   1996
618.1'75—dc21
DNLM/DLC
for Library of Congress   97-34442
                                                CIP

British Library Cataloguing in Publication Data

Progress in the management of the menopause
    1. Menopause 2. Menopause – Hormone therapy
    I. Wren, Barry G.
    618.1'75
    ISBN 1-85070-799-5

The photograph used for the cover design, of an osteoporotic vertebral body,
has been reproduced by kind permission of
Professor Lis Mosekilde, University of Aarhus, Denmark

Typeset by H&H Graphics, Blackburn, Lancs.
Printed and bound by Butler & Tanner Ltd., Frome and London, UK

Contents

List of principal contributors

N. Albery
Japan Amarant Society
31 Avenues Princess Grace
Monte Carlo
Monaco

T. Aso
Tokyo Medical and Dental University
School of Medicine
1-5-45 Bunkyo-ku
Tokyo 113
Japan

E. E. Baulieu
Unité sur les Communications Hormonales
INSERM U 33
80 rue du Général Leclerc
94276 Le Kremlin-Bicêtre Cedex
France

M. P. Brincat
Department of Obstetrics & Gynaecology
St. Luke's Hospital, Medical School
   (University of Malta)
Gwardamangia
Msida MSD 06
Malta

H. M. Buckler
Department of Endocrinology & Diabetes
Manchester University
Hope Hospital
Stott Lane
Salford
Manchester M6 8HD
UK

K. Carlström
Department of Obstetrics and Gynecology
Huddinge University Hospital
S-141 86 Huddinge
Sweden

A. Collins
Psychology and Psychiatry Section
Department of Clinical Neuroscience
Karolinska Institute
S-171 76 Stockholm
Sweden

S. R. Davis
The Jean Hailes Foundation
291 Clayton Road
Clayton
Victoria 3168
Australia

B. de Lignières
Necker Hospital
149 Rue De Sevres
75015 Paris Cedex 15
France

M. Dören
Universitäts-Frauenklinik Münster
Albert-Schweitzer-Str. 33
D-48129 Münster
Germany

S. V. Drew
The Surgery
12 The Green
Rowlands Castle
Hampshire PO9 6BX
UK

E. F. Eriksen
University Department of Endocrinology
   & Metabolism
Aarhus Amtssygehus
Klokkerbakken 73
DK-8000 Aarhus C
Denmark

J. M. Foidart
Department of Biology
University of Liege
Pathology Tower (B23)
Sart Tilman
B-4000 Liege
Belgium

I. S. Fraser
Sydney Centre for Reproductive Health
    Research
Department of Obstetrics & Gynaecology
University of Sydney
NSW 2006
Australia

M. Gambacciani
Department of Obstetrics and Gynecology
    "P. Fioretti"
University of Pisa
Via Roma 35
56100 Pisa
Italy

L. M. Garcia-Segura
Instituto Cajal (CSIC)
Avenida Doctor Arce 37
28002 Madrid
Spain

A. R. Genazzani
Department of Obstetrics & Gynecology
University of Pisa
Via Roma 35
56100 Pisa
Italy

L. J. G. Gooren
Department of Endocrinology
AZVU
PO Box 7075
1007 MB Amsterdam
The Netherlands

G. I. Gorodeski
Department of Obstetrics & Gynecology
University MacDonald Women's Hospital
11100 Euclid Ave.
Cleveland, OH 44106
USA

A. Graziottin
Casa di Cura del Policlinico
Via Dezza 48
Milan
Italy

J. C. Grimwade
Ultrasound (O&G) and Menopause Units
Monash Medical Centre
246 Clayton Road
Clayton
Victoria 3168
Australia

J. R. Guthrie
Key Centre for Women's Health
The University of Melbourne
211 Grattan Street
Carlton
Victoria 3053
Australia

V. W. Henderson
Department of Neurology (GNH-5641)
University of Southern California
School of Medicine
1200 North State Street
Los Angeles
CA 90033-1084
USA

H. Honjo
Department of Obstetrics and Gynecology
The Kyoto Prefectural University of Medicine
Kawaramachi, Hirokoji
Kamikyo Ku
Kyoto 602
Japan

C. L. Hughes
CMCRC, Department of Comparative
    Medicine
The Bowman Gray School of Medicine
Wake Forest University
Medical Center Boulevard
Winston-Salem, NC 27157-1040
USA

J. R. Jalbuena
4898 Pasay Road
Dasmarinas Village
Makati
The Philippines

S. R. Johnson
Department of Obstetrics and Gynecology
University of Iowa College of Medicine
206 CMAB
Iowa City
Iowa 52242
USA

V. C. Jordan
Robert H. Lurie Cancer Center
Northwestern University Medical School
Olson Pavilion 8256
303 E. Chicago Avenue
Chicago, IL 60611-3008
USA

M. Lachowsky
Service Gyn-Obs
Hôpital Bichat
Université Paris VII
75018 Paris
France

A. H. MacLennan
Department of Obstetrics and Gynaecology
University of Adelaide
Women's and Children's Hospital
72 King William Road
North Adelaide
SA 5006
Australia

W. McCarthy
McCarthy Management Pty Ltd
6/1 Thomson Street
Darlinghurst
NSW 2010
Australia

C. A. Morse
Department of Primary Health Care Practice
RMIT University
Bundoora West
Melbourne, Victoria 3038
Australia

Li. Mosekilde
Department of Cell Biology
Institute of Anatomy
University of Aarhus
DK-8000 Aarhus C
Denmark

T. Moskovic
University Hospital of Gynecology and
    Obstetrics
"Narodni Front"
Department of Menopause and Family
    Planning
Narodnog fronta 62
11000 Beograd
Yugoslavia

A. O. Mueck
University Hospital
Department of Obstetrics and Gynecology
Section Clinical Pharmacology
Schleichstrasse 4
D-72076 Tuebingen
Germany

Y. Muscat Baron
Department of Obstetrics & Gynecology
St. Luke's Hospital, Medical School
    (University of Malta)
Gwardamangia
Msida MSD 06
Malta

E. A. Musgrove
Cancer Research Program
Garvan Institute of Medical Research
St. Vincent's Hospital
384 Victoria Street
Darlinghurst, Sydney
NSW 2010
Australia

S. Palacios
Instituto Palacios
Gynaecological Clinic & Metabolism Research
C/Jorge Juan 36 1° izq
28001 Madrid
Spain

J. H. Pickar
Clinical Research
Wyeth-Ayerst Research
PO Box 8299
Philadelphia
PA 19101-8299
USA

A. Pines
Department of Medicine "T"
Tel Aviv-Elias Sourasky Medical Centre
Ichilov Hospital
6 Weizman Street
Tel-Aviv 64239
Israel

R. L. Prince
Department of Medicine
University of Western Australia
4th Floor, G Block
Sir Charles Gairdner Hospital
Nedlands, WA 6009
Australia

S. Punyahotra
Royal Irrigation Hospital
Parkkred
Nonthaburi 11120
Thailand

D. W. Purdie
Centre for Metabolic Bone Disease
Hull Royal Infirmary
Anlaby Road
Hull HU3 2RW
UK

J. D. Ringe
Medizin Klinik 4
Klinikum Leverkusen
University of Cologne
D-51375 Leverkusen
Germany

P.-J. Roberts
Seven Brooks Medical Centre
21 Church Street
Atherton M46 9DE
UK

J. Russo
Breast Cancer Research Laboratory
Fox Chase Cancer Center
7701 Burholme Avenue
Philadelphia, PA 19111
USA

E.-M. Rutanen
Department of Obstetrics and Gynecology
Helsinki University Central Hospital
Haarmaninkatu 2
SF-00290 Helsinki
Finland

L. A. Salamonsen
Prince Henry's Institute of Medical Research
PO Box 5152
Clayton
Victoria 3168
Australia

G. Samsioe
Department of Obstetrics and Gynecology
Lund University Hospital
S-221 85 Lund
Sweden

K. Schenck-Gustafsson
Karolinska Institute and Hospital
Department of Cardiology
S-171 76 Stockholm
Sweden

E. Seeman
Endocrine Department
Austin & Repatriation Medical Centre
Heidelberg
Studley Road
Melbourne 3084
Australia

B. B. Sherwin
McGill University
Department of Psychology and Dept Ob/Gyn
Stewart Biological Sciences Building
1205 Dr Penfield Avenue
Montreal
Quebec H3A 1B1
Canada

R. Sitruk-Ware
Department of Endocrinology
Hopital Saint-Antoine
Paris
France

M. Smith
Suite 46 Mount Medical Centre
146 Mounts Bay Road
Perth 6000
Australia

S. K. Smith
Department of Obstetrics and Gynaecology
University of Cambridge
Addenbrooke's Hospital
Cambridge CB2 2SW
UK

E. R. Somerville
Department of Neurology
Westmead Hospital
Westmead, NSW 2145
Australia

T. D. Spector
Department of Rheumatology
St. Thomas' Hospital
Lambeth Palace Road
London SE1 7EH
UK

P. H. Stern
Department of Molecular Pharmacology and
    Biological Chemistry S-215
Northwestern University Medical School
303 E. Chicago Ave.
Chicago, IL 60611
USA

J. C. Stevenson
Wynn Department of Metabolic Medicine
Imperial College School of Medicine at the
    National Heart & Lung Institute
21 Wellington Road
London NW8 9SQ
UK

J. J. W. Studd
Fertility and Endocrinology Centre
The Lister Hospital
Chelsea Bridge Road
London SW1W 8RH
UK

W. H. Utian
Department of Obstetrics & Gynecology
University Hospitals of Cleveland
11100 Euclid Avenue
Cleveland, Ohio 44106
USA

A. Vermeulen
Section of Endocrinology
Department of Internal Medicine
University Hospital, De Pintelaan 185
9000 Ghent
Belgium

A. Viitanen
Orion Corporation
Orion Pharma
PO Box 65
SF-02101 Espoo
Finland

S. Wasti
Department of Obstetrics and Gynecology
Aga Khan University
Stadium Road
PO Box 3500
Karachi 74800
Pakistan

N. S. Weiss
School of Public Health and Community
    Medicine
Department of Epidemiology SC36
University of Washington, Box 357236
Seattle
Washington 98195
USA

G. Wilcox
Department of Endocrinology and Diabetes
Ewen Downie Metabolic Unit
Alfred Hospital
Commercial Road
Prahran
Victoria 3181
Australia

B. G. Wren
Sydney Menopause Centre
Royal Hospital for Women
Barker Street
Randwick
NSW 2031
Australia

H. J. Wright
Burson-Marsteller Limited
24–28 Bloomsbury Way
London WC1A 2PX
UK

Foreword

Introduction

Following the International Menopause Society Meeting in Stockholm in 1993, Sydney was selected as the venue for the 1996 Conference. I was nominated as Chairman of the Scientific Program, and over 3 years our committee designed a scientific program which included world experts in a wide variety of disciplines related to the menopause. We included Pharmaceutical Companies into the official program as well as many branches of medicine which impacted on the health and quality of life of both men and women. The meeting was an outstanding success with 3500 delegates and 700 associates. The venue on Sydney Harbour was a delight for all to see and from the Opening Ceremony in the Opera House to the closing session there was only one common complaint. There were so many excellent programs running concurrently that delegates could not get to hear all they wished to attend.

To overcome the problem of a surfeit of excellence, most of the invited speakers have submitted their papers for publication and Parthenon Publishing has produced this excellent book so that delegates can now browse through the papers at their leisure.

This book is a collection of the finest presentations of the 8th International Menopause Society Conference in Sydney in November 1996, and I am pleased to recommend it to all those who were not in attendance as well as for those who were there. I would like to thank Parthenon Publishing, the hard-working staff who have compiled and published this edition, but mostly I would like to thank the contributors who have submitted their various chapters.

It was a pleasure to edit this book and I am proud to be associated with its publication

Barry G. Wren, MD, BS, MHPEd., FRACOG, FRCOG
Chairman Scientific Committee
Editor of Proceedings

Menopause: a modern perspective from a controversial history

1

W. H. Utian

Introduction

The purpose of this paper is to convey one message – all women should have the right to postmenopausal wellness, and it is the responsibility of the medical profession to make it happen.

Exactly 20 years ago in June 1976, 165 people of varying disciplines and backgrounds, but all with one common interest, the female menopause, gathered in the resort town of La Grande Motte in the south of France to attend the First International Congress on the Menopause. The discussions were clustered around subjects like defining the climacteric syndrome, endocrinology of menopause, psychosocial aspects, and estrogen therapy in relation to bones, lipids and endometrial cancer. Representing 22 countries, there were some 40 contributions. While menopause was defined, there was virtually no focus on women's healthcare delivery.

Two decades later in Sydney, Australia, at the Eighth International Menopause Society meeting, there are almost 20 times as many participants from over double the number of countries. The enormously expanded program includes topics such as epidemiological studies, management of the well menopausal woman, possible reduction of the risk of developing new breast cancer, the consequences of longevity, the media and the menopause, and alternative therapies – all representing a dramatic change of focus.

This is a record of phenomenal growth and development. The events leading to that first meeting, the establishment of the International Menopause Society (IMS), the journal *Maturitas,* the evolution of research and health care relating to the menopause, and the future role of the IMS within that context are the topics covered by this paper.

Above all, I stand before you as the outgoing IMS President to pay tribute to the memory of Pieter van Keep, to recall some special moments during our years of close friendship, and to challenge you all to continue the dreams we developed almost 25 years ago.

History: where we were

Attitudes to menopause

The major milestones in the history of menopause provide a fascinating background to the understanding of current attitudes and the prediction of future trends in the management of this event through which all women will inevitably pass.

'Menopause' is a word of multiple meanings. It was once the subject of taboo, but now almost in danger of overexposure. Once neglected, it is now recognized by multiple groups as the entry to a 'market'. The result is a new level of confusion and even exploitation in the minds of the health profession and the public alike.

Menopause as a life event was recognized far back in history. Aristotle (384–322 BC) noted menstruation to cease at age 40 years, and references to the cessation of the age of fertility continue to pepper the literature over the next 2000 years[1]. The Greek words *men* and *pausis* were first utilized to describe the cessation of menstruation, although a Latin basis can also be argued[2]. *Climacteric* appears to be of Greek derivation representing the word for ladder or steps of a ladder.

The review of the attitudes expressed in the literature over the last century makes one wonder whether women were meant to be climbing up or down the ladder! Viewpoints in one extreme were particularly negative; in the other extreme there were some balanced observers attempting to define the normality or universality of the phenomenon of menstrual cessation.

Colombat de L'Isere in a chapter on 'Change of Life' in his *Treatise on the Diseases of Females* (1845)[3] stated:

'Compelled to yield to the power of time, women now cease to exist for the species, and henceforward live only for themselves.'

Further, he stated

'She now resembles a dethroned queen, or rather a goddess whose adorers no longer frequent her shrine. Should she still retain a few courtiers, she can only attract them by the charm of her wit and the force of her talents.'

Charles Meigs, in a letter to his class in 1848 entitled 'Change of Life'[4] asked

'What has she to expect save gray hairs, wrinkles, the gradual decay of these physical and personal attractions, which heretofore have commanded the flattering image of society . . . The pearls of the mouth are become tarnished, the hay-like odor of the breath is gone, the rose has vanished from the cheek, and the lily is no longer the vain rival of the forehead or neck. The dance is preposterous, and the throat no longer emulates the voice of the nightingale'[4].

There are numerous other examples of similar negative attitudes.

The association of menopause and symptoms was also noted long ago. John Leake in 1777 attempted to explain the cessation of menstrual blood flow through a Harveian mechanism, namely, insufficient pumping force through the blood vessels. He also noted the association between menopause, vaginal atrophy and bladder symptoms[5]. It was a British physician, Edward Tilt, in one of the first full-length books on the subject, who noted that 'Women at the change of life are frequently affected with cancer, gout and rheumatism', and also noted that 'Well localized nervous affection sometimes occurs at this critical epoch'[6].

It is only fair to note in passing that men were not immune to writings of the late 19th and early 20th century. An example comes from Syvanus Stall writing in 1901 in *What a Man of 45 Ought to Know*[7] – 'It is usually at the age of 50 or 60 that the generative function becomes weakened. It is at this period that man, elevated to the sacred character of paternity, and proud of his virile power, begins to notice the power decreased, and does so almost with a feeling of indignation. The first step towards feebleness announces to him, unmistakably, that he is no longer the man he was.'

On the other hand, some remarkably astute comments were made by physicians who were really attempting to present the menopause in a positive light and as a natural event. For example, Tilt made the following observation: 'The change of life does not give talents but it often imparts a firmness of purpose to bring out effectively those that are possessed, whether it be to govern a household, to preside in a drawing room, or to thread and unravel political entanglements'[6]. Borner in 1887, over 100 years ago, expressed this point of view best in a statement almost as fresh as the day it was written[8]:

'The climacteric, or so-called change of life in women, presents without question, one of the most interesting subjects offered to the physician, and especially to the gynecologist, in the practice of his profession. The phenomena of this period are so various and changeable, that he must certainly have had a wide experience who has observed and learned to estimate them all. So ill-defined are the boundaries between the physiological and the pathological in this field of study, that it is highly desirable in the interest of our patients of the other sex, that the greatest possible light should be thrown upon this question.'

The narrow boundary between normal physiology and pathology had not been fully defined nearly 100 years later. Nor had the many negative and largely unsubstantiated statements ceased to be made as evidenced by the following examples.

In 1963, 'A large percentage of women . . . acquire a vapid cow-like feeling called a 'negative state'. It is a strange endogenous misery . . . the world appears as though through a gray veil, and they live as docile, harmless creatures missing most of life's values'[9].

In 1963, 'The menopausal woman is not normal; she suffers from a deficiency disease with serious sequelae and needs treatment'[10].

In 1966, 'Often busy mothers or energetic careerists who are unwilling or unprepared to acknowledge the termination of the reproductive phase of their lives and the inception of a new era are thrown into considerable turmoil by this event'[11].

In 1967, 'Many women are leading an active and productive life when this tragedy strikes. They are still attractive and mentally alert. They deeply resent what to them, is a catastrophic attack upon their ability to earn a living and enjoy life'[12].

Management of menopause

Historical treatments were aimed either at attempting to cure specific diseases which were claimed to be associated with menopause, or to alleviation of psychological symptoms which were likewise blamed on 'this critical time of life' (Leake, 1777)[5,13]. They varied from blood-letting to purgatives, from crushed powdered penis of the ass to raw eggs. Leake recommended 'At meals she may be indulged with a half of pint of old clear London Porter or a glass of rhenish wine'.

Clearly perimenopause by the late 19th century had been recognized as a potential syndrome, and orthodox and unorthodox treatments were applied. Again, men were not immune from the concept of a 'male climacteric', and Haller and Haller reported 'Whether real or imaginary, permanent or temporary, sexual impotency was a source of great anxiety for the nineteenth century male and his apprehensions furnished a lucrative market for unscrupulous quacks, clairvoyants, mesmerizers, natural healers, faith-curers, anatomical museums and layers-on-hand in his search for his recovery of his sexual powers'[14]. Nothing seems to be different today!

The concept of treatment was, however, about to heat up. In early 1896, exactly 100 years ago, three published reports represent the first on a new concept, the 'dawn of hormone replacement therapy'[15]. Separately, three groups in Germany reported trials to alleviate menopause-related symptoms by means of substitution with ovarian therapy[15].

Butenandt, a Nobel Prize winner for this work, succeeded with other research workers in 1929 in isolating and obtaining in pure form a hormone from the urine of pregnant women which was eventually to be called estrone[16]. The structural formulae of this and related hormones were worked out by Butenandt (1930) and others.

A logical development in the expanding history of glandular therapy was the substitution of the newly available estrogens in place of crushed ovaries and the like. By the early 1930s many reports began to appear on the use of 'amniotin' for hot flushes, sweats, nervousness and libido[17]. This form of treatment became popular from the early 1960s onwards, under the general description of estrogen replacement therapy. Initially, reports of this new therapy, the era of 'feminine forever', followed a similar pattern. They generally began with extremely negative statements about the menopause, which were then followed by dramatically positive descriptions for reversal of such effects by the treatment, invariably claiming the properties to be age-preventing. A classic example from this period is the following:

'At the age of 50 there are no ova, no follicles, no theca cells, no estrogen – truly a galloping catastrophe. The timely admini-stration of natural estrogens plus an appropriate progestogen to middle-aged women will prevent the climacteric and menopause – a syndrome that seems unnecessary for most of the women in the civilized world. The estrogenic treatment of older women will inhibit osteoporosis and thus help to prevent fractures, as long as they continue healthful activities and appropriate diets. Breasts and genital organs will not shrivel. Such women will be much more pleasant to live with and will not become dull and unattractive'[23].

It must be emphasized that at this time, although menopause was equated with a disease, and the specific treatment involved one medication or other, already the first ideas for preventive care were emerging.

A personal odyssey

This year 1996 represents the 30th anniversary of the author's personal professional involve-ment with menopause, and whose interest in the subject virtually coincided with the publication by Robert Wilson of his book *Feminine Forever*. A complete survey of the menopause literature up to 1966 seemed very inadequate. Late that year, just before Christian Barnard completed the historic first human transplant at the Groote Schuur Hospital in Cape Town, South Africa, the present author started a menopause research clinic with the initial interests of clarifying what the menopause really was, and to define the proper place of hormone replacement therapy. The Menopause Clinic, probably the world's first, proved to be the ideal situation to achieve this purpose, and within a relatively short time the first results of the clinic's studies began to be reported in the medical literature.

Working and publishing research reports in the late 1960s and early 1970s in a remote place like Cape Town was very much like throwing stones into a pond and hoping a ripple would return. In April 1973 a letter was received from Pieter A. van Keep, MD, Director-General of the International Health Foundation (IHF) based in Geneva, Switzerland, inviting research collaboration and telling of his early social studies on menopause. I had heard neither of him or the IHF but was delighted to discover another 'menopausologist'. By coincidence, I was about to travel to Europe the next month. I therefore responded requesting some time with him in Geneva. In later years, Pieter shared an internal memo he circulated within the Foundation – 'Does this Wulf Utian think that the IHF is a travel agency'?! Nonetheless, a date and time were set for my visit, and the result was quite extraordinary.

Pieter met me at Geneva airport, explained somewhat sheepishly that he had a light day at the office, would show me some of Geneva, and then we would meet Guus, his wife, for dinner.

The day turned out quite different. It was, when the history of menopausology was written, a true milestone. It was also the beginning of an instant and remarkable friendship that lasted until van Keep's premature death on June 17th, 1991, after the Bangkok IMS meeting. During the course of that initial brainstorming day the idea of a menopause club was conceptualized, to be a friendly organization which would draw together the few people world-wide with an interest in the subject of menopause to a series of meetings planned for Geneva under the auspices of the IHF. Of course, this club was later to become the IMS in November, 1978. There would most certainly be a need for some sort of newsletter or journal to act as a vehicle for news and new findings; this was the original concept later to become *Maturitas* in 1978. We spoke of holding gatherings in exotic places such as the Bahamas, Sri Lanka or Hawaii, the meetings ultimately to be the IMS congresses. Above all this author's basic and clinical science research approach melded well with van Keep's psycho-social interests. We spoke of a new concept of healthy women care, an idea for enhanced quality years for women by primary preventive health care, utilizing menopause as a positive entry point. This latter dream is yet to be achieved, and will be discussed further below.

Over the next 3 years we met several times and corresponded furiously – ideas for an advisors' panel on estrogens and menopause for the IHF, the establishment of an independent estrogen/menopause research unit sponsored by the IHF, an 'International Reference Center for menopause research', an International Menopause Congress in 1976 at La Grande Motte and an 'International Society for the Study of the Climacteric and Postmenopause', to be launched in 1978.

Those 3 years were difficult ones: an adversarial event with the apartheid South African government had made several people advise that the present author's continuing career in South Africa was jeopardized and 1976, just before the Soweto riots, saw a relocation to the United States.

The move to Case Western Reserve University and University Hospitals of Cleveland in 1976 coincided with the development of a major controversy regarding hormone treatment after menopause. The 'estrogen forever' attitude of the late 1960s and early 1970s had been transformed to a fear of uterine cancer after the publication of some medical research studies in late 1975. Moreover, the power of the media, the influence of a youth-oriented culture, the attention of the consumerists, the well-expressed feelings of the feminists, the inconsistent attitudes of different governmental agencies, the medical profession's fear of potential malpractice litigation and numerous other factors, had obviously combined to cause confusion in the minds of many providing health care and for women approaching menopause. They could no longer feel absolutely sure that they knew what it was all about or what they could or should do about it.

The research world, too, was confused, and this was evidenced at the First International Menopause conference at La Grande Motte in 1976. It was clear to all attendees that better information and forums for presenting data were necessary, and that an International Menopause Society was essential.

In retrospect, it seems remarkable that in the short space of time between 1973 and 1978 so much could have happened – notably, the founding of the IMS, the launch of *Maturitas*, the beginnings of national menopause societies and the recognition and development of meaningful menopause-related research, almost unthinkable at that fateful meeting back in 1973. We now need to carefully consider our current status organizationally and in the delivery of appropriate health care.

Where we are

Population trends

The 'baby boom' that followed the Second World War has had a continuous affect on society. The ranks of the baby boom children born between 1946 and 1960 are now exerting considerable power. After decades of the expanding influence of a youth-oriented culture, a slow but inexorable change is taking place that is impacting on many facets of the way of life and for the needs of health-care delivery.

Life expectancy at birth for most countries continues to increase[18,19]. The incidence and death rates of a whole range of diseases increases with age, outstanding examples represented by coronary heart disease[20], lung cancer and prevalence of diabetes mellitus[20]. Many of these problems are being accelerated and impacted on by preventable factors. Most pernicious of these is cigarette smoking, a dangerous habit or addiction still increasing in frequency in far too many countries of the world[20].

Role of menopause

Today we recognize menopause to be a time of normal physiological change often coinciding with a changing family- or work-environment. The menopause transition is extremely variable within and across cultures. The complexity of hormonal, psycho-sociocultural and aging factors produces a varied symptomatology and long-term health outcomes. Consequently untangling the relationship between menopause, aging, disease and behavioral change has been plagued with methodological difficulties.

Currently, in most parts of the world, distribution of health care is through a 'crisis care model'. Thus patients develop symptoms, or manifest disease, are seen through acute care centers and may then enter chronic care. In this instance, the system waits for the development of a problem and then attempts treatment, much of which is 'salvage' and not really cure. Under this care model, the elderly spend far too many years of their expected life span living with disease-related disability.

The new paradigm for health care is the 'preventive model'. Only a systematic process of screening and preventive care programs can spare our institutions and societies from an escalating financial and social burden.

Under these circumstances the menopause represents both an important signal in the chronological life cycle and a physiological event to be considered from a medical perspective. That is, of the potential diseases that may impact on a women beyond menopause, some may be coincidental or age-related and some might be related to perimenopausal endocrine changes. From a preventive health perspective, however, appropriate screening for all potential diseases, irrespective of potential causation, needs to be introduced in a cost-effective manner.

With this approach it is apparent that once risk factors are identified, preventive care programs need to be introduced and monitored. Some of these programs may be non-specific but beneficial, for example smoking cessation, exercise, diet modification; others might be more specific dependent on the inherent causal relationship, for example hormone replacement therapy (HRT) for menopausal hormone-related effects.

Menopause clinics, as currently established, are a good first step towards a preventive health-care paradigm; but they too are dependent upon patients seeking the services of the clinic[13].

A vast literature already exists relating to all these aspects, but what role should the International Menopause Society play in this?

International Menopause Society now

First, consider where the IMS is now. The IMS is currently an international society of 652 individual members from 43 countries. 'Article 2' of the statutes declares the objectives of the Society shall be to:

(1) Promote the study of all aspects of the climacteric in both men and women;

(2) Organize, prepare, hold and participate in international meetings and congresses on subjects related to objective (1); and

(3) Advance the interchange of research plans and experience between individual members of the Society.

Review of 'Article 2 – Objectives' shows a limitation to the potential activities and goals of the organization. The objective of promotion of study of the subject, organizing international meetings and advancing interchange of research plans and experience are being adequately met, but the next millennium is going to require far more than this.

To achieve additional objectives there is also a need to change the organs of the Society and make it truly representative of its international membership. This is being achieved by adding a third body (organ), namely, beyond the general assembly and executive committee, there will be a Council of Affiliated Menopause Societies. The result will be to bring in representation from every country in which there is a local menopause organization affiliated with the IMS. At present there are 15 national societies affiliated with the IMS. With this enhancement of the IMS structure, what should we really plan and activate for the future?

The future

From a general perspective, the major challenge we face is to reduce mortality and morbidity in an aging population. Prolongation of life is not an essential, but enhancement of quality of life is. As no country can afford the escalating burden of paying for increased numbers of older people with problems like osteoporosis, heart disease, cancer and Alzheimer's disease, national primary preventive health-care programs as a matter of public health policy are the obvious solution.

Given that menopause is a clear event in the human life cycle, we have here a fortunate alarm system for the individual to become involved in a preventive health program for the rest of her life. How should the health system be structured to meet this need?

The diversity of health systems world-wide, accessibility to health care by individuals and resources available, negate the possibility of 'one solution fits all'. The principle for provision of care and the requirements or specifics of such care should, however, be universal.

A primary requirement is a political and social acceptance of the need to make universal preventive health care for women after menopause a matter of public health policy. Next is a need for definition and development of the appropriate infrastructure to provide preventive screening and follow-up. Such a system would require a satisfactory level of primary-care health delivery fully supported by a tertiary-care back-up system. As the ability to deliver the appropriate preventive care is set in place, national menopause awareness and education programs need to be activated. Providers need factual guidelines and clinical care paths for cost-effective health delivery while consumers need to be made aware of the programs and be stimulated to utilize them.

The evolving managed care phenomenon in the United States, while certainly presenting major problems, has on the other hand stimulated thinking towards new directions for health-care delivery. On a micro-scale, the Cleveland model for University Hospitals Health System (UHHS) serves as one example. UHHS will essentially become one of three provider organizations in the tri-county area around Cleveland. Each will be responsible for about one-third of covered lives in an area of about 3 million people. Within UHHS, the University Hospitals serve as the tertiary-care delivery system and center for development of clinical guidelines, education programs and research. The tri-county area surrounding the hospital has a network of primary-care offices and primary-care surgery centers and hospitals.

Managed care involves a 'rationing' of resources, or at the very least, a method for co-ordinating delivery on a cost-effective basis. Prevention of escalation of future costs drives a need to reduce the incidence of major diseases and thus the need for expensive in-hospital services. Hence, the rapid evolution from a 'crisis care' delivery system to one more balanced between both crisis- and preventive-care paradigms, becomes cost-effectiveness driven.

Success for such a system of health care mandates development of education programs, screening guidelines and 'treatment care-paths'. There is no reason why these systems, as they are developed, cannot be expanded into a proforma for a national, or indeed, an international health policy, applicable in all countries, rich or poor. It is this background that drives the present author's vision for the role of the IMS in the future.

Expanded role for the International Menopause Society

The IMS needs to expand its role beyond simply supporting a 3-yearly scientific meeting. The new objectives should include activities such as:

(1) Screening/treatment guidelines;

(2) Public/national health policy advocacy;

(3) Information clearing house – for and between national societies.

Screening/treatment guidelines If the IMS membership accepts the concept of long-term primary preventive health care as a social and national priority and obligation, there follows a need for clear recommendations on cost-effective screening tests and interventions, medical and psycho-social. Even if not every country can support or afford such programs, minimal ideal guidelines need to be set.

The Executive Committee and the Council of Affiliated Menopause Societies should jointly and urgently develop a mechanism for sharing of information and developing comprehensive guidelines for clinical preventive services. These guidelines will have to take into account cost-effectiveness analysis, the ethical implications of such recommendations, national variations, socio-cultural differences and availability of resources.

The IMS should be in the position ultimately to provide recommendations for clinical practice on preventive interventions not only for menopause-related target conditions, but also for those to which a postmenopausal population is at risk irrespective of cause. These interventions should include screening tests, counseling interventions, immunization and pharmaco–prophylactic regimens. An example of the guidelines that could be developed or enhanced are those produced by the US Preventive Services Task Force[21].

Public/national health policy The IMS at this time has extremely limited resources, both financial and in terms of personnel. A liaison committee should therefore be developed to draw in support and representation for each national society as well as between various international organizations, especially those such as the World Health Organization (WHO), International Red Cross and United Nations Educational, Scientific and Cultural Organization (Unesco). The IMS could play the role of catalyst, co-ordinator and provider to national societies of material developed by the international committee on public health policy and preventive health care.

At the very least, the IMS should have an advocacy role for postmenopausal women at the international level, and an ability to back national societies with information and guidelines as they attempt to foster change at a local level within their own national boundaries.

The new Council of Affiliated Menopause Societies should assume as its first and immediate challenge the development of an international policy mission statement and a mechanism to develop policy and guidelines on an ongoing basis.

Information clearing house The explosion in modern technology and information systems makes access to current scientific research far simpler and more effective for virtually any investigator irrespective of their domicile. There is therefore little role or possibility for the IMS to provide the basis for a scientific information resource.

The IMS role should rather be to develop a clearing house for items such as national guidelines, committee consensus statements and national policy decisions or legislation. This material should be instantly accessible to any national organization seeking to develop their own version of clinical guidelines and care paths, prospective legislation documents or policy statements.

An expanded role as a clearing house of current international and cross-cultural research activities could also be contemplated.

Conclusions

Over 60 years ago, Maranon, in the preface to his book *The Climacteric (The Critical Age)*[22] wrote:

> 'In considering the menopause, we face a curious fact. The newly graduated physician has scarcely more than a vague idea of what the state is and what it signifies in human physiology and pathology. If you turn to the literature for an amplification of these vague, general ideas, you will have a hard time finding a comprehensive and modern study of climacteric transition . . . yet the problem of menopause comes up every day, every hour, in the professional work of every physician.'

Until the mid 1960s, there continued to exist in the medical literature a remarkable lack of established scientific data relating to human climacteric. During recent years much necessary information has been presented by leading specialists in the field through workshops and conferences, and in journals and texts. Many gaps in our knowledge still exist.

The single biggest challenge to health care of the perimenopausal woman lies not in further defining the condition nor in the elucidation of better forms of treatment, although both are obviously necessary. Rather, the issue is the delivery of currently acceptable levels of postmenopausal health care to the entire population at risk, in all countries of the world.

A critical gap exists in the area of preventive medicine for women of middle age. Traditional 'menopause clinics' have been dismally unsuccessful in initiating broad programs of preventive medicine, although their research roles have been extremely productive and justify their further existence. The establishment of new 'climacteric centers' is highly cost-productive unless that role can be expanded into one of co-ordinator of regional preventive programs. Achievement of the dream of wide-scale introduction of preventive health-care services to a properly informed public is certain to be successful in reducing morbidity to older women, as was the introduction years ago of proper prenatal care in reducing death and disability related to childbirth.

Over 20 years ago van Keep, the present author and others dreamed of something big, an international menopause club, with a journal and a regular congress in exotic places. These dreams have been realized. Were Pieter with me here today, I am confident that he would have had a vision with me for even greater things, all leading to prevention of disease and enhancement of quality of life for all women after menopause.

My journey on the 'menopause road' has been exciting and personally rewarding. Once lonely, it is now crowded with memories, good friends, colleagues and co-workers from every corner of the world. It is with extremely mixed emotions that I stand down this week as President of our Society and pass on the baton to the next generation. I hope you will expand the dream, the vision and the motivation. It is all worth the effort.

God bless and God speed!

References

1. O'Dowd, M. and Philipp, E. E. (1994). *The History of Obstetrics and Gynecology*, pp. 317–28. (New York: Parthenon Publishing)
2. Wilbush, J. (1979). La menespausie – the birth of a syndrome. *Maturitas*, 1, 145–51
3. Colombat de L'Isere, M. (1845). Treatise on the Diseases of Females. Translated by Meigs, C. D. (Philadelphia, PA: Lea and Blanchard)
4. Meigs, C. D. (1848). Females and their Diseases: a Series of Letters to his Class, p. 444. (Philadelphia, PA: Lea and Blanchard)
5. Leake, J. (1777). Chronic or Slow Diseases Peculiar to Women. (London: Baldwin)
6. Tilt, E. J. (1857). *The Change of Life in Health and Disease.* (London: Churchill)
7. Stall, S. (1901). *What a Man of 45 Ought to Know.* (Philadelphia, PA: London)
8. Borner, E. (1887). The menopause. In *Cyclopaedia of Obstetrics and Gynecology*, Vol. II. (New York: William Wood)
9. Wilson, R. A. and Wilson, T. A. (1963). The fate of the non-treated postmenopausal woman. A plea for the maintenance of adequate estrogen from puberty to the grave. *J. Am. Geriatr. Soc.*, 11, 347
10. Wilson, R. A., Brevetti, R. E. and Wilson, T. A. (1963). Specific procedures for the elimination of the menopause. *West. J. Surg. Obstet. Gynecol.*, 71, 110
11. Davis, M. E. (1966). Modern management of menopausal patient. *Can. Med. Digest*, 33, 39
12. Rhoades, F. P. (1967). Minimizing the menopause. *J. Am. Geriatr. Soc.*, 15, 346
13. Utian, W. H. (1980). *Menopause in Modern Perspective.* (New York: Appleton Century Crofts)
14. Haller, J. S. and Haller, K. M. (1974). The Physician and Sexuality in Victorian America. (Urbana, IL: Illinois University Press)
15. Kopera, H. (1991). The dawn of hormone replacement therapy. *Maturitas*, 13, 187–8
16. Butenandt, A. (1930). Uber die Reindarstellung des Follikel-hormons aus Schwangerenharn. *Z. F. Physiol. Chem.*, 191, 127
17. Geist, S. H. and Spielman, F. (1932). The

therapeutic value of amniotin in the menopause. *Am. J. Obstet. Gynecol.*, **23**, 697–707
18. National Center for Health Statistics (1994). *Life Expectancy*. Health United States, 1993. (Hyattsville, MD: Public Health Service)
19. US Congress, Office of Technology Assessment (1992). *The Menopause, Hormone Therapy, and Women's Health*, OTA-BP-BA-88. (Washington, DC: US Government Printing Office)
20. The Jacobs Institute of Women's Health (1995). *The Women's Health Data Book*. (Washington, DC: The Jacobs Institute of Women's Health)
21. US Preventive Services Task Force (1996). *Guide to Clinical Preventive Services*. (Baltimore, MD: Williams and Wilkins)
22. Maranon, G. (1929). *The Climacteric (The Critical Age)*. (St Louis, MI: Mosby)

1

Plenary papers

Politics of the menopause: my body, my life, my choice

2

N. Albery

I am a peculiar Japanese, born and raised in Japan but a British subject by marriage, now living in Monaco and roaming ubiquitously inside Europe. However, had I been an insider Japanese, thinking and behaving the way it was expected of me, could I have dared and founded the Japan Amarant Society as I did 6 years ago? I doubt it very much. If menopause remained the last taboo until only recently even to the American baby-boomers, one could imagine how much more of a taboo it would be in a society still very much governed by the Confucian maxim: if there is something stinking, put a lid on it.

Equally, if my social and economic existence depended entirely on Japanese society and its goodwill, should I question Japan's medicopolitical system as frankly as I do? I had better not; but my usefulness as an outsider has been my speaking out loud what the insiders would not and could not dare, so I consider it my duty to rush in where Japanese angels fear to tread.

My own menopause hell (koneki-jigoku)

First, I start from where it all began with my own menopause, about which, like too many women of my generation, I knew nothing and noticed nothing as I had my uterus and one ovary removed when I was aged 42 years at the American Hospital in Paris. With hindsight I believe I plunged into my menopausal disarray the moment my husband was diagnosed to be dying from an inoperable cancer. After his death I completely fell apart, mentally as well as physically. Then one day, my maid, a saucy

French woman about my age, lifted her skirt to show me a smart transparent patch on her bottom and said; 'Perhaps Madame too needs this?' How lucky that I happened to be living in the country where the end of reproductivity is not considered the end of femininity.

My mother had either forgotten or been too embarrassed to talk about menstruation soon enough; I had already suffered a nasty shock of imagining myself slowly bleeding to death at the age of 12 years. Thirty-six years later, I was once again caught unawares by my body's biological change; and to think that, had I understood my body's aging process and coped with it by hormone replacement therapy (HRT) in time, I could have assisted my dying husband with far more strength, calm and courage! The sense of remorse still torments me and has been the driving force behind my Amarant Society of Japan activities. I want my generation of Japanese women to be the last to enter menopause ignorant, unprepared or prejudiced to their own detriment by too much misinformation and taboo.

When I wrote an article on my menopausal decline and the resurrection from it by HRT (the first time, I believe, that hormone replacement therapy was reported in a non-medical publication in Japan), I had to beg, bully and cajole an old school friend working for a woman's magazine to publish the article, and she in turn had to fight against her colleagues who feared that an article on such a depressing, off-putting subject might damage the magazine's circulation.

That was 6 years ago, and since then the unstoppable trend of Japanese living longer, and once ill taking longer to die has accelerated beyond all imagination. Books with titles like *Shouldn't Parents Die in Good Time for Children?* or *How to Die Smart* flood the bookshops. The word which only a few years ago no one could pronounce, *kotsu so shô shô*, or osteoporosis, has become a household word. The predominantly male gynecologists, whose prestige and income mainly used to derive from obstetrics and infertility treatment, are so alarmed by the dizzy fall in natality that they are obliged to turn their attention to the hitherto neglected market of middle-aged women. With a very high level of literacy in Japan, newspapers and magazines have done much in removing the Confucian lid from the menopause and familiarizing people with the idea of HRT.

Such background changes helped increase membership of the Amarant Society and each time our existence was mentioned somewhere, hundreds of letters came pouring into our office. I read them, and was flabbergasted. Of course, there were many letters of gratitude and immense relief, but the majority of them told me that I, an uprooted Japanese, had grossly misjudged the country's health system and its working realities. Japan, reputedly so advanced in high technology and science, had a health care system quite unadapted, even hostile to caring for women during and after menopause. I felt guilty that I had been advocating HRT in Japan, where the obstacles to a safe and lasting HRT seemed to be rooted in the rigid bureaucratic system itself. What could a well-meaning but insignificant grass-root organization like ours effectively do?

Bureaucrats and I

When in despair, I make a point of going to the top, in this case to *Koseishô*, the Ministry of Health and Welfare. I pulled all the available strings and managed to obtain an audience with the Minister himself, who, with a selfless generosity seldom encountered in Japanese politics, arranged for me a meeting with his top bureaucrat and two officials in charge of geriatric welfare, saying: 'A politically appointed minister like me has such an ephemeral life in

office to be of real help . . .' To the three dignitaries I recklessly proposed: 'I have done my best, but have come to the limit. But Amarant enjoys a good name and an ongoing momentum. Please couldn't you exploit them somehow? Why not an Amarant section inside the local government's adult education system or family planning network? Perhaps create a chain of health co-operatives for women after menopause?' There was a dead silence, then I heard: 'What is Amarant in substance but your concept, your zeal and a thousand or so members? As for the hormone remedy, it needs a far-reaching examination.' Deciphered, this officialese would mean: 'Amarant? No thanks. HRT? Let's wait and see.'

Undaunted, I continued: 'The ancient Chinese believed that medicine is for still-healthy people, and the doctor's job to keep them in their not-yet-ill state for as long as possible. In today's jargon: preventive medicine. Our concept is the same, and HRT, probably the most cost-effective and humane gift to women in the late 20th century, is an integral part of this concept. Tell me, what is your concept behind 'the bedridden zero campaign' that I hear a lot about?'

The reply: 'In order to significantly reduce the number of bedridden, our new concept is to make them more active, rather than passive. Instead of keeping them permanently in bed, we'll encourage them to exercise and walk twice daily.'

'Can they walk?' I asked.

'Not really, but nurses will help.'

I left the Ministry, determined to continue our small, ramshackle campaign: to teach women to take charge of their body and life and future whilst they still can; to become aware of their political power and demand changes in the medical system, so that they will not be walking the crowded airless hospital corridor, hanging from the nurses' shoulders like wet laundry!

To achieve this we need international help for the following reasons. Ruth Benedict said in her book *The Chrysanthemum and the Sword* that Japan's is a culture of shame. An oversimplification perhaps, but as far as the politics is concerned, she has been proved right time and again. Our political leaders will be moved to take action and allow changes more readily by the mounting criticism and pressures coming from abroad than by their own voters. In other words, they succumb when they feel ashamed enough in the international arena. I feel squeamish about exploiting such underhand tactics, but with only 3 years ahead of us to the next International Menopause Congress in Yokohama, I have decided to wash the dirty family laundry here and now. Many Japanese may find this the height of bad taste, but something must change, and change quickly.

HRT realities in Japan

If you ask me, 'Would you have continued with your HRT, had you begun it in Japan?' I will have to answer, 'No, how could I, with only two types of estrogen available?'

Until autumn 1995 when at long last Oestraderm® passed the tests, only estriol and Premarin® had been approved; and at present, of the three, only estriol is officially approved for treating osteoporosis, therefore the one and only to be officially reimbursed by the state for this purpose. As for progestogens, plenty have been approved, but not for the treatment of menopause symptoms. Further, only the acute symptoms of estrogen deficiency are to be covered by health insurance but not when they are considered chronic, nor for prevention. One can easily imagine that such inflexible rules force many compassionate doctors to lie (especially when the expensive tests are involved) in order to help alleviate the financial burden on low-income patients, then live in fear of the official inspections,

These are roughly today's realities surrounding the available hormones and the treatment of menopause in the land where 80% of women during and after menopause suffer varying degrees of estrogen deficiency, 22% of them severely; therefore the potential number of women in need of HRT may easily surpass the total population of Austria or of Switzerland,

and in the not too distant future, perhaps, of both together.

From my own experience I believe that HRT must be an *à la carte* treatment, individually adjusted with the subtlest nuances. I suffered discouraging side-effects as I had to cope with the dosage intended for occidental women; but luckily, living as I did in Europe, I could switch and change till I found my ideal type, namely, gel.

At the first menopause workshop we organized in Tokyo in 1992, I asked the hormonophobic female audience 'To which type of female hormone will you feel the least fear and resistance?' The overwhelming majority raised hands for the transdermal type, more particularly, to the gel form. Inspired by this reaction and also seeing too many women panic at some perfectly predictable side-effects, listen to their old-school general practitioners (GPs), abandon HRT and return to the typical Japanese round of shiatsu, accupuncture, moxibustion, kigon, thermal bath, and endlessly so on, I telephoned the French gel maker and begged him to have the product marketed in Japan. His response was blunt: 'Sorry, not interested. Your ministry's approval system is too cumbersome, financially too onerous, and too time-consuming.'

Who are the losers? Japanese women. So, I approached a leading domestic pharmaceutical firm, suggesting that they either buy the patent or enter into a joint venture to produce such a tried-and-tested hormonal preparation.

'Not interested. The price range set by the ministry for this type of medicine is much too low' was the answer. To my naive question: 'Isn't it wonderful that it's so cheap?' came the retort: 'A daily requirement of both estrogen and progestogen combined comes to a mere ¥50. Do you suppose that will tempt us let alone doctors to recommend HRT?'

Here we stumble on another fundamental problem: under the current system the doctor's remuneration chiefly comes from tests conducted on the premises and the medicine he directly hands out to his patient, rationed for up to 2 weeks only for one visit. Neither his

14

diagnostic talent, experience, compassion nor the time he spends on counseling is taken into consideration over and above the legally set limit, currently ¥2400 (US$21) for the first consultation and thereafter, ¥700 (US$6), a price of a cup of coffee in a hotel lobby, whether he listens to a whining patient for 3 or 30 min, whether he is a professor or someone who started practicing last week. Is it surprising then that we read in letter after letter the same old complaint: 'Before hustling me out with a bag full of medicine, he did not once look at me!'

When we questioned 359 women in our own survey, 'How long did you go on visiting one branch of medicine after another before you finally discovered that your trouble was due to menopause?' the average length of such frustrating wandering or to put it crudely, passing the buck of time-consuming middle-aged women, came to 64 months, a big chunk out of a lifetime.

A so-called *fachidioten* syndrome this may be, each specialist being brilliantly isolated in his own field, but the fact that the doctor's counseling is so unjustly rewarded must be largely responsible for this lamentable statistic and what is commonly known as an 'in-and-out-in-3-minute' consultation.

Understandably, the number of private menopause clinics is growing. This is good news for those who can afford ¥50 000 or more for an hour-long first consultation with the rare privilege of being able to obtain an appointment in advance. However, what about the large majority who cannot afford such luxury?

'Tell me: what am I taking?'

Hormone replacement therapy without adequate explanation is disastrous to patients' compliance, but there is yet another hurdle even to those determined to stay with HRT: this is the fact that the loose tablets sold directly by the treating doctors carry no name, no indication of components and come without instructions or precautions for use. All that is read on each tablet is a row of letters and numbers, much like what one sees on the number-plate of a car. Regularly we receive letters containing sample tablets of astonishing varieties with a plea: 'Tell me. What am I taking?'

Unidentifiable tablets are one thing, but worse is when treatment involves injections. Many seemingly mature and coherent women come to me and whisper: 'What do you think is happening to me? Thick black hair is growing on queer places, and my voice . . .' and so on. When I whisper back: 'Male hormone', they are speechless, looking nauseated. Most of them thought it was some sort of fortifying vitamin injection.

'Why didn't you find out before it was inside your one and only body?'

'But he is my doctor. How can I offend him by questioning what he does for me?' is the usual exchange.

Japanese women of all ages tend to see the extension of partriarchal omnipotence and authority in their treating doctors, especially their GPs, and coyly try to be the doctor's pet patient. This may explain the high rate of HRT drop-outs and the stubborn hormonophobia amongst those who parrot their GPs' prejudice and ignorance. So, women are partly to blame for the unintended virilism, but still I cannot help wondering why the Ministry of Health and Welfare, otherwise so pathologically cautious and fault-finding, approved such esoteric cocktails, composed of estrone, testosterone, androstenedione, androstenediol, thyroxin, and so on.

Urogenital neglect

When I read the report that, due to eating so many soya-bean products, Japanese women suffered far less menopausal symptoms, I thought: 'If it were so, the splendid vegetable estrogen must be bypassing the huge majority of the Japanese urogenitalia.'

Reading from a letter written by a 56 year-old housewife: 'I'm so embarrassed and ashamed to bring this up, but I am in despair. Please, how can I possibly obtain the hormone pessaries made in Europe, the photograph of which accompanied your recent article? That area has been painfully inflamed and infected almost non-stop since my hysterectomy operation at the age of 44. The itching pain is often like a bad burn. Passing urine is sheer agony and often I cannot hold it till I get to the toilet. I tried everything from talcum powder to bicarbonate of soda solution, even mentholatum. My husband nags and complains that I am a rotten useless wife; so, feeling guilty, I accept him from time to time, but afterwards I bleed and burn and suffer for days. A month ago I finally went to consult a gynecologist in the nearest city, suffering great discomfort from having to sit with my legs pressed together for 2 hours each way on a train and a bus. The doctor laughed and said in front of a young nurse: "Still doing it at 56? Try abstinence," and gave me anti-fungal ointment and tranquilizer.'

This is by no means an exceptionally gory or sad urogenital letter amongst so many that I have read. In fact some women are so desperate that they resort to stealing. At each of the Amarant Menopause Workshops we organized in major cities from Hiroshima in the south to Yamagata in the northeast, we exhibited as many and varied hormonal medicines as I could obtain in Europe, spread out on one or two large tables in the lobby, set against one small table with the meagre collection available in Japan, as a visual protest. Soon we began noticing that most of the vaginal pessaries and creams were missing after the meeting and have been obliged since to tape these particular exhibits onto the table tops to discourage theft.

When I did discover that one estriol vaginal tablet has been approved by the Ministry but that this godsend tablet, being dry and hard and square, needs to be inserted by the doctor, I urged the manufacturer to turn it into a user-friendly, slippery lozenge. 'Alas,' he said. 'Even to change the form of presentation, the Ministry's approval will take 6 years and will cost too much to justify the operation.'

It is no wonder, therefore, that in Japan the manufacture of incontinence panties is thriving. Every time I see their prominent advertisement, boasting a new deodorizing device, I think of bedridden geriatric patients, helped out of bed and made to walk under the slogan of 'down to zero the bedridden!' To my mind, both symbolize the defeat of the health care system that mops up only after it has leaked.

If the medical system designed exclusively for illness and injury but not for prevention or check-ups on the one hand, and the traditional medical ethic of life-preserving and prolonging at all costs on the other remains in force, then Japan's proud longevity will be a misery, for many even a curse.

A 74-year old war-widow wrote to me: 'Please help. I want to try this thing, HRT. I live alone and my monthly income from both old-age and war widow pensions comes to only ¥60 000. I must, therefore, keep my mobility, my brain and cheerfulness till the very end of my life.' I was immensely moved and encouraged by the letter. Japanese women, despite all their cultural and social impediments, can and are changing, even the pre-war generation, forced to do so by the less and less caring younger generations.

When I go home to Japan and see those old women, bent in half, necks horizontally sticking out of their chests, painfully crawling up the staircase like squashed crabs, I am horrified and indignant. Those women were the young mothers and widows during and immediately after the war who gave their own rationed food to their children and husbands returning from the war; and today in the affluent and overfed Japan they, on whose sacrifice a part of the so-called Economic Miracle was built, are the geriatrics bedridden from strokes or osteoporosis or Alzheimer's disease, and accused of the destruction of home and family life.

This too common and frequent disaster, called *katei no hokai*, is today on everyone's lips, and is what their daughters and/or daughters-in-law, i.e. women of my generation and the first wave of baby-boomers, dread more than the next earthquake.

This is no exaggeration, although I admit, it may be difficult for someone living on a vast continent with an ample living space to imagine to what degree the fabric of family life could be damaged, and how intolerable the interpersonal stress and friction could become when even one bedridden patient is added to a family of three or four, living in a space of 60 or 70 m².

When I created the motto for the Amarant Society of Japan, 'My Body, My Life, My Choice' the general reaction was: 'Isn't the repetition of my, my, my a bit too aggressive? It may put off many whose help you might need one day.' I refused to tone it down. I wanted to emphasize to whom the body, the life and the choice belonged. For too long a Japanese woman has delegated the onerous task of choosing to men, to her elders and to social mores. But as she confronts her menopause with 30, even 40 years looming behind it, if she wishes to secure longevity with quality of life and a passage to death with dignity, then she must choose and bear the weight of her choice. Whether she chooses to go on HRT or not, it is her government's duty and far-sighted wisdom to make sure that a safe, accessible and *à la carte* HRT, the medicine of choice, is within reach of every woman.

Selective estrogen receptor modulators as a new postmenopausal prevention-maintenance therapy

3

V. C. Jordan, J. I. MacGregor and D. A. Tonetti

Introduction

Estrogen administration, as a hormone replacement in postmenopausal women, provides benefit by reducing cardiovascular disease[1], osteoporosis[2], Alzheimer's disease[3] and postmenopausal symptoms[4]. However, estrogen causes an increased detection of endometrial cancer[5] and there is concern that breast cancer is not prevented[6]. In contrast, the antiestrogen tamoxifen has revolutionized the treatment of breast cancer and provided a survival advantage for thousands of node-positive and node-negative breast cancer patients[7]. The drug is listed by the World Health Organization as an essential drug for the treatment of breast cancer and it is the currently most prescribed cancer medicine. What is remarkable about tamoxifen is the observation that the drug lowers cholesterol[8] and it is already known to reduce fatal myocardial infarction if given for at least 5 years[9]. Additionally tamoxifen maintains bone density in postmenopausal women[10] but like estrogen, tamoxifen causes an increased detection of endometrial cancer[11]. Most importantly, laboratory[12] and clinical data on a reduction in contralateral breast cancer in patients[7] demonstrate that tamoxifen could prevent breast cancer in high-risk women.

This paper describes the progress that is being made to evaluate tamoxifen as a preventive treatment for breast cancer and then describes the new strategy that is being implemented to discover selective estrogen receptor modulators that could be used as prevention-maintenance therapies in post-menopausal women. The goal is to retard the development of osteoporosis, coronary heart disease, breast and endometrial cancer in women over the age of 50 years.

Progression towards a prevention-maintenance therapy

Tamoxifen is being tested as an agent for the prevention of breast cancer in three large clinical trials because (1) there is clear evidence of potential efficacy, (2) there are ancillary physiological benefits and (3) the toxicities are modest compared with the development of breast cancer. In 1986, Powles and co-workers[13–16] at the Royal Marsden Hospital in London, started to recruit high-risk women who would receive either tamoxifen or placebo for up to 8 years. This Vanguard Study is now closed and 2018 women are enrolled. The group is a mixture of pre- and postmenopausal women who are also being evaluated for the effects of tamoxifen on bone density, circulating cholesterol and gynecological effects[15,16]. Overall, tamoxifen has a beneficial effect on bone maintenance and lowers circulating cholesterol in postmenopausal women, but in premenopausal women, as one would expect, there is a slight decrease in bone density and there is no effect on cholesterol measurements. The study group has made a rigorous investigation of gynecological changes but found very little effect from tamoxifen other than an increase in polyps[15].

The Vanguard Study has now been opened up to general recruitment throughout the

United Kingdom, Australia and New Zealand. The recruitment goal is 20 000 women to be randomized to tamoxifen or placebo for 5 years.

In the United States and Canada, the National Surgical Adjuvant Breast and Bowel Project is completing recruitment to a study of pre- and postmenopausal high-risk women. The current design of the clinical trial is shown in Figure 1. Indeed the volunteers have been shown to be of such high risk, the original goal of 16 000 women randomized to either tamoxifen or placebo for 5 years has been reduced to 13 000 women. It is believed that a definitive answer to the question of whether tamoxifen has worth for the prevention of breast cancer in high-risk women can be answered by 1999. Ancillary studies are also evaluating cardiovascular risk and the development of osteoporosis. Every woman is also being examined with annual endometrial sampling to determine the actual change in the detection of endometrial pathologies in treatment and control groups.

Finally, a study of tamoxifen as a preventive treatment is ongoing in Italy. Women over the age of 45 years with no risk factors, but who have already undergone a hysterectomy, are being recruited to determine the decrease in breast cancer with 5 years of therapy. Currently 5000 women have been randomized but the target is 20 000 volunteers. Overall it is clear that by the year 2000 there will be adequate data to support or reject the use of tamoxifen to prevent breast cancer in high-risk women. However, the majority of breast cancer is sporadic and the affected women are usually not associated with high-risk factors. This reasoning leads to the suggestion of a more generalized strategy to prevent breast cancer in postmenopausal women.

A new strategy

It is not possible to predict precisely who will develop breast cancer or indeed when the event will occur. Based on studies in animals it appears that the carcinogenic insult occurs

Potential participants

> 60 years old – with/without risk factors
35–59 years old – with risk factors

- LCIS
- 1° relative with breast cancer
- breast biopsies
- atypical hyperplasia
- over 25 years old before birth of first child
- no children
- menarche before age 12

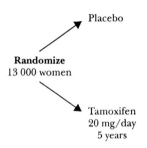

Figure 1 National Surgical Adjuvant Breast and Bowel Project – National Cancer Institute trial to test the worth of tamoxifen to prevent breast cancer in women. Women between the ages of 35 and 59 years have to present with risk factors to produce a cumulative risk equivalent to the risk for a 60-year-old woman. Recruitment of participants was completed in 1997 and results evaluating the worth of tamoxifen to prevent breast cancer will be available in 1999. LCIS, lobular carcinoma *in situ*

early in life before puberty[17]; therefore any prevention strategy later in life really prevents promotion. It is clear that a very broad strategy is required as a women's health issue if a general decrease in the incidence of breast cancer is to be achieved. To address this problem, in 1989 we suggested[18] that a new approach to the prevention of breast cancer could be achieved by developing agents to prevent osteoporosis and coronary heart disease in women. We wrote 'Important clues have been garnered about the effects of tamoxifen on bones and lipids so it is possible that derivatives could find targeted applications to retard osteoporosis or atherosclorosis. The ubiquitous application of novel compounds to prevent diseases associated with the progressive changes after menopause, may, as a side-effect, significantly retard the development of breast cancer.' This was the start of a search for targeted antiestrogens to prevent diseases of the menopause in women[19-21].

Design of an ideal targeted agent

The now extensive clinical and laboratory database about tamoxifen makes it possible to envision the properties of an ideal antiestrogen to provide the optimal clinical effects (Figure 2). The agent should exhibit estrogenic effects in the central nervous system (CNS) and on endothelial cells to improve mood and decrease the frequency of postmenopausal symptoms. Similarly the agent should have estrogen-like actions in the liver to lower low-density lipoprotein (LDL) cholesterol and raise high-density lipoprotein (HDL) cholesterol. This effect should translate to decreased atherosclerosis and coronary heart disease. It is now possible to design an agent to be free from DNA adducts in laboratory models so that there are no concerns about carcinogenesis

during prolonged treatment. This is an important aspect of the design of a new agent because indefinite therapy will be required to maintain bone density and prevent osteoporosis.

In contrast to the targeted estrogenic effects of the new agent, the compound should demonstrate inhibitory effects on growth and carcinogenesis in the uterus and breast so that there will be a decreased incidence of endometrial and breast cancer. Although there are many new compounds that exhibit the majority of properties needed in an ideal targeted antiestrogen, there is important new evidence to support a rational approach to drug design. We will survey the possible mechanisms for target site specificity before we consider the current status of strategies already in clinical trial.

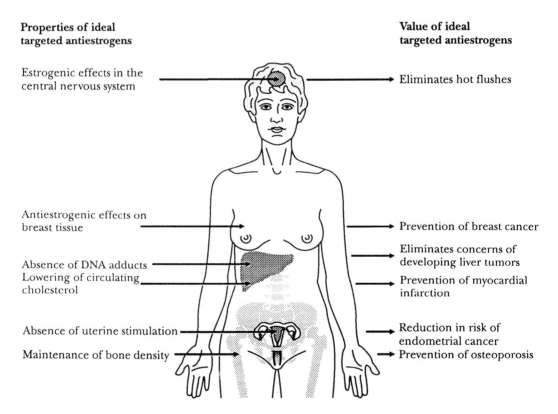

Properties of ideal targeted antiestrogens

Estrogenic effects in the central nervous system

Antiestrogenic effects on breast tissue

Absence of DNA adducts
Lowering of circulating cholesterol

Absence of uterine stimulation

Maintenance of bone density

Value of ideal targeted antiestrogens

Eliminates hot flushes

Prevention of breast cancer

Eliminates concerns of developing liver tumors

Prevention of myocardial infarction

Reduction in risk of endometrial cancer

Prevention of osteoporosis

Figure 2 The design of a new target site specific drug to stimulate or inhibit estrogenic responses selectively in target tissues; the novel agent will have the potential to control the development of several diseases associated with the menopause

Scientific basis for target site specificity

The history of pharmacology is filled with examples of the use of drugs to elucidate the complex organization of signal transduction throughout the body. Targeted blocking drugs have helped to classify adrenergic receptors into α and β (1 and 2) types and to classify histamine receptors into H-1 and H-2 types. Additionally the cholinergic system is organized into muscarinic and nicotinic receptors based on a clear-cut pharmacological classification. With this past experience as a guide, the unusual properties of non-steroidal antiestrogens have raised the possibility that these compounds could be powerful tools to elucidate the organization of the estrogenic responses throughout the body.

At the subcellular level it is now known that there is target site localization of different receptor molecules. The conventional estrogen receptors have been recognized for 30 years but a novel estrogen receptor (ER)-β[22] has just been described (Figure 3). Alternatively, inhibitory or stimulatory factors could be located in different tissues that ultimately control whether a ligand receptor complex will be an inhibitory or stimulatory signal. These associated proteins are a topic of intense investigation[23]. Finally the genes in a target tissue may be activated or blocked specifically because a receptor ligand complex binds differentially to sites in a targeted promoter region. A raloxifene response element has been described in the promoter region of the transforming growth factor (TGF)-β gene that might be responsible for differential bone stimulation[24] (Figure 4). With all these possibilities, the actions of a targeted agent could be the result of one of several or all mechanisms.

Strategies to develop a novel prevention-maintenance therapy

Since there is emerging evidence to support the view that compounds can be found to initiate target site-specific selectivity, clinical studies are

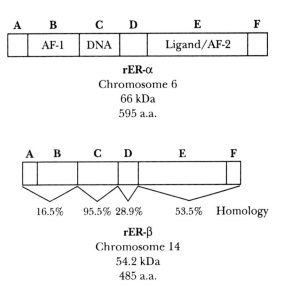

Figure 3 Comparison of the functional domains of rat estrogen receptor (rER)-α and the percentage homology with rER-β. AF, activating function; a.a., amino acids

Vitellogenin A2 estrogen response element

GGTCA CAG TGACC

Putative raloxifene response element (RRE) in TGF-β3 promoter

–38
TGGGAGGGAG *GTATAAA*TT TCAGCAGAGA

+1
GAAATAGAGA AAGCAGTGTG TGTGCATGTG

+35
TGTGTGTGTG AGAGAGAGAG GGAGAGGAGC

+75
GAGAGGGAGA GGGAGAGGGA GAGAGAGAAA

+110
GGGAGGGAAG CAGAGAGTCA AGTCCAAG

Figure 4 Comparison of the consensus estrogen response element (above) and the raloxifene response element (RRE) (below) that differentially regulate raloxifene action. RRE is shown in bold type, TATA sequence is shown in italics and GT repeat sequence is underlined. TGF-β3, transforming growth factor-β3

under way to exploit current knowledge. Two approaches can be taken at this point. Toxicologically safe target site specific agents are being examined in clinical trial to determine how successfully they fit the criteria described in Figure 2. An alternative approach would be to find an agent that will selectively complement the advantageous physiological effects of estrogen. The two approaches will briefly be described.

Target site specific agents

The pharmaceutical industry has synthesized and tested thousands of novel antiestrogens and estrogens over the past 40 years. Numerous new compounds are now being tested for the treatment of breast cancer[25] but select agents are being developed further for the treatment of osteoporosis. Droloxifene or 3-hydroxytamoxifen (Figure 5) maintains bone density in the ovariectomized rat[26] and is currently being tested as a treatment for osteoporosis in postmenopausal women. The drug has been tested extensively as a treatment for breast cancer[27] and there is no evidence of the formation of DNA adducts in laboratory models[28] or of the induction of tumors in rat liver[29].

Raloxifene (Figure 5), originally named keoxifene, was initially shown to maintain bone density in ovariectomized rats[30] and prevent rat mammary carcinogenesis[31]. Raloxifene has subsequently been studied extensively in the laboratory to confirm the actions on bone[32–34] but also to demonstrate that circulating cholesterol is reduced[32]. Perhaps of importance is the observation that raloxifene has only a modest estrogenic action in the rodent uterus[35], and it may be of advantage to develop an agent that has a less estrogenic effect on the growth of pre-existing endometrial carcinomas.

The biological effects of raloxifene in the laboratory rat are summarized in Figure 6 and the clean toxicological profile has encouraged the international testing of raloxifene as a treatment and ultimately as a preventive of osteoporosis in postmenopausal women.

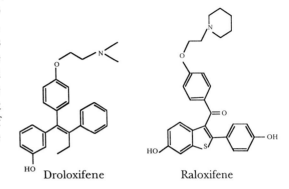

Figure 5 Formulae of droloxifene and raloxifene; two compounds that not only the have potential to prevent osteoporosis but also prevent breast cancer

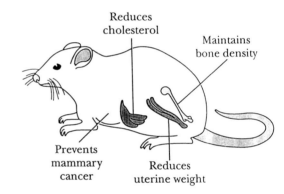

Figure 6 Biological actions of raloxifene in the rat

Combination therapeutics: binary approach

Although the idea of selective or targeted compounds is extremely attractive, it may not be possible to mimic precisely all of the beneficial actions of estrogen in the brain. Indeed it may not immediately be possible to evaluate the actions of targeted compounds on the development of Alzheimer's disease; however, it will be possible to establish an impact on changes in mood or in menopausal symptoms that may be CNS-dependent. If the quality-of-life issues are too complex to resolve satisfactorily, then another strategy is possible.

One approach to solve the problem would be to design an agent that has all the beneficial effects of a targeted antiestrogen in the periphery but which fails to penetrate the blood–brain barrier. The simultaneous administration of postmenopausal estrogen supplementation such as Premarin® would complement the prevention-maintenance therapy but provide all the benefits of estrogen in the CNS.

A novel quarternized tamoxifen (Figure 7) has recently been shown to produce tamoxifen-like effects in the periphery but not to penetrate the CNS[36]. Clearly tamoxifen may not be the ideal molecule to examine because of the potential for DNA adducts in rat liver, but the concept should be pursued with other compounds like raloxifene. An investigation of new compounds administered in combination with estrogen could result in a new prevention-maintenance therapy based on a combination of drugs. This binary approach would synthesize an appropriate range of estrogenic effects in the patient.

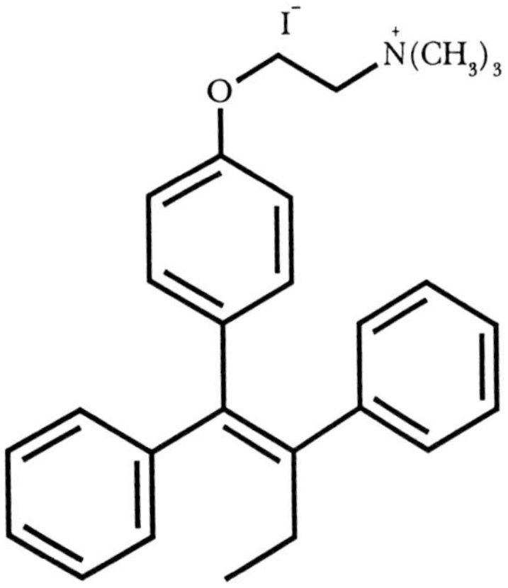

Figure 7 Formula of tamoxifen methiodide

Conclusions

There are now exciting opportunities to develop a new prevention-maintenance therapy for postmenopausal women. These strategies hold the promise of retarding the development of osteoporosis, coronary heart disease, breast and endometrial cancer. An understanding of the molecular events involved in the target site specific effects of estrogen through a novel ER-β system, or the selective activation of genes by antiestrogen through novel response elements, provides a basis for new drug discovery in the future. However, for the present, the well-documented clinical effects of estrogen coupled with the expanding database

for tamoxifen has laid the foundation for the current clinical trials with raloxifene. Clinical studies with a large population of post-menopausal women will soon establish the efficacy of the drug to treat and prevent osteoporosis and ancillary studies will confirm the actions to prevent breast cancer and coronary heart disease. Raloxifene is the first of a whole series of new agents that hold the potential to revolutionize the approach to disease prevention in the majority of postmenopausal women.

Acknowledgements

We thank Henry Muenzer for completing the diagrams and the Lynn Sage Breast Cancer Foundation for supporting our program. Jennifer MacGregor is supported by DAMD 17-94-J-4466 in our Department of Defense Breast Cancer Training Program.

References

1. Grodstein, F. and Stampfer, M. (1995). The epidemiology of coronary heart disease and estrogen replacement in postmenopausal women. *Prog. Cardiovasc. Dis.*, **38**, 199–210

2. Lindsey, R. and Tohme, J. F. (1990) Oestrogen treatment of patients with established postmenopausal osteoporosis. *Obstet. Gynecol.*, **76**, 290–5

3. Tang, M. X., Jacobs, D., Stern, Y., *et al.* (1996). Effect of oestrogen during menopause on risk and age at onset of Alzheimer's disease. *Lancet*, **348**, 429–32

4. Sherwin, B. B. (1996). Hormones, mood, and cognitive functioning in postmenopausal women. *Obstet. Gynecol.*, **87**, 20S–6S

5. Cohen, C. J. and Rahaman, J. (1995).

Endometrial cancer. Management of high risk and recurrence including the tamoxifen controversy. *Cancer*, **76**, 2044–52

6. Steinberg, K. K., Thacker, S. B., Smith, S. J. *et al.* (1991). A meta-analysis of the effect of estrogen replacement therapy on the risk of breast cancer. *J. Am. Med. Assoc.*, **265**, 1985–91

7. Early Breast Cancer Trialists' Collaborative Group (1992). Systemic treatment of early breast cancer by hormonal, cytotoxic or immune therapy. *Lancet*, **339**, 1–15, 71–85.

8. Love, R. R., Wiebe, D. A., Newcomb, P. A. *et al.* (1991). Effects of tamoxifen on cardiovascular risk factors in postmenopausal women. *Ann. Intern. Med.*, **115**, 860–4

9. McDonald, C. C. and Stewart, H. J. for the Scottish Breast Cancer Committee (1991). Fatal myocardial infarctions in the Scottish adjuvant tamoxifen trial. *Br. Med. J.*, **303**, 435–7

10. Love, R. R., Mazess, R. B., Barden, H. S., Epstein, S. *et al.* (1992). Effects of tamoxifen on bone mineral density in postmenopausal women with breast cancer. *N. Engl. J. Med.*, **326**, 852–6

11. Assikis, V. J., Neven, P., Jordan, V. C. and Vergote, I. (1996). A realistic clinical perspective of tamoxifen and endometrial carcinogenesis. *Eur. J. Cancer*, **32A**, 1464–76

12. Jordan, V. C. (1993). A current view of tamoxifen for the treatment and prevention of breast cancer. *Br. J. Pharmacol.*, **110**, 507–17

13. Powles, T. J., Hardy, J. R., Ashley, S. E., Farrington, G. M. *et al.* (1989). A pilot trial to evaluate the acute toxicity and feasibility of tamoxifen for prevention of breast cancer. *Br. J. Cancer*, **60**, 126–33

14. Powles, T. J., Tillyer, C. P., Jones, A. L. *et al.* (1990). Prevention of breast cancer with tamoxifen – an update on the Royal Marsden pilot program. *Eur. J. Cancer*, **26**, 680–4

15. Powles, T. J., Jones, A. L., Ashley, S. E. *et al.* (1994). The Royal Marsden Hospital pilot tamoxifen chemoprevention trial. *Breast Cancer Res. Treat.*, **31**, 73–82

16. Powles, T. J., Hickish, T., Kanis, J. A., Tidy, A. and Ashley, S. (1996). Effect of tamoxifen on bone mineral density measured by dual-energy X ray absorptiometry in healthy premenopausal and postmenopausal women. *J. Clin. Oncol.*, **14**, 78–84

17. Jordan, V. C. and Morrow, M. (1993). An appraisal of strategies to reduce the incidence of breast cancer. *Stem Cells*, **11**, 252–62

18. Lerner, L. J. and Jordan, V. C. (1990). Development of antiestrogens and their use in breast cancer (8th Cain Memorial award lecture). *Cancer Res.*, **50**, 4177–89

19. Jordan, V. C. (1995). Alternate antiestrogens and approaches to the prevention of breast cancer. *J. Cell. Biochem.*, **22** (Suppl.), 51–7

20. Tonetti, D. A. and Jordan, V. C. (1996). Targeted antiestrogens to treat and prevent diseases in women. *Mol. Med. Today*, **2**, 218–23

21. Tonetti, D. A. and Jordan, V. C. (1996). Design of an ideal hormone replacement therapy for women. *Mol. Carcinogensis*, **17**, 108–11

22. Kuiper, G. G. J. M., Enmark, E., Pelto-Huikko, M., Nilsson, S. and Gustafsson, J.-A. (1996). Cloning of a novel estrogen receptor expressed in rat prostate and ovary. *Proc. Natl. Acad. Sci. USA*, **93**, 5925–30

23. Baniahmad, C., Nawaz, Z., Banaihmad, A., Gleeson, M. A. G., Tsai, M.-J. and O'Malley, B. W. (1995). Enhancement of human estrogen receptor activity by SPT6: a potential coactivator. *Mol. Endocrinol.*, **9**, 34–43

24. Yang, N. N., Venugopalan, M., Hardikar, S. and Glasebrook, A. (1996). Identification of an estrogen response element activated by metabolites of 17β-estradiol and raloxifene. *Science*, **273**, 1222–4

25. Gradishar, W. J. and Jordan, V. C. (1996). The clinical potential of new antiestrogens. *J. Clin. Oncol.*, in press

26. Ke, H. Z., Simmons, H. A., Pirie, C. M., Crawford, D. T. and Thompson, D. D. (1995). Droloxifene, a new estrogen antagonist/agonist, prevents bone loss in ovariectomized rats. *Endocrinology*, **136**, 2435–41

27. Raushning, W. and Pritchard, K. I. (1994). Droloxifene, a new antiestrogen: its role in metastatic breast cancer. *Breast Cancer Res. Treat.*, **31**, 83–94

28. White, I. N. H., deMatteis, F., Davies, A., *et al.* (1992). Genotoxic potential of tamoxifen and analogues in female Fischer 344/n rats, DBA/2 and C57BL/6 mice and in human MCL-5 cells. *Carcinogenesis*, **13**, 2197–203

29. Hasman, M., Rattel, B. and Loser, R. (1994). Preclinical data for droloxifene. *Cancer Lett.*, **84**, 101–16

30. Jordan, V. C., Phelps, E. and Lindgren, J. U. (1987). Effect of antiestrogens on bone in castrated and intact female rats. *Breast Cancer Res. Treat.*, **10**, 31–5

31. Gottardis, M. M. and Jordan, V. C. (1987). The antitumor action of keoxifene and tamoxifen in the N-nitrosomethylurea-induced rat mammary carcinoma model. *Cancer Res.*, **47**, 4020–4

32. Black, L. J., Sato, M., Rowley, E. R. *et al.* (1994). Raloxifene (LY139481 HCl) prevents bone loss and reduces serum cholesterol without causing uterine hypotrophy in ovariectomized rats. *J. Clin. Invest.*, **93**, 63–9

33. Evans, G. L., Bryant, H. U., Magee, D., Sato, M. and Turner, R. T. (1994). The effects of raloxifene on tibia histomorphometry in ovariectomized rats. *Endocrinology*, **134**, 2283–8

34. Sato, M., Kim, J., Short, L. L., Szemenda, C.W. and Bryant, H. U. (1995). Longitudinal and cross-sectional analysis of raloxifene effects on tibiae from ovariectomized rats. *J. Pharmacol. Exp. Ther.*, **272**, 1251–9

35. Black, L. J., Jones, C. D. and Falcone, J. F. (1983). Antagonism of estrogen action with a new benzothiophene-derived antiestrogen. *Life Sci.*, **32**, 1031–6

36. Biegon, A., Brewster, M., Degani, H., Pop, E., Somjen, D. and Kaye, A. M. (1996). A permanently charged tamoxifen derivative displays anticancer activity and improved tissue selectivity in rodents. *Cancer Res.*, **56**, 4328–31

Media and menopause

W. McCarthy

It is a misconception that menopause is frequently mentioned in the media and that the main issues for discussion will therefore be about perceived bias and the integrity of the information source. In retrospect this misconception reflects the author's own interests and biases. Menopause does not take center stage in the media and if informed discussion is required, the medical profession will need to take a leadership position.

In the course of searching for information it was decided that preliminary assumptions should be tested in a more structured way and for 2 weeks in May 1996 three major metropolitan newspapers, two national newspapers, a weekly news magazine with many contributing columnists and six monthly magazines marketed to women were monitored. The total circulation figures would be in excess of 3 million, a meaningful demographic figure in a population of 18 million Australians. We were looking for editorials, news coverage, columns and advertisements. Simultaneously we monitored life-style programs on television and radio, again with large audiences.

The 2-week slice into the media very strongly indicated that menopause is not newsworthy: there was not a great deal of material to analyze. In fact, there was only one mention of menopause during that period. Since that period in May to the date of writing this paper four further articles on menopause have been found in the press. One was a particularly intriguing article on the use of hormone replacement therapy for the male menopause suggesting that at least this is newsworthy: it received a full-page feature in the *Sydney Morning Herald.*

So the question is, should menopause be newsworthy? If the answer is yes how is it to be framed? Is it to be a medical story or is it to be more than that, a story about health and longevity? Whose voices will be heard? Are they to be the women's, are they to be medical practitioners', or both together?

Hopefully the great example of newsworthiness in 1975 will not be repeated. This was an interview by Jane Brody of a San Francisco gynecologist who gave her a headline that journalists dream about when he responded to her question relating to menopause by saying: 'I think of menopause as a deficiency disease like diabetes.'

By contrast, an Australian prize-winning program maker was asked for her advice to medical practitioners who wish to communicate with the media about menopause. She said, 'Before you do, search in your hearts about your feelings about aging women. Books won't help. It is the conversation that women need, for so often they fear they are being patronized as though they are seen as a person who's already lived a life. Men fear older women and their neediness.' We might expand that to say society fears older women and their neediness, and yet it is this neediness which is often being expressed when presenting to a physician with symptoms of menopause.

Regrettably, little seems to have changed in the media since 1977 when Paula Weideger wrote in her book *Menstruation and Menopause,*

'Women in this society don't want to get old for many reasons. We do not want to face the implications of ageing and therefore refuse to face the image of ourselves as having aged. Menopause and ageing are not dreadful diseases or conditions. In part, these beliefs are a result of rather wild rumours about the troubles of menopause, and in part they are a realistic reflection of the social position of older women in our society.

Menopause is feared because it is associated with being old. The more one embraces the belief that motherhood is holy and fertility golden, the greater the conviction that menopause is the corrosive end to all that is desirable and worthwhile.

Once menopause is identified as the end to the best time of life, it naturally looms as a life crisis and its impending occurrence exerts formidable pressures on younger women.

Fifty or 60 years ago the image of a glowing, feminine fertility and a dreary painful menopause may have been a terrible burden for many women. But menopause was in all probability an event that took place shortly before one's death.'

Today most women will live one-third of their lives after menopause, so if physicians are to look at communicating with the media about menopause, it is perhaps important to recognize that they must look at menopause in the social context of female aging and sexuality. Returning to well-read books written over the last two decades it is astonishing to see how frequently menopause was seen as a medical construction and how rarely was a holistic approach adopted.

The media in many ways will reflect those messages or search out news stories, and such coverage is more likely to be about the virtue or otherwise of hormone replacement therapy, or the relationship, if any, where menopausal depression was claimed as a reason for murder. There will be little about menopause and sexuality.

Derek Llewellyn-Jones' book *Everywoman* has sold a great number of copies and must have significantly influenced both our journalists and our society to an extent. While advocating the end of the myth that a woman's sexuality and her sexual capacity and desire diminishes as she grows older, his section on menopause states in an encouraging way: 'An older woman who is single or widowed should not feel guilty if she has sexual desires. These can be satisfied if she can find a man to whom she can relate.' Is that a threat? Does it exclude relationships with women? Further he says: 'She can still enjoy sexuality by masturbating and should feel neither shame nor guilt, nor embarrassment if she does. It is a normal healthy activity.' This sounds just like advice given to adolescents when the present author was a sex educator in the 1970s. Nowhere is there the suggestion of relationships with same-sex or younger partners, a now socially observable phenomenon.

Understanding Human Sexual Inadequacy by Belliveau and Richter was again a widely read book which paraphrased much of Masters and Johnson's work. The aging female fared a little better here as it was acknowledged that she, like the aging male, usually has a shorter orgasmic phase and experiences the same slowing process and hormone deprivation. However, this information is not to be found in the media.

So the first issue is the message: can we trust our physicians to be our reference point and advisers for life after menopause? Can they collectively reassure the media that women who are seeking advice about the management of menopause will find physicians who offer both clinical advice, reassurance and attention to their neediness.

A larger challenge is presented to male practitioners. Can mature male practitioners distance themselves from their particular domestic circumstances when offering advice to the peer group of their partners?

There is no prior generation whose longevity stretches so far into the future. Many women do not have careers and are now looking forward to one-third of their life with no direct responsibility for children and possibly no partner, which can be very frightening. The story that needs to be communicated to the media is how the medical profession is managing this challenge.

Is it possible to reframe public issues? In short, yes. Some of the successful case studies are offered here.

A good example across the world over the last three decades is the story of the women's movement. Originally called women's liberation it then became the second stage women's movement. The movement progressed to being about the rights of women and the case of women for social justice, and its main concern is now probably closer to the changing role of women in society. This is a story that has been told with many voices since the early 1970s and the media has responded to the plurality of those voices and political perspectives. Women are newsworthy. In a very short period of time women have reframed the debate about themselves.

The story of female circumcision came out of Africa in the 1970s, and was brought to the attention of world media by activist women. In 1980 in Copenhagen a brave Egyptian woman doctor called Nawal-el-Sadawi called for a ban on female circumcision. By 1995 female circumcision had become genital mutilation and a proper concern of international health: this is a significant reframing.

The issue of family planning was once only about contraception and prior to that, in Australia, about racial hygiene. Over three decades family planning has been reframed and is now about choice, human sexuality, women's health and reproductive rights, and increasingly about men's health and reproductive rights. Physicians who are associated with family planning are seen as high-integrity sources of information. This was not always the case.

Smoking was once fashionable and even role-modelled by doctors on television.

These shifts do not happen accidentally. As the paradigms move the key players learn to use the media to tell their stories. Getting through to the editorial page is one of the great challenges in the media and to do that one needs to know how editorials are created. This requires an understanding of the routines of news gathering and determination of news selection. The media feed off each other for news stories. If a story runs in a prestigious newspaper or is featured in a prestigious radio or television slot, the other media will approach for new angles on the story.

Similarly, professional journals are story sources for journalists. An individual can help by calling the journal and offering a background briefing and, in this way, establish themselves as a resource of integrity and information. Contribution of a guest piece can be offered, paraphrasing any scientific data.

Creating columns in high-circulation magazines is another effective way of telling the story. When the present author was managing information and media at Family Planning Australia, we ourselves wrote most of the columns in women's magazines on sex and relationships, i.e. the agony columns were written to Family Planning practitioners who were seen as high-quality listeners capable of responding to readers' questions, a perfect communication process.

Letters to the editor remain an effective form of media release. To be published requires an adherence to simplicity but it can be a valuable entry into a debate. Sometimes criticism of a colleague's approach to an issue may be necessary, but if the criticism is newsworthy and has high integrity that is acceptable.

Journalists can be very suspicious of people with agendas. In that category they include drug companies, politicians and organizations responsible for the issue being investigated, for example health departments. Good journalists, however, will always speak to a variety of sources and one individual will not be the only source. It must be made clear whether a discussion is on or off the record.

Journalists do not react well to PR companies about which they are mostly cynical. They will accept the free lunch but are sceptical, as they should be, about the public relations companies trying to influence them regarding the coverage of an issue. However, it should be noted that innovative PR companies have reframed themselves. They are now called issues' management communications companies and many of the major public health issues across the world are being managed by such communication companies. It would be useful for many physicians to establish a relationship with them.

So what can a physician do to develop a better relationship with the journalist? It is important to treat the craft of the journalist with respect. Like any group of professionals, journalists have standard operating procedures. It is important to respect deadlines, respect objectivity and follow up on promises; reporters are not necessarily friends or enemies, and media etiquette should be based on mutual respect.

In summary, the challenge for physicians is to present a collegiate view that managing menopause is about partnerships of equality and respect. As women face lives far longer than they ever dreamt of they need respect, support and understanding from their physicians. That is a good story for the physician to tell.

Bibliography

Advocacy Institute, Washington DC (1991). *Getting Through to the Editorial Page.* (Adapted for Australian Context by Chapman, S.)

Belliveau, F. and Richter, L. (1975). *Understanding Human Sexual Inadequacy.* (London: Hodder & Stoughton Ltd.)

Chapman, S., McCarthy, S. and Lupton, D. (1995). *Very Good Punterspeak – How Journalists Construct the News on Public Health,* Research Monograph No. 1, Centre for Health Advocacy and Research, University of Sydney

Friedan, B. (1994). *The Fountain of Age.* (London: Vintage)

Hailes, J. (1980). *The Middle Years,* Amcal Health Information Series. (Melbourne: Pitman Publishing)

Llewellyn-Jones, D. (1978). *Everywoman. A Gynaecological Guide for Life,* 2nd edn. (London: Faber & Faber)

Mackenzie, R. (1984). *New Zealand Women's Health Series – Menopause.* (Auckland: AH & AW Reed Ltd.)

Pertschuk, M., Wilbur, P. and the Advocacy Institute, Washington, DC (1991). *Media Advocacy – Strategies for Reframing Public Debate.* Short Courses in Public Health Advocacy, Australia (entered by Chapman, S.)

Seaman, B. and Seaman, G. (1981). *Women and the Crisis in Sex Hormones.* (New York: Bantam Books)

Weideger, P. (1977). *Menstruation and Menopause.* (Melbourne: Penguin Books)

Dietary soy phytoestrogens and the health of menopausal women: overview and evidence of cardioprotection from studies in non-human primates

5

C. L. Hughes, J. M. Cline, J. K. Williams, M. S. Anthony, J. D. Wagner and T. B. Clarkson

Introduction

Phytoestrogens are naturally occurring constituents of many plants. Legumes are particularly rich in estrogenic isoflavones and coumestans while grains are rich in estrogenic lignans. Isoflavones affect mammalian physiology via several mechanisms including estrogen-receptor agonism and possible antagonism, plus receptor-independent antioxidant properties and inhibition of several enzymes involved in cell-signaling and proliferation. Since several chronic diseases of menopausal women (including breast cancer, colon cancer and arteriosclerotic cardiovascular disease) in 'Western' nations are much less prominent in Pacific Rim nations where traditional diets include substantial intake of soy foods rich in isoflavones, the strengthening hypothesis is that intake of these non-nutritive dietary phytochemicals accounts for these differences in disease occurrence. Ongoing studies at several centers around the world are assessing the biological bases for the growing enthusiasm regarding the potential beneficial role of these compounds in reducing risk of disease in menopausal women.

Due to the remarkable demographic differences in rates of chronic 'Western' diseases in Japan versus North America, we have initiated studies to determine whether the prominence of soy in the Asian diet could account for these findings. In particular, we hypothesized that the soy isoflavones might act as estrogens or mixed estrogen agonists/antagonists in the cardiovascular system to protect against coronary artery atherosclerosis in women. We currently have in progress large studies in both ovariectomized non-human primates and perimenopausal women that will determine some of the major effects of dietary soy isoflavones on lipid metabolism, coronary artery atherosclerosis, bone metabolism and menopausal symptomatology. Results to date indicate remarkable beneficial changes in plasma lipoprotein levels and coronary artery vasodilatation. Additionally, our preliminary results from rats and non-human primates show antagonism of estrogen-induced proliferation of both endometrium and mammary epithelium, and encourage us to characterize the effects of isoflavones on these tissues and on disease processes common to these sites.

Structure and occurrence of phytoestrogens

Dietary phytoestrogens are naturally-occurring constituents of plants that elicit estradiol-like effects in one or more target tissues in animals. Nearly 70 years ago, it was noted that certain plants could induce estrus in animals[1]. Subsequently, after adoption of bioassay methods that assessed vaginal or uterine effects of putative estrogens, over 300 plants were found to possess some degree of estrogen-like activity[1,2]. These phytoestrogens are predominantly from two chemical classes (coumestans and isoflavones) and their metabolites, such as equol. The isoflavones and the coumestans have 15-carbon structures similar to the 17-carbon structure of estradiol-17. The richest sources of isoflavones among foodstuffs are legumes and grains, with soy content of the isoflavones genistein, daidzein and their conjugates in the order of 0.5–3 mg/g of soy protein. For human health considerations, a focus on the isoflavones from soybeans is justifiable owing to the facts that consumption of soybeans and soyfood products is increasing[3] and soybeans are the major source of genistein and daidzein in human diets[4].

In human beings dietary phytoestrogens are readily absorbed, circulate in the plasma and are excreted in the urine[5-7]. The plasma levels range up to hundreds of nmol/l in persons consuming diets that are rich in these compounds[8].

Mechanisms of action of phytoestrogens in mammals

Estradiol-like effects can be produced by these compounds, and the impact of these actions of phytoestrogens on the reproductive physiology of mammals can be quite prominent[9-11]. Multiple studies in rats and mice show uterotrophic effects which may be estrogenic or antiestrogenic in nature depending upon the experimental design. Extensive studies in sheep demonstrate either transient or permanent alterations in the female genital tract including morphological and biochemical changes of the cervix[12] and the uterus[13,14] which can credibly explain reversible and irreversible loss of fertility. Limited trials in women[15,16] and monkeys[17,18] suggest that phytoestrogens elicit minimal estrogenic effects on the maturation of vaginal epithelium, and do not antagonize the actions of steroidal estrogens on the vagina. On the other hand, stimulation of some estrogen-dependent histochemical and histomorphometric markers in the uterus by dietary steroidal estrogens is diminished by

Table 1 Possible mechanistic categories of phytoestrogen action in mammals

---

Phytoestrogens may

Have pharmacokinetic and metabolic effects that alter production, patterns of secretion, distribution or metabolism of endogenous sex hormones

Act as agonist at estrogen receptors

Act as antagonist (or mixed agonist/antagonist) at estrogen receptors

Have non-receptor-mediated estradiol-like actions (as agonist or antagonist)

Have no action on particular target tissues or processes

Have effects on particular target tissues or processes that involve non-estrogenic mechanisms. In this case, several possibilities are known for isoflavones

---

concurrent inclusion of soy phytoestrogens in the diet[19]. The implication is that the pattern of effect may not be simply that of a weak estrogen agonist. Although these phytochemicals might affect mammalian reproductive physiology solely by mimicry of estradiol via estrogen receptors, there is no *a priori* justification for assuming that all mammalian reproductive effects of these compounds will be estrogen receptor-mediated, or that observed effects will necessarily be limited to mechanisms that are known to be affected by steroidal estrogens. The possible mechanistic categories are summarized in Table 1.

'Classical' estrogen receptor-dependent activity

Many different phytoestrogens have been shown to bind the estrogen receptors and affect nuclear translocation[20]. Soy isoflavones have long been recognized as 'phytoestrogens'[21]. Most isoflavones act as weak estrogens *in vivo*[22] and *in vitro*[23]. Genistein binds with approximately 1/250th of the affinity of estradiol to the estrogen receptor (ER)[24]. Such low-affinity binding might explain observations that suggest mixed estrogen agonist/antagonist properties of phytoestrogens[25].

Table 2 Receptor-mediated estrogenic mechanisms distinct from classical estrogen receptor (ER)

Estrogen-related receptors
DNA sequences of two estrogen-related receptors (ERR1 andERR2) are distinct from both ER-α and ER-β but have a high degree of sequence homology[26]. ERR1 has been implicated in regulation of expression of at least one estrogen-responsive gene (lactoferrin)[27,28]. Specific putative ERR1 or ERR2 ligands have not been identified

Estrogen receptor β
Recently a second ER was identified, shares high homology with the classical ER (ER-α) and binds several known estrogens with high affinity[29]

Heat shock protein 90 (HSP 90) and aryl hydrocarbon receptor (AhR)
HSP90 is a chaperone protein that modulates AhR[30,31] and ER activity[32]. In the case of the AhR, isoflavones inhibit phosphorylation of HSP90, thus inhibiting dissociation of HSP90 from the receptor and inhibiting transcription of AhR-responsive genes. A comparable effect may occur with the ER

Membrane binding
Estradiol appears to be a ligand for the truncated form of the epidermal growth factor receptor (c-erb-B-2)[33]. Extremely rapid induction (within 10 s) of protein tyrosine phosphorylation by estradiol in MCF-7 cells suggests a membrane-mediated effect[34]

'Non-classical' receptor-dependent activities

Several possibilities other than the ER exist which might function as alternative receptor-mediated mechanisms for manifestation of phytoestrogen action (see Table 2). A specific mechanistic alternative to the ER offers the possibility of rectifying some of the phenomenological differences between observed effects of phytoestrogens and more traditional ER agonists. Furthermore, since phytoestrogens are not endogenous ligands *per se* within animals, these compounds may not act exclusively through a single mechanism.

After the fashion of the retinoic acid receptor family, DNA sequences have been identified that are distinct from the classical 'ER-α' but have a high degree of sequence homology[26,29]. These three receptors, estrogen-related receptors 1 and 2 (ERR1 and ERR2) and ER-β, belong to a subfamily of the nuclear receptor superfamily, the steroid hormone/thyroid hormone superfamily. The receptor ERR1 has been implicated in regulation of expression of at least one estrogen-responsive gene (lactoferrin)[27]. Recent studies have shown that ERR1 binds upstream from the estrogen response element (ERE) for lactoferrin and that mutations at the ERR1 binding site result in a reduction in ER-mediated response[35].

While it is of interest to note that ERR1 and ERR2 appear to exhibit constitutive activity in the absence of an exogenous ligand[36], these two 'orphan' receptors have not yet been well-characterized, and specific putative ligands have simply not been identified. Estrogen receptor-β has been shown to bind classical estrogen-receptor ligands but with relative affinities that are distinct from those observed with the classical ER-α[29]. Estradiol-like compounds such as phytoestrogens could be ligands for these or other unidentified 'orphan' receptors.

There is growing evidence of important actions of isoflavones upon heat shock protein 90 (HSP90). This chaperone protein modulates the activity of both aryl hydrocarbon receptor (AhR)- and ER-mediated events[37]. The most complete studies suggest that isoflavones inhibit phosphorylation of HSP90[30,31], thus inhibiting release of HSP90 from the AhR and in turn inhibiting receptor-mediated transcription of AhR-responsive genes.

Extremely rapid effects (response in seconds) of estrogens on target tissues have been described in some studies. Since membrane binding of estradiol has been shown for the c-erb-B-2 protein which is closely related to the epidermal growth factor (EGF) receptor[33], other putative estrogens might act in a similar fashion to influence target tissue growth or differentiation.

Receptor-independent actions of isoflavones

Isoflavones have been shown to have multiple effects on cellular and biochemical processes that are known to be important in normal mammalian physiology. These actions of isoflavones are summarized in Table 3. Prominent among these are effects on cell proliferation and tyrosine kinases.

Genistein suppresses the growth of several tumor cell types in culture, such as tumor cells derived from gastrointestinal tract including stomach and colon[38] as well as from breast[39–41]. Genistein also decreases the expression of the oncogene c-*myc* in, and inhibits proliferation of, two different colon cancer cell lines[42]. It appears that the antiproliferative effects of the isoflavones override proliferative tendencies arising from any estrogenic actions, as shown by an increased proliferation of breast cancer cells *in vitro* at low (estrogenic) doses of genistein[43], and inhibition of proliferation at higher doses[44].

Genistein modulates signal transduction by alteration of kinase activity, and affects growth-factor action. Genistein is a specific inhibitor of tyrosine protein kinases[45,49], which in turn play an important role in mediating signal transduction events for growth factors such as epidermal growth factor, insulin, platelet-derived growth factor and insulin-like growth factors. Genistein has been shown to inhibit dioxin-induced downregulation of the inhibitory transforming growth factor-β (TGF-β) in hepatoma cells, presumably by its tyrosine kinase-inhibiting activity[56]. Furthermore, since there is evidence of antagonism of steroidal estrogen actions by isoflavones[57], the report[34] of extremely rapid induction (within 10 s) of protein tyrosine

Table 3 Cellular and biochemical actions of isoflavones that are presumably receptor-independent

---

Isoflavone genistein inhibits
Proliferation[38–44]
Tyrosine kinases[45]
DNA topoisomerases I and II[46]
Aromatase[47]
17β-hydroxysteroid oxidoreductase[48]
Ribosomal S6 kinase[49]
Formation of reactive oxygen species[50–53]

Isoflavone genistein stimulates
Apoptosis [54]
Prostaglandin H synthase[55]

---

phosphorylation by estradiol in human breast cancer cells (MCF-7), suggests that the antagonistic actions of isoflavones could be independent of the classical ER-mediated transcriptional mechanism.

Initial evidence from non-human primate studies

Cynomolgus monkeys (*Macaca fascicularis*) have several advantages as models for human beings. We have a large database for, and much experience with this species, particularly involving hormonal issues and postmenopausal animals. A particular strength of the monkey model is that it provides distinct advantages for evaluating the reproductive tissues. Female macaques are similar to women in many aspects of repro-ductive physiology and anatomy. Macaques have a distinct menarche and menopause, at about 3 and 20 years of age, respectively. They have a 28-day menstrual cycle, with a hormonal profile similar to that of women. Their endometrial responses to endogenous and exogenous hormones parallel those of women. Since cynomolgus macaques are similar to women in many aspects of repro-ductive physiology and anatomy, we have used the ovariectomized macaque as a model for menopausal women to investigate the effects of hormone treatments on intermediate markers of cancer risk in the breast and endometrium.

Effects of soy isoflavones on lipids and coronary artery atherosclerosis

We have completed an initial study in a small group of non-human primates to assess the potential cardioprotective actions of dietary soy isoflavones[58]. In this experiment with a 6-month crossover design, 27 monkeys were fed a moderately atherogenic diet containing soy protein that had either previously undergone extraction of the isoflavones, or soy protein with the normal isoflavone content still intact. Plasma low-density lipoprotein plus very low-density lipoprotein (LDL + VLDL) cholesterol was markedly reduced and total plasma cholesterol: high-density lipoprotein (HDL) cholesterol ratios were significantly lowered in both males and females during the isoflavone-intact diet phase. By organ weights and limited assessment of hormone levels, no reproductive system effects were found.

We have further studied the effects of these dietary soy isoflavones on markers of risk of coronary artery atherosclerosis in two additional groups of non-human primates. In an ongoing study[59], surgically postmenopausal (ovariectomized) monkeys are fed a moderately atherogenic diet, and the protein source is soy isolate. A control group is fed the soy isolate from which the isoflavones have been ethanol-extracted (< 0.17 mg isoflavones/g protein), a Soy (+) group is fed the soy isolate with its isoflavones intact (~1.7 mg isoflavones/g protein) and a conjugated equine estrogens (CEE) group is fed the isoflavone-extracted soy isolate to which CEE are added to approximate a human dose of 0.625 mg/day. Soy (+) has a beneficial effect on plasma lipid concentrations that is primarily on the LDL components, which secondarily results in lower total plasma cholesterol concentrations (see Table 4). Additionally, we have found that soy isoflavones, like CEE and other steroidal estrogens, enhance dilatory responses of atherosclerotic coronary arteries to acetylcholine[60] and reduce aortic cholesterol ester content[61].

In a third study (in this instance in young male monkeys), we have distinguished the relative contributions of the protein moiety versus the isoflavones for cardioprotection[62]. We studied young cynomolgus macaque males fed a moderately atherogenic diet and randomized into three groups. The groups differed only in the source of dietary protein, being either casein/lactalbumin (Casein, $n = 23$), soy protein with the isoflavones intact (Soy(+), $n = 26$), or soy protein with the isoflavones extracted (Soy(−), $n = 28$). The diets were fed for 14 months (see Table 5)[62]. Coronary artery atherosclerosis prevalence, the proportion of

Table 4 Mean plasma lipid and lipoprotein concentrations in surgically menopausal adult cynomolgus macaques[59]. Soy(+), diet containing soy protein with normal content of soybean estrogenic isoflavones; CEE, diet containing soy protein with isoflavones predominantly depleted and conjugated equine estrogens added equivalent to a woman's daily dose of 0.625 mg/day

	Control ($n = 41$)	Soy(+) ($n = 56$)	CEE ($n = 41$)	p value Con. vs. Soy(+)	p value Con. vs. CEE	p value Soy(+) vs. CEE
TPC (mg/dl)	391	340	334	0.01	0.008	NS
TG (mg/dl)	30	33	49	NS	0.0001	0.0001
HDLC (mg/dl)	66	70	54	NS	0.002	0.0001
LDLC + VLDLC (mg/dl)	325	272	278	0.02	0.05	NS
TPC/HDLC	8.02	6.25	9.04	NS	NS	0.01

TPC, total plasma cholesterol; TG, triglycerides; HDLC, high-density lipoprotein cholesterol; LDLC, low-density lipoprotein cholesterol; VLDLC, very low-density lipoprotein cholesterol; NS, not significant

each group with intimal thickness greater than or equal to one-half of the medial thickness, was 73% for the Casein group, 64% for Soy(–), and 45% for Soy(+). Testicular weights were unaffected by the phytoestrogens. The beneficial effects of soy protein on cardiovascular disease appear to be primarily mediated by the isoflavone component. Our results strongly suggest that dietary soy phytoestrogens will be shown to provide important cardioprotective benefits in human beings.

Effects of soy isoflavones on mammary gland and endometrium

Another critical goal of our research is to determine the effects and mechanisms by which dietary soy isoflavones may act to protect against breast and endometrial cancer in women. We have initiated studies in monkeys that feature dietary trials of these compounds to determine the potential influence of dietary soy isoflavones on these cancers in women.

In a recent study of hormonal replacement therapy and its alternatives[63], adult surgically postmenopausal female macaques were treated continuously with either estradiol (E_2), soy protein isolate containing the normal content of isoflavones (Soy (+)), or E_2 + Soy (+) for 6 months. Test compounds were administered in the diet at doses equivalent on a caloric basis to 1 mg/woman per day for estradiol and 148 mg/woman per day for soy isoflavones. Proliferation was assessed by histopathological, morphometric and immunohistochemical means in endometrium and mammary gland. In the endometrium, E_2 induced endometrial hyperplasia. Soy(+) alone did not induce endometrial hyperplasia. Endometrial thickness and gland area (as a percentage of total endometrial area) were increased by E_2 and E_2 + Soy (+). The effects of E_2 were partially antagonized by Soy (+) (manifested as decreased Ki-67 staining). In the mammary gland, E_2 induced mammary-gland hyperplasia. Soy (+) alone did not induce mammary-gland hyperplasia. Mammary-gland proliferation was induced by E_2 and E_2 + Soy (+). Soy (+) significantly antagonized Ki-67 proliferation-marker induction by E_2 in the mammary gland. These results indicate that in this model, dietary soy isoflavones have antiproliferative effects in the endometrium and mammary gland of E_2-treated primates, supporting the

Table 5 Mean plasma lipid and lipoprotein concentrations and coronary artery atherosclerosis extent in young male cynomolgus macaques[59,62]. Casein, diet containing casein and lactalbumin as protein sources; Soy(+), diet containing soy protein with normal content of soybean estrogenic isoflavones; Soy(–), diet containing soy protein with isoflavones predominantly depleted; CAA extent, coronary artery atherosclerosis extent is cross-sectional area of intimal lesions averaged for three coronary arteries. Means are adjusted for baseline covariates and comparisons were done by ANCOVA. Atherosclerosis evaluations were carried out on 11 monkeys per group

				p value		
	Casein	Soy(–)	Soy(+)	Casein vs. Soy(–)	Casein vs. Soy(+)	Soy(–) vs. Soy(+)
TPC (mg/dl)	457	427	307	0.32	< 0.0001	0.0001
HDLC (mg/dl)	39	47	58	0.04	< 0.0001	0.002
LDLC + VLDLC (mg/dl)	416	380	251	0.29	< 0.0001	0.0001
CAA extent (mm²)	0.13	0.06	0.02	0.16	0.003	0.05

TPC, total plasma cholesterol; HDLC, high-density lipoprotein cholesterol; LDLC, low-density lipoprotein cholesterol; VLDLC, very low-density lipoprotein cholesterol

Table 6 Summary of soy isoflavone effects on cardiovascular, mammary and endometrial sites in cynomolgus macaques: implications for risk of human diseases

Site/effect	Study subjects	Implied impact on risk for human disease
Lipids and lipoproteins	ovariectomized adult females	improved profile suggests lower risk of atherosclerosis
Lipids and lipoproteins	young males	improved profile suggests lower risk of atherosclerosis
Coronary artery vasomotion	ovariectomized adult females	improved vasodilatation suggests lower risk of atherosclerosis
Aortic cholesterol content	ovariectomized adult females	diminished content suggests lower risk of atherosclerosis
Coronary artery intimal area	young males	reduced plaque area suggests lower risk of atherosclerosis
Endometrium	ovariectomized adult females	lack of proliferation and reduction of steroidal estrogen-induced proliferation suggest lower risk of endometrial cancer
Mammary gland	ovariectomized adult females	limited proliferation and reduction of steroidal estrogen-induced proliferation suggest lower risk of breast cancer

notion that these dietary estrogenic soy isoflavones have a beneficial antagonistic (protective) effect on these target tissues regarding cancer risk.

Conclusions and future research

Dietary phytoestrogens affect many physiological processes in mammals. The estrogenic isoflavones are particularly relevant for human health concerns. At present, the emerging impression for menopausal women is enthusiasm regarding potential benefit on risk of several chronic 'Western' diseases (e.g. breast and endometrial cancers and cardiovascular disease) (Table 6).

We are presently continuing studies of the cardioprotective effects of soy isoflavones in non-human primates and in women. Individual projects include a prospective trial in perimenopausal women, mechanistic experiments in small groups of non-human primates and a long-term dietary trial in 189 surgically menopausal female monkeys to compare a diet rich in soy isoflavones to one essentially devoid of isoflavones. In the non-human dietary trial, lipid, hormonal and bone densitometry effects will ultimately be correlated with pathological outcomes of coronary artery atherosclerosis, bone histomorphometry, breast and uterine pathology and histomorphometry. To date, our preliminary results from experiments in non-human primates show distinct evidence of beneficial cardioprotective effects. Results indicative of antagonism of estrogen-induced proliferation of both endometrium and mammary epithelium provide a strong basis for optimism regarding the role of these compounds in the health of menopausal women.

Acknowledgements

This work is supported in part (T.C.) by Program Project Grant PO 1 HL45666, National Institutes of Health, Bethesda, MD. Soy protein isolates are provided by Protein Technologies, Inc., St. Louis, MO.

References

1. Bradbury, R. B. and White, D. C. (1954). Oestrogens and related substances in plants. *Vitamin Horm.*, **12**, 207–33

2. Farnsworth, N. R., Bingel, A. S., Cordell, G. A., Crane, F. A. and Fong, H. H. S. (1975). Potential value of plants as sources of new antifertility agents. II. *J. Pharm. Sci.*, **64**, 717–54

3. Messina, M. and Messina, V. (1991). Increasing use of soyfoods and their potential role in cancer prevention. *J. Am. Diet. Assoc.*, **91**, 836–40

4. Franke, A. A., Custer, L. J., Cerna, C. M. and Narala, K. (1995). Rapid HPLC analysis of dietary phytoestrogens from legumes and from human urine. *Proc. Soc. Exp. Biol. Med.*, **208**, 18–26

5. Adlercreutz, H., Fotsis, T., Lampe, J., Wahala, K., Makela, T., Bronow, G. and Hase, T. (1993). Quantitative determination of lignans and isoflavonoids in plasma of omnivorous and vegetarian women by isotope dilution gas chromatography–mass spectrometry. *Scand. J. Clin. Lab. Invest.*, **53** (Suppl. 215), 5–18

6. Morton, M. S., Wilcox, G., Wahlqvist, M. L. and Griffiths, K. (1994). Determination of lignans and isoflavonoids in human female plasma following dietary supplementation. *J. Endocrinol.*, **142**, 251–9

7. Xu, X., Harris, K. S., Wang, H.-J., Murphy, P. A. and Hendrich, S. (1995). Bioavailability of soybean isoflavones depends upon gut microflora in women. *J. Nutr.*, **125**, 2307–15

8. Adlercreutz, H., Markkanen, H. and Watanabe, S. (1993). Plasma concentrations of phyto-oestrogens in Japanese men. *Lancet*, **342**, 1209–10

9. Cheng, E., Story, C. D., Yoder, L., Hale, W. H. and Burroughs, W. (1953). Estrogenic activity of isoflavone derivatives extracted and prepared from soybean oil meal. *Science*, **118**, 164–5

10. Biggers, J. D. and Curnow, D. H. (1954). Oestrogenic activity of subterranean clover. *Biochem. J.*, **58**, 278–82

11. Cheng, E. W., Yoder, L., Story, C. D. and Burroughs, W. (1955). Estrogenic activity of some naturally occurring isoflavones. *Ann. NY Acad. Sci.*, **61**, 652–9

12. Adams, N. R. (1995). Organizational and activational effects of phytoestrogens on the reproductive tract of the ewe. *Proc. Soc. Exp. Biol. Med.*, **208**, 87–91

13. Tang, B. Y. and Adams, N. R. (1981). Oestrogen receptors and metabolic activity in the genital tract after ovariectomy of ewes with permanent infertility caused by exposure to phytoestrogens. *J. Endocrinol.*, **89**, 365–70

14. Tang, B. Y. and Adams, N. R. (1982). Properties of nucleic acids in the uteri of ewes with clover disease and the effect of oestrogen after ovariectomy. *Aust. J. Biol. Sci.*, **35**, 527–31

15. Wilcox, G., Wahlqvist, M. L., Burger, H. G. and Medley, G. (1990). Oestrogenic effects of plant foods in postmenopausal women. *Br. Med. J.*, **301**, 905–6

16. Baird, D. D., Umbach, D. M., Lansdell, L., Hughes, C. L., Setchell, K. D. R., Weinberg, C. R., Haney, A. F., Wilcox, A. J. and McLachlan, J. A. (1995). Dietary intervention study to assess estrogenicity of dietary soy among postmenopausal women. *J. Clin. Endocrinol. Metab.*, **80**, 1685–90

17. Hughes, C. L., Tansey, G., Cline, J. M. and Lessey, B. (1995). Estrogenic, anti-estrogenic and non-estrogenic effects of phytoestrogens in reproductive tissues from female primates. *Third International Conference on Phytoestrogens*, Little Rock, AR, December, abstr.

18. Cline, J. M., Paschold, J. C., Anthony, M. S., Obasanjo, I. O. and Adams, M. R. (1996). Effects of hormonal therapies and dietary soy phytoestrogens on vaginal cytology in surgically postmenopausal macaques. *Fertil. Steril.*, **65**, 1031–5

19. Tansey, G., Krummer, A., Hughes, C. L., Cline, J. M. and Walmer, D. (1997). Effects of dietary soy phytoestrogens on the uterus of ovariectomized rats. *Proc. Soc. Exp. Biol. Med.*, in press

20. Martin, P. M., Horwitz, K. B., Ryan, D. S. and McGuire, W. L. (1978). Phytoestrogen interaction with estrogen receptors in human breast cancer cells. *Endocrinology*, **103**, 1860–7

21. Price, K. R. and Fenwick, G. R. (1985). Naturally occurring estrogens in foods – a review. *Food Add. Contam.*, **2**, 73–106

22. Bickoff, E. M., Livingston, A. L., Hendrickson, A. P. and Booth, A. N. (1962). Relative potencies of several estrogen-like compounds found in forages. *Agr. Food Chem.*, **10**, 410–12

23. Markiewicz, L., Garey, J., Adlercreutz, H. and Gurpide, E. (1993). *In vitro* bioassays of non-steroidal phytoestrogens. *J. Steroid Biochem. Mol. Biol.*, **45**, 399–405

24. Miksicek, R.J. (1994). Interaction of naturally occurring nonsteroidal estrogens with expressed recombinant human estrogen receptor. *J. Steroid Biochem. Mol. Biol.*, **49**, 153–60

25. Verdeal, K., Brown, R. R., Richardson, T. and Ryan, D. S. (1980). Affinity of phytoestrogens for estradiol binding proteins and effect of

coumestrol on growth of 7,12-dimethylbenz[a] anthracene induced rat mammary tumors. *J. Natl. Cancer Inst.*, **64**, 285–90

26. Giguere, V., Yang, N., Segui, P. and Evans, R. M. (1988). Identification of a new class of steroid hormone receptors. *Nature (London)*, **331**, 91–4

27. Liu, Y., Yang, N. and Teng, C. T. (1993). COUP-TF acts as a competitive repressor for estrogen receptor-mediated activation of the mouse lactoferrin gene. *Mol. Cell. Biol.*, **13**, 1836–46

28. Yang, N., Shigeta, H., Shi, H. and Teng, C. T. (1996). Estrogen-related receptor, hERR1, modulates estrogen receptor-mediated response of human lactoferrin gene promoter. *J. Biol. Chem.*, **271**, 5795–804

29. Kuiper, G. G. J. M., Enmark, E., Pelto-Huikko, M., Nilsson, S. and Gustafasson, J.-A. (1996). Cloning of a novel estrogen receptor expressed in rat prostate and ovary. *Proc. Natl. Acad. Sci. USA*, **93**, 5925–30

30. Gradin, K., Whitelaw, M. L., Toftgard, R., Poellinger, L. and Berghard, A. (1994). A tyrosine kinase-dependent pathway regulates ligand-dependent activation of the dioxin receptor in human keratinocytes. *J. Biol. Chem.*, **269**, 23800–7

31. Poellinger, L., Whitelaw, M. L., McGuire, J., Anotsson, C., Pongratz, I., Lindebro, M., Kleman, M. and Gradin, K. (1995). Regulation of dioxin receptor function by genistein and phytoantiestrogens. *Third International Conference on Phytoestrogens*, Little Rock, AR, December, abstr.

32. Nathan, D. F. and Lindquist, S. (1995). Mutational analysis of Hsp90 function: interactions with a steroid receptor and a protein kinase. *Mol. Cell. Biol.*, **15**, 3917–25

33. Matsuda, S., Kadowaki, Y., Ichino, M., Akiyama, T., Toyoshima, K. and Yamamoto, T. (1993). 17β-estradiol mimics ligand activity of the c-erbB2 protooncogene product. *Proc. Natl. Acad. Sci. USA*, **90**, 10803–7

34. Migliaccio, A., Pagano, M. and Auricchio, F. (1993). Immediate and transient stimulation of protein tyrosine phosphorylation by estradiol in MCF-7 cells. *Oncogene*, **8**, 2183–91

35. Shi, H., Shigeta, H., Yang, N., Fu, K. and Teng, C. (1996). Human estrogen-related receptor 1 gene: identification of multiple transcripts and promoter usage. *1996 Triangle Conference on Reproductive Biology*, Chapel Hill, NC, January, abstr.

36. Lydon, J. P., Power, R. F. and Conneely, O. M. (1992). Differential methods of activation define orphan subclasses within the steroid/thyroid receptor superfamily. *Gene Expr.*, **2**, 273–83

37. Nathan, D. F. and Lindquist, S. (1995).

38. Yanagihara, K., Ito, A., Toge, T. and Numoto, M. (1993). Antiproliferative effects of isoflavones on human cancer cell lines established from the gastrointestinal tract. *Cancer Res.*, **53**, 5815–21

39. Naik, H. R., Lehr, J. E. and Pienta, K. J. (1994). An *in vitro* and *in vivo* study of antitumor effects of genistein on hormone refractory prostate cancer. *Anticancer Res.*, **14**, 2617–19

40. Barnes, S. (1995). Effect of genistein on *in vitro* and *in vivo* models of cancer. *J. Nutr.*, **125** (Suppl.), 777S–83S

41. Barnes, S. and Peterson, T. G. (1995). Biochemical targets of the isoflavone genistein in tumor cell lines. *Proc. Soc. Exp. Biol. Med.*, **208**, 103–8

42. Heruth, D. P., Wetmore, L. A., Leyva, A. and Rothberg, P. G. (1995). Influence of protein tyrosine phosphorylation on the expression of the c-*myc* oncogene in cancer of the large bowel. *J. Cell. Biochem.*, **58**, 83–94

43. Mäkelä, S., Davis, V. L., Tally, W. C., Korkman, J., Salo, L., Vihko, R., Santii, R. and Korach, K. (1994). Dietary estrogens act through estrogen receptor-mediated processes and show no antiestrogenicity in cultured breast cancer cells. *Environ. Health Perspect.*, **102**, 572–8

44. Peterson, T. G. and Barnes, S. (1991). Genistein inhibition of the growth of human breast cancer cells: independence from estrogen receptors and the multi-drug resistance gene. *Biochem. Biophys. Res. Commun.*, **179**, 661–7

45. Akiyama, T., Ishida, J., Nakagawa, S., Ogawara, H., Watanabe, S., Itoh, N., Shibuya, M. and Fukami, Y. (1987). Genistein; a specific inhibitor of tyrosine-specific protein kinase. *J. Biol. Chem.*, **262**, 5592–5

46. Okura, A., Arakawa, H., Oka, H., Yoshinari, T. and Monden, Y. (1988). Effect of genistein on topoisomerase activity and on the growth of [val 12]Ha-ras-transformed NIH 3T3 cells. *Biochem. Biophys. Res. Commun.*, **57**, 183–9

47. Gangrade, B. K., Davis, J. S. and May, J. V. (1991). A novel mechanism for the induction of aromatase in ovarian cells *in vitro*: role of transforming growth factor alpha-induced protein tyrosine kinase. *Endocrinology*, **129**, 2790–2

48. Mäkelä, S., Poutanen, M., Lehtimäki, J., Kostian, M. L., Santti, R. and Vihko, R. (1995). Estrogen-specific 17β-hydroxysteroid oxidoreductase type 1 (E.C. 1.1.1.62) as a possible target for the action of phytoestrogens. *Proc. Soc. Exp. Biol. Med.*, **208**, 51–9

49. Linassier, C., Pierre, M., LePeco, J.-B. and Pierre,

J. (1990). Mechanisms of action in NIH-3T3 cells of genistein, an inhibitor of EGF receptor tyrosine kinase activity. *Biochem. Pharmacol.*, **39**, 187–93

50. Wei, H. C., Freakel, K., Bowen, R. and Barnes, S. (1993). Inhibition of tumor promoter-induced hydrogen peroxide formation *in vitro* and *in vivo* by genistein. *Nutr. Cancer*, **20**, 1–12

51. Wei, H., Bowen, R., Cai, Q., Barnes, S. and Wang, Y. (1995). Antioxidant and antipromotional effects of the soybean isoflavone genistein. *Proc. Soc. Exp. Biol. Med.*, **208**, 124–30

52. Wei, H. C., Cai, Q. Y., and Rahn, R. O. (1996). Inhibition of UV light- and Fenton reaction-induced oxidative DNA damage by the soybean isoflavone genistein. *Carcinogenesis*, **17**, 73–7

53. Cai, Q.Y. and Wei, H.C. (1996). Effect of dietary genistein on antioxidant enzyme activities in SENCAR nude mice. *Nutr. Cancer*, **25**, 1–7

54. Kiguchi, K., Glesne, D., Chubb, C. H., Fujiki, H. and Huberman, E. (1994). Differential induction of apoptosis in human breast tumor cells by okadaic acid and related inhibitors of protein phosphatases 1 and 2A. *Cell Growth Differ.*, **5**, 995–1004

55. Degen, G. H. (1990). Interaction of phytoestrogens and other environmental estrogens with prostaglandin synthase *in vitro*. *J. Steroid Biochem.*, **35**, 473–9

56. Lee, D. C., Barlow, K. D. and Gaido, K. W. (1996). The actions of 2,3,7,8 tetra-chlorodibenzo-p-dioxin on transforming growth factor-2 promoter activity are localized to the TATA box binding region and controlled through a tyrosine-kinase-dependent pathway. *Toxicol. Appl. Pharmacol.*, **137**, 90–9

57. Folman, Y. and Pope, G. S. (1966). The interaction in the immature mouse of potent oestrogens with coumestrol, genistein and other utero–vaginotrophic compounds of low potency. *J. Endocrinol.*, **34**, 215–25

58. Anthony, M. S., Clarkson, T. B., Hughes, C. L., Morgan, T. M. and Burke, G. L. (1996). Soybean isoflavones improve cardiovascular risk factors without affecting the reproductive system of peripubertal rhesus monkeys. *J. Nutr.*, **126**, 43–50

59. Hughes, C. L., Williams, J. K., Anthony, M. S. and Clarkson, T. B. (1996). Dietary soy phytoestrogens and cardiovascular disease: evidence from studies in nonhuman primates. *Women and Heart Disease Satellite Meeting to the 8th International Congress on the Menopause,* Melbourne, Australia, October, November, abstr.

60. Honore, E. K., Williams, J. K., Anthony, M. S. and Clarkson, T. B. (1997). Soy isoflavones enhance coronary vascular reactivity in atherosclerotic female macaques. *Fertil. Steril.*, **67**, 148–54

61. Wagner, J. D., Cefalu, W. T., Anthony, M. S., Litwak, K. N., Zhang, L. and Clarkson, T. B. (1997). Dietary soy protein and estrogen replacement therapy improve cardiovascular risk factors and decrease aortic cholesterol ester content in ovariectomized cynomolgus monkeys. *Metabolism*, in press

62. Anthony, M.S., Clarkson, T.B. and Bullock, B.C. (1996). Soy protein versus soy phytoestrogens (Isoflavones) in the prevention of coronary artery atherosclerosis of cynomolgus monkeys. *Circulation*, **94** (Suppl.), I-265, abstr. 1548

63. Foth, D. and Cline, J. M. (1997). Effects of mammalian and plant estrogens on mammary glands and uteri of macaques. *Am. J. Clin. Nutr.*, in press

Estrogens and dementia: a clinical and epidemiological update

6

V. W. Henderson

Introduction: overview of Alzheimer's disease and vascular dementia

The term dementia refers to the loss of cognitive (mental) abilities, where the mental decline is of sufficient magnitude as to interfere with occupational or social activities, or to impede the conduct of day to day affairs. Dementia is the most feared and devastating accompaniment of aging. Although there are many forms of dementia, the most frequent cause by far is Alzheimer's disease. The second most common cause is that attributed to cerebrovascular disease (stroke), and together Alzheimer's disease and vascular dementia account for approximately four-fifths of all dementia. While this article considers possible estrogen effects on both of these common causes of dementia, the focus is on estrogen and Alzheimer's disease.

The key symptom of Alzheimer's disease is a defect in long-term episodic memory – the ability to learn new information that can be recalled after a delay of several minutes or longer. Although semantic memory – memory for over-learned general information such as word names – is also affected, a disturbance in semantic memory is usually not the initial symptom, and semantic memory is less severely disrupted early in the disease course. Episodic memory loss in Alzheimer's disease is linked to severe pathological changes within hippocampal and parahippocampal structures of the medial temporal lobes[1] and to a deficiency in the neurotransmitter acetylcholine[2]. Semantic memory loss reflects more widely distributed pathology within the association cortex of the cerebral hemispheres.

Other cognitive and behavioral alterations are common in this illness. Visuospatial impairments, for example, are implied when patients become lost in their own home or are unable to copy simple line drawings[3]. A depressed mood[4] and other behavioral disturbances are observed in some patients.

Pathologically, Alzheimer's disease is manifest by the accumulation of neurofibrillary tangles within vulnerable neurons of the central nervous system and by the abundance of neuritic plaques in the neuropil between nerve cell bodies. A typical neuritic plaque consists of a central core of β-amyloid protein surrounded by distended nerve cell processes (neurites). An inflammatory process is suggested by the colocalization within the plaque of microglia and reactive astrocytes, together with cytokines, complement proteins, and acute phase reactants[5,6].

Alzheimer's disease is etiologically heterogeneous. It is likely that different genetic and environmental factors interact to culminate in the characteristic clinical and pathological features of this disorder. However, except for age and family history, there are few firmly established risk factors[7]. Recently delineated genetic mutations are etiologically linked to uncommon forms of this illness that present before age 60 years[8]. The risk of Alzheimer's disease is also strongly influenced by polymorphisms of apolipoprotein E, a plasma lipid transport protein encoded by chromosome 19[9]. There are three common apolipoprotein E alleles: ε2, ε3 and ε4, and the ε2 and ε4 variants differ from the ε3 wild type by a single amino acid. Persons with at least one copy of the ε4 allele have a lifetime risk of Alzheimer's disease of about 29%, whereas without an ε4 allele, the lifetime risk is only about 9%[10]. Possession of the ε4 allele is associated with increased β-amyloid deposition and neurofibrillary tangle formation in the cerebrum[11,12].

The presence of the ε4 allele of apolipoprotein E is neither sufficient nor necessary for the development of Alzheimer's disease[13,14], and later-onset dementia is rarely attributed to genetic mutations known to cause symptoms in the fourth, fifth, and sixth decades of life. Another important observation is that many identical twins are discordant for Alzheimer's disease[15,16]. Together, these facts imply that there must be non-genetic factors – perhaps many such factors – that cause Alzheimer's disease, or that modify the risk of Alzheimer's disease through interactions in a multifactorial model that includes environmental as well as genetic contributions. Evidence is accumulating that for women one such exogenous factor may relate to postmenopausal estrogen deprivation.

Ischemic stroke elevates the risk of dementia[17], where dementia is usually attributed to the accumulation of multiple infarcts in subcortical and cortical regions of the cerebral hemispheres and in the brain stem. Appropriately, the typical form of vascular dementia is referred to as multi-infarct dementia. Whereas Alzheimer's disease symptoms are almost imperceptible at their onset, vascular dementia is more often characterized by the abrupt onset of cognitive impairments. Symptoms progress in a stepwise fashion, contrasting with the more gradual worsening of Alzheimer's disease. Although the cognitive profiles can differ in these two dementing disorders, vascular dementia is usually distinguished on the basis of its saltatory clinical course, associated signs of focal neurological disturbance (e.g. hemiparesis), and brain imaging studies that confirm the presence of infarction. The most important risk factor for vascular dementia is hypertension[18]. Interestingly, the ε4 allele of apolipoprotein E may be linked to a greater risk of cerebrovascular disease[19], in addition to its more firmly established association with Alzheimer's disease.

Gender differences and dementia

In contrast to dementia caused by stroke where men are affected more often than women, the age-specific prevalence of Alzheimer's disease is higher for women than for men[20]. Incidence studies are less conclusive, but several suggest that the incidence of Alzheimer's disease is also higher for women than for men[21-23]. Although sex differences in Alzheimer's disease pathology have not been systematically examined, the risk of Alzheimer's disease conferred by the apolipoprotein E ε4 allele appears to be greater for women[13,24,25].

Cognitive abilities of healthy men and women taken as a group are quite similar, but men tend to score better on some visuospatial and mathematical reasoning tasks, and women tend to perform better on certain verbal tasks[26,27]. One perspective is that putative sex-associated differences in patterns of neuronal connectivity within the brain might contribute to performance differences on female-advantaged and male-advantaged tasks. The cerebral hemispheres of women are conjectured to be more bilaterally (or diffusely) organized for certain skills, whereas men's cerebral hemispheres are more unilaterally (or asymmetrically or focally) organized[28,29]; such differences in neuronal organization might lead to gender differences in the risk of Alzheimer's disease or in the expression of Alzheimer's disease symptoms[30].

Estrogen and behavior

Estrogen effects are not limited to sexual and reproductive behaviors. In ovariectomized rats, estrogen replacement enhances both sensorimotor performances[31] and learning[32,33]. Human cognitive abilities may also be influenced by sex steroids. In a study of cross-gender hormone therapy in transsexual men and women[34], estrogen and testosterone appeared to exert reciprocal effects in different areas of cognitive functioning. Although measurable effects are small, a woman's cognitive skills vary during the course of the menstrual cycle[35–38] and verbal memory may be enhanced by hormone replacement therapy after the menopause[39–41]. Interestingly, among patients with Alzheimer's disease, women tend to perform worse than men on naming tasks[30,42], a pattern opposite to that typically reported for healthy adults[43].

In addition to effects on cognition, estrogen may enhance mood and subjective well-being in the perimenopausal and postmenopausal period[44–48]. The manner in which estrogen affects mood is uncertain but may involve interactions with noradrenaline or serotonin[49–52], neurotransmitters that have been implicated in depression.

Estrogen and brain function

Mature mammalian neurons do not divide, and in the adult nervous system there is no precursor pool from which to replace lost nerve cells. However, neuronal circuits are continually remodeled as synaptic connections are formed, relinquished and later re-established. Gonadal steroids play important roles in this dynamic process. Perhaps through interactions with growth and neurotrophic factors[53–55], estrogen can potentiate the extension of neuronal processes, promote the formation of synapses between nerve cells, and alter the composition of neuronal circuits[56–60].

Estrogen influences a number of neurotransmitter systems, and many neurons in the adult central nervous system possess estrogen receptors. For example, estrogen receptors are found in basal forebrain neurons that use the neurotransmitter acetylcholine[61], and basal forebrain cholinergic neurons are heavily affected by pathological alterations of Alzheimer's disease[2]. These neurons supply cholinergic input to large regions of the hippocampus and neocortex, and in female rats

estradiol increases cholinergic markers in the basal forebrain and its projection target areas[62,63]. Some estrogen effects on cholinergic neurons may be mediated through low-affinity receptors for nerve growth factor[61].

Other estrogen effects could also enhance general brain function. Estrogen increases cerebral blood flow[64,65]. In addition, estrogen augments the cerebral uptake and utilization of glucose[66,67], the primary energy substrate of the brain.

Estrogen and Alzheimer's disease

Estrogen levels plummet after the menopause[68], and as described above this change in hormonal milieu has the capacity to impact on brain function. There are also other ways in which estrogen deprivation might theoretically influence the development or manifestations of a neurodegenerative disorder such as Alzheimer's disease.

The large amyloid precursor protein can be cut at alternative sites to yield smaller degradation products. Estradiol *in vivo* promotes the breakdown of the amyloid precursor protein to soluble fragments less likely to aggregate as β-amyloid[69]. Moreover, antioxidant properties of estrogen[70,71] may serve to blunt neurotoxic effects of β-amyloid fragments that do form[72,73]. Estrogen also reduces circulating levels of apolipoprotein E[74–76], although the impact of such a reduction on Alzheimer's disease pathology is unknown. Finally, inflammatory responses are implicated in certain aspects of neuritic plaque formation[5,77] and estrogen may mitigate this process[78,79].

Estrogen and the risk of Alzheimer's disease: epidemiological studies

It is useful to distinguish between therapeutic strategies designed to prevent the onset of Alzheimer's disease among persons who are not currently demented, and treatment designed to improve dementia symptoms once the illness has manifested itself through memory loss and other symptoms. It does not necessarily follow that factors that reduce the risk of Alzheimer's disease will also ameliorate dementia symptoms, nor is it logically essential that symptomatic therapy given presymptomatically will prevent or postpone the onset of disease. There is evidence that estrogen may be relevant to both of these therapeutic approaches.

Several factors are associated with a lower risk of Alzheimer's disease[7]. One of these is postmenopausal estrogen replacement therapy. Compared to elderly women without dementia, women with Alzheimer's disease are significantly less likely to be current users of estrogen[80-82]. For example, in a voluntary cohort recruited for a longitudinal clinical and autopsy study of aging and dementia, Henderson and colleagues[81] found that of 7% of 143 women with Alzheimer's disease were current estrogen users, as compared to 18% of 92 non-demented elderly controls (odds ratio = 0.31, 95% confidence interval = 0.14 to 0.76). Analyses were retrospective, but there were no discernible differences in the use of other prescription drugs, and women in each group were equally likely to have undergone surgical procedures that could have influenced physicians' decisions to prescribe estrogens. Similar results are reported by others[80,82]. Although these studies support the view that estrogen replacement in the menopause decreases the risk of Alzheimer's disease, the lower frequency of estrogen usage might simply reflect physicians' unwillingness to prescribe a discretionary medication for demented patients. It is therefore important to consider estrogen usage before the onset of dementia symptoms.

Stronger support for the estrogen hypothesis comes from studies where information on a woman's use of estrogen was obtained prospectively, before some study participants became demented. The Leisure World retirement community cohort in southern California was established by postal survey in the early 1980s. The 8879 women in this upper middle-class cohort self-reported their past and current use of estrogen replacement therapy at the time of enrollment, before the development of dementia[83,84]. Among cohort members who subsequently died, diagnoses suggestive of Alzheimer's disease were listed on death

certificates of 248 women. Five controls without mention of these diagnoses were matched to each of these cases by birth date and death date within 1 year. In this nested case–control study, the risk of developing Alzheimer's disease among estrogen users was about one-third less than among those who never used estrogens (odds ratio = 0.65, 95% confidence interval = 0.49 to 0.88)[84]. This risk decreased significantly with increasing dose of the longest used oral estrogen and with increasing duration of any estrogen use. Although Alzheimer's disease is almost certainly under-reported on death certificate records, any resulting bias would probably have reduced the likelihood of detecting any effect of hormone replacement.

Different conclusions were reached in a Seattle study, where computerized pharmacy records of 107 women diagnosed with Alzheimer's disease were compared to records of control subjects without dementia[85]. As in the Leisure World study, the risk of an Alzheimer's disease diagnosis was reduced by about 30% when analyses were confined to women who had previously used oral estrogens, but in the Seattle study the magnitude of reduction was not statistically significant, and no risk reduction at all was apparent when other types of estrogen preparation were also considered. More recently, oral estrogen use was evaluated among participants in the New York City cohort reported by Tang and colleagues[86]. One hundred and sixty-seven incident cases of Alzheimer's disease were identified, and among estrogen users, the risk of Alzheimer's disease was reduced by over one-half (odds ratio = 0.40, 95% confidence interval = 0.22 to 0.85). Risk reductions were apparent in women who did and did not possess a copy of the ε4 allele of apolipoprotein E.

Estrogen and Alzheimer's disease symptoms: clinical studies

In the past decade, several clinical trials have considered effects of oral estrogen replacement on symptoms of women diagnosed with Alzheimer's disease[87-92]. All have been small (no more than 15 treated women), and in most instances outcome measures were limited to brief cognitive rating instruments.

Fillit and co-workers[87] treated seven demented women for 6 weeks with low doses of estradiol. Three subjects improved on brief measures of attention, orientation, mood and social interaction. The estrogen-responsive women had evidence of osteoporosis and lower baseline serum estrogen levels. Honjo and associates[88] treated seven women with Alzheimer's disease with conjugated estrogens. Over the 6-week course, six patients showed significant improvements on one cognitive assessment instrument, and five improved on a second brief instrument. Six untreated patients showed no improvement over the 6-week course. Ohkura and colleagues[92] compared 15 untreated women with Alzheimer's disease to 15 patients given conjugated estrogens for 6 weeks. Women receiving estrogen performed better on brief cognitive instruments, and they showed improvements in mood, cerebral blood flow and electroencephalographic slowing. In a separate study[90] of conjugated estrogens given for 6 weeks, the same authors reported improvement in three cognitive measures for six demented out-patients but not for five more severely impaired in-patients. Ohkura and co-workers[91] also reported a longer open-label study of conjugated estrogens involving 20 women with Alzheimer's disease. After 5 months, better cognitive performance on one of two brief measures distinguished treated women from those who had been untreated.

In the only placebo-controlled double-blind study published to date, Honjo and associates[89] compared conjugated estrogens with placebo for 3 weeks. Scores on three cognitive instruments increased significantly over baseline for seven demented women given conjugated estrogens but not for seven control subjects.

Each of these treatment studies concludes that oral estrogen improves Alzheimer's disease symptoms in some treated women. The lack of randomization or blinding in most estrogen trials, however, continues to suggest the need for caution in deciding whether estrogen is indeed efficacious for dementia symptoms.

What target symptoms putatively benefit from estrogen replacement? Referring to scores derived from a large neuropsychological battery, Henderson and colleagues[93] found that women with Alzheimer's disease who were receiving hormone replacement therapy performed better on a broad spectrum of cognitive tasks than a matched group of women with Alzheimer's disease not receiving estrogen. However, the sample size was small (nine demented women were receiving estrogen while 27 women with Alzheimer's disease were not), and not all comparisons were statistically significant. Differences favoring estrogen users were greatest on a naming (semantic memory) task, suggesting that estrogen in Alzheimer's disease may have differential effects on different cognitive domains. In this study, cognitive differences were not associated with changes in mood[93], so cognitive benefits in these women could not be attributed simply to estrogen effects on mood.

Estrogen interactions with cholinergic systems of the brain may be particularly relevant to Alzheimer's disease. Profound cholinergic deficits occur in Alzheimer's disease, and reductions in central acetylcholine transmission clearly affect learning and memory[2,94]. In the United States, the only drug approved by the Food and Drug Administration for Alzheimer's disease symptoms is tacrine, a centrally active anticholinesterase that retards the inactivation of acetylcholine. Several large randomized trials have shown significant, but modest, cognitive benefits for Alzheimer's disease patients able to tolerate the drug. A recent retrospective analysis of data from one such large tacrine intervention trial[95] found that women using oral estrogen replacement at entry and subsequently randomized to tacrine performed significantly better on the primary cognitive outcome measure than women receiving placebo[96]. Women in the tacrine arm who were not taking estrogens performed comparably with those in the placebo group.

The number of estrogen users in this trial was quite small and estrogen use was not randomized, but these observational findings support the contention that some estrogen effects in Alzheimer's disease may be mediated through the cholinergic system. Future randomized controlled trials should specifically consider additive or synergistic effects of estrogen and an agent that boosts central cholinergic activity.

Estrogen and vascular dementia

Cerebral infarction is the primary mechanism of multi-infarct dementia, and it is reasonable to assume that if estrogen lowers the risk of stroke then it should impact favorably on the risk of vascular dementia. However, effects of estrogen on the risk of vascular dementia or on symptoms of patients with this form of dementia have not yet been reported. Estrogen replacement does reduce the progression of atherosclerotic changes in the carotid arteries[97], an important risk factor for cerebral infarction. However, despite convincing data that postmenopausal estrogen replacement lowers the risk of cardiovascular disease[98–100], it remains unclear whether estrogen also affects the risk of cerebrovascular disease[99,101].

Conclusions

The mean age of menopause is about 51 years, and most women will spend one-third of their adult life in a state of estrogen deprivation. Estrogen undoubtedly affects the brain and brain function, and there are substantial reasons to consider whether postmenopausal estrogen loss may be related to dementia in later life. With regard to a woman's risk of developing Alzheimer's disease, the evidence to date is suggestive but not compelling that estrogen replacement can reduce risk. Concerning the symptomatic amelioration of the woman with Alzheimer's disease, published treatment studies are at best preliminary, although findings to date are consistent with the hypothesis that estrogen may be of some benefit. There is strong evidence that estrogen is protective against cardiovascular disease in women, but the potential role of estrogen in the prevention or treatment of dementia attributed to cerebrovascular disorders remains largely unexplored.

Acknowledgements

This work was supported in part by National Institute of Health (NIH) grant AG05142. Some material in this article has been previously published[102,103].

References

1. Hyman, B. T., van Hoesen, G. W., Damasio, A. R. and Barnes, C. L. (1984). Alzheimer's disease: cell-specific pathology isolates the hippocampal formation. *Science*, **225**, 1168–70
2. Coyle, J. T., Price, D. L. and DeLong, M. R. (1983). Alzheimer's disease: a disorder of cortical cholinergic innervation. *Science*, **219**, 1184–90
3. Henderson, V. W., Mack, W. and Williams, B. W. (1989). Spatial disorientation in Alzheimer's disease. *Arch. Neurol.*, **46**, 391–4
4. Rovner, B. W., Broadhead, J., Spencer, M., Carson, K. and Folstein, M. F. (1989). Depression and Alzheimer's disease. *Am. J. Psychiatry*, **146**, 350–3
5. McGeer, P. L. and McGeer, E. G. (1995). The inflammatory response system of brain: implications for therapy of Alzheimer and other neurodegenerative diseases. *Brain Res. Rev.*, **21**, 195–218
6. Strauss, S., Bauer, G., Ganter, U., Jonas, U., Berger, M. and Volk, B. (1992). Detection of interleukin-6 and α2-macroglobulin immuno-reactivity in cortex and hippocampus of Alzheimer's disease patients. *Lab. Invest.*, **66**, 223–30
7. Graves, A. B. and Kukull, W. A. (1994). The epidemiology of dementia. In J. C. Morris (ed.) *Handbook of Dementing Illnesses*, pp. 23–69. (New York: Marcel Dekker)
8. Pericak-Vance, M. A. and Haines, J. L. (1995). Genetic susceptibility to Alzheimer disease. *Trends Genet.*, **11**, 504–8

9. Strittmatter, W. J., Saunders, A. M., Schmechel, D., Pericak-Vance, M., Enghild, J., Salvesen, G. S. and Roses, A. D. (1993). Apolipoprotein E: high-avidity binding to β-amyloid and increased frequency of type 4 allele in late-onset familial Alzheimer disease. *Proc. Natl. Acad. Sci. USA*, **90**, 1977–81

10. Seshadri, S., Drachman, D. A. and Lippa, C. F. (1995). Apolipoprotein E ε4 allele and the lifetime risk of Alzheimer's disease. *Arch. Neurol.*, **52**, 1074–9

11. Ohm, T. G., Kirca, M., Bohl, J., Scharnagl H., Gross, W. and März, W. (1995). Apolipoprotein E polymorphism influences not only cerebral senile plaque load but also Alzheimer-type neurofibrillary tangle formation. *Neurosci.*, **66**, 583–7

12. Polvikoski, T., Sulkava, R., Haltia, M., Kainulainen, K., Vuorio, A., Verkkoniemi, A., Niinistö, L., Halonen, P. and Kontula, K. (1995). Apolipoprotein E, dementia, and cortical deposition of β-amyloid protein. *N. Engl. J. Med.*, **333**, 1242–7

13. Farrer, L. A., Cupples, L. A., van Duijn, C. M., Kurz, A., Zimmer, R., Müller, U., Green, R. C., Clarke, V., Shoffner, J., Wallace, D. C., Chui H., Flanagan, S. D., Duara, R., St George-Hyslop, P., Auerbach, S. A., Volicer, L., Wells, J. M., van Broeckhoven, C., Growdon, J. H. and Haines, J. L. (1995). Apolipoprotein E genotype in patients with Alzheimer's disease: implications for the risk of dementia among relatives. *Ann. Neurol.*, **38**, 797–808

14. Kukull W. A., Schellenberg, G. D., Bowen, J. D., McCormick, W. C., Yu, C.-E., Teri, L., Thompson, J. D., O'Meara, E. S. and Larson, E. B. (1996). Apolipoprotein E in Alzheimer's disease risk and case detection: a case–control study. *J. Clin. Epidemiol.*, in press

15. Nee, L. E., Eldridge, R., Sunderland, T., Thomas, C. B., Katz, D., Thompson, K. E., Weingartner, H., Weiss, H., Julian, C. and Cohen, R. (1987). Dementia of the Alzheimer type: clinical and family study of 22 twin pairs. *Neurology*, **37**, 359–63

16. Small, G. W., Leuchter, A. F., Mandelkern, M. A., La Rue, A., Okonek, A., Lufkin, R. B., Jarvik, L. F., Matsuyama, S. S. and Bondareff, W. (1993). Clinical neuroimaging, and environmental risk differences in monozygotic female twins appearing discordant for dementia of the Alzheimer type. *Arch. Neurol.*, **50**, 209–19

17. Tatemichi, T. K., Desmond, D. W., Mayeux, R., Paik, M., Stern, Y., Sano, M., Remien, R. H., Williams, J. B. W., Mohr, J. P., Hauser, W. A. and Figueroa, M. (1992). Dementia after stroke: baseline frequency, risks, and clinical features in a hospitalized cohort. *Neurology*, **42**, 1185–93

18. Ueda, K., Kawano, H., Hasuo, Y. and Fujishima, M. (1992). Prevalence and etiology of dementia in a Japanese community. *Stroke*, **23**, 798–803

19. Pedro-Botet, J., Sentí M., Nogués, X., Rubiés-Prat, J., Roquer, J., D'Olhaberriague, L. and Olivé, J. (1992). Lipoprotein and apolipoprotein profile in men with ischemic stroke: role of lipoprotein (a), triglyceride-rich lipoproteins, and apolipoprotein E polymorphism. *Stroke*, **23**, 1556–62

20. Jorm, A. F., Korten, A. E. and Henderson, A. S. (1987). The prevalence of dementia: a quantitative integration of the literature. *Acta Psychiatr. Scand.*, **76**, 465–79

21. Mölsä, P. K., Marttila, R. J. and Rinne, U. K. (1982). Epidemiology of dementia in a Finnish population. *Acta Neurol. Scand.*, **65**, 541–52

22. Katzman, R., Aronson, M., Fuld, P., Kawas, C., Brown, T., Morgenstern, H., Frishman, W., Gidez, L., Eder, H. and Ooi, W. L. (1989). Development of dementing illnesses in an 80-year-old volunteer cohort. *Ann. Neurol.*, **25**, 317–24

23. Payami, H., Zareparsi, S., Montee, K. R., Sexton, G. J., Kaye, J. A., Bird, T. D., Yu, C. E., Wijsman, E. M., Heston, L. L., Litrt, M. and Schellenberg, G. D. (1996). Gender difference in apolipoprotein E-associated risk for familial Alzheimer disease: a possible clue to the higher incidence of Alzheimer disease in women. *Am. J. Hum. Genet.*, **58**, 803–11

24. Poirier, J., Davignon, J., Bouthillier, D., Kogan, S., Bertrand, P. and Gauthier, S. (1993). Apolipoprotein E polymorphism and Alzheimer's disease. *Lancet*, **342**, 697–9

25. Corder, E. H., Saunders, A. M., Strittmatter, W. J., Schmechel, D. E., Gaskell, P. C., Small, G. W., Roses, A. D., Haines, J. L. and Pericak-Vance, M. A. (1993). Gene dose of apolipoprotein E type 4 allele and the risk of Alzheimer's disease in late onset families. *Science*, **261**, 921–3

26. Halpern, D. F. (1992). *Sex Differences in Cognitive Abilities*, 2nd. edn. (Hillsdale, NJ: Lawrence Erlbaum)

27. Jarvik, L. F. (1975). Human intelligence: sex differences. *Acta Genet. Med. Gemellol.*, **24**, 189–211

28. McGlone, J. (1980). Sex differences in human brain asymmetry: a critical survey. *Behav. Brain Sci.*, **3**, 215–63

29. Shaywitz, B. A., Shaywitz, S. E., Pugh, K. R., Constable, R. T., Skudlarski, P., Fulbright, R. K., Bronen, R. A., Fletcher, J. M., Shankweiler, D. P., Katz, L. and Gore, J. C. (1995). Sex differences in the functional organization of the brain for language. Nature (London), **373**, 607–9

30. Henderson, V. W. and Buckwalter, J. G. (1994). Cognitive deficits of men and women with Alzheimer's disease. *Neurology*, **44**, 90–6

31. Becker, J. B., Snyder, P. J., Miller, M. M., Westgate, S. A. and Jenuwine, M. J. (1987). The influence of estrous cycle and intrastriatal estradiol on sensorimotor performance in the female rat. *Pharmacol. Biochem. Behav.*, **27**, 53–9

32. Singh, M., Meyer, E. M., Millard, W. J. and Simpkins, J. W. (1994). Ovarian steroid deprivation results in a reversible learning impairment and compromised cholinergic function in female Sprague–Dawley rats. *Brain Res.*, **644**, 305–12

33. O'Neal, M. F., Means, L. W., Poole, M. C. and Hamm, R. J. (1996). Estrogen affects performance of ovariectomized rats in a two-choice water-escape working memory task. *Psychoneuroendocrinology*, **21**, 51–65

34. Van Goozen, S. H. M., Cohen-Kettenis, P. T., Gooren, L. J. G., Frijda, N. H. and Van de Poll N. E. (1995). Gender differences in behaviour: activating effects of cross-sex hormones. *Psychoneuroendocrinology*, **20**, 343–63

35. Kimura, D. and Hampson, E. (1994). Cognitive pattern in men and women is influenced by fluctuations in sex hormones. *Curr. Dir. Psychol. Sci.*, **3**, 57–61

36. Hampson, E. (1990). Variations in sex-related cognitive abilities across the menstrual cycle. *Brain Cognit.*, **14**, 26–43

37. Phillips, S. M. and Sherwin, B. B. (1992). Variations in memory function and sex steroid hormones across the menstrual cycle. *Psychoneuroendocrinology*, **17**, 497–506

38. Krug, R., Stamm, U., Pietrowsky, R., Fehm, H. L. and Born, J. (1994). Effects of menstrual cycle on creativity. *Psychoneuroendocrinology*, **19**, 21–31

39. Kampen, D. L. and Sherwin, B. B. (1994). Estrogen use and verbal memory in healthy postmenopausal women. *Obstet. Gynecol.*, **83**, 979–83

40. Robinson, D., Friedman, L., Marcus, R., Tinklenberg, J. and Yesavage, J. (1994). Estrogen replacement therapy and memory in older women. *J. Am. Geriatr. Soc.*, **42**, 919–22

41. Phillips, S. M. and Sherwin, B. B. (1992). Effects of estrogen on memory function in surgically menopausal women. *Psychoneuroendocrinology*, **17**, 485–95

42. Ripich, D. N., Petrill S. A., Whitehouse, P. J. and Ziol, E. W. (1995). Gender differences in language of AD patients: a longitudinal study. *Neurology*, **15**, 299–302

43. Ganguli, M., Ratcliff, G., Huff, F. J., *et al.* (1991). Effects of age, gender, and education on cognitive tests in a rural elderly community sample: norms from the Monongahela Valley Independent Elders Survey. *Neuroepidemiology*, **10**, 42–52

44. Schneider, M. A., Brotherton, P. L. and Hailes, J. (1977). The effect of exogenous oestrogens on depression in menopausal women. *Med. J. Aust.*, **2**, 162–3

45. Sherwin, B. B. (1988). Affective changes with estrogen and androgen replacement therapy in surgically menopausal women. *J. Affect. Disord.*, **14**, 177–87

46. Ditkoff, E. C., Crary, W. G., Cristo, M. and Lobo, R. A. (1991). Estrogen improves psychological function in asymptomatic postmenopausal women. *Obstet. Gynecol.*, **78**, 991–5

47. Best, N. R., Rees, M. P., Barlow, D. H. and Cowen, P. J. (1992). Effect of estradiol implant on noradrenergic function and mood in menopausal subjects. *Psychoneuroendocrinology*, **17**, 87–93

48. Gerdes, L. C., Sonnendecker, E. W. W. and Polakow, E. S. (1982). Psychological changes effected by estrogen–progestogen and clonidine treatment in climacteric women. *Am. J. Obstet. Gynecol.*, **142**, 98–104

49. Greengrass, P. M. and Tonge, S. R. (1974). The accumulation of noradrenaline and 5-hydroxytryptamine in three regions of mouse brain after tetrabenazine and iproniazid: effects of ethinyloestradiol and progesterone. *Psychopharmacologia*, **39**, 187–91

50. Ball P., Knuppen, R., Haupt, M. and Breuer, H. (1972). Interactions between estrogens and catechol amines. III. Studies on the methylation of catechol estrogens, catechol amines and other catechols by the catechol-O-methyltransferases of human liver. *J. Clin. Endocrinol. Metab.*, **34**, 736–46

51. Sar, M. and Stumpf, W. E. (1981). Central noradrenergic neurones concentrate ^{3}H-oestradiol. *Nature (London)*, **289**, 500–2

52. Cohen, I. R. and Wise, P. M. (1988). Effects of estradiol on the diurnal rhythm of serotonin activity in microdissected brain areas of ovariectomized rats. *Endocrinology*, **122**, 2619–25

53. Miranda, R. C., Sohrabji, F. and Toran-Allerand, C. D. (1993). Presumptive estrogen target neurons express mRNAs for both the neurotrophins and neurotrophin receptors: a basis for potential developmental interactions of estrogen with neurotrophins. *Mol. Cell. Neurosci.*, **4**, 510–25

54. Sohrabji, F., Miranda, R. C. and Toran-Allerand, C. D. (1994). Estrogen differentially regulates estrogen and nerve growth factor receptor mRNAs in adult sensory neurons. *J. Neurosci.*, **14**, 459–71

55. Shughrue, P. J. and Dorsa, D. M. (1993). Estrogen modulates the growth-associated protein GAP-43 (neuromodulin) mRNA in the rat preoptic area and basal hypothalamus. *Neuroendocrinology*, **57**, 439–47

56. Chung, S. K., Pfaff, D. W. and Cohen, R. S. (1988). Estrogen-induced alterations in synaptic morphology in the midbrain central grey. *Exp. Brain Res.*, **69**, 522–30

57. Toran-Allerand, C. D. (1991). Organotypic culture of the developing cerebral cortex and hypothalamus: relevance to sexual differentiation. *Psychoneuroendocrinology*, **16**, 7–24

58. Woolley, C. S. and McEwen, B. S. (1993). Roles of estradiol and progesterone in regulation of hippocampal dendritic spine density during the estrous cycle in the rat. *J. Comp. Neurol.*, **336**, 293–306

59. Lustig, R. H. (1994). Sex hormone modulation of neural development *in vitro. Horm. Behav.*, **28**, 383–95

60. Keefe, D., Garcia-Segura, M. and Naftolin, F. (1994). New insights into estrogen action on the brain. *Neurobiol. Aging*, **15**, 495–7

61. Toran-Allerand, C. D., Miranda, R. C., Bentham, W. D. L., Sohrabji, F., Brown, T. J., Hochberg, R. B. and MacLusky, N. J. (1992). Estrogen receptors colocalize with low-affinity nerve growth factor receptors in cholinergic neurons of the basal forebrain. *Proc. Natl. Acad. Sci. USA*, **89**, 4668–72

62. Luine, V. (1985). Estradiol increases choline acetyltransferase activity in specific basal forebrain nuclei and projection areas of female rats. *Exp. Neurol.*, **89**, 484–90

63. Gibbs, R. B. and Pfaff, D. W. (1992). Effects of estrogen and fimbria/fornix transection on p75NGFR and ChAT expression in the medial septum and diagonal band of Broca. *Exp. Neurol.*, **116**, 23–39

64. Belfort, M. A., Saade, G. R., Snabes, M., Dunn, R., Moise, K. J. Jr, Cruz, A. and Young, R. (1995). Hormonal status affects the reactivity of the cerebral vasculature. *Am. J. Obstet. Gynecol.*, **172**, 1273–8

65. Ohkura, T., Teshima, Y., Isse, K., Matsuda, H., Inoue, T., Sakai, Y., Iwasaki, N. and Yoshimasa, Y. (1995). Estrogen increases cerebral and cerebellar blood flows in postmenopausal women. *Menopause*, **2**, 13–18

66. Bishop, J. and Simpkins, J. W. (1992). Role of estrogens in peripheral and cerebral glucose utilization. *Rev. Neurosci.*, **3**, 121–37

67. Namba, H. and Sokoloff, L. (1984). Acute administration of high doses of estrogen increases glucose utilization throughout brain. *Brain Res.*, **291**, 391–4

68. Burger, H. G. (1996). The endocrinology of the menopause. *Maturitas*, **23**, 129–36

69. Jaffe, A. B., Toran-Allerand, C. D., Greengard, P. and Gandy, S. E. (1994). Estrogen regulates metabolism of Alzheimer amyloid β precursor protein. *J. Biol. Chem.*, **269**, 13065–8

70. Niki, E. and Nakano, M. (1990). Estrogens as antioxidants. *Meth. Enzymol.*, **186**, 330–3

71. Mooradian, A. D. (1993). Antioxidant properties of steroids. *J. Steroid Biochem. Mol. Biol.*, **45**, 509–11

72. Behl, C., Davis, J. B., Lesley, R. and Schubert, D. (1994). Hydrogen peroxide mediates amyloid β protein toxicity. *Cell*, **77**, 817–27

73. Sagara, Y., Dargusch, R., Klier, F. G., Schubert, D. and Behl, C. (1996). Increased antioxidant enzyme activity in amyloid β protein-resistant cells. *J. Neurosci.*, **16**, 497–505

74. Kushwaha, R. S., Foster, D. M., Barrett, P. H. R., Carey, K. D. and Bernard, M. G. (1991). Metabolic regulation of plasma apolipoprotein E by estrogen and progesterone in the baboon (*Papio* sp). *Metabolism*, **40**, 93–100

75. Applebaum-Bowden, D., McLean, P., Steinmetz, A., Fontana, D., Matthys, C., Warnick, G. R., Cheung, M., Albers, J. J. and Hazzard, W. R. (1989). Lipoprotein, apolipoprotein, and lipolytic enzyme changes following estrogen administration in postmenopausal women. *J. Lipid Res.*, **30**, 1895–906

76. Muesing, R. A., Miller, V. T., LaRosa, J. C., Stoy, D. B. and Phillips, E. A. (1992). Effects of unopposed conjugated equine estrogen on lipoprotein composition and apolipoprotein-E distribution. *J. Clin. Endocrinol. Met.*, **75**, 1250–4

77. Bauer, J., Ganter, U., Strauss, S., Stadtmüller, G., Frommberger, U., Bauer, H., Volk, B. and Berger, M. (1992). The participation of interleukin-6 in the pathogenesis of Alzheimer's disease. *Res. Immunol.*, **143**, 650–7

78. Ershler, W. B. (1993). Interleukin-6: a cytokine for gerontologists. *J. Am. Geriatr. Soc.*, **41**, 176–81

79. Horowitz, M. C. (1993). Cytokines and estrogen in bone: anti-osteoporotic effects. *Science*, **260**, 626–7

80. Birge, S. J. (1994). The role of estrogen deficiency in the aging central nervous system. In Lobo, R. A. (ed.) *Treatment of the Postmenopausal Woman: Basic and Clinical Aspects*, pp. 153–7. (New York: Raven Press)

81. Henderson, V. W., Paganini-Hill, A., Emanuel, C. K., Dunn, M. E. and Buckwalter, J. G. (1994). Estrogen replacement therapy in older women: comparisons between Alzheimer's disease cases and nondemented control subjects. *Arch. Neurol.*, **51**, 896–900

82. Mortel, K. F. and Meyer, J. S. (1995). Lack of postmenopausal estrogen replacement therapy and the risk of dementia. *J. Neuropsychiatr. Clin. Neurosci.*, **7**, 334–7

83. Paganini-Hill, A. and Henderson, V. W. (1994). Estrogen deficiency and risk of Alzheimer's disease in women. *Am. J. Epidemiol.*, **140**, 256–61

84. Paganini-Hill, A. and Henderson, V. W. (1996).

Estrogen replacement therapy and risk of Alzheimer's disease. *Arch. Intern. Med.*, **156**, 2213–17

85. Brenner, D. E., Kukull, W. A., Stergachis, A., van Belle, G., Bowen, J. D., McCormick, W. C., Teri, L. and Larson, E. B. (1994). Postmenopausal estrogen replacement therapy and the risk of Alzheimer's disease: a population-based case-control study. *Am. J. Epidemiol.*, **140**, 262–7

86. Tang, M.-X., Jacobs, D., Stern, Y., Marder, K., Schofield, P., Gurland, B., Andrews, H. and Mayeux, R. (1996). Effect of oestrogen during menopause on risk and age at onset of Alzheimer's disease. *Lancet*, **348**, 429–32

87. Fillit, H., Weinreb, H., Cholst, I., Luine, V., McEwen, B., Amador, R. and Zabriskie, J. (1986). Observations in a preliminary open trial of estradiol therapy for senile dementia-Alzheimer's type. *Psychoneuroendocrinology*, **11**, 337–45

88. Honjo, H., Ogino, Y., Naitoh, K., Urabe, M., Kitawaki, J., Yasuda, J., Yamamoto, T., Ishihara, S., Okada, H., Yonezawa, T., Hayashi, K. and Nambara, T. (1989). *In vivo* effects by estrone sulfate on the central nervous system – senile dementia (Alzheimer's type). *J. Steroid Biochem.*, **34**, 521–5

89. Honjo, H., Ogino, Y., Tanaka, K., Urabe, M., Kashiwagi, T., Ishihara, S., Okada, H., Araki, K., Fushiki S., Nakajima, K., Hayashi, K., Hayashi, M. and Sakaki, T. (1993). An effect of conjugated estrogen to cognitive impairment in women with senile dementia – Alzheimer's type: a placebo-controlled double blind study. *J. Jpn. Menopause Soc.*, **1**, 167–71

90. Ohkura, T., Isse, K., Akazawa, K., Hamamoto, M., Yaoi, Y. and Hagino, N. (1994). An open trial of estrogen therapy for dementia of the Alzheimer type in women. In Berg, G. and Hammar, M. (eds.) *The Modern Management of the Menopause: a Perspective for the 21st Century*, pp. 315–33. (New York: Parthenon Publishing)

91. Ohkura, T., Isse, K., Akazawa, K., Hamamoto, M., Yaoi, Y. and Hagino, N. (1994). Low-dose estrogen replacement therapy for Alzheimer disease in women. *Menopause*, **1**, 125–30

92. Ohkura, T., Isse, K., Akazawa, K., Hamamoto, M., Yaoi, Y. and Hagino, N. (1994). Evaluation of estrogen treatment in female patients with dementia of the Alzheimer type. *Endocr. J.*, **41**, 361–71

93. Henderson, V. W., Watt, L. and Buckwalter, J. G. (1996). Cognitive skills associated with estrogen replacement in women with Alzheimer's disease. *Psychoneuroendocrinology*, **21**, 421–30

94. Bartus, R. T., Dean, R. L., Beer, B. and Lippa, A. D. (1981). The cholinergic hypothesis of geriatric memory dysfunction. *Science*, **217**, 208–17

95. Knapp, M. J., Knopman, D. S., Solomon, P. R., Pendlebury, W. W., Davis, C. S. and Garcon, S. I. (1994). A 30-week randomized controlled trial of high-dose tacrine in patients with Alzheimer's disease. *J. Am. Med. Assoc.*, **271**, 985–91

96. Schneider, L. S., Farlow, M. R., Henderson, V. W. and Pogoda, J. M. (1996). Effects of estrogen replacement therapy on response to tacrine in patients with Alzheimer's disease. *Neurology*, **46**, 1580–4

97. Espeland, M. A., Applegate, W., Furberg, C. D., Lefkowitz, D., Rice, L. and Hunninghake, D. (1995). Estrogen replacement therapy and progression of intimal–medial thickness in the carotid arteries of postmenopausal women. *Am. J. Epidemiol.*, **142**, 1011–19

98. Stampfer, M. J. and Colditz, G. A. (1991). Estrogen replacement and coronary heart disease: a quantitative assessment of the epidemiologic evidence. *Prevent. Med.*, **20**, 47–63

99. Grodstein, F., Stampfer, M. J., Manson, J. E., Colditz, G. A., Willett, W. C., Rosner, B., Speizer, F. E. and Hennekens, C. H. (1996). Postmenopausal estrogen and progestin use and the risk of cardiovascular disease. *N. Engl. J. Med.*, **335**, 453–61

100. Ettinger, B., Friedman, G. D., Bush, T. and Quesenberry, C. P. Jr (1996). Reduced mortality associated with long-term postmenopausal estrogen therapy. *Obstet. Gynecol.*, **87**, 6–12

101. Falkeborn, M., Persson, I., Terent, A., Adami, H. O., Lithell, H. and Bergstrom, R. (1993). Hormone replacement therapy and the risk of stroke: follow-up of a population-based cohort in Sweden. *Arch. Intern. Med.*, **153**, 1201–9

102. Henderson, V. W. and Paganini-Hill, A. (1995). Estrogens and Alzheimer's disease. In Asch, R. and Studd, J. (eds.) *Progress in Reproductive Medicine*, pp. 185–93. (New York: Parthenon Publishing)

103. Henderson, V. W. (1997). Estrogen replacement therapy and Alzheimer's disease. In Whitehead, M. (ed.) *The Prescriber's Guide to Hormone Replacement Therapy*. (New York: Parthenon Publishing)

Menopause transition

C. A. Morse

7

Introduction

For several decades in Western society widespread beliefs have prevailed that mid-aged women undergo considerable and debilitating experiences as they pass through the menopausal transition. Yet many women report they have found their actual experiences to be more tolerable and manageable than they had expected[1,2]. The well-designed large community-based studies in the last decade from Australia, Britain, North America and Scandinavia have provided little substantive support that the negative predictions apply to most mid-aged women[3-7]. However, it is important to recognize that within these large cohort studies, a proportion of women do seek help for a wide range of troublesome experiences and that not all women undergo a relatively benign passage with only transient disturbance. The natural transition to menopause occurs for most women between the ages of 45 and 55 years with a mean age of about 50–51 years. This onset has not changed for at least two centuries and appears to be unrelated to age at menarche, socioeconomic factors or body mass index (BMI).

For methodological precision, the changes which women undergo during their transition to menopause are best considered in discrete phases. These have been described in several studies during the past thirty years[5,8,9] and are well known. Women are considered premenopausal if they report no changes to menstrual frequency or flow during the prior months; any changes to flow and/or frequency during the same time span is classified as perimenopausal; and 12 consecutive months of amenorrhea is the internationally accepted definition of postmenopause. Women who undergo surgical removal of the uterus with or without oophorectomy are designated as surgically menopausal.

Help-seeking women

Understandably, distressed women seek help from general practitioners and specialist clinics, and the different studies of women presenting for help reveal very similar symptom profiles. These typically include: vasomotor and general physical discomforts (hot flushes, sweats, aches, pains, headaches, weight gain, urinary dysfunction, fatigue, skin problems); sexual difficulties (low desire, response, orgasmic capability); negative moods (depression, anxiety, irritability, tension); and cognitive problems (forgetfulness, distractibility, low concentration)[6,10-13]. Findings from the Melbourne Women's Midlife Health Study[14] revealed that treatment-seekers reported more complaints from all categories of symptoms than did non-utilizers of services. Of 1606 women, help-seeking women were found to a be a non-homogeneous group of two distinctive subcategories. Approximately 24% used health services for prevention-related purposes while 52% sought help for problem-related reasons, and these two subgroups of treatment-seekers had very different symptom profiles. Significant differences favoring the prevention-related utilizers were: being engaged in work (part/full-time), reporting fewer general somatic and vasomotor symptoms, higher well-being, lower self-reported stress or history of premenstrual syndrome (PMS) complaints.

A prior history of menstrually related problems, such as PMS-type complaints, has been identified in several studies[3,4,7,15] as a predictor of subsequent perimenopausal symptom reporting. A new report from the longitudinal phase of the Melbourne Women's Midlife Health Study[16] reveals that significant relationships are to be found between premenstrual physical and psychological complaints and perimenopausal symptom experience. Prior PMS complainants reported significant negative moods, skeletal, digestive and general somatic symptoms during menopause transition compared to women without a PMS-type history, but not more vasomotor complaints including hot-flush frequency, cardiopulmonary or respiratory symptoms. These findings support the notion of increased vulnerability in certain women which predates the onset of menopause transition and is predictive of a more troubled climacteric[17,18].

Biological changes

The wide range of symptoms attributed to menopause onset and progression affects most body systems. These symptoms can be clustered into broad categories of vasomotor instability, cardiopulmonary, skeletal, respiratory, digestive, general somatic symptoms, mood and behavioral changes[3,5,19]. While many of the complaints are reported by women whose menstrual cycles are still continuing, the magnitude of symptoms seems to increase throughout the transition from premenopause to postmenopause, with the perimenopausal phase as the most symptomatic. From the large studies world-wide, similar symptom profiles across the transition have been reported and complaints seem to be directly linked to women's changing menstrual status, which is underpinned by the shifting hormonal milieu.

Endocrinological profile

Data reported from the Melbourne Women's Midlife Health Study[20] show that both age and body mass index (BMI) exert significant effects within each menstrual category throughout the menopause transition. An age-related increase occurred in follicle-stimulating hormone (FSH), decreases were apparent in inhibin, estradiol (E_2)

and testosterone (T), with no age-dependent changes in sex hormone-binding globulin (SHBG) or free androgen index. Similarly, the effects of BMI, across all menstrual categories, were that FSH, E_2, inhibin, T and SHBG all decreased slightly whereas free androgen index increased. After age and BMI effects were corrected, the most impressive change was in FSH the levels of which increased with age across all menstrual groups. In women whose cycles had undergone obvious change in both flow and frequency, levels were 53% higher than in those with unchanged menstrual status ($p < 0.0005$) and in the completed postmenopausal group levels were 253% higher ($p < 0.0001$). Both E_2 and inhibin, when age- and BMI-adjusted, were lower in women who had not menstruated for 3 months or longer and levels continued to decrease the longer the women went without a menstrual bleed, with mean E_2 and inhibin levels being one-half of those observed in women with unchanged menstrual status.

Burger and colleagues[20] suggest these findings support the conclusion that E_2 and inhibin are important feedback hormones, and that their decline approximates equally to FSH increases with age and reducing ovarian function. Richardson and co-workers[21] previously reported evidence for an accelerated loss of follicle numbers leading to their ultimate depletion in women over the age of 40 years, so the rising FSH level is regarded as providing a sensitive index of this decline. The Melbourne data indicate also that women may return to a regular menstrual cycle status for many months before the advance of further menstrual irregularities[20], so single measurements of serum FSH in women aged 45 years and over are regarded as of little true diagnostic value given the very wide range of observed values.

Vasomotor symptoms

Vasomotor instability giving rise to hot flushes and sweating episodes and vaginal atrophy are the key complaints attributed directly to the menopause, termed the 'true' symptoms of the climacteric[22]. They are commonly associated with a range of diverse complaints including dizziness, palpitations, headaches and nausea.

Hot flushes appear to originate within the central nervous system in the anterior hypothalamus[23] and have been clearly linked to a transient lowered thermoregulatory set point which activates the heat-loss responses of sweating and increased peripheral blood flow[24]. Thermographic studies have shown the occurrence of actual temperature changes of up to 5 K in the peripheral skin[25]. Hot flushes may be discrete, self-limiting episodes of up to 3–6 min in duration, or longer experiences lasting up to 1 h or more. They invariably occur with the pulsatile pituitary release of luteinizing hormone (LH). It is also proposed that catecholamine release in the same brain areas provides the link between LH release and hot-flush occurrence.

Ginsberg and colleagues[26] noted that menopausal women seeking help who complained of flushing, had a significantly higher forearm blood flow than a group of non-flushing age-matched women although there were no significant differences in blood pressure between the groups. Other studies support the idea that stress effects influence hot-flush frequency[27,28], and significantly lower levels of plasma β-endorphins have been observed at the onset of flushes[29]. It has also been proposed that many factors impact on and influence hot-flush symptom experiences[27], including time of day, alcohol and caffeine use and anxiety proneness.

Although hot flushes seem to emanate directly from the changing hormonal profile they are by no means universally reported. Transcultural variations in menopausal symptom reporting are well documented[30,31], linked to sociocultural factors that influence symptom perception and reporting biases. Alternatively, cross-cultural differences in symptom experience may be due to racial biological variability. This issue clearly requires further examination.

Sexual changes

General declines in incidence and frequency of intercourse in aging married couples have been reported many times since Kinsey's major study[32]. Cross-sectional studies generally attest to decreasing orgasmic ability, coital frequency and lowered sexual interest during the two decades from 45 years to 65 years[33,34]. These changes in women's sexual response are related both to age and menopausal endocrine status. Some are less clearly directly attributable to menopause and may be due to the aging partner's physical and/or psychological incapacities, while many reported sexual problems have been shown to predate the climacteric[35,36].

The clear biological effects of menopause transition on women's sexuality include reduced basal vaginal-fluid production, an estrogen-dependent process[37,38] which occurs in direct relation to menopausal status. The reduction of vaginal fluid results not only in vaginal discomfort and even trauma during sexual intercourse, but also a woman's level of sexual arousal tends to be judged by the amount and ease of vaginal lubrication achieved. Thus, vaginal dryness, dyspareunia and perceived low sexual response are all linked and presented as problems for treatment by menopausal women seeking help.

A substantial body of research from the social sciences reveals that major causes of sexual problems in women and men arise from the quality of the marital and sexual relationship[39]. Influential factors include the general level of enjoyment of sexual activities, satisfaction with their frequency, the degree of affection for the partner, the level of knowledge and sensitivity by partners regarding the woman's sexual wants and desires[40,41], and the level of confident assertiveness of women to freely express their sexual wants and dissatisfactions.

In dysfunctional sexual partnerships, unassertive women are more likely to comply with requests for intercourse and submit when they are sexually uninterested[42], resulting in limited genital arousal and a learned reinforcement of negative attitudes towards intercourse and sexual activities. Conversely, sexually assertive women report higher levels of sexual desire, orgasmic frequency and greater satisfaction with both the sexual and marital relationships[43].

A lack of effective communication on sexual wants, desires and activity between partners contributes to dysfunctional dissatisfying sexual relations[44]. In heterosexual couples, mid-aged men who experience their own erectile and ejaculatory problems may withdraw from their female partners to protect their own self-esteem. The women in turn interpret that withdrawal as a rejection of them, construed as due to being unattractive, undesirable and not sexually arousing. Lesbian couples also experience sexual difficulties in midlife and beyond, and these will be multiplied if both women in the partnership are undergoing menopause transition simultaneously.

Data on the sexual experiences of 1979 women in the Melbourne Women's Midlife Health Study[3] showed that 62% reported no change in sexual interest over the previous 12 months, 31% reported a decline and 6.6% reported an increase. Decline in interest related to the male partner's lack of interest, ill health or long periods of absence. Overall, findings revealed that the natural menopause transition is associated with declining sexual intercourse frequency and increasing discomfort on intercourse during the transition from pre- to postmenopause. However, surprisingly, women using hormone replacement therapy (HRT) were the group most likely to report changed sexual interest. Of the 124 women using HRT, many women reported increased frequency of intercourse, but paradoxically, they were also the ones most likely to report unusual pain on intercourse.

Psychological changes

The advent of menopause has been linked to many and varied psychological consequences in mid-aged women. These include negative moods, low self-confidence and self-esteem, increased reports of stress and poor ability to cope. These changes are generally regarded as secondary to the hormonal alterations[4,45,46]. The recent well-designed studies from around the world show no significant support for the view that psychological problems can be attributed directly to the effects of the natural menopause transition (e.g. Busch and colleagues[47]). Where poor psychological well-being has been reported, this was related to: long-term adverse physical-health conditions resulting in restricted physical activity[5]; stressful relationships with others; multiple overwhelming roles; past problematic histories of menstrual distress[15,48]; treatment-seeking for problem-related issues[14,49]; socioeconomic status and lack of gainful employment[4]; vulnerable women with long-standing previous psychiatric diagnoses[18]; users of HRT[50]; and those women with a history of premenstrual-related moods, with or without physical problems[7,15,16,51].

From these sources, reports of negative moods, stress and poor psychological status clearly emanate from socially based sources of causality that interact with episodes of menstrual function change.

These findings provide strong support for the notion that menopausal transition cannot be held responsible for the adverse psychological symptoms presented by those mid-aged women who seek help for troublesome experiences. Instead, it appears that 'self-fulfilling prophecies' operate, where women undergoing menopause who either fear the onset of adverse changes or expect minimal disturbances, tend to report matching experiences.

Cognitive function in menopausal women

A proportion of mid-aged women seek help and treatment for changes to mental processing capabilities, forgetfulness, poor concentration, distractibility and problem-solving difficulties. This disturbance in brain functions is at present being attributed to the hormonal changes that occur during menopause transition and after, and reflects long-standing scientific beliefs that intellectual abilities are gender-specific, influenced from intrauterine life and across the life span by differential hormonal influences.

Though the primary ovarian steroids have been credited with influencing a wide range of mental functions and resultant behaviors, a large body of research undertaken to date reveals that distinct hormonal influences on intellectual capacities in otherwise well-functioning individuals is not well supported and that evidence is slight for direct effects on behaviors (e.g. testosterone-aggression/estrogen-passivity hypotheses).

Some researchers have considered whether the more stable and low hormonal milieu found in oophorectomized postmenopausal women can explain symptom reports of poor memory, concentration loss and deficits in decision-making and problem-solving ability, and proposals are emerging that 'rescue' with hormone therapies will reverse this trend[52,53]. Kampen and Sherwin[54] reported that some specific effects were achieved on verbal memory skills in 28 healthy postmenopausal volunteers taking estrogen replacement therapy (ERT). Compared with 43 untreated controls the ERT users performed significantly better on immediate and delayed paragraph recall. There were no significant group differences on other tests of language, spatial or attention skills and the changes, though statistically significant, do not necessarily have direct implications for daily living in otherwise well-functioning women.

A large population-based study[55] of aged women, 65–95 years, living in California, evaluated whether ERT delayed or prevented cognitive function loss. Results indicated no compelling evidence for an estrogen effect on cognitive functions. The findings from this comprehensive study are persuasive although the large age range and differential survival over the 20-year span may have obscured some effects.

While common methodological flaws can be identified in these initial studies, more work is clearly needed to identify the exact mechanisms whereby the inevitable hormonal changes during menopause transition exert the full range of their potential effects, and further, whether all women are at risk equally, and what specific conditions interact with hormonal change to determine cognitive dysfunctions.

Lifestyle factors

Finally, several researchers have drawn attention to life-style factors as major issues influencing the quality of women's menopausal transition[5,7,15,17,51,56]. Socioeconomic status, employment, diet, substance use (alcohol, nicotine), life events and physical activity all impact on women's midlife health prior to, and during, the menopause transition. Research suggests that an earlier menopausal onset seems to be related to long-term cigarette smoking, previous short menstrual cycle length (< 26 days), parity and race[57,58]. Several of the large community-based studies carried out around the world all implicate long-term cigarette smoking as a major factor influencing menopausal health.

The Massachusetts' Women's Health Study[57] reported that current smokers underwent a significantly earlier menopause than non-smokers of almost 2 years (mean 48.89 vs. mean 50.56 years). The Healthy Women Study[59] found that cigarette smoking was the major factor linked to adverse health status, chronic disease, higher intake of saturated fats and alcohol and lower dietary fibre, vitamins and minerals when current smokers were compared with never smokers and ex-smokers. The current and former smokers consumed 50% more alcohol than never smokers, suggesting a strong relationship between the behaviors supporting use of the two substances; and less physical energy was expended by the smokers compared with the ex-smokers, who increased their exercise levels after giving up smoking. From these findings, smokers appear to be largely passive managers of their health.

In the longitudinal phase (L1 to L4) from the Melbourne Women's Midlife Health Study, Guthrie and colleagues[56] have reported that better self-rated health was associated with being engaged in the paid work-force, either for part-time or full-time hours, and regular general exercising. Being an exerciser was linked to fewer reports of skeletal problems, a lower incidence of chronic disease and headaches and a rise in high-density lipids.

Conclusions

It is clearly apparent that the menopause transition does not impact on all women equally. For many women, the experience is minimal with transient effects, if any; for others it heralds the onset of significant ill health with long-term adverse outcomes. It is clear that a biological hormonal explanation alone cannot account adequately for all the wide range of symptoms that women report. For a comprehensive understanding, as with many other human experiences, it is imperative that menopause be considered within the multi-factorial complex of interactive factors from biosocial, psychophysiological, sociocultural and psychosocial sources. As well, menopausal women should not be regarded as one homogeneous group as they clearly are not. It is important to take into account women's past history of psychophysical health experiences which are brought to bear on their menopausal changes; the ways they dealt with earlier health changes and challenges in terms of coping; their typical ways of experiencing and expressing distress and discomfort; and how they perceive their own health and mental well-being in relation to their life activities and important relationships. Each of these aspects will determine to a considerable extent how women respond to the impact of their menopause transition. From the rapid growth

of research during the last 20 years, although much has been uncovered about the nature of women's midlife health experiences through the menopausal transition, controversies and uncertainties remain to be explored and solved. The optimal way forward is to proceed through multi-disciplinary interactive research and the careful evaluation of treatment outcomes.

When presented with women's complaints of vasomotor, sexual, mood, behavioral or cognitive problems the common response by many clinicians is to prescribe HRT as a cure-all for these multifarious changes that emerge in relation to the menopause transition. Although estrogen appears to have a direct effect on ensuring genital comfort (vaginal lubrication, vaginal cytology, bladder neck and urethra) and reducing hot-flush frequency, there is less consistent support for the role of hormones (as estrogen and progesterone) in stimulating sexual desire or enhancing orgasmic frequency and satisfaction.

We still need to conduct careful treatment studies utilizing strong methodologies other than double-blind cross-over designs, of outcomes over the short and long terms, from both qualitative and quantitative perspectives. Also, we need to compare differing treatment modalities that include hormones and other drugs with psychological therapies, complementary therapies and total life-style behavioral management. Only in these ways will we become more able to identify the 'true' nature of changes due to menopause transition and assist women to experience their later years of life in optimal ways.

References

1. Neugarten, B. L. and Kraines, R. J. (1963). Menopausal symptoms in women of various ages. *Psychosom. Med.*, **273**, 266–73
2. Leiblum S. R. and Swartzman, L. C. (1985). Women's attitudes toward the menopause: an update. *Maturitas*, **8**, 47–56
3. Dennerstein, L., Morse, C. A., Burger, H., Green, A., Hopper, J. and Ryan, M. (1993). Menopausal symptomotology; the experience of Australian women. *Med. J. Aust.*, **159**, 232–6
4. Hunter, M., Battersby, R. and Whitehead, M. (1986). Relationships between psychological symptoms, somatic complaints and menopausal status. *Maturitas*, **8**, 217–28

5. McKinlay, J. B., McKinlay, S. M., and Brambilla, D. (1987). The relative contributions of endocrine changes and social circumstances to depression in mid-aged women. *J. Health Soc. Behav.*, **28**, 345–63

6. Matthews, K. A., Wing, R. R., Kuller, L. H., Meilahn, E. N. and Kelsey, S. F. (1991). Influences of natural menopause on psychological characteristics and symptoms of mid-aged healthy women. *J. Cons. Clin. Psychiatry*, **58**, 345–51

7. Holte, A. and Mikkelson, A. (1991). Psychosocial determinants of menopausal complaints. *Maturitas*, **13**, 193–203

8. Jaszmann, L. (1969). The perimenopausal symptoms. *Med. Gynecol. Soc.*, **4**, 268–77

9. Treloar, A. E. (1974). Menarche, menopause and intervening fecundability. *Hum. Biol.*, **46**, 89–107

10. Anderson, E., Hamburger, S., Liu, J. H. and Rebar, R. W. (1987). Characteristics of menopausal women seeking medical assistance. *Obstet. Gynecol.*, **156**, 428–33

11. Farrell, E., Morse, C. A. and Varnavides, K. (1987). The prevalence of menopausal symptoms; a multidisciplinary approach. Presented at *5th International Congress on Menopausal Research*, Sorrento, Italy, October

12. Egeland, G. M., Kuller, L. H., Mathews, K. A., Kelsey, S. F., Cauley, J. and Guzick, D. (1991). Premenopausal determinants of menopausal estrogen use. *Prevent. Med.*, **20**, 343–9

13. Sherwin, B. B. (1994). Sex hormones and psychological functioning in post-menopausal women. *Exp. Gerontol.*, **29**, 423–30

14. Morse, C. A., Smith, A., Dennerstein, L., Green, A., Hopper, J. and Burger, H. (1994). The treatment-seeking woman at menopause. *Maturitas*, **18**, 161–73

15. Collins, A. and Landgren, B.-M. (1995). Reproductive health, use of oestrogen and experience of symptoms in perimenopausal women: a population-based study. *Maturitas*, **20**, 101–11

16. Morse, C. A., Guthrie, J. R., Dudley, E. and Dennerstein, L. (1996). Relationships between premenstrual syndrome and perimenopausal experiences. *Psychosom. Med.*, submitted

17. Greene, J. G. (1990). Psychosocial influences and life events at the time of the menopause. In Formanek, R. (ed.) *The Meaning of Menopause; Historical, Medical and Clinical Perspectives*, pp. 79–115. (New Jersey: The Analytic Press)

18. Stewart, D. E. and Boydell, K. M. (1993). Psychologic distress during menopause: associations across the reproductive life cycle. *Int. J. Psychiatr. Med.*, **23**, 157–62

19. Kaufert, P. and Syrotuik, J. (1981). Symptom reporting at the menopause. *Soc. Sci. Med.*, **15e**, 173–84

20. Burger, H. G., Dudley, E. C., Hopper, J. L., Shelley, J. M., Green, A., Smith, A., Dennerstein, L. and Morse, C. A. (1995). The endocrinology of the menopausal transition: a cross-sectional study of a population-based sample. *Clin. Endocrinol. Metab.*, **80**, 3537–45

21. Richardson, S. J., Senikas, V. and Nelson, J. F. (1991). Follicular depletion during the menopausal transition: evidence for accelerated loss and ultimate exhaustion. *J. Clin. Endocrinol. Metab.*, **65**, 1231–5

22. Utian, W. (1980). *Menopause in Modern Perspective; a Guide to Clinical Practice.* (New York: Appleton-Century-Crofts)

23. Rebar, R. W. and Spitzer, I. B. (1987). The physiology and measurement of hot flushes. *Am. J. Obstet. Gynecol.*, **156**, 1284–8

24. Kronenberg, F., Cote, L. J., Linkie, D. M., Dyrenfurth, I. and Downey, J. A. (1984). Menopausal hot flashes: thermoregulatory, cardiovascular, and circulating catecholamine and LH changes. *Maturitas*, **6**, 31–43

25. Schneider, H. P. G. (1986). The climacteric syndrome. In Greenblatt, R. B. (ed.) *A Modern Approach to the Perimenopausal Years*, pp. 39–56. (Berlin: Walter de Gruyter)

26. Ginsburg, J., Hardiman, P. and O'Reilly, B. (1989). Peripheral blood flow in menopausal women who have hot flushes and in those who do not. *Br. Med. J.*, **298**, 1488–90

27. Gannon, L., Hansel, S. and Goodwin, J. (1987). Correlates of menopausal hot flashes. *J. Behav. Med.*, **10**, 277–85

28. Swartzman, L. C, Edelberg, R. and Kemmann, E. (1990). Impact of stress on objectively recorded menopausal hot flushes and on flush report. *Health Psychol.*, **9**, 529–45

29. Tepper, R., Neri, A., Kaufman, H., Schoenfeld, A. and Ovadia, J. (1987). Menopausal hot flushes and plasma B-endorphins. *Obstet. Gynecol.*, **70**, 150–2

30. Swartzman, L. C., Edelberg, R. and Kemmann, E. (1990). The menopausal hot flush: symptom reports and concomitant physiological changes. *J. Behav. Med.*, **13**, 15–30

31. Kronenberg, F. (1990). Hot flashes: epidemiology and physiology. In Flint, M. and Utian, W. (eds.) *Multidisciplinary Perspectives on the Menopause*, pp. 52–86. (New York: Academy of Sciences)

32. Kinsey, A. C. (1953). *Sexual Behavior in the Human Female.* (Philadelphia, PA: W. B. Saunders)

33. Pfeiffer, R. E, Verwoendt A. and Davis, G. C. (1972). Sexual behaviour in middle life. *Am. J. Psychiatry*, **128**, 1262–7

34. Hallstrom, T. (1973). *Mental Disorder and Sexuality in the Climateric*. (Copenhagen: Scandinavian Books)

35. McCoy, N. and Davidson, J. (1985). A longitudinal study of the effects of menopause on sexuality. *Maturitas*, **7**, 203–10

36. Sarrel, P. M. and Whitehead, M. (1985). Sex and menopause: defining the issues. *Maturitas*, **7**, 217–24

37. Riley, A. J. (1991). Sexuality and the menopause. *J. Sex. Marital Ther.*, **6**, 135–46

38. Semmens, J. P. and Wagner, G. (1982). Oestrogen deprivation and vaginal function in post-menopausal women. *J. Am. Med. Assoc.*, **248**, 445–8

39. McCabe, M. P. (1994). The influence of the quality of relationship on sexual dysfunction. *Aust. J. Marital Fam.*, **15**, 2–8

40. Snyder, D. K. and Berg, P. (1985). Determinants of sexual dissatisfaction in sexually distressed couples. *Arch. Sex. Behav.*, **12**, 237–46

41. Pietropinto, A. (1986). Male contribution to female sexual dysfunction. *Med. Asp. Hum. Sex.*, **20**, 84–91

42. Hoch, Z., Safir, M. P., Peres, G. and Shepner, J. (1981). An evaluation of sexual performance: comparison between sexually dysfunctional couples. *J. Sex. Marital Ther.*, **7**, 195–206

43. Hurlbert, D. F. (1991). The role of assertiveness in female sexuality: a comparative study between sexually assertive and sexually non-assertive women. *J. Sex. Marital Ther.*, **17**, 183–90

44. Bachman, G. A. and Leiblum, S. (1991). Sexuality in sexagenarian women. *Maturitas*, **19**, 43–50

45. Morse, C. A. and Dennerstein, L. (1989). Psychosocial aspects of the climacteric. In Demers, L. M., McGuire, J. L., Phillips, A. and Rubinow, D. R. (eds.) *Premenstrual, Post-Partum and Menopausal Mood Disorders*, pp. 179–92. (Baltimore: Urban and Schwarzenberg)

46. Greene, J. G. and Cooke, D. (1980). Life stress and symptoms at the climacteric. *Br. J. Psychiatry*, **136**, 486–91

47. Busch, C. M., Zonderman, A. B. and Costa, P. T. (1994). Menopausal transition and psychological distress in a nationally representative sample. *J. Aging Health*, **6**, 209–28

48. Holte, A. (1992). Influences of natural menopause on health complaints; a prospective study of healthy Norwegian women. *Maturitas*, **14**, 127–41

49. Stewart, D. E., Boydell, K., Derzko, C. and Marshall, V. (1992). Psychologic distress during the menopausal years in women attending a menopause clinic. *Int. J. Psychiatr. Med.*, **22**, 213-20

50. Matthews, L. H., Wing, K. A., Kuller, R., Meilahn, E. N. and Kelsey, S. F. (1991). Influences of natural menopause on psychological characteristics and symptoms of mid-aged healthy women. *J. Cons. Clin. Psychol.*, **58**, 345–51

51. Hunter, M. S. (1993). Predictors of menopausal symptoms: psychosocial aspects. *Baill. Clin. Endocrinol. Metab.*, **7**, 33–45

52. Sherwin, B. B. (1988). Estrogen and/or androgen replacement therapy and cognitive functioning in surgically menopausal women. *Psychoneuroendocrinology*, **13**, 345–57

53. Phillips, S. M. and Sherwin, E. (1992). Effects of estrogen on memory function in surgically menopausal women. *Psychoneuroendocrinology*, **17**, 485–95

54. Kampen, D. L. and Sherwin, B. B. (1994). Estrogen use and verbal memory in healthy post-menopausal women. *Obstet. Gynecol.*, **83**, 979–83

55. Barrett-Connor, E. and Kritz-Silverstein, D. (1993). Estrogen replacement therapy and cognitive function in older women. *J. Am. Med. Assoc.*, **269**, 2637–41

56. Guthrie, J. Dennerstein, L., Dudley, E. C., Burger, H. G., Hopper, J. L., Green, A. and Morse, C. A. (1996). Lifestyle approach to management of the menopause. Presented at *8th World Congress on the Menopause*, Sydney, November.

57. Brambilla, D. J. and McKinlay, S. N. (1989). A prospective study of factors affecting the age at menopause. *J. Clin. Epidemiol.*, **42**, 1031–9

58. Whelan, E. A., Sandler, D. P., McConnaughey, D. R. and Weinberg, C. R. (1990). Menstrual and reproductive characteristics and age at natural menopause. *Am. J. Epidemiol.*, **131**, 625–32

59. Perkins, K. A., Rohay, J. and Meilahn, E. N. (1993). Diet, alcohol and physical activity as a function of smoking status in middle aged women. *Health Psychol.*, **12**, 410–15

New delivery systems for hormone replacement therapy

8

I. S. Fraser and Y. Wang

Introduction

Delivery systems are 'devices' designed to modify release of a drug in some specific way, usually at a controlled rate over a specific period of time. They are usually understood to be devices which prolong the action of the released drug and improve the convenience of administration. Examples of these systems have been in general use for many years, and one familiar example in the field of hormone replacement therapy is the series of compressed crystalline estradiol subdermal implants marketed by the Organon Company (Oss, The Netherlands).

Delivery systems offer a range of advantages in certain situations in terms of improved efficacy, safety, ease and convenience, and in many communities have high acceptability. There is a measure of urgency to develop improved choices, because of the rapidly increasing worldwide awareness of the need for many women to use postmenopausal hormone replacement therapy (HRT) for preventive indications over very many years. There is also good evidence that the beneficial effects of HRT wear off within a few years of stopping medication. In this situation, compliance becomes a matter of over-riding importance, and any measures which can be taken to assist women with long-term use will be worthwhile. There is currently substantial evidence that most women who start taking HRT do not continue in the long term[1,2].

The increasing need for long-term postmenopausal hormone replacement therapy

There are still many in modern society who regard hormone replacement therapy as unnatural and unnecessary, and indeed even harmful, for long-term use[3]. The present authors would challenge these individuals to consider the menopause in a different light in our complex and demanding modern society. In more primitive human societies few women ever lived to see menopause, and there was no need to develop specific health maintenance mechanisms for this phase of life. In an evolutionary sense the human species has not developed specific mechanisms to cope with the extraordinarily rapid pace of change in the structure and health of modern society, and the altered demands which these have placed on reproductive function and on multiple organ function in old age. The steady increase in longevity in all countries means that increasing numbers of women will be living a substantial portion of their lives after the menopause.

There is a high level of morbidity in the postmenopausal phase of life, and recent data suggest that 60–80% of health costs are spent on people who are within 6 months of the end of their lives. With increasing numbers of women in this phase of life it may become impossible to finance adequate care of all their health problems from the earnings of the smaller workforce. Anything which can be done to improve overall community health in this age group will be enormously valuable to individuals and communities. There is steadily increasing evidence to indicate that long-term HRT improves general health, and reduces morbidity and mortality so convincingly that those with some risk factors for the problems which may develop as a consequence of estrogen withdrawal in the postmenopause should all be on HRT. In order to achieve widespread usage of HRT it is essential that it is made as appealing and easy to use as possible, and a move towards increasing the availability and appeal of the newer developments in long-acting delivery seems to be one of the most promising avenues for further progress.

Definition of a delivery system

In its broadest sense, a delivery system is any device which modifies release of a drug, but in common usage it is taken to mean a device which prolongs drug release and maintains it at a more constant rate than normal oral ingestion. Delivery systems come in a wide range of forms for releasing drugs into many different body compartments. The possible routes for HRT include slow-release oral tablets, transdermal, subcutaneous, intramuscular, transvaginal and intrauterine administration. There is now considerable experience with a number of systems capable of releasing estrogens, progestogens and androgens in various combinations for hormone replacement therapy.

The pharmacokinetic aim of most delivery systems for HRT is to achieve release rates close to zero-order, which should result in relatively constant blood levels over prolonged periods of time. It is hypothesized that this pattern of release is most likely to result in optimum symptom relief at minimum blood levels with minimal side-effects and metabolic effects, although there is little substantive evidence that this is really the case. The systems which come closest to achieving zero-order release are generally those which are truly long-acting and are non-biodegradable with a rate-limiting

membrane, such as the vaginal rings and intrauterine hormone-releasing systems. Transdermal systems have the potential to come close, but the 3–4-day systems still have a modified first-order profile with a substantial initial peak.

Need for delivery systems

Most people find the frequent taking of any medication to be a real problem unless they have well-regulated lives where remembering the next dose is triggered by some regularly occurring event. In modern society the increasing complexity of most individuals' lives makes frequent dosage a difficult dilemma, hence prolonged duration of action is one of the major advantages of delivery systems. Other attributes of delivery systems which begin to meet some of the needs of many HRT users include tailored and constant release rates, ease of use, some user control, low blood levels of active steroids, usually reduced side-effects, avoidance of the first-pass effect of metabolism through the liver, high acceptability and high continuation rates of usage.

No system is perfect, and disadvantages include the need for careful counseling about optimal usage, ongoing supervision and high cost compared with tablets. There is also an overt suspicion by the media and the general public about high technology in health and about 'hormone' therapy in particular. This translates into increased recourse by the public to medicolegal activity and solution by the court system when a perceived problem arises. A number of serious legal problems have arisen with high technology systems used for other indications, including contraception, and it is a matter of considerable urgency that strategies are developed by manufacturers and health providers for identifying and avoiding possible target areas. This may be a vain hope, since numerous lawyers in North America, Europe and Australia have now become expert at identifying and exploiting any avenue of possible litigation in 'growth areas' related to health. The delivery systems are a prime target because they have prolonged duration of action, usually involve high technology (which is often vulnerable), involve close medical supervision, cause some side-effects (like every treatment) and have a higher cost than older oral drugs.

Currently available systems

Unfortunately, there is no uniformity of availability of different systems in different countries, and no country has full availability of all systems and few have access to all routes of delivery at the present time. It is to be hoped that the current major restructuring within the international pharmaceutical industry should lead to more rapid introduction of new technologies on a global scale in the future. Parallel changes in international harmonization of drug regulatory evaluations should also expedite some of the ponderous bureaucracy for which this field of human endeavor is noted.

Transdermal delivery

This is currently the most active field for HRT delivery system research and system refinement. Several different systems are marketed and numerous different systems are under development, utilizing different types of technology with various combinations of steroids over different device life spans and with different adhesives[4]. Skin-patch delivery systems are usually called transdermals since the drug reservoir remains outside the skin. Steroid-containing gels which are massaged into the skin are often referred to as percutaneous systems, where the skin itself acts as a partial, temporary reservoir. Transdermal delivery occurs mainly by passive diffusion of lipid-soluble substances through lipophyllic spaces between keratinized cells of the stratum corneum[5].

Transdermal patches have excellent potential to approach zero-order release of steroids, and the 7-day matrix patches closely approximate this following a small initial peak[6,7]. The twice-weekly reservoir patches have a release profile which is more complex with a very rapid initial rise within 3–4 h followed by a slower rise to a second peak at 48 h, and then a gradual decline to low levels at 96 h[6,7]. The 7-day patches maintain higher and more constant blood levels to the end of their planned therapeutic duration of action, although both systems have high and similar clinical efficacy. One of their disadvantages is the high and costly technology involved in their development and manufacture. A variety of differing technologies is involved in the manufacture of different patches, and the systems exhibit a range of different constructions to store and control the release of the active ingredients[4].

Major interest in the transdermal approach has focused on plastic patches which can be engineered to deliver relatively precise dosages, although there are also a number of percutaneous steroid-delivering gel systems available. The gels require the woman to apply a carefully measured amount of an alcohol-based steroid-containing gel onto the abdominal skin once a day. When used correctly, these systems deliver approximately equivalent daily amounts of estradiol into the body and are highly effective at symptom relief[8]. Some women find this approach very appealing, but they appear to be in a minority.

Several differently constructed skin patches are available. These can be broadly divided into two groups: reservoir patches and matrix patches. The original system (Estraderm®; Ciba-Geigy, Basel) is a 3–4-day reservoir patch containing 400 µg of estradiol dissolved in an alcohol-based gel enclosed in a permeable membrane, backed by impermeable plastic and framed by an adhesive strip. The overall area of the patch is 18 cm² (of which 10 cm² releases drug) and it is designed to release approximately 50 µg of estradiol per 24 h. The matrix patches usually involve a technology such as that developed by the 3M Corporation where the steroid is incorporated into a non-ethanol adhesive matrix. These patches are ultrathin (less than 0.5 mm), translucent, two-layer, non-reservoir film laminates with a protective liner attached to the adhesive surface, and are constructed of elastomeric materials which are capable of some stretch. The rate of drug delivery is controlled by diffusion through the skin, rather than by use of a rate-limiting membrane as in the reservoir patches[9].

The matrix patches incorporate 300–400 µg of estradiol into a 12.5–30 cm^2 surface area for a daily 50 µg release rate. Larger surface areas will deliver higher daily release rates. Mean serum levels of estradiol of around 90–120 pmol/l can be expected during use of the 50-µg patches, with approximately double the concentration (180–210 pmol/l) from the 100-µg patches. Serum estrone levels are very similar to those of estradiol, which is much lower than would be expected after oral administration. A number of comparative studies have been carried out to demonstrate the similarities and differences between different transdermal systems[7,10,11]. These tend to confirm that the matrix patches have a number of advantages over reservoirs, and that the newer adhesives are more effective and less likely to cause side-effects.

Several combination estrogen–progestogen patches are being brought on to the market to provide a full range of choices to rival oral preparations. These can either be used in a standard sequential manner or as a continuous combined preparation[12]. Considerable activity is also being directed towards the development of clinically useful androgen-releasing patches.

Transdermal estradiol-releasing (and combination) systems are highly effective at relieving the full range of menopausal symptoms[13–16], and are probably as effective as oral HRT in preventing the longer-term effects of menopause, such as osteoporosis[17]. The latest 7-day patches probably do this at lower mean serum levels of estradiol than oral preparations or early patches because of the relatively constant blood levels over prolonged periods of time[18]. This low-dose concept should also apply to vaginal rings and non-biodegradable implants.

Side-effects are relatively minor apart from the well-recognized problem of local allergic skin irritation which occurs in 15–40% of women with the original alcohol-based reservoir patches[19]. This side-effect still occurs with the more recent pressure-sensitive adhesives in the latest 7-day patches, but is probably less than 10% overall[6,18]. Nevertheless, this side-effect is a major disincentive to use of these systems especially in hot and humid countries, where this problem is perceived to be worse. There is evidence that occlusion of the skin by an impermeable plastic backing may cause sweat-duct blockage and microbial proliferation in some women, contributing to the local reaction[20]. Some women dislike the minor accumulation of skin debris and dirt on the rim of adhesive around the 7-day patches. Other side-effects, such as breast tenderness, headaches and nausea, have always been minor and transient. The only other significant problem with this type of delivery system is premature detachment, which increases the cost (and the inconvenience) if it occurs with any frequency. Metabolic changes are usually less than those demonstrated with oral preparations[13,15,19,21], although some studies have demonstrated more 'beneficial' lipid changes with certain oral combinations[22].

Acceptability of transdermal systems is high in most cultures[10], and this has encouraged the confidence of the several manufacturers who are in the process of bringing a wide range of different estrogen, estrogen–progestogen and androgen patches to the market.

Subdermal implants

Subcutaneous hormone implants have been in regular use for the control of menopausal symptoms since their first use by Bishop in London in 1938. Estradiol- and testosterone-releasing implants were extensively pioneered by Greenblatt in the 1940s and 1950s, and more recently by Studd and colleagues[23]. These biodegradable implants all consist of fused, crystalline steroid in a single compressed pellet which erodes very slowly at the surface following insertion, to release the active hormone into the subcutaneous fat. The implants come in different sizes (e.g. 20 mg, 50 mg and 100 mg of estradiol) in order to provide different durations of action, but durations and blood levels vary very widely depending on individual rates of metabolism. This is the biggest disadvantage of these simple, effective and completely biodegradable implants. Other disadvantages include the great difficulty in removing the implants following insertion if intolerable side-effects supervene (which is very unusual), and the need to provide regular moderate-dosage progestogen exposure for women who retain their uterus. These implants have been used particularly in hysterectomized women[24].

The pharmacokinetics varies considerably from woman to woman, and some experience very high initial blood levels (greater than 1000 pmol/l) which gradually decline over periods of many months, or occasionally years[25]. Blood levels tend to increase steadily over a period of 3 years or more[26]. The high blood levels of estradiol give excellent symptom relief, although recurrence of atypical vasomotor and headache symptoms with the onset of the decline in estradiol levels from their initial peak in some women is occasionally a problem. With use of higher-dosage implants a small number of women develop a type of tachyphylaxis[27,28] where they require progressively higher and higher estradiol blood levels (with more frequent implant insertions) to maintain good symptom relief. Low-dose (20 mg) implants have been used with considerable success on a long-term basis to prevent osteoporosis[29,30].

Subdermal testosterone implants have been used extensively for androgen replacement in hypogonadal males, but their use in women has been more controversial. In recent years, there has been increasing agreement that they have an important and effective place in the management of low libido in women with depressed testosterone levels after menopause, who have not improved with estradiol alone[31]. They should always be used in conjunction with estrogen (usually also given by implant), to reduce the incidence of androgenic side-effects associated with the high free testosterone level which occurs when serum estradiol and sex hormone-binding globulin levels are low.

It is clear that there is a place for the development of a non-biodegradable silastic-type estradiol implant, which will provide much lower (150 pmol/l) serum levels on a constant, zero-order basis, and which will avoid the problems of symptom recurrence at high, but declining, serum levels, and of tachyphylaxis. Much lower serum levels will also be more easily opposed by lower doses of progestogen. Easy removal of a single non-biodegradable implant would also simplify the timing of reinsertion. A single implant releasing 50 µg of estradiol per day could be designed to provide a 2-year life span. Such systems are still in the early stages of design and trial, but would seem to have an important place in the overall future range of HRT choices.

Intramuscular injections

Injections of estrogenic preparations or combinations of estrogen and progestogen esters have been used for many years for the relief of postmenopausal symptoms, but most of the preparations suffer from a short duration of action and the need for frequent injections. They also result in very high early blood levels and a variable duration of action. A few combinations can be given at 6–8-week intervals[32], and the progestogen-only preparation, depot medroxyprogesterone acetate, has been used for symptom relief at 12-week intervals[33]. This is not regarded as a promising route for future HRT delivery systems.

Menopausal vaginal rings

Vaginal ring delivery systems for hormone replacement therapy are not nearly as advanced as their counterparts for contraceptive use, although paradoxically the only hormone-releasing vaginal ring currently marketed anywhere in the world is an ultralow-dose postmenopausal estradiol-releasing ring. This delivery system has the potential to provide great flexibility of dosage, and has considerable appeal to many women. Rings can easily be designed to provide a wide range of release rates, and estradiol-17β is relatively well absorbed across the vaginal mucosa. It is also feasible to design combination rings, simultaneously releasing varying dosages of estradiol and progesterone (or a progestogen) which can be used in cyclical, sequential or continuous regimens.

This approach has high acceptability for many women, provided that they are comfortable about touching their genitalia. The main appeal is that the woman herself has complete control of the method in relation to insertion and removal, if she wishes. Long-term compliance is such a problem with most HRT regimens that a convenient long-acting system such as a vaginal ring is very attractive to both providers and users. The only marketed ring is an ultralow-dose estradiol-releasing system (Estring®; Pharmacia, Sweden), which is designed for the management of local urogenital symptoms, and not for systemic HRT. This vaginal ring releases estradiol at a constant rate of 5–10 μg/day (mean 8 μg/day) over a 3 month period. Higher-dose estradiol-releasing rings for systemic HRT delivery are in the early stages of development, and are being designed to release between 50 and 200 μg of estradiol per day. Cyclical usage will be recommended for perimenopausal women or for those who wish to have a withdrawal bleed. Continuous usage will be for those who are clearly postmenopausal and do not wish to have regular withdrawal bleeds.

The ultralow-dose estradiol ring is capable of producing a high level of relief from hypoestrogenic vaginal symptoms and some urinary symptoms. This ring is designed for use without an opposing progestogen, because the release rate is so low. Initial absorption of estradiol through the very thin atrophic postmenopausal vaginal mucosa is rapid and measurable estradiol levels can be detected in serum, but once some vaginal mucosal thickening has occurred the systemic absorption of estradiol is so low that elevations of serum estradiol cannot be measured, and subsequent endometrial proliferation is very uncommon[34,35].

Symptomatic improvement in vaginal dryness, dyspareunia, pruritis, dysuria and urgency with this remarkably low estradiol exposure, is accompanied by major improvements in all objective signs of vaginal atrophy including vaginal mucosal pallor, petechiae, friability, dryness, and in mucosal maturation values and indices for vaginal cytology[34–37]. These studies have demonstrated that this system is as effective as, but much more acceptable than, several vaginal creams and pessaries releasing estrogens. In a large multicenter Australian trial comparing Estring with Premarin® vaginal cream, 131 women were treated with Estring over a 3-month period[35]. Mild breakthrough bleeding or spotting only occurred in 6% of ring users, mainly during the very early absorption period before thickening of the vaginal mucosa. Some superficial vaginal erythema was noted at the ring site after removal in 8% of women, but no cases of abrasion or ulceration were detected. Of 11 Estring treatment withdrawals, nine women complained of nausea, headache, abdominal pain, backache, urinary infection or vulval discomfort, and only two women experienced spontaneous expulsion on several occasions[35]. The ultralow-dose estradiol delivery system was graded excellent or good by 84% of Estring users, and by only 43% of cream users. Of the 27 women using Estring who had previously used an estrogen vaginal cream, all preferred Estring to previous cream use[35]. Ongoing clinical trials are currently involved in comparing this ring with twice-weekly use of small biodegradable vaginal tablets releasing 25 μg estradiol (Vagifem®; Novo Nordisk) over a 12-month period of continuous use. Preliminary results confirm that both therapeutic approaches are symptomatically effective with minimal side-effects, no ulcerative effects on the vaginal mucosa or any increase in ultrasonically determined endometrial thickness. Most women prefer the convenience of the ring, but a small number find it unsuitable because of a tendency for expulsion during defecation.

Higher-dose rings aimed at relief of vasomotor symptoms appear to be highly effective in early clinical trials and have the potential to perform in an equivalent manner to skin patches releasing estradiol and progesterone. Comparisons of these systems have not yet been performed. Preliminary pharmacological data indicate that rings delivering 160 µg and 80 µg of estradiol per day will produce mean serum levels of approximately 200–250 pmol/l and 140–160 pmol/l respectively. These levels should be highly effective in alleviating climacteric symptoms and protecting against bone loss and cardiovascular disease. Combination estradiol–progesterone menopausal vaginal rings for systemic HRT are currently in the early stages of clinical development, and should provide a valuable addition to the range of vaginal delivery systems.

These systems are likely to fulfil an increasingly important role for HRT in most societies in the future, as the vaginal route becomes more widely recognized as an appropriate route for treatment delivery. Acceptability of the vaginal approach to hormone delivery is high in contraceptive users[38], and preliminary indications suggest that this will also be true for HRT users.

Intrauterine systems

It has been suggested that intrauterine delivery of a low dose of progestogen might be an excellent means of protecting the endometrium against the excessive proliferative effects of unopposed estrogen, without causing some of the unwanted side-effects of systemic progestogens. Preliminary experience with a levonorgestrel-releasing intrauterine system (Levonova/Mirena®; Leiras, Finland) appears to confirm this promise. This system was designed as a long-acting contraceptive (5–7 years), but has also proven to be an effective treatment for menorrhagia. The dosage chosen for these indications was a 20-µg daily release rate, and this results in some absorption with measurable circulating levels of around 500 pmol/l. This is highly effective at protecting the endometrium in HRT users[39,40], but it appears probable that equally effective

protection can be provided by 10-µg or even 5-µg daily release[41]. At these dosages when combined with oral estradiol valerate, the system remained highly effective at protecting the endometrium, inducing amenorrhea, relieving postmenopausal symptoms and producing beneficial changes in circulating lipids[41]. At the 20-µg dosage, lipid effects were similar to those seen with oral levonorgestrel and were less beneficial[41,42]. The 20-µg device is relatively wide for insertion into the postmenopausal uterus, and it is to be hoped that reduction of dosage to 5 µg will allow a more slimline version to be manufactured.

New delivery systems

The present systems are still far from ideal. They exhibit a range of appealing attributes, but all still exhibit a number of disadvantages. Since these systems each offer a variety of different attributes, there is a real need to continue development of all approaches. In order to allow women to reach optimal usage of HRT through informed choice it is important that relevant choices with differing appeal are provided.

It was calculated that there were around 40 new HRT preparations under development in 1995[43]. The majority of these were transdermal formulations, but a quarter were oral, and the remainder were vaginal, sublingual and intranasal systems. It is unclear whether the popularity of this commercial research investment is an indication of fashion or an indication of logical emphasis on the most rational approaches! There are a substantial number of needs in further HRT delivery system development:

(1) The need for greater personal choice;

(2) The need to reduce or eliminate present disadvantages, e.g. use problems such as loss of skin adhesion with patches or vaginal ring expulsion, side-effects;

(3) The need for greater flexibility and control of dosage;

(4) The need to make really long-term use much easier, for example with 5-year systems analogous to those used in contraception;

(5) The need to maximize efficacy.

A wide range of technologies needs to be explored further, to achieve acceptable solutions for the needs of widespread, long-term HRT usage in increasingly aging populations. There are some indications of a commercial recognition that further investment of venture capital in this field will eventually achieve a substantial return, despite the long lead times and the risk of unforeseeable pitfalls.

The long term

There is an overwhelming need for manufacturers and providers of long-acting menopausal delivery systems to avoid the types of problem being artificially manufactured by lawyers around long-acting contraceptives in the USA and UK. The archaic present-day legal system is becoming totally inappropriate for dealing with the real problems occurring with modern medical treatments, and needs a major overhaul. Recently, only about 12% of the

awards made by the courts against the Detroit Medical Center in 1992–94 actually reached the plaintiff, the majority going to court expenses, legal and witness fees[44]. No system can continue to sustain a ponderous and self-serving bureacracy which consumes 88% of the 'venture capital' in order to provide a minimal amount of compensation to the 'victim'. It would be devastating indeed if the huge amount of scientific effort and clinical care and concern which has gone into the development of these new and improved technical approaches to the delivery of HRT, is 'torpedoed' in the same way that the legal machine has targeted the subdermal contraceptive implant, Norplant® in the USA.

These delivery system approaches have the potential for enormous benefit to mankind, need to be developed carefully, tested thoroughly and provided by well-trained health professionals to a well-informed public. In order to use the increasing range of types of HRT optimally there is a real need for the public to become better informed about the different choices. The public needs to be educated, in the broadest sense, about how to find out information for itself, and how to discriminate the quality of information.

References

1. Ravnikar, V. A. (1987). Compliance with hormone therapy. *Am. J. Obstet. Gynecol.*, **156**, 1332–4
2. Harris, R. E., Laws, A., Reddy, V. M., King, A. and Haskell, W. (1990). Are women using postmenopausal estrogens? A community survey. *Am. J. Publ. Health*, **80**, 1266–8
3. Greer, G. (1991). *The Change.* (London: Hamish Hamilton)
4. Balfour, J. A. and Heel, R. C. (1990). Transdermal estradiol: a review of its pharmacodynamic and pharmacokinetic properties, and therapeutic efficacy in the treatment of menopausal complaints. *Drugs*, **40**, 561–82
5. Kligman, A. M. (1984). Skin permeability: dermatological aspects of transdermal drug delivery. *Am. Heart J.*, **108**, 200–8

6. Gordon, S. F. (1995). Clinical experience with a seven-day estradiol transdermal system for estrogen replacement therapy. *Am. J. Obstet. Gynecol.*, **173**, 998–1004
7. Baracat, E., Haidar, M., Castelo, A., Tufik, S., Rodriguez de Lima, G., Vieira, J. G. H., Peloso, U. and Casoy, J. (1996). Comparative bioavailability study of a once-a-week matrix versus a twice-a-week reservoir transdermal estradiol delivery systems in postmenopausal women. *Maturitas*, **23**, 285–92
8. Scott, R. T. J. K., Ross, B., Anderson, C. and Archer, D. F. (1991). Pharmacokinetics of percutaneous estradiol: a cross-over study using a gel and a transdermal system in comparison with oral micronized estradiol. *Obstet. Gynecol.*, **77**, 758–64
9. Knepp, V. M. (1987). Transdermal drug delivery:

problems and possibilities. *Crit. Rev. Ther. Drug Carrier Syst.*, **4**, 13–32

10. Transdermal HRT Investigators Group (1993). A randomised study to compare the effectiveness, tolerability and acceptability of two different transdermal estradiol replacement therapies. *Int. J. Fertil.*, **38**, 5–11

11. Pornel, B., Genazzani, A. R., Costes, D., Dain, M. P., Lelann, L. and Vandepol, C. (1995). Efficacy and tolerability of Menorest 50 compared with Estraderm TTS50 in the treatment of postmenopausal symptoms. A randomised, multicentre, parallel group study. *Maturitas*, **22**, 207–18

12. Oosterbaan, H. P., van Buuren, A. H. J. A. M., Schram, J. H. N., van Kempen, P. J. H., Ubachs, J. M. H., van Leusden, H. A. I. M. and Beyer, G. P. J. (1995). The effects of continuous combined transdermal oestrogen–progestogen treatment on bleeding patterns and the endometrium in postmenopausal women. *Maturitas*, **21**, 211–19

13. Padwick, M. L., Endacott, J. and Whitehead, M. I. (1985). Efficacy, acceptability and metabolic effects of transdermal estradiol in the management of postmenopausal women. *Am. J. Obstet. Gynecol.*, **152**, 1084–91

14. Place, V. A., Power, M., Darley, P. E., Schenkel, L. and Good, W. R. (1985). A double-blind comparative study of Estraderm and Premarin in the amelioration of postmenopausal sumptoms. *Am. J. Obstet. Gynecol.*, **152**, 1092–9

15. Selby, P. L., McGarrigle, H. H. G. and Peacock, M. (1989). Comparison of the effects of oral and transdermal oestradiol administration on oestrogen metabolism, protein synthesis, gonadotrophin release, bone turnover and climacteric symptoms in postmenopausal women. *Clin. Endocrinol.*, **30**, 241–9

16. Studd, J. W. W., McCarthy, K., Zamblera, D., Burger, H. G., Silberberg, S., Wren, B., Dain, M. P., Le Lann, L. and Vandepol, C. (1995). Efficacy and tolerance of Menorest compared to Premarin in the treatment of postmenopausal women. A randomised, multicentre, double-blind, double-dummy study. *Maturitas*, **22**, 105–14

17. Field, C. S., Ory, S. J., Wahner, H. W., Hermann, R. R., Judd, H. L. and Riggs, B. L. (1993). Preventive effects of transdermal estradiol on osteoporotic changes after surgical menopause: a two-year placebo-controlled trial. *Am. J. Obstet. Gynecol.*, **168**, 114–21

18. Speroff, L., Whitcomb, R. W., Kempfert, N. J., Boyd, R. A., Paulissen, J. B. and Rowan, J. P. (1996). Efficacy and local tolerance of a low-dose, 7-day matrix estradiol transdermal system in the treatment of menopausal vasomotor symptoms. *Obstet. Gynecol.*, **88**, 587–92

19. Utian, W., (1987). Transdermal estradiol overall safety profile. *Am. J. Obstet. Gynecol.*, **156**, 1335–8

20. Uchegbu, I. F. and Florence, A. T. (1996). Adverse drug events related to dosage forms and delivery systems. *Drug Safety*, **14**, 39–67

21. Fox, J., George, A. J., Newton, J. R., Parsons, A. D., Stuart, G. K., Stuart, J. and Sturdee, D. W. (1993). Effect of transdermal oestradiol on the haemostatic balance of menopausal women. *Maturitas*, **18**, 55–64

22. Schram, J. H. N., Boerrigter, P. J. and The, T. Y. (1995). Influence of two hormone replacement therapy regimens, oral oestradiol valerate and cyproterone acetate versus transdermal oestradiol and oral dydrogesterone, on lipid metabolism. *Maturitas*, **22**, 121–30

23. Thom, M., Collins, W. P. and Studd, J. W. W. (1981). Hormonal profiles in postmenopausal women after therapy with subcutaneous implants. *Br. J. Obstet. Gynaecol.*, **88**, 426–33

24. Staland, B. (1978). Treatment of menopausal oestrogen deficiency symptoms in hysterec-tomised women by means of 17-beta-oestradiol pellet implants. *Acta Obstet. Gynecol. Scand.*, **57**, 281–5

25. Alder, E. M., Bancroft, J. and Livingstone, J. (1992). Estradiol implants, hormone levels and reported symptoms. *J. Psychosom. Obstet. Gynaecol.*, **13**, 223–35

26. Barlow, D. H., Abdalla, H. I., Roberts, A. D. G., Al Azzawi, F., Leggate, I. and Hart, D. M. (1986). Long-term hormone implant therapy – hormonal and clinical effects. *Obstet. Gynecol.*, **67**, 321–5

27. Gangar, K., Cust, M. and Whitehead, M. I. (1989). Symptoms of oestrogen deficiency associated with supraphysiological plasma oestradiol concentrations in women with oestradiol implants. *Br. Med. J.*, **299**, 601–2

28. Garnett, T., Studd, J. W., Henderson, A., Watson, N., Savvas, M. and Leather, A. (1990). Hormone implants and tachyphylaxis. *Br. J. Obstet. Gynaecol.*, **97**, 917–21

29. Naessen, T., Persson, I., Adami, O., Bergstrom, R. and Bergkvist, L. (1990). Hormone replacement therapy and the risk of first hip fracture. A prospective, population-based cohort study. *Ann. Intern. Med.*, **113**, 95–103

30. Naessen, T., Persson, I., Thor, L., Mallmin, H., Ljunghall, S. and Bergstrom, R. (1993). Maintained bone density at advanced ages after long-term treatment with low-dose oestradiol implants. *Br. J. Obstet. Gynaecol.*, **100**, 454–9

31. Burger, H. G., Hailes, J., Nelson, J. and Menelaus, M. (1987). Effect of combined implants of oestradiol and testosterone on libido in postmenopausal women. *Br. Med. J.*, **294**, 936–7

32. Frigo, P., Eppel, W., Asseryanis, E., Sator, M.,

Golaszewski, T., Gruber, D., Lang, C. and Huber, J. (1995). The effects of hormone substitution in depot form on the uterus in a group of 50 perimenopausal women – a vaginosonographic study. *Maturitas*, **21**, 221–5

33. Bullock, J. L., Massey, F. M. and Gambrell, R. D. (1975). Use of medroxyprogesterone acetate to prevent menopausal symptoms. *Obstet. Gynecol.*, **46**, 165–74

34. Henriksson, L., Stjernquist, M., Boquist, L. Alander, U. and Selinus, I. (1994). A comparative multicenter study of the effects of continuous low-dose estradiol released from a new vaginal ring versus estriol pessaries in postmenopausal women with symptoms and signs of urogenital atrophy. *Am. J. Obstet. Gynecol.*, **171**, 624–32

35. Ayton, R. A., Darling, G. M., Murkies, A., Farrell, E. A., Weisberg, E. and Fraser, I. S. (1996). A comparative study of safety and efficacy of continuous low-dose estradiol released from an intravaginal ring versus conjugated equine estrogen vaginal cream in the treatment of postmenopausal urogenital atrophy. *Br. J. Obstet. Gynaecol.*, **103**, 351–8

36. Holmgren, P., Lindskog, M. and von Schoultz, B. (1989). Vaginal rings for continuous low-dose release of oestradiol in the treatment of vaginal atrophy. *Maturitas*, **11**, 55–63

37. Smith, P., Heimer, G., Lindskog, M. and Ulmsten, U. (1993). Oestradiol-releasing vaginal ring for treatment of postmenopausal urogenital atrophy. *Maturitas*, **16**, 145–54

38. Weisberg, E., Fraser, I. S., Mishel, D. R. Jr, Lacarra, M. and Bardin, C. W. (1995). The acceptability of a combined oestrogen– progestogen contraceptive vaginal ring. *Contraception*, **51**, 39–44

39. Schmidt, G., Andersson, S. B., Nordle, O., Johansson, C. J. and Gunnarsson, P. O. (1994). Release of 17-beta-oestradiol from a vaginal ring in postmenopausal women: pharmacokinetic evaluation. *Gynecol. Obstet. Invest.*, **38**, 253–60

40. Raudaskoski, T. H., Tomas, E. I., Paakari, I. A., Kaupilla, A. J. and Laatikainen, T. J. (1995). Transdermal oestrogen with a levonorgestrel-releasing intrauterine device for climacteric complaints: clinical and endometrial responses. *Am. J. Obstet. Gynecol.*, **172**, 114–19

41. Wollter-Svensson, L. P., Stadberg, E., Andersson, K., Mattsson, L. A., Mattsson, V., Odlind, V. and Persson, I. (1995). Intrauterine administration of levonorgestrel in two low doses in HRT. A randomised clinical trial during one year: effects on lipid and lipoprotein metabolism. *Maturitas*, **22**, 199–205

42. Raudaskoski, T. H., Tomas, E. I., Paakari, I. A., Kauppila, A. J. and Laatikainen, T. J. (1995). Serum lipids and Lipoproteins in post-menopausal women receiving transdermal oestrogen in combination with a levonorgestrel-releasing intrauterine device. *Maturitas*, **22**, 47–54

43. Nachtigall, L. E. (1995). Emerging delivery systems for estrogen replacement: aspects of transdermal and oral delivery. *Am. J. Obstet. Gynecol.*, **173**, 993–7

44. Ransom, S., Dombrowski, M. P., Shephard, R. and Leonardi, M. (1996). The economic cost of the medico-legal tort system. *Am. J. Obstet. Gynecol.*, **174**, 1903–9

The consequences of longevity

M. Lachowsky

Longevity is life, longevity is living and living longer: longer than what? Does mankind have a specified time to spend on earth, with individuals living their different ages, or is each human being living his own allotted time? This may well be an important issue as we do not know the duration of our life spans, but we do know there is a beginning, already duly recorded, and there will be an end, maybe already recorded somewhere. There is no infinity there, rather a full-stop, but without either a when or a where.

This awareness of death is one of the privileges man has over animal, but is it a privilege? It could be, rendering priceless that evanescent and fragile possession we may lose even without our knowledge. It should be, so why is one part of mankind always inventing new devices to maim or kill, battling against a life others are trying hard to protect and lengthen? We have to live knowing eternity is not for us, although sometimes in the spring of youth we tend to forget it. Later, some of us call for help and need to reach for metaphysical or religious heights, referring to that valley of tears as being a station, the only possible antechamber to the unknown other world, a space with no limit and no end, and a time without time.

Time seems to have always been humanity's great interrogation, and perhaps its even greater anxiety. Chronos keeps eating his children as our sophisticated watches keep nibbling at our life account, without ever giving us the exact balance. The only inkling is age and its weighty numbers, but even that is not an absolutely reliable datum. Children die, and grandparents add a third digit to their age.

Longevity used to mean the duration of life, but now we hear it as meaning longer than life, longer than we could hope for at the end of our finishing 20th century. These 'great expectations' seem amply justified by today's happenings. The dream of being allowed a bigger quota of years is nowadays a reality, as long as we do not forget it is still a privilege, given solely to those richer parts of the globe where we have the chance – as astonishing as it is unmerited – to have alighted. What makes it even more of a chance, or a lottery, is that we still do not know in advance to whom this privilege may or may not have been given. It goes without saying that science is trying to make it less of a hazard and more of a necessity, hoping to decode the genetic status which would lead to a general status.

We all understand that longevity does not mean immortality, but that is one part of the problem. 'Die, we do the rest', proclaimed an American undertaker's motto. Changing it to 'live, we do the rest' could be a good way to express what everybody expects in order to enjoy longevity. After all, why not simply say that doctors and scientists are proud to play a role, and a major one, in this new state of affairs; but are they always happy, and are their fellow human beings always happy with their newly found bonus?

Is it a bonus? Maybe that is the question, the core of the discussion. It certainly cannot be anything less as far as quantity is concerned. Life has always seemed so short that one has to hurry not to let it bypass you or pass you by. That rapid passing of time was and is food for thought to the poet and the philosopher. Each in his own way urges man to put those fleeting hours to good use, even if that good use does not have the same meaning for all. More often than not, in the poet's book, man presses woman to give in to passion, before he eventually takes his vows elsewhere, or before she gets too old even to remember how she and everything else around them was desirable and enjoyable. Have we changed so much since Ronsard wrote his *Sonnets to Hélène*; do we not still call our young times the good old times?

'Aye, there's the rub...' says young Hamlet. The tissue of life is not of the same fabric all along; persons and circumstances change, weighed down as they all are by that same time which passes alternately too slowly and too quickly. Life is threaded with different colors: those of our ups and downs, of our gains and our losses, full of right and wrong, or of tears and laughter, sometimes for the same reasons. That is what longevity is all about. If it meant staying forever happy and healthy, we would not have given it a second thought, and would simply enjoy it rather than discuss it.

As usual, things are not that simple, and there is not just one aspect to the matter but many, as many cofactors as in any severe disease, although it is quite understood that if longevity does not always induce ease, it certainly cannot be taken for a disease. Ease or disease, anyway it is far from an easy notion, more of a new problem arising – as often today – from our ever-increasing progress and discoveries. We live longer and we will live even longer, but how and what for, 'that is the question'?

That brings us to the real issue, or put in an even more provocative way: what or where is the sense of that addition to the subtractions that age is entering on everyone's personal computer? Will it only cause a multiplication of ills, all in all a loss in an operation no raider would ever contemplate, the odds being what they are?

What is the use of quantity if it does not rhyme with quality, that quality of life so often spoken of nowadays, as if it really was a new demand? This is a new concept perhaps, needing sociology for its definition and medicine for its obtention, a concept already included in the World Health Organization (WHO) definition of health, where well-feeling is as necessary as well-being, both being of concern to medical doctors. Let us remember that in ancient China, the role of doctors was to prevent rather than cure, sickness being

considered as a failure and leaving the practitioner open to punishment. It is true that much more recently, at the time of the French revolution, Saint-Just said that 'Happiness is a new idea in Europe.' By now it is not an idea any longer, it is everybody's wish, and it might be the new way to put that old demand, this label of quality without which there seems to be no point to an increase of quantity.

However, what lies underneath these old and new formulations? Is a life of quality similar for everybody, does it have the same meaning and does it cover identical needs or desires in all of us? Certainly not, apart from basic necessities, and that might well be what makes it so difficult to define. Let us express it as the intertwining of 'sense and sensibility' – as Jane Austen so aptly put it – that gives us the will and the strength, the desire and the drive to go on as long as possible, to deal with pleasure with that longevity which is our own life. Maybe the wishes we usually express at the New Year actually represent what we expect of a 'good' life: health and a wealth of love and friendship, meaning a body that will stay as reliable as the people around us, be they family or friends. This becomes all the more important to alleviate the fear that can turn the gift of longevity into the worst poison, the fear of the dreaded impairments of age and even worse, of aging alone. What if longevity left you stranded, in a world where nobody needs you or where few know you? It might well be what used to be called 'a fate worse than death'.

Anyway, all the above is true; it has already happened. Fresh new statistics from all over the world show us how, despite the violence of man and nature, old people keep getting older. In a society where youth is the major value and aging the greatest sin, it does seem strange to sing the praise of years. It should be a feat and not a defeat to manage to go on living in our dangerous end of century, but it is usually more appreciated on paper than socially. It is also true that health-care professionals have a great responsibility in this recent state-of-the-art, especially as gynecologists, caring for women, the 'second sex' as Simone de Beauvoir named them in the 1950s.

Women, in fact, used to survive fewer years than men. Their direct link to life made them an easier prey for death, which not so long ago was still lurking around the four-poster beds as well as in the hospital wards. Women paid a heavy ransom for that extraordinary privilege, the power of bringing new lives into the world. The literature is full of those big families sired by one man and cared for by at least two women, hemorrhaging or infected wombs being then part of women's legacy.

There have been changes, however: men have worked at making childbirth less dangerous as well as less painful, and women have been offered the gift of choosing their time for motherhood and the gift of love and sex without the perennial fear of unwanted pregnancy. 'Make love, not war' could have been their motto when so many died or were maimed for life, because nothing was too terrible when trying to get rid of a menacingly tell-tale embryo. Birth-control and family planning are part of today's woman's life, and of her expected longevity. But what of her man's longevity? Has it also made his life easier and added years to his time? It should have, with a healthier companion, a happier one, more present at his side, more free to accompany and sustain him while less burdened by womanly troubles, and much more attuned to his earthly needs. It could have, especially now, when even menopause and its wake of unpleasantness has almost given way before medicine's assaults: but has it? To be honest, it does not seem so. Statisticians as well as doctors confirm that men fare less well nowadays, losing a few years to womankind, and maybe feeling somewhat left aside by that new surge of tender and loving care gynecologists are bestowing on their patients. The word 'patients' is wrong and misleading; there is no sickness there but rather a way to get help before it is needed, before age has taken its toll; a custom-made replacement therapy in a sup-portive environment which is now the rule . . . for those women who so desire.

Men sometimes feel when looking at their sixtyish spouses that nothing is being done for them. What if androgens were suddenly not so much of a bargain? Leaving him more open to accidents, with less protected arteries and heart, even if wars now make fewer differences between the lines and the genders, man's life appears more at risk. Although if he escapes with his life, what about his shorter life-expectancy; does it really make a difference other than mathematically? Yes, but only if this relatively small package of older days can actually be something to live for, with enough brain and legs left to enjoy them and fellowmen and women with whom to share them, thus turning something old into something new, that famous new longevity which got lost along with paradise. However, let us not forget how long our biblical ancestors are reported to have survived those quite difficult times, lacking very much our domestic and health services. If Sarah conceived so late in life, does it not mean Abraham was still in full glory?

Longevity means living longer, but do we want it at any price, and whatever the condition? As a matter of fact, we are not consulted but just informed, a little like those roses that have long been cultivated for their beauty and longevity although losing their soul, or rather their perfume, in the process. Researchers are now trying to give them their fragrance back, hoping not to diminish their longevity. Fragrance for flowers or charm for human beings, whatever we call the ways to attract interest and love, maybe this is the salt of life. However, our society still has to accept that age and aging is not a shame, in a world which is not getting any younger either. Longevity is like life itself; it is new and old, it brings and it takes, and it is full of promises but also fraught with risks. How can we live longer without getting older; the modern Sphinx enigma?

Bibliography

Bruckner, P. (1995). *La Tentation de l'Innocence.* (Paris: Grasset et Fasquelle)

Launois, R. and Régnier, F. (eds.) (1992). *Décision Thérapeutique et Qualité de Vie.* (Paris: John Libbey, Eurotext)

Mermet, G. (1996). *Tendances 96.* (Paris: Larousse)

Alternative to hormone replacement therapy for menopausal management: possible role of Kampo medicine

10

T. Aso, T. Koyama, H. Kaneko and M. Seki

Introduction

Hormone replacement therapy (HRT) has been widely used in perimenopausal medical care, especially in the USA, Canada and Australia. As a result of a recent survey by Intercontinental Medical Statistics, it is reported that more than 30% of women between the ages of 40 and 65 years in these three countries have been prescribed HRT, and the percentage of women taking HRT is increasing year by year. Even though the net percentages of women taking HRT in the UK, France and Japan are smaller than those of the aforementioned three countries, the same increasing trends are observed.

By extensive evaluation of the risks and benefits of HRT, the apparent positive effects of HRT in cardiovascular diseases, osteoporosis and fractures, and reduction of vasomotor and urogenital symptoms have been indicated. In addition, recent studies have revealed favorable effects of HRT on brain function, and preventive effects on dementia and Alzheimer's disease. Conversely, the estimated relative risks in women taking HRT show that breast cancer and endometrial cancer under unopposed estrogen replacement therapy are the major hazards of HRT. Due to the risks and benefits of currently available HRT mentioned above, one has to recognize its limitations for medical care, and alternatives for treating women who have absolute contraindications such as breast and endometrial cancers are needed. Even for some women bearing myoma or benign breast diseases, HRT has to be occasionally discontinued. In cases showing sustained inexplicable genital bleeding there always exists a risk of malignant alteration of endometrial tissue which cannot be definitely excluded by clinical examination. Both patients and physicians want to be released from the fear of hazards associated with HRT. Although every woman is entitled to her own opinion regarding treatment for estrogen deficiency, a certain number of women are convinced that the administration of female sex hormones after menopause is not natural or physiological. Thus, various kinds of management to meet the needs of all perimenopausal individuals and at all times during this period are required.

Regimens are available to prevent or improve particular individual problems in perimenopause, for example, vasomotor symptoms, bone resorption and cardiovascular diseases. However the complexity of disorders which occur simultaneously in perimenopausal women cannot be totally managed by such methods. Hormone replacement therapy is expected to be beneficial for conditions caused by estrogen deficiency in perimenopausal women, and the effects of treatment should be long-lasting and general rather than targeting a particular organ or function. As an attempt to introduce other candidates that may play similar roles to that of HRT in perimenopausal medical care, the possibility of Kampo medicine is discussed in this paper.

Basic aspects of Kampo medicine

Kampo medicine has been developed on the basis of traditional Japanese culture[1]. The unique conceptual system and procedures to interpret and treat the causes and states of disorders and diseases have been established upon the accumulation, organization and systematization of massive amounts of clinical experience[2].

One of the basic concepts of Kampo medicine is that the normal mental and physical conditions can be maintained on the balance of *Qi*, *Ketsu* and *Sui*. *Qi* has functions but is not identified as a material. It encompasses mental nervous activity, especially the appetite for food and the actual process of digesting and absorbing nutrients. When *Qi* is rushing to the head, flashing, headaches, palpitation and sweating are induced. Conversely, in the state of depressed *Qi*, depression, neurotic symptoms and loss of appetite, so-called stagnated *Qi* symptoms are observed. It can be pointed out that most of these signs are included in the so-called climacteric symptoms.

Ketsu, which means 'blood', is a general term not only referring to blood but also having the meanings of hormones, autonomic nervous system and other regulatory functions of the internal environment. The function of *Ketsu* is under the control of *Qi*. It may be suggested that the relationship and interaction between *Qi* and *Ketsu* is comparable with the feedback mechanism of Western medicine. In cases with stagnation of *Ketsu*, blood congestion causes purpura, hemorrhagic tendency, cold sensation in lower extremities and menstrual disorders.

Sui means water or body fluid. It encompasses overall water metabolism and various functions related to defense mechanisms, such as immune systems. In the state of stagnation of *Sui*, abdominal 'gurgling', diarrhea, edema, joint pain and dizziness are frequently observed.

As the mind and body are considered to be inseparable and interrelated in Kampo medicine, an individual is always diagnosed as a whole organism, and the ultimate goal of treatment is to maintain the systemic homeostasis. These concepts of Kampo medicine are extremely important when health care is carried out for perimenopausal women and also the elderly.

Practice of Kampo medicine

Classification of mental and physical states

In order to practise Kampo medicine, the conceptual classification of mental and physical conditions, confirmation of *Sho*, should be understood. Since the selection of a Kampo formula is done on the basis of the current *Sho*, the proper classification of *Sho* is essential. The *Sho* does not necessarily correspond to the name of a disease used in Western medicine. It is an expression for a state of disease determined by assessing the pattern of symptoms, the stage of the disease state and the degree of stamina.

In Kampo medicine, subjects are classified into two groups of *Sho* named *Yin* and *Yang*. The subjects classified as *Yin* show comparatively depressed vital responses, and those in the *Yang* state express comparatively accelerated responses. The vital responses referred to here are body temperature, pulse and respiratory status, sharpness of movement, pattern response to external stress and so forth.

Another classification of *Sho* is carried out which mainly depends on the current degree of stamina of the body. In this classification, 'deficient' means lacking stamina and a state of depressed physiological functions. 'Excessive' is the state showing considerable stamina and accelerated physiological functions, and 'intermediate' is the state between 'deficient' and 'excessive'.

In the procedures to assess mental and physical state, *Sho* are confirmed by the following four methods:

(1) By questioning, chief complaints, subjective symptoms, history of the current illness and family history are analyzed;

(2) By observation, complexion, appearance of the tongue and condition of the skin are examined visually;

(3) By listening, the pitch of voice, breathing, retention of water in the stomach and so forth are assessed using sense of hearing;

(4) By palpation, the sense of touch is used to examine the conditions of pulse and abdomen.

Table 1 Questionnaire to assess *Sho* (mental physical state). Self-rated scores for each question are added to give a total score. 'In between' also includes unanswered questions

Question	Yes	In between	No
1. Are you a muscular type?	6	3	0
2 Are you of solid build?	6	3	0
3. Are you lustrous-complexioned?	8	4	0
4. Is your abdomen still elastic and tight?	8	4	0
5. Are you usually not troubled by overeating?	6	3	0
6. Do you rather eat rapidly?	6	3	0
7. Do you feel discomfort when not having a daily bowel movement?	6	3	0
8. Are you usually not bothered excessively by hot or cold weather?	6	3	0
9. Is it rare for you to have a chilly sensation in the extremities?	6	3	0
10. Are you an active type?	6	3	0
11. Is it rare for you to feel tired in comparison with other people?	6	3	0
12. Is your voice rather strong?	8	4	0
13. Can you readily perform your daily tasks?	8	4	0
14. Would you rather take a bitter stomachic?	6	3	0
15. Is it rare for you to sweat at night?	8	4	0

An example of a questionnaire used to assess *Sho* and to select prescription of Kampo medicine is shown in Table 1. According to results of the self-rated scoring, women who have a total score of less than 40 are classified as 'deficient', and those with a score of 65 or more are 'excessive'. The term 'intermediate' is used to describe women with a score between 40 and 64.

Prescription of Kampo medicine

The prescription of Kampo medicine is called *Ho* which means the combination of several herbs. The kinds of raw herbs and the amount of each herb in a particular formula have been arranged and determined by experience accumulated in the classic texts[2,3]. Effects produced by Kampo formulae are a synthesis of the various interactions of the constituent substances, and the overall effects are different from the combined effects of individual raw herbs. Some of the Kampo formulae which have been frequently used for climacteric disorders according to classification of the *Sho* are depicted in Table 2. The raw herbs and their major chemicals contained in three representative Kampo formulae named *Toki-shakuyaku-san*,

Keishi-bukuryo-gan and *Hachimi-jio-gan* which have been commonly prescribed for women with climacteric symptoms are summarized in Table 3. To date, more than 140 formulae have been approved for clinical use in Japan. In the process of manufacturing Kampo preparations, strict quality inspections at every stage are carefully conducted in order to supply the formulae to a high quality and with constant efficacy.

Effects of Kampo medicine

Various clinical effects of Kampo medicine, not only on climacteric disorders, have been reported. The results of a clinical study in which the Kampo formula *Keishi-bukuro-gan* was used are depicted in Figure 1. In this study[4], women complaining of climacteric symptoms and also demonstrating elevated serum triglyceride levels greater than 150 mg/dl were enrolled. After 3 months of ingestion of this formula, both the Kupperman index and the triglyceride levels decreased significantly. The Kampo formula Toki-shakuyaku-san exhibits marked beneficial effects in cases suffering from senile vaginitis[5].

In addition to local and specific effects, general and systemic improvements have been

Table 2   Representative Kampo prescriptions for climacteric disorders, their *Sho* scores and clinical features

Prescription	Score	Features
Toki-shakuyaku-san	0–40	Used for rather feeble women of any age with irregularity of menstruation
Kami-shoyo-san	20–50	For relief of psychoneurological symptoms such as shoulder stiffness and easy fatigability as well as for reactivation of ovarian functions. Used primarily for women in their 30th to 50th years
Hachimi-jio-gan	20–60	For relief of lumbar pain, numbness and pollakiuria, and used primarily for those in age bracket from menopause to senility
Nyoshin-san	40–75	Used for patients with prolonged hot flushes and dizziness
Keishi-bukuryo-gan	50–100	For women of sturdy build, with irregularity of menstruation and shoulder stiffness
Tokaku-joki-to	65–100	For patients with relatively greater body strength, suffering from hot flushes, shoulder stiffness and/or constipation

Table 3   Components of three Kampo formulae commonly prescribed for climacteric disorders

Formula	Components	Daily dose (g)
Toki-shakuyaku-san	paeoniae radix	4.0
Pulvis paeoniae et angelicae	atractylodis lanceae rhizoma	4.0
	alismatis rhizoma	4.0
	angelicae radix	3.0
	hoelen	4.0
	cnidii rhizoma	3.0
Keishi-bukuryo-gan	cinnamomi cortex	3.0
Pilulae hoelen et cinnamomi	paeoniae radix	3.0
	persicae semen	3.0
	hoelen	3.0
	moutan radix	3.0
Hachimi-jio-gan	rehmanniae radix	6.0
Formula rehmanniae et octo-medicamentorum	corni fructus	3.0
	dioscoreae radix	3.0
	alismatis rhizoma	3.0
	hoelen	3.0
	moutan cortex	2.5
	cinnamomi cortex	1.0
	aconiti tuber	0.5

provided by Kampo medicine. The clinical course of a postmenopausal woman treated by Kampo medicine is summarized in Table 4. She was 51 years of age and reached menopause 2 years before start of therapy. Her complaints were sleep disturbance, loss of stamina and cold sensation in extremities. The pretreatment evaluations revealed that the simplified

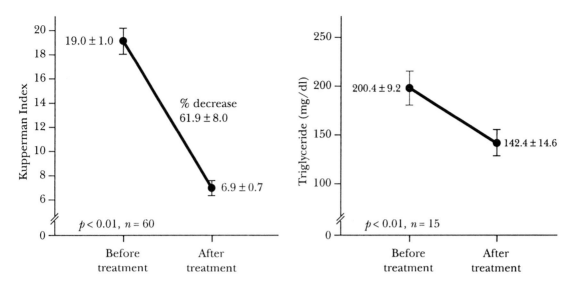

Figure 1 Effects of Kampo formula *Keishi-bukuryo-gan* on climacteric symptoms (Kupperman index) and serum triglyceride levels. Values expressed as mean ± SE. Data from reference 5

Table 4 Clinical course of 51-year-old woman treated by Kampo medicine. Age of menopause 49 years; three pregnancies, two children; height 159 cm; body weight 59 kg. Chief complaints: sleep disturbance, loss of stamina, cold sensation in extremities. Kampo formulae prescribed: *Kami-kihi-to* 5.0 g/day, *Gissha-jinki-gan* 5.0 g/day

	Months of treatment											
	2	*4*	*6*	*8*	*10*	*12*	*14*	*16*	*18*	*20*	*22*	*24*
S M I	88	64	—	52	—	47	—	—	54	38	—	36
Sho	18	20	—	18	—	24	—	—	28	32	—	30
T-chol (mg/dl)	232	—	—	230	—	222	—	—	204	—	—	194
TG (mg/dl)	204	—	—	74	—	130	—	—	148	—	—	126
BMD (g/cm²)	0.821	—	—	—	—	0.832	—	—	—	—	—	0.846

SMI, simplified menopause index; *Sho*, score of Kampo medicine; T-chol, serum total cholesterol; TG, triglyceride; BMD, bone mineral density

menopause index was 88, *Sho* score was 18, serum total cholesterol level was 232 mg/dl, triglyceride was 204 mg/dl and bone mineral density (BMD) at L2–4 was 0.821 g/cm². She complained of severe climacteric symptoms and her *Sho* was classified as *Yin* and 'deficient'. The laboratory data indicated a total cholesterol level at the upper limit of the normal range, elevated triglyceride and decreased BMD. Two kinds of Kampo formulae were selected for her, based on the results of the confirmation of *Sho*

and the subjective and objective findings. After 8 months of treatment, the climacteric symptoms were improved and triglyceride levels decreased to the normal range. After 2 years, further improvement of the subjective symptoms was obtained; normal laboratory data and increased BMD were detected. No adverse effect was observed during the treatment.

An increasing number of experimental approaches have been made to elucidate the background of the clinical effects of Kampo

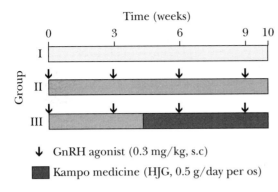

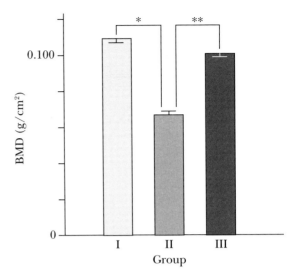

Figure 2 Experimental protocol of study on effects of *Hachimi-jio-gan (HJG)* on bone metabolism in hypoestrogenic, female Sprague–Dawley rats. GnRH, gonadotropin-releasing hormone

Figure 3 Bone mineral density (BMD) of rats in three experimental groups of Figure 4. Values expressed as mean ± SE. *$p < 0.05$; **$p < 0.005$

medicine[6]. The results obtained from a study evaluating the effects of the Kampo formula *Hachimi-jio-gan* on the bone metabolism of hypoestrogenic rats, are reported below. In this study, the rats were given gonadotropin-releasing hormone (GnRH) agonist to induce hypoestrogenic state. As shown by the experimental protocol in Figure 2, the rats of group I were the control, the group II rats were injected with GnRH 0.3 mg/kg of body weight every 3 weeks, and the rats of group III were given *Hachimi-jio-gan* 0. 5 g/day after the second injection of GnRH. All rats were sacrificed after 10 weeks of treatment. The bone mineral contents, measured by the dual energy X-ray absorptiometry (DEXA) method, of the group II rats treated by GnRH alone, were significantly depressed, but administration of the Kampo formula to group III rats could prevent such a decrease (Figure 3). The findings of contact microradiogram of the tibial metaphysis frontal sections of these three groups indicated that osteopenia induced in group II was restored by Kampo medicine in group III (Figure 4). The findings of texture analysis of the tibial diphysis transverse sections of the three groups revealed a statistically significant difference in bone area and width, between groups II and III (Figure 5). The bone-formation parameters investigated by the fluorescent photomicrograph method indicated that the mineralizing surface and

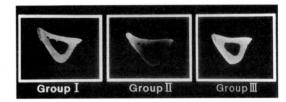

Figure 4 Findings of contact microradiogram of tibial metaphysis frontal sections of rats in three experimental groups of Figure 4

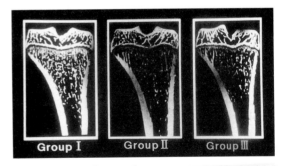

Figure 5 Findings of texture analysis of tibial diphysis transverse sections of rats in three experimental groups of Figure 4

mineral apposition rates were greater in group III, treated by GnRH and Kampo formula, than those of group II, the hypoestrogenic rats treated by GnRH alone. These results strongly suggest the positive involvement of Kampo medicine in the restoration of bone metabolism associated with hypoestrogenic conditions.

Summing up the clinical experience and experimental results, it is convincing that Kampo medicine can provide a variety of beneficial effects on the disorders that commonly appear in perimenopause.

Conclusion

Kampo medicine has unique concepts which are different from those of Western medicine. It seems to be difficult and unacceptable for physicians who have been trained in Western medicine to treat patients by Kampo medicine exclusively. In practice, patients in Japan today are diagnosed and treated from both the Western medicine and Kampo aspects. In the process of selection of Kampo formulae, a Western medical diagnosis is initially conducted by clinical examination and then the pattern of symptoms, the *Sho* manifesting in the patient's whole body, is evaluated by traditional Kampo diagnostic methods. Needless to say, many aspects of Kampo medicine still need to be explored. A scientific explanation for the unique Kampo diagnosis, efficacy and safety are to be evaluated. Research must also be conducted into the origins of the raw herbs, their active ingredients and their mechanisms of action.

It should be emphasized that the treatment objectives of modern medicine have been changing to the extent that maintenance and improvement of quality of life are now included as a key objective. It is hoped that Kampo medicine will play an important role, not only in climacteric medicine as an alternative to HRT, but also in improving the welfare of people all over the world.

Acknowledgement

This study was supported by a Research Grant from the Japan Ministry of Health and Welfare (1995).

References

1. Yamamura,Y. (1988). The history of Kampo medicine and its development in modern Japan. In Hosoya,E. and Yamamura,Y. (eds.) *Recent Advances in the Pharmacology of Kampo Medicine*, pp. 3–13. (Amsterdam, Princeton, Hong Kong, Tokyo and Sydney: Excerpta Medica)

2. Veith, I. (1966). *The Yellow Emperor's Classic of Internal Medicine*. (Berkeley and Los Angeles: University of California Press)

3. Terasawa, K. (1993). *Kampo, Japanese-Oriental Medicine. Insights from Clinical Cases*. (Tokyo: KK Standard McIntyre)

4. Maruo, T. (1993). Kampo medicine for climacteric disorders. *World Obstet.Gynecol.*, **45**, 167–76 (in Japanese)

5. Sakamoto, S., Kudo, H. and Suzuki, S. (1996). Pharmacotherapeutic effects of *Toki-shakuyaku-san* on leukorrhegia in young women. *Am. J. Chinese Med.*, **24**, 165–8

6. Hosoya, E. and Yamamura, Y. (1997). *Recent Advances in the Pharmacology of Kampo Medicine.* (Amsterdam, Princeton, Hong Kong, Tokyo and Sydney: Excerpta Medica)

2

Reports of epidemiological trials

A European trial on secondary prevention of cardiovascular disease 11

K. Schenck-Gustafsson

During the past decades, about 75 mostly observational and epidemiological studies have been published in the area of primary and secondary prevention of cardiovascular disease by estrogens. However, most of the studies were conducted in selected groups of the general population. Eighty-eight reviews in this area have also been published, i.e. more reviews than original articles.

In November 1996, the Swedish Council on Technology Assessment in Health Care[1] reported on all aspects of treatment with estrogens. Concerning prevention of cardiovascular disease, a total of 28 articles were chosen because they fulfilled generally accepted scientific criteria. Eighteen of these related to cardiovascular disease and 10 to stroke. Of the nine cohort studies of cardiovascular disease and estrogen replacement therapy (ERT) one came from Europe, but of the nine case–control studies of cardiovascular disease, none came from Europe. Only four of these 18 studies were secondary preventive, and in addition with retrospectively chosen patients. In the area of stroke and ERT, 10 studies fulfilled the criteria; only two came from Europe. A predominant number of all these studies originated from California. In summary, the above mentioned 18 studies showed a 35–45% reduction of morbidity and mortality in cardiovascular disease induced by estrogen treatment. Concerning stroke and ERT, neither positive nor negative effects were reported by the 10 stroke-related studies. Some of these studies also included estrogens in combination with progestins.

However, all these observational studies share a major flaw, that is that the women who take estrogens are more healthy than women who do not. Estrogen users have a lower risk of death from almost all causes including cancers and other diseases with no possible biological relationship to estrogens. The studies with the lowest relative risks for deaths from coronary heart disease also have the lowest risk for cancer deaths. Unintended selection of healthy women may explain these findings, and may also contribute to an exaggerated estimate of a cardioprotective effect. A better health profile has been shown to be present even before women are prescribed estrogens. Women who have recently stopped hormone replacement therapy (HRT) have higher relative risks for all causes of death, indicating cessation of treatment when risk factors or early disease become manifest.

Probably it is very difficult to correct for all the potential biases in analyzing observational data. Also, combining the results of the observational studies in meta-analyses may even be misleading. If there is a systemic bias in study data, then combining the data of all studies ascribes a significance level to the bias, but does not deal with the basic question. Currently, we simply cannot tell from the observational studies whether there is a real benefit of estrogens on coronary heart disease or what the size of an effect might be. As most of the studies are carried out in the United States there might be a substantial difference between women in Europe and women in the USA. It is well known for example that hysterectomy is more common in the USA compared with Europe. The type of estrogen used differs between Europe and the USA. In Europe 17-β estradiol is the most frequently used drug but in the USA it is conjugated estrogens. Also the addition of gestogens is not quite as common in the United States as in Europe. Whether socioeconomics and religion play a role to explain the differences is still unclear.

The only way to obtain reliable information is through randomized controlled clinical studies, which if large enough will eliminate the possibility that differences between study groups account for the results. Even though insufficient for public health recommendations, the observational data are certainly strong enough to justify the need for trials of clinical outcomes.

What are the Swedish habits? Looking at all women born in 1942 in Stockholm, about 50% of them had HRT. The total figure for the whole country has increased from about 8–10% to 20–25%. This indicates that women born in the 1940s demand HRT the most. A recently performed study from Gothenburg[2] sent a questionnaire to all Swedish gynecologists and one-third of the general practitioners in Sweden. From replies it appeared that 55% of the gynecologists and 19% of the general practitioners gave their patients HRT. Interestingly, 83% of the female gynecologists and 72% of the female general practitioners took HRT themselves. Among the doctors, 86% of the male gynecologists and 68% of the male general practitioners gave HRT to their wives. With reference to indications, 66% of the gynecologists in Sweden thought that prevention of coronary heart disease was a relative or absolute indication for estrogen treatment. This figure obviously reflects that at least the gynecologists believe very much in HRT and its cardioprotective role. The sales figures for HRT in Sweden (when low-dose estrogens are excluded) have increased from about 16 million Swedish crowns in 1987 to about 175 million Swedish crowns in 1995.

There is a substantial amount of biological evidence that estrogens will have an effect on the cardiovascular system. One mediator is the positive estrogen effect on the lipids. Another mediator is the positive effect on the vessel wall where nitric oxide is probably involved. The potential favorable effects on fibrinogen and plasminogen by estrogen may well also explain the positive effects on arterial cardiovascular disease. The slight increase in risk of venous thromboembolism may be explained by an increase in factor X and factor VII and a decrease in antithrombin III.

Treatment suggested by favorable epidemiological associations or effects on intermediate biological outcomes may not confirm clinical benefit. The disappointing and even alarming result of recent trials of β-carotene, and meta-analysis of trials of short-acting calcium-channel blockers as well as nitrates are good examples. Because of their inherent weaknesses, further observational studies or trials of intermediate biological outcome will not answer the important questions: HRT will reduce coronary heart disease incidence, but what is the overall benefit and risk of long-term use? to what extent do the benefits and risks apply to older women? should most postmenopausal women be prescribed HRT? what about long-term compliance and the pharmacokinetics of the different hormone regimens for older patients and other special groups? are there different effects for conjugated estrogens and other types of estrogens? what are the roles of different administrations, for example patches or tablets? what type of schedule should be used – continuous combined or cyclic? and how much spacing out?

Only randomized trials of sufficient size and duration and with clinical outcomes can answer the above questions. Such trials are being conducted in the USA, currently: HERS (Heart and Estrogens–Progestins Replacement Studies) and WHI (Women's Health Initiative). In Europe the British Medical Research Council has financed Wisdom (Medical Research Women's International Study of Long Duration Estrogen after Menopause). These studies will not produce results until the years 2000, 2006 and 2012. In the interim we will have to prescribe estrogens for cardiovascular disease prevention. There are for the moment better proven treatment alternatives, for example diet, smoking cessation, cholesterol-lowering medication, blood-pressure control, low-dose aspirin and beta blockers. There is an urgent need to find answers through these randomized placebo-controlled trials and there is a special need also to conduct more trials not only in the USA, but also in Europe.

References

1. Andersson, K., Mattson, L. A. and Milson, I. (1996). *Lancet*, **348**, 130

2. The Swedish Council on Technology Assessment in Health Care (1996). Treatment with estrogen. Report no. 131, November

The Women's Health Initiative

12

S. R. Johnson

The Women's Health Initiative (WHI) is an ambitious research program currently in progress, sponsored by the United States National Institutes of Health (NIH) and the United States Congress. The WHI was originally conceived to address the relative deficit of research regarding the major medical problems experienced by postmenopausal women, and to provide definite evidence regarding the efficacy of selected, commonly used prevention strategies. The WHI employs two strategies to meet these goals. First, an observational cohort was established. The purpose of the observational cohort is to provide the opportunity to study a wide variety of disorders utilizing nested case–control studies. The second strategy was to conduct randomized controlled clinical trials to determine the efficacy of the selected prevention strategies.

Planning for this project began at the NIH in the mid 1980s[1]. It was felt that a primary prevention trial was warranted. Two initial NIH-sponsored studies paved the way including the Postmenopausal Estrogen Progestins Intervention Trial[2–4] and the Women's Health Trial[5]. These studies supported the idea that postmenopausal women could be effectively recruited and could maintain hormone replacement therapy and/or a low-fat diet for up to 3 years.

Four major causes of morbidity and mortality in postmenopausal women were selected as primary outcomes: coronary heart disease, osteoporosis-associated fractures, breast cancer and colorectal cancer. The rationale for these choices is straightforward. Coronary heart disease is the leading cause of death among women over 65 years of age and accounts for approximately 30% of all-causes mortality in women. Thirty per cent of women experience osteoporosis-related fractures and these are a significant cause of morbidity, including loss of independence in elderly women. Breast and colorectal cancer are among the top three causes of cancer and related mortality in women in the United States. In addition, the risk of each of these may be affected by two of the intervention strategies selected for study.

The Women's Health Initiative is the largest clinical study ever mounted. The budget is approximately US$625 000 000, and 40 clinical recruiting centres will recruit a total of 164 500 participants, 100 000 to the observational cohort and an additional 64 500 to the clinical trials. The total length of the study from beginning of recruiting to close-out is approximately 15 years. Figure 1 illustrates the overall timetable of the trial. The total follow-up period is scheduled to last 12 years. However,

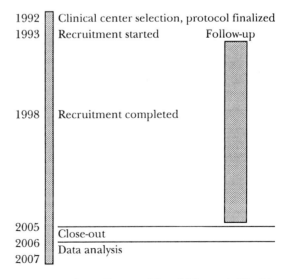

Figure 1 Overall timetable of Women's Health Initiative (WHI) trial

because women will be recruited over 12 years and closed out together in 1 year, the average duration of study intervention is 9 years.

The recruiting approach for the WHI is illustrated in Figure 2. The primary recruiting strategy is to appeal directly to potential participants through the media, direct mail and meetings with relevant groups of women. In general, recruiting will not be done through clinical sites, thus enhancing the generalizability of the ultimate study results. One deficiency of most American clinical trials is that the subjects have been largely healthy Caucasian women of relatively high socioeconomic status. It is the aim of the WHI to recruit a broadly representative sample of American postmenopausal women so that the results of the trial will be widely generalizable. Basic eligibility inclusion criteria include age 50–79 years and postmenopausal status with or without a uterus. Women are excluded if they have a competing health risk that is likely to predict a life span of less than 3 years, or if significant adherence or retention problems are likely. The WHI also aims to focus on older postmenopausal women, a group not often studied. To that end, approximately 60% of the cohort will be over 65 years of age. In addition, the program plans to include approximately 30% of non-white participants. To increase the chance of meeting this goal several clinical centers were selected to specifically target minority-group recruitment.

The observational study has been designed to provide a large cohort of women, and nested case–control studies can be performed. Participants in the observational study will come from women who express interest in the clinical trial but either are found to be ineligible or are

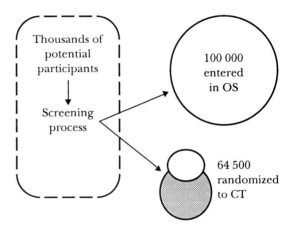

Figure 2 Recruiting approach for Women's Health Initiative (WHI). OS, observational cohort; CT, clinical trial

uninterested after learning what is involved. Observational-study participants will each complete a battery of written questionnaires to establish baseline-risk information, and will donate blood to storage from which various biomarkers can be measured as needed.

Each woman will be contacted by mail at regular intervals to collect information about outcomes of interest. In addition, a subsample of women will return to the clinical center for additional measurements in later years of the trial. To illustrate the potential value of the observational study Table 1 shows the expected number of events in this cohort for each of the four major disease end-points. The hypothesis to be tested in the observational study will encompass a wide variety of illnesses beyond the four disease end-points. Currently, for example, plans include various cancers, the various arthritides, urinary incontinence and other forms of cancer, and all-cause mortality. To

Table 1 Expected number of events in observational study cohort for each of four major disease end-points

Year of study	Total deaths (n)	Coronary heart disease (n)	Breast cancer (n)	Colorectal cancer (n)	Osteo-related fractures (n)
3	5000	1500	1000	500	3300
6	11 000	4200	2000	1100	7000
9	18 200	6700	3100	1800	11 200

summarize the method plan, women with outcomes of interest will be matched with women in the cohort who have not developed that disease. Then the two groups can be compared on a variety of prospectively measured risk factors and biomarkers including genetic markers.

The overall clinical trial design is illustrated in Figure 3. Three separately powered studies will be conducted but with some plan to overlap them. There will be an overlap of about 20% between the dietary modification and hormone replacement therapy studies. All women in the calcium/vitamin D study will be recruited from among women already enrolled in one of the other two trials.

The essential feature of these clinical trials is the use of clinical end-points. Many clinical trials of preventive therapies for chronic diseases have employed what are often called intermediate or 'surrogate' end-points. These are typically biological risk factors such as lipids for coronary heart disease. The problems with this approach are that first, favorable alterations in specific risk factors do not necessarily predict a change in occurrence of the actual clinical disease. Second, many important disorders such as most cancers do not have good biological markers, so that intermediate marker end-point studies are simply not feasible.

The Women's Health Initiative clinical trials are primary prevention trials. This means that the aim is to determine whether women without the disease of interest can be prevented from developing the disease. In contrast, secondary prevention trials investigate whether various interventions can prevent recurrences of a disease.

The dietary modification trial will examine the effect of a low-fat diet on the occurrence of breast and colorectal cancer and secondarily on coronary heart disease. Women will be randomized to either their usual diet, or a program that will train them to ingest a diet consisting of 20% fat calories and 7% saturated fat and an increased amount of fiber represented by increased servings of fruits, vegetables and grains. The intervention will be

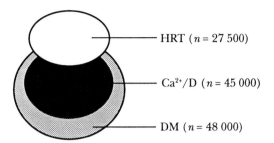

Figure 3 Overall Women's Health Initiative (WHI) clinical trial design. HRT, hormone replacement therapy; Ca^{2+}/D, calcium/vitamin D; DM, dietary modification

implemented by an active, intensive group-education process over the first year of the study. In this process, women will be trained to self-monitor their dietary fat intake on a daily basis, and both to prepare meals with the appropriate content and to select meals when they are eating out. Although women are not blinded to their study-arm assignment, all outcomes will be ascertained by investigators who are blinded to the study groups. The power of the dietary modification arm to detect clinically significant changes in the three outcomes of interest is shown in Table 2.

The calcium/vitamin D study is designed to study the effects of 1000 mg of calcium and 400 mg of vitamin D versus placebo on the occurrence of hip fractures. Secondary outcomes include all other factors and colorectal cancer. There is epidemiological evidence that ingestion of calcium supplements in particular may protect against the development of colorectal cancer at approximately the 40% level. There have been

Table 2 Power of dietary modification trial to detect clinically significant reduction in incidence (effect) of breast cancer, colorectal cancer and coronary heart disease

Disease	Effect (%)	Power (%)
Breast cancer	14	86
Colorectal cancer	20	90
Coronary heart disease	14	86

no randomized clinical trials to date of calcium/ vitamin D to study the clinical end-point of hip fracture for calcium supplements, although there is substantial evidence that calcium has a beneficial effect on bone mineral density. Table 3 shows the power of the WHI to establish a clinically significant benefit for hip fracture and colorectal cancer.

The hormone replacement trial will investigate whether the use of hormone replacement therapy protects against coronary heart disease. The secondary end-point will be hip fracture. In addition, in this arm of the trial we will research into whether hormone replacement therapy has an adverse effect on breast cancer incidence. The rationale for performing a primary prevention trial of hormone replacement therapy is that, to date, virtually all data that support the cardioprotective effects of hormone replacement therapy are based on observational evidence, or on small clinical trials which have used surrogate end-points. This would be the first primary prevention trial to study actual cardiac clinical events. In addition, there is very little evidence examining the effects of combined estrogen–progestin therapy.

The intervention in the hormone replacement therapy will be stratified by uterine status. Women who have a uterus will be randomized to either placebo or conjugated estrogen, 0.625 mg and medroxyprogesterone acetate, 2.5 mg each taken daily. Women without a uterus will be randomized to receive either the conjugated estrogen, 0.625 mg preparation or placebo. Table 4 shows the power in the hormone replacement therapy arm for the primary and secondary end-points. The power to detect the difference in an increase in breast cancer is somewhat limited. Observational studies have suggested that 10–15 years of estrogen use may be required before

Table 3 Power of calcium/vitamin D trial to detect clinically significant reduction in incidence (effect) of hip fracture and colorectal cancer

Disease	Effect (%)	Power (%)
Hip fracture	25	97
Colorectal cancer	30	85

Table 4 Power in hormone replacement therapy arm of trial to identify reduction in primary and secondary end-point conditions (effect), plus power to detect increase in incidence (effect) of breast cancer

		Power (%)	
Disease	Effect (%)	ERT	PERT
Coronary heart disease	35	92	96
Hip fracture	35	79	86
Breast cancer	30	51	
		(80 if 5 more years follow-up)	

ERT, estrogen replacement therapy; PERT, progestin/estrogen replacement therapy

any increase in breast-cancer risk is noted. The trial plans to follow women for an additional 5 years after discontinuation of study medication, and we will be particularly interested in examining breast-cancer incidents in this cohort. If we are able to achieve good follow-up for 5 years our power to detect an increase in breast cancer will rise to approximately 80%.

The trial is on schedule to be completed. As of the fall of 1996, with 2 years of recruitment remaining, 70% of the total clinical trial cohort has been recruited. When analyzed, this study will provide answers to critical clinical questions.

References

1. Rossouw, J. E., Finnegan, L. P., Harlan, W. R. *et al.* (1995). The evolution of the Women's Health Initiative: perspectives from the NIH. *J. Am. Med. Women's Assoc.*, **50**, 50–5

2. Espeland, M. A., Bush, T. L., Mebane-Sims, I., Stefanick, M. L., Johnson, S., Sherwin, R. and Waclawiw, M. (1995). Rationale, design and conduct of the PEPI Trial. *Contr. Clin. Trials*, **16**, 3S–19S

3. Johnson, S., Mebane-Sims, I., Hogan, P. E. and Stoy, D. B. (1995). Recruitment of post-menopausal women in the PEPI Trial. *Contr. Clin. Trials*, **16**, 20S–35S

4. The Postmenopausal Estrogen/Progestin Interventions (PEPI) Trial (1995). Effects of estrogen or estrogen/progestin regimens on heart disease risk factors in postmenopausal women. *J. Am. Med. Assoc.*, **273**, 199–208

5. White, E., Shattuck, A. L., Kristal, A. R. *et al.* (1992). Maintenance of a low-fat diet: follow-up of the Women's Health Trial. *Cancer Epidemiol., Biomarkers and Prevention*, **1**, 315–23

3

Management of the well menopausal woman

Management of a well menopausal woman: the role of menopause clinics

13

M. Smith

Introduction

The word 'menopause' needs no definition. 'Clinic', from the Greek word 'klinikos', literally means 'pertaining to a bed'. So, in a sense, to talk about a clinic as a place for management of the well menopausal woman appears inappropriate. It is important to conserve hospital beds, not fill them unnecessarily.

A more modern definition is 'one of a number of outpatient sections of a hospital for the specialized treatment of particular conditions and diseases'. Even this may be too restrictive: the author believes that the word 'center' needs to replace the word 'clinic' and that perimenopausal or midlife well women should be the target population. So 'menopause clinics' should be interpreted as 'midlife centers'. Hopefully, around menopause clinicians' attitudes will not be too clinical – clinical attitudes being defined medically as 'involving professional knowledge, not affected by emotions'.

It is well known that menopause can be emotional and emotive and that care of women around this time needs to be sensitive to psychological as well as physical needs. Menopause is a natural, physiological event; it can be used by physicians as a time of opportunity to enrol women in health maintenance but quality of life[1] as well as quantity of life should be the goal. Menopause is the end of reproduction but it can be the beginning of re-creation of the woman herself, the beginning of a positive time when a good health program can be initiated. There has been a tendency to focus on the physical aspects of this.

Quoting Speroff and Byyney[2]: 'All physicians who interact with women at this time of menopause have a wonderful opportunity and therefore a significant obligation. Medical intervention at this time of life offers women years of benefit from preventive health care. This represents an opportunity which should be seized.' Such language has drawn a less than positive response from some women, for example Germaine Greer. Many well women feel wary of the so-called 'medicalization of the menopause'.

Screening and maintenance of wellness

The emphasis in this paper will be on disease prevention, but talking specifically about the 'well' woman, not normally a medical priority since medicine has for so long concentrated on treatment of illness or disease rather than the promotion of 'wellness' (lack of disease). It is important that wellness is maintained – disease prevention is the medical approach to this ideal. Clinics should not be run only for those already affected, although medical models often lean this way.

Prevention is still, far too often, approached through illness management. For example, Calcitriol, one of the recognized medications for osteoporosis, has been shown to protect against bone loss, in a fine study by Tilyard and colleagues[3]. In Australia this drug, which is expensive, carries a recognized benefit on authority which reduces the cost to the patient only for those patients who have already sustained a fracture with minimal trauma (e.g. a grandmother hugged by her children or grandchildren who breaks a rib, or an elderly woman who trips lightly yet breaks a hip). This is too late for prevention!

How can osteoporosis be best diagnosed before fracture occurs, rather than after the event? Can osteoporosis be prevented? Can fracture be prevented? Should bone density be measured in all women? Can osteoporosis be predicted on clinical factors only? Ribot and co-workers[4] concluded that 'Direct bone densitometry remains indispensable to assess osteoporosis since risk factors alone are not sufficient for accurate delineation of either low or normal bone density'. If bone densitometry is an essential screening tool in all clinics, what is the cost/benefit ratio? This appears not to have been evaluated so far[5]. This and similar questions may be best answered in a well women's screening clinic.

Similarly, mammography needs to be carried out before clinical signs have developed. In Australia this screening service is provided free for women over 50 years of age, every 2 years. On request, women aged 40–49 years can also avail themselves of this free service and women with a strong family history of breast cancer may have a yearly mammogram from age 35. If a midlife clinic is the ideal place to provide screening services for well women, it is also a place of referral for women with menopause problems which a general practitioner may not feel able or willing to handle.

It makes sense that such a clinic be attached to a public teaching hospital so that teaching, research and patient treatment can be combined with all the allied services, both screening and diagnostic. Again, those components of such a clinic that attend to quality of life for the well woman should be emphasized.

Value and benefits of menopause clinics

Wolff Utian, former International Menopause Society (IMS) President, who set up the first research clinic on menopause in the world at Groote Schur Hospital in 1969, set out the value and benefits of menopause clinics at the 3rd World Menopause Conference in 1981[6]. The present author believes his statements are still relevant. He talked about 'centralization and control of hormone replacement therapy', and 'interdisciplinary long-term collaborative research as the main aims and goals of dedicated menopause clinics'.

Utian listed the benefits as follows:

(1) Well women's clinic – providing medical checkup and information;

(2) Screening programs for breast cancer, diabetes, hypertension, osteoporosis, thyroid disease;

(3) All menopause experience gathered in one center;

(4) All medical and paramedical specialties available for referral, e.g. endocrine, internal medicine, psychiatry, sociology;

(5) Hormone therapy controlled and evaluated and long term benefit/risk ratio more effectively observed;

(6) Centralization of care – which is cost-effective;

(7) Broad educational programs with the opportunity to change societal attitudes;

(8) Small or large group counseling and self-help programs can be initiated and directed on a wide geographic basis;

(9) Research a major and vital component with which to provide effective management, e.g. long-term evaluation of effects of various hormone replacement therpay regimes.

He thus included a well women's clinic as part of the larger menopause clinic. The present author thinks that the other way around is appropriate, with the main aim of a midlife center being screening, illness detection and prevention, and education of women psychologically as well as physically, to give good quality of life; hence the menopause clinic has the definite but smaller role of menopause treatment (especially hormone replacement therapy).

It is true that only long-term prospective, randomized controlled trials will be able to answer the vital questions that are raised about the safety of hormone therapy. It would cause immense distress if, as a result of therapy to prevent heart disease and osteoporosis administered to the majority of women as a preventive exercise, not only the incidence of breast cancer increased but also the death rate from this[7].

Unfortunately, there is a media bias towards sensation and bad news, so the lay public does not often receive a balanced account. A midlife center plays a crucial role in disseminating accurate and appropriate information.

Side-effects of hormone therapy, though not life-threatening, are quite co:nmon. Risks, while not common, may be lethal. The approach – that menopause is a normal physiological (aging) event so that hormone therapy can be viewed as 'meddlesome, unnecessary and possibly dangerous' must be evaluated for the individual. After all, presbyopia is also a normal aging process but it is doubtful that many individuals refuse to use glasses on this account!

We do need to talk about 'hormone-responsive' rather than 'hormone-dependent' disease since the latter suggests causation especially for breast cancer. Thus a midlife center has an important role in giving appropriate, up-to-date information to many women as well as in assessing individuals. Women may come with or without symptoms and be given full assessment and screening (including psychological/psychiatric assessment).

Practical considerations

In Australia general practitioners (GPs) are the linchpins of the medical system. Since they have a wide range of disciplines to cover and specialists are only available on referral from a general practitioner, a menopause clinic offers a useful meeting place where the GP can be trained and supported.

Free-standing private clinics are very costly to maintain, thus a menopause clinic in each region is an appropriate way to manage menopause for both symptomatic and well women[8-10].

At the IMS Conference in Florida, 1987, Notelowitz spoke of such clinics existing for service, education and research. He favors a holistic approach with paramedical disciplines such as dietetics, physiotherapy and psychotherapy an integral part of the preventive and treatment program.

Scope and purpose of clinics

The following should be considered in the establishment of a menopause clinic:

(1) Base – hospital or outside;

(2) Staffing – medical, paramedical, other;

(3) Data gathering – universal or particular, information sheets, computerization;

(4) Methods of informing the public of the existence and purpose of the clinic;

(5) Educational and outreach programs;

(6) Research role;

(7) Clinical operation;

(8) Co-existing disciplines: mammography and related breast services; bone densitometry; urodynamics; laboratory, biochemistry, pathology, etc.; physiotherapy.

Hidden benefits – discovery of occult disease

Any screening program for so-called well women will of course turn up a small percentage of occult disease, e.g thyroid disorder, diabetes, osteoporosis and breast disorders including cancer. If the range of menopause clinics is extended to include perimenopausal women (35–50 years), hormone-related hidden diseases will be discovered in time for prevention of sequelae.

As younger women have understood the importance of their own hormones both in wellness and illness, they are reporting more minor menstrual disturbances which may be related to progesterone rather than estrogen deficiency. In this area, the work of Prior[11-13] in Canada opens new vistas. Exercise amenorrhea and its link with osteoporosis is well understood but the idea that relative or absolute progesterone deficiency in women at all ages may lead to reduction in premenopausal peak bone loss is not so well known, and offers exciting challenges in the prevention of osteoporosis.

Summary – future possibilities

Menopause clinics have an important role in our communities, both for symptomatic and asymptomatic women.

The focus should be broadened to include perimenopausal women (from 35 to 50 years) since hormone changes in their age group may be precursors for premenopausal osteoporosis.

The role of education for quality of life as well as screening for quantity of life makes the main need for well women that of a midlife center containing a menopause clinic rather than the other way around.

References

1. Daly, E., Gray, A., Barlow, D., McPherson, K., Roche, M. and Vessey, M. (1993). Measuring the impact of menopausal symptoms and quality of life. *Br. Med. J.*, **307**, 836–40
2. Speroff, L. and Byyney, R. L. (1990). *A Clinical Guide for the Care of Older Women*, pp. 15–16. (Baltimore: Williams and Wilkins)
3. Tilyard, M. W., Spears, G. F. S., Thomson, J. and Dovey, S. (1992). Treatment of post menopausal osteoporosis with Calcitriol or calcium. *N. Engl. J. Med.*, **326**, 357–61
4. Ribot, C., Pouilles, J. M., Bonneu, M. and Tremollieres, F. (1992). Assessment of the risk of postmenopausal osteoporosis using clinical factors. *Clin. Endocrinol.*, **36**, 225–8
5. Melton, L. J. (1990). Screening for osteoporosis. *Ann. Intern. Med.*, **112**, 516–28
6. van Keep, P. A., Utian, W. H. and Vermeulen, A. (eds.) (1981). The Controversial Climacteric. Report of the *3rd International Congress on the Menopause*, Ostend, June, pp. 147–61. (Lancaster: MTP Press)
7. Colditz, G. A., Hankinson, S. E., Hunter, D. J., Willett, W. C., Manson, J. E., Stampfer, M. J., Hennekins, C., Rosner, B. and Speizer, F. E. (1995). The use of estrogens and progestins and the risk of breast cancer in postmenopausal women. *N. Engl. J. Med.*, **332**, 1589–93
8. Hay, A. G., Bancroft, J. and Johnstone, E. C. (1994). Affective symptoms in women attending a menopause clinic. *Br. J. Psychiatry*, **164**, 513–16
9. MacLennan, A. H. (1993). Running a menopause clinic. *Baill. Clin. Endocrinol. Metab.*, **7**, 243–53
10. Milner, M., Barr ʃ-Kinsella, C., Short, M. and Harrison, R. F. (1990). Setting up a specialist menopause clinic in Ireland: the initial experience. *Maturitas*, **16**, 71–7
11. Prior, J. C., Vigna, Y. M., Schechter, M. T. and Burges, A. E. (1990). Spinal bone loss and ovulatory disturbance. *N. Engl. J. Med.*, **323**, 121–7
12. Prior, J. C. (1990). Progesterone as a bone-trophic hormone. *Endocr. Rev.*, **11**, 386–98
13. Prior, J. C. (1989). Trabecular bone loss is associated with abnormal luteal phase length: endogenous progesterone deficiency may be a risk factor for osteoporosis. *Int. Proc. J.*, **1**, 70–3

A psychological approach to the management of menopause

14

A. Collins

Menopause as a deficiency disease

The hormonal changes in the perimenopausal phase are well documented. However, the attitude to menopause and its treatment has varied over time. At present there continues to be considerable controversy among physicians concerning the role of hormone replacement therapy and whether this period in women's lives should be regarded as a deficiency disease requiring pharmacological or hormonal intervention, or whether it should be considered as a normal transition in women's development.

The concept of menopause as a disease that should be treated with hormone replacement is based on ideas originating in Wilson's book *Feminine Forever* which was published in the United States[1]. This book emphasized the deficiency disease model of menopause, and suggested that all women be treated with hormones to alleviate symptoms. The notion that all menopausal symptoms are associated with estrogen deficiency has received further support from clinical studies of women attending menopause clinics. The implication arising from this viewpoint is that menopause is an estrogen deficiency state which needs to be substituted. Women should consult a doctor to diagnose their menopausal state, and the focus should be treatment of all menopause-related symptoms with hormonal replacement therapy, a trend which has been conceptualized as medicalization of the menopause[2]. The biomedical model has also influenced women's views of menopause and created a disease-orientation, help-seeking and perhaps more negative stereotyping among women. In the

1980s medical attention shifted to the long-term effects of decreased estrogen on the cardiovascular system and bone density. The emphasis is on hormone replacement therapy for most women to prevent osteoporosis and cardiovascular disease. The biomedical model, while stimulating clinical research into the effects of estrogen on different bodily systems, has many opponents, particularly among feminist writers.

Menopause as a developmental phase

According to an alternative view menopause is a stage in women's development, a natural transition. Menopause has been characterized as a period of great psychosocial change. Notman described such developmental transitions as presenting women with the opportunity for personal growth and restructuring[3]. It can also be a threat to the balance they have accomplished during earlier phases of their lives. The way women cope will be decisive for their quality of life. To date there is very little research based on the developmental model, and further study of the psychological changes associated with menopause and the menopausal years is urgently needed.

Factors that have been considered important in the menopausal transition are loss of child-bearing capacity and feminine attributes. Psychoanalytic writers such as Deutsch[4], painted a dark picture of menopause as a period of decline and loss. Several authors have suggested that the empty nest is the most crucial transition for midlife women. More recently, writers such as Crafoord have emphasized that this stage can be seen as an individuation process which is characterized by the gradual development of greater independence from the pre-Oedipal parental figures casting their shadow, as well as an increasing independence from a partner[5]. Representing clinical psychology, McCain conceived of menopause as a major developmental event in a woman's life[6]. Rather than a negative phase to be endured or alleviated, menopause is seen as an empowering experience that women can use for personal growth. McCain goes beyond a discussion of menopausal symptoms to analyze some of the deep emotional and spiritual significance of this phase in women's lives.

Menopause can be seen as a developmental phase in women's lives requiring adjustment, with a potential for turmoil, low self-esteem and periods of self-doubt. However, many women find strength from going through such a process, and experience a stronger sense of identity with increased maturation and self-esteem.

What is the menopausal syndrome?

Earlier research suggested that there is a menopausal syndrome, a group of symptoms occurring together at menopause. The concept of a menopausal syndrome is in agreement with the deficiency-disease theory, and assumes that physical as well as psychological symptoms are caused by decreased estrogen levels.

A more recent approach has focused on analysis of different symptoms and description of particular symptoms that are related to hormones, and identification of factors other than biological that can help explain the development of symptoms. It has become clear that much of our knowledge of menopause is based on small clinical studies of women attending menopause clinics for their symptoms[7-9]. It has become increasingly important to consider the methodological problems associated with research on menopause in order to obtain objective information about this phase of life. Better designed studies of population-based samples that are followed over

a number of years are needed. Such studies will yield more reliable knowledge of how women generally cope with the transition to menopause. Recent epidemiological studies have shown that menopause is not such a negative event for women in general[10]. Although natural menopause is associated with increased reports of vasomotor symptoms, it does not have a significant effect on mood or mental health.

Influence of psychosocial factors

Parallel to the hormonal changes occurring at midlife, a whole range of psychosocial changes take place. These changes include both positive and negative aspects and may influence how women feel about themselves. Factors such as marital status, education, occupation, general health, social support, personality variables, coping style and attitudes have been shown to affect women's health during transition to menopause.

Attitude to menopause and aging is a central aspect that has been shown to influence symptom reporting[11]. In a longitudinal population-based study of 150 women residing in the Stockholm area, we found that hormonal status played a relatively minor role in explaining most symptoms. Factor analysis of symptom ratings completed by the women each year yielded ten independent factors explaining 56% of the variance. Multiple regression analyses of background factors showed that only vasomotor symptoms, memory problems and joint pain were significantly associated with menopausal status. Other symptoms such as negative mood, decreased sexual interest, vaginal dryness and urogenital symptoms were more strongly related to a negative attitude to menopause and aging, lifestyle such as smoking and lack of exercise, experience of life stress, dissatisfaction with work role, presence of physical complaints and presence of vasomotor symptoms. It seems particularly important to identify the factors that contribute to symptoms occurring at menopause, since many of them can be modified by psychosocial interventions and lifestyle changes.

Personality variables were also found to correlate with symptom dimensions. Anxiety-proneness was significantly correlated with negative mood, vasomotor symptoms and decreased sexual desire. In an earlier study[12] we found an association between menopausal symptoms and anxiety-proneness, detachment and psychasthenia as measured by the Karolinska Scales of Personality. Psychological symptoms were also correlated with an external locus of control, i.e. a feeling that external forces determine important events in one's life.

Perception of work role

Very little research has addressed women's work role. The underlying assumption has been that women do not invest as much as men in their work, and that they are more involved in family life and childrearing. Although the majority of women have joined the workforce, paid employment has not been considered as central in women's lives, and there is very little discussion about self-esteem and identity derived from this role[13]. In the current debate concerning women's multiple roles and their effect on women's health, some writers have predicted that women who work full-time will suffer from stress-related illness such as hypertension and heart disease to the same extent as men. However, there is strong evidence to show that employment *per se* has a positive effect on women's health[14,15]. Women who are in paid work are generally in better health than home-makers. Multiple roles are beneficial for women. Baruch found that women derived an increased self-esteem and a feeling of mastery from their work[16]. Barnett and Baruch have shown that there is a constant interaction between the private sphere and work role, and that stresses in one sphere will carry over to the other but will also be buffered by satisfaction and rewards in the other roles[17].

In the longitudinal study that we are conducting in Stockholm we have addressed the issue of work role in terms of women's perception of work role and the importance they attach to their work. The data were collected during the 3rd and 4th year of the longitudinal follow-up. The women's responses to the questions pertaining to work were content analyzed, and based on these results the women were categorized into two groups. Group 1 included those women who always thought their work was stimulating and important, and those women who in the last few years thought work was more important than before. This group was called 'work more important'. Group 2 included women whose family role always had been more important, and women who in the last few years felt less involvement in their work and who wanted to cut back. This group was labeled 'work less important'. Comparing the health profile of these two groups, we found that group 1 (work more important) had a more favorable health profile in terms of a lower systolic blood pressure, their body weight was lower and their blood lipid profile was more favorable: they had significantly lower total cholesterol and low-density lipoprotein levels than the women who were not so involved in their work.

Level of education was not associated with workrole attitude. The women held a whole range of occupations but the large majority (66%) were employed in female-dominated areas such as service type jobs, daycare, clerical work, etc. Twenty per cent held professional jobs and 5% were employed in unskilled jobs; 3% were unemployed at the fourth follow-up.

The results showed that women from very different walks of life can find reward and satisfaction in their jobs, and the most important dimensions of the work role include being able to use one's skills and competence and the experience of fulfilling an important task. It is interesting that stress at work or lack of social support did not contribute to a more negative attitude to work. Work stress, such as monotonous work with constant deadlines as well as long working hours and physically heavy work, was distressing to a proportion of the women.

A number of women had made changes in their lives by changing careers, taking on new responsibility or devoting time to additional job training. These women ranked amongst those who scored highest in job satisfaction and happiness, and said that they had never been more satisfied with their lives. The results do not support Sarrel's view that menopausal symptoms interfere with working capacity, or that women quit their jobs because of menopausal symptoms or that they view their work in more negative term[18]. None of the women reported that menopausal symptoms negatively affected their work efficiency, and menopausal status did not contribute to a more negative workrole attitude. On the contrary, many women reported that work had become more important since the children left home or became more independent.

Conclusions

Our results indicate that hormonal factors play a relatively minor role in menopausal symptomatology, and that psychosocial factors, lifestyle as well as attitude to menopause and work role, are far more important for women's health during the perimenopausal years.

Workrole identity and satisfaction with work role seem to be of particular importance for women's well-being. Attitudes to menopause and to aging also influence symptom reporting. A more positive attitude predicts less frequent symptoms. Similar results were reported by Avis and McKinlay[11].

Attitudes to aging particularly as far as women are concerned need to change. We need to view the life span differently and encourage a more even distribution of workforce participation among women. Many women feel that it is too late to change their situation. At the same time there is a marked sex segregation in the job market. Many of the jobs that women in this age group hold are highly stressful with little opportunity for growth. These are the very conditions that affect their health in a negative way, increasing the risk of stress-related disease. We should encourage women to change careers, to quit 'dead-end' jobs, to realize their ambitions, to take on new responsibilities and to develop work identities of their own. These changes will promote well-being and good health for women during the transitional years.

References

1. Wilson, R. (1996). *Feminine Forever.* (New York: M. Evans)
2. Kaufert, P. (1982). Myth and the menopause. *Sociol. Health Illness,* **4**, 141–65
3. Notman, M. (1979). Midlife concerns of women: implications of the menopause. *Am. J. Psychiatr.,* **136**, 1270–4
4. Deutsch, H. (1945). The climacterium. In *The Psychology of Women.* (New York: Green & Stratton)
5. Crafoord, K. (1988). Individuation from a life cycle perspective. *Kvinnovetenskaplig Tidskrift,* **1**, 44–55
6. McCain, M. (1991). *Transformation through Menopause.* (New York: Bergin and Garvey)
7. McKinlay, J. B., McKinlay, S. M. and Brambilla, D. J. (1987). Health status and utilisation behavior associated with menopause. *Am. J. Epidemiol.,* **125**, 110–21
8. Holte, A. (1991). Prevalence of climacteric complaints in a presentative sample of middle-

aged women in Oslo. *J. Psychosom. Obstet. Gynecol.,* **12**, 303–17
9. Dennerstein, L., Smith, A. M., Morse, C., Burger, H., Green, A., Hopper, J. and Ryan, M. (1993). Menopausal symptoms in Australian women. *Med. J. Aust.,* **159**, 232–6
10. Matthews, K., Wing, R., Kuller, L., Meilahn, E. and Kelsey, S. (1990). Influences of natural menopause on psychological characteristics and symptoms of middle-aged healthy women. *J. Consult. Clin. Psychol.,* **58**, 345–51
11. Avis, N. and McKinlay, S. M. (1991). A longitudinal analysis of women's attitude toward the menopause: results from the Massachusetts Women's Health Study. *Maturitas,* **13**, 65–79
12. Collins, A., Hanson, U. and Eneroth, P. (1983). Post-menopausal symptoms and reponse to hormonal replacement therapy: influence of psychological factors. *J. Psychosom. Obstet. Gynecol.,* **2**, 227–33
13. Barnett, R. and Baruch, G. B. (1978). Women

in the middle years: a critique of research and theory. *Psychol. Women Q.*, **3**, 187–97

14. Waldron, I. and Jacobs, J. A. (1989). Effects of multiple roles on women's health. Evidence from a longitudinal study. *Women Health*, **15**, 3–19

15. Barnett, R. and Rivers, C. (1996). *She Works, He Works* (San Francisco: Harper & Collins)

16. Baruch, G. B. (1984). The psychological wellbeing of women in the middle years. In Baruch, G. B. and Brooks-Gun, J. (eds.) *Women in Midlife*, pp.161–80. (New York: Plenum Press)

17. Barnett, R. and Baruch, G. (1987). Gender, social role and distress. In Barnett, R. and Baruch, G., (eds.) *Gender and Stress*, pp.122–43. (New York: Free Press)

18. Sarrel, P. (1991). Women, work and menopause. In Frankenhaeuser, M., Lundberg, L. and Chesney, M. (eds.) *Women, Work and Stress*, pp.225–36. (New York: Plenum Books)

Lifestyle approach to management of the menopause   15

J. R. Guthrie, L. Dennerstein, P. R. Ebeling, J. D. Wark, E. C. Dudley, J. L. Hopper, A. Green and H. G. Burger

Introduction

This paper seeks to determine what lifestyle factors contribute to the maintenance of health during the menopausal transition. Two questions must be asked in order to investigate the lifestyle approach to managing the midlife woman. First, what are the optimal health outcomes for menopausal/midlife women? Second, what are the factors which are associated with these outcomes?

Data from the Melbourne Women's Midlife Health Project (MWMHP) are used to provide the lifestyle management strategies for the midlife woman. This project incorporated both a cross-sectional study of 2000 randomly selected Australian-born women aged 45–55 years in 1991 and a longitudinal study of 494 of these women who were still menstruating in 1991. Information is presented from the cross-sectional (XS) and longitudinal study (L1 to L4), which included five interviews conducted annually by trained interviewers. The first interview was conducted by telephone, the subsequent four interviews were in the women's homes when physical measurements and blood were also taken. Information about nutrition and physical activity were obtained at baseline (XS) and in the 3rd longitudinal year of the study (L3) by self-administered questionnaires, which were returned by post. Bone mineral density of the hip and spine was measured in the Bone Densitometry Unit, Department of Medicine, Royal Melbourne Hospital.

During the study period, menopausal status was subject to change. Women either remained pre- or perimenopausal, or became peri- or postmenopausal, or took hormone replacement therapy. Women were classified as: premenopausal if there was no change in menstrual frequency or flow in the prior 12 months; perimenopausal if menses occurred in the prior 12 months but there were changes in frequency or flow (the Melbourne Women's Midlife Health Project is currently revising these definitions) or both; postmenopausal if no menses occurred in the prior 12 months and the respondent had not undergone hysterectomy and/or bilateral oophorectomy. Women who were taking (or had taken) hormone replacement therapy during the study were placed in a separate group.

Health outcomes

To describe the healthy midlife woman three different health outcomes are defined: (1) optimal self-rated health, i.e. the woman who continually rates her health as better than the health of her peers; (2) optimal bone health, i.e. the woman who has high bone mineral density of the hip and spine; and (3) optimal cardiovascular health, i.e. the woman who has a low cardiovascular risk profile.

Previous research has established self-rated health as a significant predictor of the use of health services[1] and it appears to be related to mortality independent of objective health status[2,3]. An increase in bone fragility occurs in women as a result of both aging and the menopause, and is characteristic of osteoporosis[4,5]. Bone mineral densitometry is an established technique for measuring this bone fragility[6]. Cardiovascular disease has also been implicated as a long-term sequela of the cessation of ovarian endocrine activity[7]. Studies[8,9] have shown that around the menopause there is an escalation in coronary risk, with an increase in low-density lipoprotein (LDL) cholesterol and a decrease in high-density lipoprotein (HDL) cholesterol. However, whether menopause *per se* or whether changes in lifestyle factors are responsible for altering the risk of coronary heart disease remains controversial[10]. Lifestyle factors which influence self-rated health, bone mineral density and cardiovascular risk factors were investigated for this paper.

Self-rated health

Participants in the Melbourne Women's Midlife Health Project were asked at each interview to rate their present health compared with other women of about the same age as: worse than most; about the same as most; better than most. Those women who rated their health as better than that of their peers at every interview were compared with the others in relation to the various lifestyle variables.

Bone mineral density

Bone mineral density (BMD) of the lumbar spine (second to fourth vertebrae) and the femoral neck was measured by dual energy X-ray absorptiometry (DEXA) using a Hologic QDR-1000 W densitometer.

Cardiovascular health

Risk factor assessment for coronary heart disease (CHD) included measures of weight, height, blood pressure, fasting blood glucose, total cholesterol, HDL cholesterol and LDL cholesterol. Australian National Heart Foundation guidelines state that total cholesterol levels greater than 5.5 mmol/l are associated with an increased risk, and greater than 6.5 mmol/l with a high risk of heart disease. HDL cholesterol should be greater than 1.19 mmol/l and LDL cholesterol levels should be less than 3.5 mmol/l. The recommended LDL/HDL ratio is between 1.0 and 4.0. Increased risk of CHD is also associated with smoking one or more cigarettes per day, having a diastolic blood pressure of greater than 95 mmHg and being overweight.

Explanatory variables

The variables used were: menopausal status; physical activity, described as leisure-time physical activity expressed as average hours or kcal per week calculated retrospectively over 12 months[11]; age at baseline; body mass index (BMI), calculated as kg/m^2; employment, coded as two categories: being on average in full or part-time paid employment, and being on average unemployed or having some part-time employment over 4 years; smoking expressed as pack years[12]; troublesome symptoms expressed as symptom factors[13]; marital status coded as two categories: continually married or living with a partner over 4 years, and single, widowed, divorced/separated or changed status over 4 years; calcium and caffeine intake; dietary fat, fruit and vegetable intake; alcohol intake; years of education completed; and experience of chronic disease (arthritis, cancer, heart disease, migraine headache, hypertension, diabetes).

Statistical analysis

Stepwise logistic regression analysis was used to compare self-rated health groups. Analysis of variance was used to compare BMD measurements and levels of cardiovascular risk factors between menopausal status groups. The associations of BMD and cardiovascular risk factors with age, BMI and lifestyle variables were analyzed by multiple linear regression. Unless otherwise noted, a nominal $p < 0.05$ level of significance was used and all statistical tests were two-tailed. Analyses were performed using SPSS for Windows.

Results

Self-rated health

After five interviews, complete data on self-rated health were obtained from 430 women, 84 (20%) of whom always rated their health as better than that of their peers. Women were more likely to continually report better self-rated health if they averaged full or part-time paid employment over the 4 years, had decreased skeletal/headache symptomatology, i.e. backaches, aches and stiff joints, headaches and migraine headaches and, also, if they spent more hours per week being physically active. There was no association of better self-rated health with menopausal status. The data set in Table 1 refers to the 334 women who returned their physical activity questionnaires. Similar results were obtained with the larger cohort (430 women) with regard to employment (odds ratio (OR) 1.84, 95% confidence interval (CI)

1.04–3.27), marital status (OR 2.56, 95% CI 1.47–4.43), skeletal symptomatology (OR 0.86, 95% CI 0.78–0.95) and chronic disease reporting (OR 2.68, 95% CI 1.58–4.55).

Fifty-one per cent of the better self-rated health group reported the existence of chronic disease compared with 78% of the others; the most common chronic diseases reported were arthritis and high blood pressure. Arthritis was reported by 35% of the best self-rated health group compared to 52% of the others, and high blood pressure by 17% of the best group and 31% of the others. Sixty per cent of the better self-rated health group had been continually married or living with a partner compared with 80% in the group who did not continually rate their health as better than their peers. There was no significant association between self-rated health and years of education completed, however employment was associated with years of education ($p < 0.0001$). Forty-two per cent of the women who averaged full or part-time employment during the study period had completed more than 12 years of education compared with 22%

Table 1 Variables associated with continually reporting self-rated health over 4 years to be better than health of peers ($n = 61$) vs. others ($n = 273$). Odds ratio (OR) and 95% confidence interval (CI) for having continually better self-rated health

Variable	Estimate of mean	SE	OR	95% CI
Paid employment				
None or some part-time	0.00	—	1.00	
Average full or part-time	0.95	0.35	2.57*	(1.29–5.12)
Marital status				
Continually married or living with a partner	0.00	—	1.00	
Single/widowed/divorced/changed category	0.74	0.34	2.09*	(1.08–4.04)
Increased skeletal/headache symptom score	−0.13	0.06	0.88*	(0.78–0.99)
Increased level of physical activity	0.35	0.15	1.40*	(1.06–1.90)
Chronic disease				
yes	0.00	—	1.00	
no	0.93	0.33	2.54**	(1.36–4.81)

*$p < 0.05$; **$p < 0.005$; SE, standard error

of those who were unemployed or had some part-time employment.

Bone density studies

A sub-group of 405 women recruited from the population sample participated in a cross-sectional bone density study. This sub-group comprised 360 women from the longitudinal cohort and 45 randomly selected naturally postmenopausal women from the cross-sectional cohort. These women had one measurement of the bone density of their hip and spine during

1992–94. Table 2 shows that, using the premenopausal group as the reference category, the postmenopausal group had lower BMD at both the lumbar spine and femoral neck ($p < 0.0005$). The women taking hormone therapy at the time of the BMD measurements had lower femoral neck BMD ($p < 0.05$). Table 3 shows the lifestyle and gynecological variables of the menopausal groups. The peri-, post- and hormone replacement therapy groups were all significantly older than the premenopausal groups. There were no significant differences in other variables.

Table 2 Mean (standard error (SE)) bone mineral density (BMD) of lumbar spine and femoral neck of pre-, peri-, postmenopausal and hormone replacement therapy (HRT) groups

Group	Lumbar spine BMD (g/cm^2)	Femoral neck BMD (g/cm^2)
Premenopausal ($n = 72$)	1.114 (0.019)	0.837 (0.013)
Perimenopausal ($n = 181$)	1.111 (0.010)	0.836 (0.009)
Postmenopausal ($n = 88$)	0.980 (0.016)***	0.758 (0.010)***
HRT ($n = 64$)	1.097 (0.021)	0.799 (0.014)*

***$p < 0.0005$, *$p < 0.05$ compared with premenopausal group

Table 3 Mean (standard error (SE))of gynecological and lifestyle variables of cohort of 405 women by pre-, peri-, postmenopausal and hormone replacement therapy (HRT) groups

Variable	Pre- ($n = 72$)	Peri- ($n = 181$)	Post- ($n = 88$)	HRT ($n = 64$)
Age (years)	49.4 (0.29)	50.7 (0.18)*	53.9 (0.26)***	53.0 (0.31)**
Body mass index (kg/m^2)	25.1 (0.5)	25.7 (0.4)	25.8 (0.5)	24.4 (0.5)
Calcium (mg/day)	940 (96)	843 (48)	873 (70)	870 (70)
Caffeine (mg/day)	337 (34)	367 (16)	363 (25)	330 (30)
Physical activity (h/week)	6.9 (0.7)	6.5 (0.6)	6.5 (0.7)	5.3 (0.6)
Oral contraceptive pill (years taken)	4.9 (0.6)	5.0 (0.4)	5.0 (0.7)	5.6 (1.0)
Parity	2.8 (0.2)	2.5 (0.1)	2.9 (0.2)	2.6 (0.1)
Ever breast fed (% yes)[†]	88%	87%	88%	93%
Months breast fed[†]	14.5 (1.8)	13.2 (1.8)	11.4 (1.5)	9.9 (1.3)
Age at menarche (years)	13.2 (0.2)	12.8 (0.1)	13.1 (0.2)	13.1 (0.2)
Years since last menstrual period	0	0	3.4 (0.3)	—
Family history of fracture (% yes)	20%	19%	29%	18%
Current smokers	10%	18%	21%	11%
Pack years[‡]	26.7 (5.0)	18.6 (1.9)	21.0 (2.9)	17.6 (3.8)

***$p < 0.0005$, **$p < 0.005$, *$p < 0.05$ compared with premenopausal group; [†]ever breast fed and months breast fed were computed only among women who reported one or more live births; [‡]pack years were computed only among women who were current or past smokers

Table 4 Multiple regression analyses of determinants of bone mineral densities in lumbar spine (LS-BMD) and femoral neck (FN-BMD) of pre-, peri- and postmenopausal groups combined, $n = 341$; coefficients (standard errors) given

	Age	Body mass index	Menopausal status
LS-BMD	−0.0032 (0.0031)	0.0074 (0.0015)***	−0.1248 (0.0259)***
FN-BMD	−0.0065 (0.0023)*	0.0068 (0.0011)***	−0.0544 (0.0197)*

$*p < 0.05$, $***p < 0.0005$

Table 5 Multiple regression analyses with age, years since menopause (YSM) and body mass index (BMI) as determinants of bone mineral densities in lumbar spine (LS-BMD) and femoral neck (FN-BMD) in postmenopausal women, $n = 88$; coefficients (standard errors) given

	Age	Years since menopause	Body mass index
LS-BMD	−0.0045 (0.0065)	−0.0159 (0.0060)*	0.0070 (0.0036)
FN-BMD	−0.0086 (0.0041)*	−0.0063 (0.0038)	0.0062 (0.0023)*

$*p < 0.05$

Table 4 shows the result of multiple regression analysis with age, BMI and menopausal status as determinants of bone mineral density (the hormone replacement therapy group being excluded from this analysis). Femoral BMD decreased with increasing age ($p < 0.05$), and increasing menopausal status ($p < 0.05$) and increased with increasing body mass index ($p < 0.0005$). Lumbar spine BMD decreased with increasing menopausal status ($p < 0.0005$) and increased with increasing body mass index ($p < 0.0005$). No significant association was found between BMD and the lifestyle or gynecological variables studied.

In the postmenopausal group the mean (SD) years from menopause were 3.40 (2.65), and the women had a mean (SD) age of 53.9 (2.4) years, range 47.8–59.0 years. Table 5 shows the results of multiple regression analyses with age, BMI and years since menopause as determinants of BMD in these women.

Cardiovascular health

During the 3rd year of the longitudinal study data on lifestyle variables and cardiovascular risk factors were collected. Considering the whole cohort, 59% had a total cholesterol level of greater than 5.5 mmol/l and 26% had a level greater than 6.5 mmol/l. With regard to other risk factors, 2.4% of the women had a diastolic blood pressure greater than 95 mmHg, 15% smoked one or more cigarettes daily, 18% had a BMI of greater than 30 kg/m^2 and 4% had a waist to hip ratio of greater than 0.85. Thirty-three per cent of the cohort recorded less than 3 h of physical activity per week. Eight per cent drank 15 or more alcoholic drinks in the week, while 38% claimed to have not had an alcoholic drink in the past 7 days. Table 6 shows the distribution of cholesterol values among pre-, peri- and postmenopausal women and hormone replacement therapy groups according to the National Heart Foundation guidelines. A greater proportion of the postmenopausal group have high-risk cholesterol levels compared with the other groups ($p < 0.05$).

Multiple regression analysis of this L3 cohort showed that LDL/HDL ratio ($p < 0.0001$), systolic ($p < 0.0001$) and diastolic ($p < 0.01$) blood pressure were all positively associated with BMI.

The dietary questionnaires were returned by 80% of the cohort and the mean (SE) dietary intakes were 48 (1) g/day of total fat, 8 (0.2)

Table 6 Distribution of cholesterol values between pre-, peri-, postmenopausal and hormone replacement therapy (HRT) groups at 3rd year of follow-up (L3)

Group	n	Total cholesterol > 5.5 mmol/l	Total cholesterol > 6.5 mmol/l	HDL < 1.19 mmol/l	LDL > 3.5 mmol/l	LDL/HDL > 4
Premenopausal	53	30 (57%)	8 (15%)	6 (11%)	26 (50%)	2 (4%)
Perimenopausal	214	122 (57%)	53 (24%)	36 (17%)	103 (48%)	14 (7%)
Postmenopausal	71	48 (68%)	26 (37%)*	7 (10%)	45 (63%)	7 (10%)
HRT	105	63 (60%)	27 (26%)	12 (11%)	52 (50%)	7 (7%)

$*p < 0.05$; HDL, high-density lipoprotein cholesterol; LDL, low-density lipoprotein cholesterol

servings per day of fruit and vegetables in winter and 13 (0.3) servings in summer. There was no difference in dietary intakes of fat or fruit and vegetables between the menopausal groups and none of these dietary measures was associated with the cardiovascular risk factors. There was no association between cardiovascular risk factors and education or employment.

Discussion

In this paper we have considered several health outcomes and the factors which are associated with these outcomes. Continually reporting self-rated health as better than one's peers is associated with the absence of skeletal symptoms, being employed, not living with a partner and exercising.

Menopausal status or hormone replacement therapy use did not directly have an impact on self-rated health reporting. These results were similar to those reported in the cross-sectional analysis of 1687 women[14] except that in the cross-sectional cohort, increasing dysphoric symptoms were associated with the likelihood of not reporting better self-rated health. During the 4 years of the study one of the most common symptoms reported was aching or stiff joints, this being a problem for almost 50% of the participants. There was no change in the prevalence of these symptoms over the 4 years of the study. Also, arthritis was the most common chronic condition, being reported at some stage during the study by 49% of the participants. Though bone and joint pain is a commonly

accepted feature of the menopause[15], there are few studies that specifically address this issue. Further studies are needed to clarify whether these problems are an effect of age or of the menopause.

In the cohort of 405 women who had their BMD measured, the postmenopausal women had significantly lower spine and hip BMD and the hormone replacement therapy group had lower BMD of the hip. As we had no measures of BMD in this latter group before they took hormones we cannot make any valid conclusions about the effects of hormone replacement therapy on BMD. Age appears to be a more significant determinant of femoral neck BMD compared with spinal BMD, whereas both sites show an effect of the menopause. The postmenopausal women had significantly lower estrogen levels than the pre- and perimenopausal women[16] and these levels are predictive of their lower BMD[17]. There was no difference in the bone densities of our pre- and perimenopausal groups, however results of studies to determine whether bone loss begins before the menopause appear discordant[15]. Our longitudinal study, now in progress, will provide a better understanding of the pattern of bone loss before, during and following the menopausal transition.

There was a positive association between BMI and BMD at both the hip and spine, and this has been documented in other cross-sectional studies[18,19]. Salamone and colleagues[20] have shown in pre- and early perimenopausal women that greater lean mass appears to be more important than fat mass in determining overall bone densities at the femoral neck and spine. This stronger association between lean mass and BMD than that for fat mass may be attributed to differences in determinants of lean mass, such as exercise history, heredity factors, estrogen levels or a combination of these factors. Our longitudinal study is including DEXA measurements of whole-body soft tissue composition and will allow us to examine changes in body composition across the menopause, and its relation to postmenopausal bone mass and the risk of developing osteoporosis.

There was no significant association between BMD and lifestyle variables in the pre-, peri- or postmenopausal women. The physical activities of our cohort were weight-bearing activities and included walking, gardening and dancing[11]. However, these activities were not the weight- or strength-training regimes described in other studies[21,22] which have been shown to maintain femoral neck and lumbar spine bone density in postmenopausal women. Nelson and co-workers[21] achieved an increase in BMD with a 12 month high-intensity strength-training program carried out for 45 min, 2 days per week. Also, our calcium intake levels may not be sufficient to show beneficial associations with BMD; certainly they were not as high as those in the successful intervention study of Reid and associates[23] in which an intake of about 1750 mg per day of calcium resulted in a marked slowing of axial and appendicular bone loss. In Australia, the recommended daily intake of calcium for postmenopausal women is 1000 mg per day and maybe this should be increased. However, in considering lifestyle strategies for the prevention of osteoporosis, not smoking, high calcium intake and weight-bearing exercise are all recommended particularly to reduce bone loss in the postmenopausal period.

High HDL-cholesterol and low LDL-cholesterol levels appear to be important in providing a protective effect from coronary heart disease[24]. Other studies have shown the benefit of exercise in midlife women in increasing HDL-cholesterol levels[25] and lowering blood pressure[26]. Although our cross-sectional analyses showed that the postmenopausal women had higher cholesterol levels, longitudinal analyses, now in progress, are looking at changes in HDL and LDL cholesterol in relation to changes in menopausal status, taking account of changes in BMI and exercise during the same period, and will provide better evidence of the association between cardiovascular risk factors, the menopause and lifestyle variables. Women in different countries have remarkably different cardiovascular death rates[27], differences that are more likely to be explained by differences in lifestyle variables than by differences in endogenous estrogen levels, and this suggests that lifestyle management will be beneficial in improving cardiovascular health.

We have previously shown[11] that BMI is inversely associated with hours of leisure-time physical activity. In view of our finding that increasing BMI was associated with increasing levels of systolic and diastolic blood pressure and an increasing LDL/HDL ratio, and the finding of others[28] that overweight is an independent predictor of cardiovascular disease, physical activity is also recommended to control excess weight. As was mentioned previously BMI is a major determinant of bone mineral density, and thus weight reduction, although beneficial from a cardiovascular point of view may have a deleterious effect on the osteoporosis-prone woman.

A combined effect of low-fat, high-fruit and -vegetable diet has been shown to decrease total cholesterol and triglycerides[29]. The average daily consumption of fat, fruit and vegetables in our population of Melbourne midlife women was already, on average, reasonably low in fat and high in fruit and vegetables, and we were unable to show any correlations between these dietary factors and blood lipid levels. A diet high in phytoestrogens is recommended as being beneficial in protecting against heart disease, osteoporosis and menopausal symptoms[30]. We are currently investigating the phytoestrogen content of the women's diets in order to see if there is a relationship between this and various health outcomes.

In conclusion, physical activity is the lifestyle behavior which is related to all three health outcomes. Increasing physical activity in midlife women can improve cardiovascular risk factors, is associated with the reporting of better self-rated health and, although our study did not show a benefit of physical activity on BMD, others have shown that it has the potential to reduce bone loss. Further study is needed to identify barriers against and motivation for increasing physical activity, for use in health promotion campaigns.

Acknowledgements

This study was supported by grants from the Victorian Health Promotion Foundation, the Public Health Research and Development Committee of the National Health and Medical Research Council (NHMRC), the Australian Dairy Corporation, the Percy Baxter Trust, the H & L Hecht Trust, the Estate of the late Daniel Scott, the Ian Potter Foundation, the Smorgan Family Trust, the Leigh and Majorie Bronwen Murray Charitable Trust and the Helen M. Schutt Trust. Dr Hopper is supported by a NHMRC Research Fellowship. The research team would like to thank Corry Garamszegi, Liz River and the field workers in the Melbourne Women's Midlife Health Project for their help and Mr Nick Balazs and the staff of the department of Chemical Pathology, Monash Medical Centre and Bahtiyar Kaymakci and Sue Cantor from the Bone Densitometry Unit, Royal Melbourne Hospital, for their technical assistance. The research team would also like to thank all the women who participated in this study.

References

1. Fylkesnes, K. and Forde, O. H. (1991). The Tromso study: predictors of self-evaluated health – has society adopted the expanded health concept? *Soc. Sci. Med.*, **32**, 141–6
2. Kaplan, G. A. and Camacho, T. (1988). Perceived health and mortality: a nine-year follow up of the human population. Laboratory cohort. *Am. J. Epidemiol.*, **117**, 292–304
3. Idler, E. L. and Angel, R. J. (1990). Self-rated health and mortality in the NHANES-I epidemiologic follow-up study. *Am. J. Publ. Health*, **80**, 446–52
4. Riggs, B. L., Wahner, H. W., Dunn, W. L., Mazess, R. B., Offord, K. P. and Melton, L. J. III (1981). Differential changes in bone mineral density of the appendicular and axial skeleton with aging. *J. Clin. Invest.*, **67**, 328–35
5. Nilas, L. and Christiansen, C. (1989). The pathophysiology of peri- and postmenopausal bone loss. *Br. J. Obstet. Gynaecol.*, **96**, 580–7
6. Riggs, B. L. and Melton, L. J. III (1986). Involutional osteoporosis. *N. Engl. J. Med.*, **314**, 1676–86
7. Kannel, W., Hjortland, M. C., McNamara, P. M. and Gordon, T. (1976). Menopause and the risk of cardiovascular disease: the Framingham Study. *Ann. Intern. Med.*, **85**, 447–52
8. Matthews, K. A., Meilahn, E., Kuller, L. H. N., Kelsy, S. F., Caggiula A. W. and Wing, R. R. (1989). Menopause and risk factors for coronary heart disease. *N. Engl. J. Med.*, **321**, 641–6
9. Jensen, J., Nilas L. and Christiansen, C. (1990). Influence of menopause on serum lipids and lipoproteins. *Maturitas*, **12**, 321–31
10. Isles, C. G., Hole, D. J., Hawthorne, V. M. and Lever, A. F. (1992). Relationships between coronary risk and coronary mortality in women of the Renfrew and Paisley survey: comparison with men. *Lancet*, **339**, 702–6
11. Guthrie, J. R., Smith, A. M. A., Dennerstein, L. and Morse, C. (1995). Physical activity and the menopause experience: a cross-sectional study. *Maturitas*, **20**, 71–80
12. Hopper, J. L. and Seeman, E. (1994). The bone density of female twins discordant for tobacco use. *N. Engl. J. Med.*, **330**, 387–92
13. Dennerstein, L., Smith, A. M. A., Morse, C. A., Burger, H. G., Green, A., Hopper, J. L. and Ryan, M. (1993). Menopausal symptoms in Australian women. *Med. J. Aust.*, **159**, 232–6
14. Smith, A. M. A., Shelley, J. M. and Dennerstein, L. (1994). Self-rated health: biological continuum or social discontinuity? *Soc. Sci. Med.*, **39**, 77–83
15. Sowers, M. R. and La Peitre, M. T. (1995). Menopause: its epidemiology and potential association with chronic diseases. *Epidemiol. Rev.*, **17**, 287–302
16. Guthrie, J. R., Ebeling, P. R., Hopper, J. L., Dennerstein, L., Wark, J. D. and Burger, H. G. (1996). Bone mineral density and hormone

levels in menopausal Australian women. *Gynecol. Endocrinol.*, **10**, 199–205

17. Johnston, C. Jr, Hui, S. L., Witt, R. M., Appledorn, R., Baker, R. S. and Longcope, C. (1985). Early menopause changes in bone mass and sex steroids. *J. Clin. Endocrinol. Metab.*, **61**, 905–11

18. Dawson-Hughes, B., Shipp, C., Sadowski, L. and Dallal, G. (1987). Bone mineral density of the radius, spine and hip in relation to per cent of ideal body weight in postmenopausal women. *Calcif. Tiss. Int.*, **40**, 310–14

19. Slemenda, C. W., Hui, S. L., Williams, C. J., Christian, J. C., Meaney F. J. and Johnston, C. C. Jr (1990). Bone mass and anthropometric measurements in adult females. *Bone Miner.*, **11**, 101–9

20. Salamone, L. M., Glynn, N., Black, D., Epstein, R. S., Palermo, L., Meilahn, E., Kuller, L. H. and Cauley, J. A. (1995). Body composition and bone mineral density in premenopausal and early perimenopausal women. *J. Bone Miner. Res.*, **10**, 1762–8

21. Nelson, M. E., Fiatarone, M. A., Morganti, C. M., Trice, I., Greenberg, R. A. and Evan, W. J. (1994). Effects of high-intensity strength training on multiple risk factors for osteoporotic fractures. A randomized controlled trial. *J. Am. Med. Assoc.*, **272**, 1909–14

22. Pruitt, L. A., Jackson, R. D., Bartels, R. L. and Lehnhard, H. J. (1992). Weight-training effects on bone mineral density in early postmenopausal women. *J. Bone Miner. Res.*, **7**, 179–85

23. Reid, I. R., Ames, R. W., Evans, M. C., Gamble, G. D. and Sharpe, S. J. (1993). Effect of calcium supplementation on bone loss in postmenopausal women. *N. Engl. J. Med.*, **328**, 460–4

24. Gordon, D. J., Probstfield, J. L., Garrison, R. J., Neaton, J. D., Castelli, W. P., Knoke, J. D., Jacobs, D. R. Jr, Bangdiwala, S. and Tyroler, H. A. (1989). High-density lipoprotein cholesterol and cardiovascular disease. Four prospective American studies. *Circulation*, **79**, 8–15

25. Owens, J. F., Matthews, K. A., Wing, R. R. and Kuller, L. H. (1992). Can physical activity mitigate the effects of aging in middle-aged women? *Circulation*, **85**, 1265–70

26. Reaven, P. D., Barrett-Connor, E. and Edelstein, S. (1991). Relation between leisure-time physical actvity and blood pressure in older women. *Circulation*, **83**, 559–65

27. Barrett-Connor, E. (1994). Heart disease in women. *Fertil. Steril.*, **62** (Suppl. 2), 127S–32S

28. Manson, J. E., Colditz, G. A., Stampfer, M. J., Willett, W. C., Rosner, B., Monson, R. R., Speizer, F. E. and Hennekens, C. H. (1990). A prospective study of obesity and risk of coronary heart disease in women. *N. Engl. J. Med.*, **322**, 882–9

29. Singh, R. B., Rastage, S. S., Niaz M. A., Ghosh, S., Singh, R. and Gupta, S. (1992). Effects of fat modified and fruit- and vegetable-enriched diets on blood lipids in the Indian diet heart study. *Am. J. Cardiol.*, **70**, 869–74

30. Knight, D. C. and Eden, J. A. (1995). Phytoestrogens – a short review. *Maturitas*, **22**, 167–75

An Asian perspective of the menopause 16

S. Punyahotra and K. Limpaphayom

Introduction

Women's experiences of menopause in Western cultures and Asian cultures have some similarities and differences. Studies from Asian countries revealed that menopause in Asian women is associated with fewer and less severe symptoms[1]. The prevalence of symptoms, particularly those related to estrogen decline, was different in these cultures. For example, Asian women have a low incidence of hot flushes. This can be confirmed by the studies of Agoestina and vanKeep[2], Lock and colleagues[3], Sukwatana and co-workers[4] and Wasti and associates[5]. Chinese women are not found to report hot flushes[6]. Symptoms unique to menopause in Japanese women are headaches, shoulder stiffness and aches in the joints[3]. Many menopausal women in Malaysia and Thailand saw no need to consult a doctor about their menopausal symptoms[4,7]. They related their health as good during their climacteric years[7]. The end of menstruation was a liberation for Indian women of the Rajput caste[8]. They looked forward to menopause and had virtually no symptoms.

In Western and industrialized societies, many studies indicate that menopause signals the beginning of a period in life when risk for diseases such as coronary heart disease (CHD) and osteoporosis begins to increase. These problems are not well documented in the developing countries, including Thailand and other Asian countries. There have been some clinical studies on CHD and osteoporosis in Thailand, but epidemiological data are unsatisfactory[9]. However, the prevalence and incidence of osteoporotic fractures are expected to increase in the near future as the number of elderly people increases[10].

Many researchers have mentioned sociocultural aspects of menopause, and that menopause may have different meanings for women of different cultural backgrounds[3,8]. Middle-aged women respond to menopause according to the beliefs of their respective cultures[3]. In Asian societies, health-care practitioners still know little about the relationship of genetics, environment, diet and some other factors which may contribute to the differences in menopausal symptoms[3]. Health intervention for well menopausal women in Asia may have to be approached differently compared with that for Western women. There is a need to understand the process by which Asian women describe, explain and experience menopause. This paper therefore, will present the story of women in Thai society in terms of their social status, lifestyle behaviors, cultural attitudes and cultural beliefs of menopause, and also will present results from a national survey of menopausal experiences of mid-aged Thai women which the Ministry of Public Health carried out in 1995.

About the country

The Kingdom of Thailand, with an area of 198 456 square miles, is located in central Southeast Asia. Geographically, Thailand is divided into four regions: the Central Plains, the North, the Northeast and the South. The population in 1996 is 59.6 million with 79% of the people living in rural areas. The annual population growth rate in 1996 is 1.1%, and women comprise half of the Thai population. The practice of family planning in 1996 is 74%. The proportion of people aged 0–14 years declined from 46.2% in 1970 to 28.8% in 1996, while that of people aged 60 years and over increased from 4.8% to 7.3%. Life expectancy at birth for males and females has been gradually increasing from 51.9 and 56.1 years respectively in 1960 to 66.6 and 71.7 years in 1996 (Table 1)[11].

Social status of women

Throughout history, women in Thai society were not recognized as having the same status as men[12]. Wives were taught to be loyal, respectful and never show anger towards their husbands. There is a Thai saying that 'men are the fore legs of the elephant and women are the hind legs'. This means the male household head is the one with the leading role in making a living to support the family, and the women follow. Frequently, a wife addresses her husband as 'pee' or elder brother[13].

Education

In general, Thai women are more rural and less educated than men (most have less than 4 years of schooling). Thai women in the past lacked educational and training opportunities, because education formerly was dependent on Buddhist monasteries[14]. The rapid economic changes in the contemporary period have transformed Thai society. Women now have better opportunities to acquire further education, to be able to work outside the home and be self-reliant as well as to be more independent. Although women may not be the official household head, they play important roles as family treasurer and financial manager in addition to their principal roles of mother and wife.

The middle years

The position of women is enhanced as they reach their middle years[15]. In non-Western societies, menopause may be defined as a transition towards a higher-status age group. Middle-aged women improve their status in three major aspects[15]: fewer restrictions, the right to exert authority over particular relatives, and the opportunity to achieve beyond the

Table 1 Thai population and vital statistics, 1996. From reference 11

Population (thousands)	59 781
male	29 873
female	29 908
Rural population (thousands)	40 902
Population under 15 years (%)	28.8
Population aged 60 years and older (%)	7.3
Annual population growth rate (%)	1.1
Practice of family planning (%)	74.0
Life expectancy at birth (years)	
male	66.6
female	71.7

household setting. This is true in Thailand. When women get older their power and authority within their families increase. Many of them attain the status of mother-in-law, and the obedience of daughters-in-law further enhances their position. Middle-aged women control the household purse and play an important role in decision-making and family management[16].

How Thai society views menopause

As in other cultures, menopause is perceived as 'the change' in Thai society. Evidence for this can be seen in the old Thai words describing menopause. The common phrase which can be generally understood as referring to menopause is 'leod cha pai – lom cha ma'. This phrase literally means 'the blood will go – the wind will come'. According to Buddhist teaching, nature is made up of four elements: earth, water, wind and fire. These four major elements are the essential ingredients of everybody[9]. The earth element is characterized as strong, heavy and unshakable; the water element is cool, calm and pleasant while the wind tends to be violent and unpredictable on some occasions; fire is characterized by hot temper, always furious or highly emotional. During menopause, unpredictable changes have long been observed in Thai women. However, the changes are believed to happen occasionally and are not expected in every woman.

Thai experiences of the menopause

More information about middle-aged Thai women and their experiences of menopause can be learnt from a national study conducted by the Ministry of Public Health in 1995[17]. It consisted of 8300 Thai women aged 40–59 years randomly selected from the general population, except Bangkok and its environs. Personnel from 12 regional health centers conducted face-to-face interviews. Within each region, 35 villages were randomly selected and within each village 20 women between the ages of 40 and 59 were randomly selected.

The survey instrument comprised questions relating to sociodemographic data including health and sexual behaviors, six questions on knowledge and five questions on attitude toward menopause, and a 21-item check-list of symptoms frequently associated with menopause. The check-list was based on the Kaufert and Syrotuik check-list modified to include common complaints related to menopause reported to the survey organizers.

Characteristic of the subjects

The average age of women in the survey sample was 49 (± 6) years. Thirty-eight per cent of them were premenopausal, 18% perimenopausal and 44% postmenopausal. The average age at first menstruation was 16 (± 1.7) years and the last menstruation was at 48 (± 4) years. Most women were agricultural workers who had attended primary school and were married with three children. The average age of the youngest child was 17 (± 6.6) years.

Summary of findings

Lifestyles and health behaviors

On the body mass index (BMI), 49% had a standard value of BMI (20–25 kg/m^2), 35% above standard and 16% below standard. Very few women smoked or drank alcohol. Most were Buddhists. Eighty-two per cent had adequate sleeping hours. Their diets consisted mainly of rice, vegetables and fruits; 55% did not drink milk, 32% sometimes drank milk and 13% drank milk regularly. Nearly 60% reported never exercising for health reasons, but most worked in the fields so could be described as physically active. About 85% reported they still had sexual relations with their husbands and only 3% complained of painful intercourse.

Knowledge

Respondents' knowledge of menopause was rated according to their response to six true or false questions. Fifty per cent scored highly on the test, 42% had a medium score and 8% a low score. Sources of knowledge on menopause were listed as first, friends and relatives, and second, self-experience. Respondents were also asked to list three symptoms of menopause. The most common responses were abnormal menstruation (15.6%), headaches (14.3%), dizziness (9.4%) and mood swings (5.7%). Only 3.8% cited hot flushes, which is the most common symptom listed in Western surveys.

Attitudes and belief

Most women (78%) believe menopause is a natural occurrence, not an ailment, and 64% believe emotional problems experienced in the menopausal years are caused by individuals' backgrounds, behaviors and situations, not because of menopause. Some women said that after menopause, the natural aging process accelerated.

Checklist of symptoms

Respondents were read a 21-item check-list of symptoms and asked to identify which ones they had experienced and which ones they found bothersome. Three per cent reported having no symptoms. The most common symptoms that respondents reported as bothersome were backaches (26%), headaches (25%), dizziness (24.7%), forgetfulness (23.8%) and joint pains (22.5%). In rank order, hot flushes ranked 10th (15.8%) and night sweats 15th (9%). About 10% of women complained of urinary problems

(Table 2). Women most likely to experience symptoms were postmenopausal. Of those with symptoms, about one-half said they would see a doctor about the symptoms, one-quarter would treat themselves and one-quarter would do nothing.

The picture of middle-aged Thai women

From this study, we can understand more about middle-aged women in Thai society. Many Thai women are in agricultural careers and are physically active. It is very common to see rural women working side by side with their husbands in the field. During the busy farm season, they are likely to work long hours in the rice field and have little time for food preparation. Most women do not smoke or drink alcohol. Their health status regarding BMI is mostly satisfactory. The majority of rural Thai women do not drink milk, which is known to be a very important source of calcium. However, they have rice, fruits and vegetables in their daily diets. The analysis of Thai food by the Department of Health showed that the traditional Thai dishes contain a lot of calcium[18]. Thai people take calcium from small fishes and green leafy vegetables (possibly high in naturally estrogenic properties). The incidence of postmenopausal osteoporosis in Thailand is in the process of being studied. However, a study on hip fractures from nine hospitals in four regions of Thailand revealed that the incidence of hip fractures was low. An average incidence was 7.05 per 100 000 women per year[19]. The average age of the patient was 74 ($\pm$ 10) years and the incidence increased with age. Sex ratio of hip fracture incidence comparing women with men was 2.23 to 1.

In Thailand, the majority of people are Buddhists. Buddhism plays an important role in shaping Thai beliefs and behaviors. Many Thai women express positive views about menopause. The Buddhist concept of the impermanence of life leads women to accept the decline of body functions that comes with age[20]. Women accept that at this age

Table 2 Percentage of respondents reporting bothersome symptoms in a previous month ($n = 8300$). From reference 17

Symptom	Frequency	%
Backache	1874	26.1
Headache	1835	25.1
Dizziness	1806	24.7
Forgetfulness	1725	23.8
Ache or stiff joint	1630	22.5
Tiredness	1490	20.2
Muscle pain	1432	19.9
Irritability	1405	19.5
Insomnia	1159	16.0
Hot flushes	1167	15.8
Shortness of breath	1040	14.7
Pins and needles in hands and feet	1049	14.2
Uncontrolled urination	688	9.6
Dry and itchy skin	667	9.0
Night sweats	667	9.0
Lower abdominal pain	645	8.9
Frequent urination	576	8.1
Depression	558	7.9
Irregular menstruation	331	4.7
Vaginal symptoms	321	4.5
Painful urination	184	2.6

menstruation stops and they naturally enter the aging period. The ideas of maintaining youth and beauty after menopause are quite rare, particularly in rural Thai women.

The health ministry survey found that Thai women are generally ill-informed about menopause. The knowledge of menopause mostly comes from the experiences of friends and relatives. Women may not recognize some symptoms as menopausal changes. In addition, many women usually connect symptoms with specific organs. For example, a woman would perceive that she has problems of heart disease by saying 'my heart is weak' when she feels perspiration, dizziness and shortness of breath. Many women do not associate those symptoms with menopause.

The major complaints in the previous month of those Thai women surveyed involved skeletal and general malaise symptoms such as back pain, diffuse extremity pain, headaches and dizziness. As many women worked in agricultural careers, they were likely to spend long hours in the field. In addition, the increase in migration of young adults to urban areas owing to the economic changes of the country has had an impact on women's lives. Many women have to bear the burden of running the farm and household alone. All this may intensify the skeletal and general malaise symptoms. However, Thai women may have low incidences of some health problems related to menopause because they smoke and drink less than their Western counterparts.

The report rate for hot flushes was markedly low compared with that of Western women. The prevalence of hot flushes was similar to that reported in other Asian women[2,3,5,6]. Women in our region get used to living and working in the hot climate. For this reason the symptom may not be reported as bothersome.

Conclusion: management of the well menopausal Asian woman

The management of the well menopausal woman in Thailand must be seen in the wider context of health care for Thai women, especially rural Thai women. In general Thai women are not particularly interested in their health. They may not acknowledge a need for preventive care. Some women may never have breast examinations or cervical cancer screenings. Many of them wait until they have symptoms and feel ill; patients may not seek medical attention until a problem is fairly advanced[21]. In rural Thailand when people become ill, they usually treat themselves first by using traditional and available herbal medicines.

Management of well menopausal women in Thai society needs to be considered carefully. In many ways, Thai women's lifestyles contribute to a protective mechanism for problems related to menopause. In developing strategies for the Thai society, it is important to retain the already positive attitudes towards menopause. The question needing to be asked is: how can we maintain traditional Thai beliefs, lifestyles, eating Thai food and living close to nature?

Recently, hormone replacement therapy has been promoted as a preventive therapy for osteoporosis and heart disease in many countries. In Thailand, infectious diseases, diseases of the digestive system, and malignant neoplasm still account for most hospital admissions. General preventive measures including health education and health promotion are most important for Thai women, providing health benefits for all, rather than being confined to prevention of hormonal deficiency problems.

References

1. Payer, L. (1990). The menopause in various cultures. In Burger, H. and Boulet, M. A. (eds.) *Portrait of the Menopause*, pp. 3–21. (New York: Parthenon Publishing)
2. Agoestina, T. and vanKeep, P. A. (1984). The climacteric in Bandung, West Java province, Indonesia. *Maturitas*, **6**, 327–33
3. Lock, M., Kaufert, P. and Gilbert, P. (1988). Cultural construction of the menopausal symptoms: the Japanese case. *Maturitas*, **10**, 317–32
4. Sukwatana, P., Meekhangvan, J., Tamrongterakul, T., Tanapat, Y., Asavarait, S. and Boonjitrpimon, P. (1991). Menopausal symptoms among Thai women in Bangkok. *Maturitas*, **13**, 217–28
5. Wasti, S., Robinson, S. C., Akhtar, Y., Khan, S. and Badaruddin, N. (1993). Characteristics of menopause in three socioeconomic urban groups in Karachi, Pakistan. *Maturitas*, **16**, 61–9
6. Tang, G. W. K. (1993). Menopausal symptoms. *J. Hong Kong Med. Assoc.*, **45**, 249–54
7. Ismail, N. N. M. (1990). A study of menopause in seven Far-Eastern countries – Malaysia. Presented at the *6th International Congress on the Menopause*, Bangkok, Thailand, October–November, abstr. 015
8. Flint, M. and Garcia, M. (1979). Cultural and climacteric. *J. Biosoc. Sci.*, **6** (Suppl.), 197–215
9. Dusitsin, N. and Snidvong, W. (1993). The Thai experience. In Berg, G. and Hammer, M. (eds.) *The Modern Management of the Menopause: a*

Perspective for the 21st century, pp. 23–33. (Casterton, UK: Parthenon Publishing)

10. Bose, K. (1996). Osteoporosis; a growing problem in Southeast Asia. *Med. Prog.*, **23**, 5–7

11. Mahidol Population Gazette, July, 1996, pp. 1–2. (Bangkok: The William and Flora Hewlett Foundation)

12. Sirisambhand, A. and Gordon, A. (1987). Rural women and changes in work pattern: the impact of a reservoir and transportation networks on three Thai villages. In Heyzer, N. (ed.) *Women Farmers and Rural Change in Asia: Towards Equal Access and Participation*, pp. 313–47. (Kuala Lumpur: Asian and Pacific Development Centre)

13. Yoddumnern-Attig, B. (1992). Conjugal and parental roles: a behavioral look into past and present. In Yoddumnern-Attig, B., Richter, K., Soonthorndhada, A., Sethaput, C. and Pramualratana, A. (eds.) *Changing Roles and Status of Women in Thailand: a Documentary Assessment*, pp. 25–35. (Bangkok: Institute for Population and Social Research, Mahidol University)

14. Dharmasakti, S. (1991). Dutiful but overburdened. In Tantiwiramanond, D. and Pandey, S. (eds.) *By Women, for Women: a Study of Women's Organizations in Thailand*, pp. 13–24. (Bangkok: Institute of Southeast Asian Studies)

15. Oswalt, W. H. (1986). *Life Cycles and Lifeways. An Introduction to Cultural Anthropology*, pp. 159–61. (Palo Alto, CA: Manfield Publishing)

16. Yoddumnern-Attig, B. (1992). Thai family structure and organization: changing roles and duties in historical perspective. In Yoddumnern-Attig, B., Richter, K., Soonthorndhada, A., Sethaput, C. and Pramualratana, A. (eds.) *Changing Roles and Status of Women in Thailand: a Documentary Assessment*, pp. 8–24. (Bangkok: Institute for Population and Social Research, Mahidol University)

17. The Department of Health (1996). *The National Study of Health Behaviors of Pre- and Post-menopausal Thai Women*. (Bangkok: The Ministry of Public Health)

18. Prateprasaen, M. (1996). Nutrition for menopausal women. Presented at the *3rd Scientific Meeting on the Menopause*, Bangkok, March

19. Siriyawongpaisal, P., Loahachareonsombat, W., Kumpoo, U., Suksawai, P., Supachutikul, A., Siriwongpairat, P., Angsachon, T., Sujaritputtangkul, S., Preechapannyakul, V., Rajatanavin, R. and Puavilai, G. (1994). A multicenter study of hip fracture in Thailand. *J. Med. Assoc. Thai.*, **77**, 488–95

20. Chirawatkul, S. (1992). The social construction of menopause in Northeastern Thailand. Presented at the *4th Tropical Health and Nutrition Conference*, Brisbane, Australia, October

21. Douglas, K.C. and Fujimoto, D. (1995). Asian Pacific elders: implications for health care providers. In Espino, D. V. (ed.) *Clinics in Geriatic Medicine*, pp.69–82. (Philadelphia: W.B. Saunders)

Dealing with the complications of HRT management

17

M. Dören

Introduction

In middle-aged women who have undergone natural menopause, there are insufficient data to draw meaningful conclusions as to whether there are specific advantages associated with any regimen or route of hormonal replacement therapy (HRT) with respect to treatment of climacteric symptoms or preventive treatment of urogenital aging, postmenopausal osteoporosis or arterial diseases. In particular, no data are available for women with premature menopause. Whether surgical menopause in younger women and premature menopause affect mineral homeostasis to the same extent as in (early) postmenopause remains to be proven. However, it is clear that oral estrogens, e.g. conjugated equine estrogens have been shown to prevent the increase in risk for coronary heart disease in women with bilateral oophorectomy. Castration apparently increases the risk of coronary heart disease[1]. Women with bilateral oophorectomy have an increased risk of 2.2 for coronary heart disease[2] (Table 1).

At appropriate doses, oral and transdermal estrogens have comparable effects on target organs if extrapolation from data generated in women with natural menopause is justified, which is apparently reasonable. Similarily it is appropriate to administer a progestational agent to women with premature menopause who have an intact uterus to protect the endometrium. Whether the administration of oral contraceptives is associated with any benefit compared to HRT remains to be proven. There is a lifetime chance of conception of 5–15% in women with premature menopause on HRT[3,4] which may be regarded as a significant advantage compared with the administration of oral contraceptives as a specific form of HRT. However, overall assessments of long-term benefits and risks of oral contraceptives in women of reproductive age[5,6] (Table 2) need to be conducted in the heterogenous subset of women with premature menopause.

Hormone replacement therapy may increase the quality of life in postmenopausal women with climacteric symptoms. Nevertheless, even if clear-cut benefits are demonstrated, women are very reluctant to accept HRT and adhere to a treatment regimen. There are virtually no data on premature menopause and compliance.

As well as the fact that the explanation of how to administer a drug is often felt to be too

Table 1 Risk of coronary heart disease: cohort of 127 000 American women aged 30–35 years. Data from reference 2

	Odds ratio (95% confidence limits)	
Type of menopause	*No treatment*	*Estrogen replacement*
Natural	1.2 (0.8–1.8)	0.8 (0.4–1.3)
Hysterectomy and bilateral oophorectomy	2.2 (1.2–4.2)	0.9 (0.6–1.6)

114

Table 2 Oral contraceptive (OC) use and risk of cancer development in American women aged 20–54 years: estimates in absolute figures per 100 000 women. Data from reference 6

	Never users	OC use > 8 years	
Breast	2.782	2.933	⇑
Cervix	425	550	⇑
Endometrium	438	241	⇓
Ovary	369	176	⇓
Liver	20	61	⇑

complicated or inconvenient, women often feel that the prescription of hormones is not natural. This is a common attitude irrespective of demographic factors such as age or education. Opinions concerning the overall benefit in an individual risk–benefit assessment of HRT differ considerably, not only within the medical community but also within the generation of women approching menopause. It has become increasingly clear that patient willingness to take and continue HRT is influenced not only by the medical community, but also by package inserts with conflicting information listing contraindications no longer existing, and increasingly by mass media. In particular, in younger women it may be difficult to explain the reasons for HRT which is 'normally' recommended for women significantly older.

Although the advantages and the possible drug-related side-effects are to be explained and discussed before initiation of treatment, there is considerable reluctance of women to start and consequently use HRT. We may consider this as an attempt to demonstrate independence from therapeutic decisions of physicians. Thus, emancipation of women may be one basic trend warranting further attention whenever the question of compliance is addressed in HRT.

The cessation of menses is an event belonging to every woman's life; many women do not consider withdrawal bleeding induced by most of the HRT regimens to be 'natural' or 'normal' after the menopausal transition. The absence of withdrawal bleeding after menopause is appreciated by a substantial majority of postmenopausal women at least in the industrialized societies. In surveys women rate bleeding as the most negative factor influencing their decision to discontinue HRT[7]. Whether the cessation of menses in premature menopause is perceived as a hazard or a convenient event has not been thoroughly investigated.

Treatment regimens and routes of administration

Oral administration of *estrogens*, mainly conjugated estrogens in the United States and estradiol (valerate) in European countries, are the most common types of HRT. The use of parenteral administration, i.e. patches and gel containing estradiol is increasing; recent data referring to the reasons for this shift point out that the feeling of women 'not to be medicated'[8] may be important. The use of a more physiological, 'natural' form of HRT may be another reason, and 'fashion' yet another. The author is not aware of any data mainly investigating compliance in relation to the profile of potential medical, physical, psychological and metabolic side-effects of the various pharmacological subgroups of estrogens in premature menopause.

Progestogens given almost exclusively to induce regular shedding of the endometrium in postmenopausal women with intact uterus may cause a considerable number of physical, psychological and metabolic side effects due to the pharmacological profile of C-21 or C-19 derivatives. Breast tenderness, bloatedness and edema are common physical side-effects, and depressive mood swings, anxiety, and increased irritability are frequent psychological side-effects seen also in young menopausal women. Endometrial effects have been extensively studied in postmenopausal women; whether results may be extrapolated to younger women with ovarian failure remains to be investigated.

Various prescribing schedules are used for combined, sequential estrogen and progestogen therapy as first-line HRT in postmenopausal women. Specific recommendations do not exist for younger women.

Opposed sequential therapy with estrogens and progestogens to minimize the risk of endometrial pathology leads to withdrawal bleeding in almost 90% of women. Alternative schemes with continuous combined estrogen and progestogen have been designed to restore or maintain amenorrhea in postmenopausal women while offering the same endometrial safety as in conventional sequential therapy. Whether this concept is valid for younger women with premature menopause has not been studied.

Large variations in the success rate to achieve amenorrhea and adherence of patients on *continuous combined HRT* are reported. The largest body of information concerns a combination of estradiol and norethisterone acetate, and conjugated equine estrogens and medroxyprogesterone acetate. In general, the frequency of bleeding episodes in early postmenopausal women is higher compared with that in late postmenopausal women. Histology after endometrial sampling showed atrophy in the range 54–65% irrespective of the occurence of uterine bleeding; correlations to pretreatment biopsies are not always available.

In prospective investigations comparing *oral and transdermal HRT* [9] the issue of compliance is addressed on the side; so far main outcome variables have focused on lipids, bone and hemostasis. In a retrospective trial comparing oral and transdermal estrogen therapy, both in combination with oral progesterone, compliance of the two regimens stratified to the different routes of administration of the estrogenic compound was not reported. However, it seems prudent to offer non-oral estrogen replacement in order to reproduce physiological serum concentrations of estradiol without increasing serum concentrations of estrone as in oral estrogen replacement. Once again, specific treatment modalities have not been studied in women with premature menopause.

Conclusions

Quality of life evaluations [10] are necessary to find HRT regimens for young women with early ovarian failure. Therefore, it seems unlikely that a 'standard regimen' will be developed to improve long-term adherence to HRT. Fears that replacement therapy might cause (breast) cancer and induce weight increase, to name only two common opinions of patients, exist also in younger women. Measurements of risk factors influencing the quality of life in postmenopausal women, e.g. the risk for osteoporotic fractures by densitometry, are probably not the way to increase compliance in younger women; only the first-line decision, but not the adherence to HRT was apparently influenced [11]. Educational programs for younger women, in particular for those with an unsuccessful history of reproduction, need to be developed not only to prevent sequelae of estrogen deficiency but to overcome the common frustration of failed reproduction.

References

1. Oliver, M. F. and Boyd, G. S. (1959). Effect of bilateral ovariectomy on coronary-artery disease and serum-lipid levels. *Lancet*, **2**, 962–4
2. Colditz, G. A., Willett, W., Stampfer, M. J., Rosner, M. J., Speizer, F. E. and Hennekens, C. A. (1987). Menopause and the risk of coronary heart disease in women. *N. Engl. J. Med.*, **316**, 1105–10
3. Alper, M. M., Jolly, E. E. and Garner, P. R. (1986). Pregnancies after premature ovarian failure. *Obstet. Gynecol.*, **67**, S59–62
4. Kreiner, D., Droesch, K., Navot, D., Scott, R. and Rosenwaks, Z. (1988). Spontaneous and pharmacologically induced remissions in patients with premature ovarian failure. *Obstet. Gynecol.*, **72**, 926–8
5. Collaborative Group on Hormonal Factors in Breast Cancer (1996). Breast cancer and hormonal contraceptives: collaborative reanalysis of individual data on 53 297 women with breast cancer and 100 239 women without

breast cancer from 54 epidemiological studies. *Lancet*, **347**, 1713–27

6. Schlesselman, J. J. (1995). Net effect of oral contraceptive use on the risk of cancer in women in the United States. *Obstet. Gynecol.*, **85**, 793–801

7. Nachtigall, L. E. (1990). Enhancing patient compliance with hormonal replacement therapy at menopause. *Obstet. Gynecol.*, **75**, S77–80

8. Cano, A. (1995). Compliance to hormone replacement therapy in menopausal women controlled in a third level academic centre. *Maturitas*, **20**, 91–9

9. Stevenson, J. C., Crook, D. and Godsland, I. F. (1993). Oral versus transdermal hormone replacement therapy. *Int. J. Fertil.*, **38**, S30–5

10. Wiklund, I., Karlberg, J. and Mattson, L.-M. (1993). Quality of life of postmenopausal women on a regimen of transdermal estradiol therapy: a double-blind placebo-controlled study. *Am. J. Obstet. Gynecol.*, **168**, 824–30

11. Rubin, S. M. and Cummings, S. R. (1992). Results of bone densitometry affect women's decisions about taking measures to prevent fractures. *Ann. Int. Med.*, **116**, 990–5

4

Hormone replacement therapy and osteoporosis

Estrogens and bone cells

18

P. H. Stern, G. Tarjan and J. L. Sanders

Although it has been recognized for a number of years that a deficiency in estrogen results in increased bone fragility, the mechanism of the effect has been elusive. It is only within the past 10 years that investigators have had the cellular models and analytical methodologies to establish that bone cells of several types possess high affinity receptors for estrogens. This was first reported in 1988 by Komm and colleagues in two osteoblast cell lines, rat ROS 17/2.8 and human HOS TE85[1] and by Ericksen and co-workers in cultured osteoblastic cells from human surgical specimens[2]. Receptors for estrogens or genes for estrogen receptors were subsequently reported in other osteoblastic cell lines[3–5], as well as in normal osteoblasts and preosteoblastic cells from other species[6–9], osteoclastic and preosteoclastic cells[10–14], osteocytes[15] and a bone endothelial cell line[16]. The density of the receptors is generally lower than in reproductive tissues, although the affinities are comparable to those in typical estrogen target tissues. This widespread presence of estrogen receptors allows for multiple options in terms of how estrogens might directly affect bone, and also for the possibility of multifaceted effects. This is especially true since normal bone remodeling requires direct actions of osteoclasts on the bone matrix, which can involve acute activation of these osteoclasts by osteoblasts, and more delayed effects on differentiation of osteoblasts and osteoclasts. Studies in the past several years have revealed a number of effects of estrogens on bone, which include effects on proliferation, on phenotypic responses and on the secretion of local factors that could be mediators of the action of estrogens. Estrogens have been observed to have inconsistent and often opposite effects on osteoblast proliferation and phenotypic responses, such as alkaline phosphatase and osteocalcin, in different studies[17–19]. Since a wide range of culture conditions, cell lines and passage numbers are represented in the data, the diversity of response may be indicative that the effects are limited to a subpopulation of the bone cells. Alternatively, the lack of a consistent response may indicate that these are not critical phenomena in the actions of estrogen to preserve bone. In osteoclasts and osteoclastic cells, the effects of estrogens on functions related to the bone resorbing activity of the cells are in the direction of inhibition, with decreased osteoclast-mediated resorption and decreases in several osteoclast lysosomal enzymes[20]. However, other investigations have failed to show effects of physiological concentrations of estrogen on osteoclastic pit formation[21].

Turning to a more intact resorbing system, bone organ cultures, it has again been difficult to demonstrate direct inhibitory effects of estrogen unless very high concentrations are used. This is a very striking observation when we consider that agents that are less effective in preventing osteoporosis *in vivo*, i.e. calcitonin and bisphosphonates, dramatically and rapidly decrease resorption in the *in vitro* models. One study in which estrogen effects were seen was that of Pilbeam and associates, in mouse calvariae[22]. Interestingly, the effect was elicited after a preculture with estrogen together with a glucocorticoid, which was added to suppress endogenous prostaglandin synthesis. Even under these conditions, the maximum response was a 20% inhibition, and the effect showed a biphasic dose-dependence. It is possible that the effect of estrogen is slow and requires longer incubation times than are practical with current organ culture models. A slow response would be consistent with the possibility that the estrogen effect is indirect, and that a suppression or increase of one or more of the many local factors affecting bone is the mediator of the response. In the same calvarial model, estrogen decreased prostaglandin production. In earlier studies, Feyen and Raisz showed that ovariectomy increased prostaglandin concentrations in bone and this was prevented by estrogen[23], implicating effects on prostaglandin production in mediating or modulating estrogen action on bone. Recently, it has been found that mRNA for the inducible prostaglandin synthase is increased by conditioned medium from oophorectomized animals[24]. Also, the effect of marrow supernatants from oophorectomized animals to stimulate resorption was prevented by indomethacin[25].

Several cytokines that increase bone resorption are elevated in the absence of estrogen. These include interleukin-1 (IL-1), tumor necrosis factor-α (TNF-α) and IL-6. Interleukin-1 production in monocytes is sensitive to estrogen status[26,27]. Treatment with an IL-1 receptor antagonist markedly inhibited the bone loss elicited by ovariectomy in rats[28]. Complete inhibition of bone loss was accomplished with the combination of an IL-1 receptor antagonist protein and a TNF-α binding protein[29]. Although the IL-1 could be produced by bone cells[30], the effect might be indirectly mediated through another cell type in the marrow. Interleukin-6 is produced by bone marrow-derived stromal cells and osteoblasts[31,32] and is a potent stimulator of osteoclast differentiation from hematopoietic progenitor cells in human marrow[33]. Interleukin-6 production is stimulated by parathyroid hormone (PTH) as well as by IL-1 and TNF-α in bone[34,35]. Estrogen decreases IL-6 production by bone marrow stromal cells and osteoblasts[36,37], whereas estrogen withdrawal in mice results in increased production of IL-6[38]. Antibodies to IL-6 decreased bone loss and osteoclast proliferation in oophorectomized mice, an effect similar to that produced by estrogen replacement[39]. An IL-6 knockout mouse was found to have an impaired response to ovariectomy, in that bone turnover was not stimulated[40]. Interleukin-6 is increased in postmenopausal women[41]. In our own organ

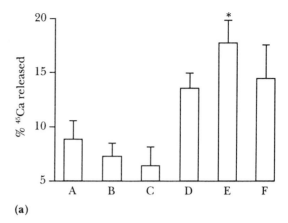

(a)

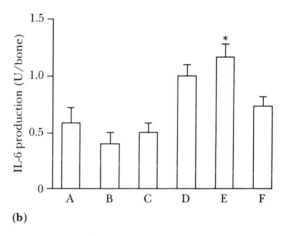

(b)

Figure 1 Effect of 17β-estradiol (E_2) on (a) parathyroid hormone (PTH)-stimulated bone resorption and (b) interleukin-6 (IL-6) production in fetal rat limb bone organ cultures; values are means $\pm$ SEM of responses from four bones per treatment. *$p < 0.05$; A, no treatment; B, E_2 0.1 nmol/l (0–72 h); C, E_2 (0–144 h); D, no treatment (0–72 h), PTH 2 nmol/l (72–144 h); E, E_2 (0–72 h), PTH (72–144 h); F, E_2 (0–72 h), PTH plus E_2 (72–144 h)

culture studies, we have found that estrogen withdrawal increases both IL-6 production and the responsiveness of the bones to the bone-resorbing effects of PTH (Figure 1). This could be a useful model for studying estrogen-deficiency bone loss, especially as it relates to IL-6.

Prostaglandin production could be part of the pathway by which IL-6 is generated in bone.

We have found that both the bone resorption and the IL-6 production elicited by IL-1 in this same bone organ culture model are inhibited by the prostaglandin synthase blocker indomethacin[42]. The bone resorbing activity in marrow supernatants from oophorectomized animals, which could be partially inhibited by an antibody to IL-6, was prevented by indomethacin[25]. There may also be a protein kinase C (PKC) signal transduction step in the production of IL-6 in osteoblasts, as we have found that down-regulation of PKC with a phorbol ester partially prevents the increase in IL-6 production elicited by PTH[43].

The growth factors are another group of local agents that could be involved in estrogen actions on bone. Transforming growth factors are of particular interest because they stimulate bone formation and inhibit resorption[44-46] and their production is increased by estrogen in both osteoblastic and osteoclastic cells[46,47]. It has recently been shown that there are several isoforms of transforming growth factor-β (TGF-β), and that TGF-β3 is the isoform specifically increased by estrogen in osteoclastic cells[48]. Although most studies have focused on either cytokines or growth factors, a recent study of SaOS-2 human osteoblastic osteosarcoma cells transfected with estrogen receptors showed that they had both increased TGF-β expression in response to estrogen, and decreased endogenous IL-6 mRNA in comparison to non-transfected cells[49].

Recent studies have examined whether similar mechanisms can explain the effects of estrogens and the antiestrogens that also inhibit bone resorption. It is particularly interesting that in oophorectomized animals, TGF-β3 production in bone is stimulated by both estrogens and antiestrogens that protect bone[50]. In recent work from our laboratory, we have been studying effects of estrogens and antiestrogens on the PKC signaling pathway, which has been shown to be affected by these hormones in reproductive tissues. We have found that in long-term cultures, there is a similar PKC isozyme response to both 17β-estradiol and the antiestrogen 4-OH tamoxifen[51].

The antiestrogens may also inhibit bone resorption by cellular mechanisms that are not shared by estrogens, including apoptotic effects on osteoclasts[21]. There may be specific effects on unique cell functions such as the osteoclast adenosine triphosphatase[52]. Again, in our organ culture systems we have a counterpart to this. Although we do not see direct inhibition of bone resorptive activity by physiologic concentrations of estrogen, the antiestrogens tamoxifen and clomiphene can rapidly inhibit resorption[53]. In further studies we have found that the antiestrogen ICI 164,384, which acts by stimulating estrogen receptor loss[54] and thus should lack estrogenic effects, also inhibits resorption. The antiestrogen ICI 164,384 does not reverse or antagonize the antiresorptive effects of tamoxifen.

In summary, bone is clearly a target tissue for estrogen. Although the mechanism of the response is unclear, it is not for lack of possibilities. The effect could be due to local factors produced by bone cells or by cells in the vicinity of bone. The existence of multiple factors that are regulated by estrogen and influence bone-cell activity could be taken as evidence for a tightly regulated system that evolved because of the importance of estrogen for bone. However, since the skeletal effects of estrogen deficiency do not appear until late in life, when they do not offer a reproductive disadvantage, it may be misleading to conclude that this complex system evolved to protect the skeleton. None the less, the local factors could offer useful targets for the prevention and treatment of osteoporosis.

Acknowledgements

The technical assistance of Shirley Foster is gratefully acknowledged. Studies from our laboratory were supported by National Institute of Health research grant AR 11262. Anti-estrogen ICI 164,384 was generously provided by Dr A. E. Wakeling, ICI Pharmaceuticals.

J. L. Sanders was supported by Predoctoral Fellowship DAMD 17-44-4145 from the Department of Defense Breast Cancer Research Program.

References

1. Komm, B. S., Terpening, C. M., Benz, D. J., Graeme, K. A., Gallegos, A., Korc, M., Greene, G. L., O'Malley, B. W. and Haussler, M. R. (1988). Estrogen binding, receptor mRNA, and biologic response in osteoblast-like osteosarcoma cells. *Science*, **241**, 81–4

2. Eriksen, E. F., Colvard, D. S., Berg, N. J., Graham, M. L., Mann, K. G., Spelsberg, T. C. and Riggs, B. L. (1988). Evidence of estrogen receptors in normal human osteoblast-like cells. *Science*, **241**, 84–6

3. Etienne, M. C., Fischel, J. L., Milano, G., Formento, P., Formento, J. L., Francoual, M., Freney, M. and Namer, M. (1990). Steroid receptors in human osteoblast-like cells. *Eur. J. Cancer*, **26**, 807–10

4. Masuyama, A., Ouchi, Y., Sato, F., Hosoi, T., Nakamura, T. and Orimo, H. (1992). Characteristics of steroid hormone receptors in cultured MC3T3-E1 osteoblastic cells and effect of steroid hormones on cell proliferation. *Calcif. Tissue Int.*, **51**, 376–81

5. Davis, V. L., Couse, J. F., Gray, T. K. and Korach, K. S. (1994). Correlation between low levels of estrogen receptors and estrogen responsiveness in two rat osteoblast-like cell lines. *J. Bone Min. Res.*, **9**, 983–91

6. Grandien, K., Backdahl, M., Ljunggren, O., Gustafsson, J. A. and Berkenstam, A. (1995). Estrogen target tissue determines alternative promoter utilization of the human estrogen receptor gene in osteoblasts and tumor cell lines. *Endocrinology*, **136**, 2223–9

7. Ikegami, A., Inoue, S., Hosoi, T., Mizuno, Y., Nakamura, T., Ouchi, Y. and Orimo, H. (1993). Immunohistochemical detection and Northern blot analysis of estrogen receptor in osteoblastic cells. *J. Bone Min. Res.*, **8**, 1103–9

8. Ohashi, T., Kusuhara, S. and Ishida, K. (1991). Estrogen target cells during the early stage of medullary bone osteogenesis: immunohistochemical detection of estrogen receptors in osteogenic cells of estrogen-treated male Japanese quail. *Calcif. Tissue Int.*, **49**, 124–7

9. Zhang, R. W., Supowit, S. C., Xu, X., Li, H., Christensen, M. D., Lozano, R. and Simmons, D. J. (1995). Expression of selected osteogenic markers in the fibroblast-like cells of rat marrow stroma. *Calcif. Tissue Int.*, **56**, 283–91

10. Oursler, M. J., Osdoby, P., Pyfferoen, J., Riggs, B. L. and Spelsberg, T. C. (1991). Avian osteoclasts as estrogen target cells. *Proc. Natl. Acad. Sci. USA*, **88**, 6613–17

11. Oursler, M. J., Pederson, L., Fitzpatrick, L., Riggs, B. L. and Spelsberg, T. (1994). Human giant cell tumors of the bone (osteoclastomas) are estrogen target cells. *Proc. Natl. Acad. Sci. USA*, **91**, 5227–31

12. Pensler, J. M., Radosevich, J. A., Higbee, R. and Langman, C. B. (1990). Osteoclasts isolated from membranous bone in children exhibit nuclear estrogen and progesterone receptors. *J. Bone Min. Res.*, **5**, 797–802

13. Westerlind, K. C., Sarkar, G., Bolander, M. E. and Turner, R. T. (1995). Estrogen receptor mRNA is expressed *in vivo* in rat calvarial periosteum. *Steroids*, **60**, 484–7

14. Fiorelli, G., Gori, F., Petilli, M., Tanini, A., Benvenuti, S., Serio, M., Bernabei, P. and Brandi, M. L. (1995). Functional estrogen receptors in a human preosteoclastic cell line. *Proc. Natl. Acad. Sci. USA*, **92**, 2672–6

15. Braidman, I. P., Davenport, L. K., Carter, D. H., Selby, P. L., Mawer, E. B. and Freemont, A. J. (1995). Preliminary *in situ* identification of estrogen target cells in bone. *J. Bone Min. Res.*, **10**, 74–80

16. Brandi, M. L., Crescioli, C., Tanini, A., Frediani, U., Agnusdei, D. and Gennari, C. (1993). Bone endothelial cells as estrogen targets. *Calcif. Tissue Int.*, **53**, 312–17

17. Ernst, M., Heath, J. K. and Rodan, G. A. (1989). Estradiol effects on proliferation, messenger ribonucleic acid for collagen and insulin-like growth factor-1, and parathyroid hormone-stimulated adenylate cyclase activity in osteoblastic cells from calvariae and long bones. *Endocrinology*, **125**, 825–33

18. Gray, T. K., Flynn, R. C., Gray, K. M. and Nabell, L. M. (1987). 17β-Estradiol acts directly on the clonal osteoblastic cell line UMR106. *Proc. Natl. Acad. Sci. USA*, **84**, 6267–71

19. Keeting, P. E., Scott, R. E., Colvard, D. S., Han, I. K., Spelsberg, T. C. and Riggs, B. L. (1991). Lack of a direct effect of estrogen on proliferation and differentiation of normal human osteoblast-like cells. *J. Bone Min. Res.*, **6**, 297–304

20. Kremer, M., Judd, J., Rifkin, B., Auszmann, J. and Oursler, M. J. (1995). Estrogen modulation of osteoclast lysosomal enzyme secretion. *J. Cell. Biochem.*, **57**, 271–9

21. Arnett, T. R., Lindsay, R., Kilb, J. M., Moonga, B. S., Spowage, M. and Dempster, D. W. (1996). Selective toxic effects of tamoxifen on osteoclasts: comparison with the effects of oestrogen. *J. Endocrinol.*, **149**, 503–8

22. Pilbeam, C. C., Klein-Nulend, J. and Raisz, L. G. (1989). Inhibition by 17β-estradiol of PTH stimulated resorption and prostaglandin production in cultured neonatal mouse calvariae. *Biochem. Biophys. Res. Commun.*, **163**, 1319–24

23. Feyen, J. H. M. and Raisz, L. G. (1987). Prostaglandin production by calvariae from sham operated and oophorectomized rats: effect of 17β-estradiol *in vivo*. *Endocrinology*, **121**, 819–21

24. Kawaguchi, H., Pilbeam, C. C., Vargas, S. J., Morse, E. E., Lorenzo, J. A. and Raisz, L. G. (1995). Ovariectomy enhances and estrogen replacement inhibits the activity of bone marrow factors that stimulate prostaglandin production in cultured mouse calvariae. *J. Clin. Invest.*, **96**, 539–48

25. Miyaura, C., Kusano, K., Masuzawa, T., Chaki, O., Onoe, Y., Aoyagi, M., Sasaki, T., Tamura, T., Koishihara, Y., Ohsugi, Y. and Suda, T. (1995). Endogenous bone-resorbing factors in estrogen deficiency: co-operative effects of IL-1 and IL-6. *J. Bone Min. Res.*, **10**, 1365–73

26. Pacifici, R., Rifas, L., McCracken, R., Vered, I., McMurtry, C., Avioli, L. V. and Peck, W. A. (1989). Ovarian steroid treatment blocks a postmenopausal increase in blood monocyte interleukin 1 release. *Proc. Natl. Acad. Sci. USA*, **86**, 2398–402

27. Pacifici, R., Brown, C., Puscheck, E., Friedrich, E., Slatopolsky, E., Maggio, D., McCracken, R. and Avioli, L.V. (1991). Effect of surgical menopause and estrogen replacement on cytokine release from human blood mononuclear cells. *Proc. Natl. Acad. Sci. USA*, **88**, 5134–8

28. Kimble, R. B., Vannice, J. L., Bloedow, D. C., Thompson, R. C., Hopfer, W., Kung, V. T., Brownfield, C. and Pacifici, R. (1994). Interleukin-1 receptor antagonist decreases bone loss and bone resorption in ovariectomized rats. *J. Clin. Invest.*, **93**, 1959–67

29. Kimble, R. B., Matayoshi, A. B., Vannice, J. L., Kung, V. T., Williams, C. and Pacifici, R. (1995). Simultaneous block of interleukin-1 and tumor necrosis factor is required to completely prevent bone loss in the early postovariectomy period. *Endocrinology*, **136**, 3054–61

30. Pivirotto, L. A., Cissel, D. S. and Keeting, P. E. (1995). Sex hormones mediate interleukin-1β production by human osteoblastic HOBIT cells. *Mol. Cell. Endocrinol.*, **111**, 67–74

31. Lowik, C. W. G. M., van der Pluijm, G., Bloys, H., Hoekman, K., Bijvoet, O. L. M., Aarden, L. A. and Papapoulos, S. E. (1989). Parathyroid hormone (PTH) and PTH-like protein (Plp) stimulate interleukin-6 production by osteogenic cells: a possible role of interleukin-6 in osteoclastogenesis. *Biochem. Biophys. Res. Commun.*, **162**, 1546–52

32. Ishimi, Y., Miyaura, C., Jin, C. H., Akatsu, T., Abe, E. and Nakamura, Y. (1990). IL-6 is produced by osteoblasts and induces bone resorption. *J. Immunol.*, **145**, 2478–82

33. Kurihara, N. C., Civin, C. and Roodman, G. D. (1991). Osteotropic factor responsiveness of highly purified populations of early and late precursors for human multinucleated cells expressing the osteoclast phenotype. *J. Bone Min. Res.*, **6**, 257–61

34. Gowen, M. and Mundy, G. R. (1986). Actions of interleukin-1, interleukin-2 and interferon-γ on bone resorption *in vitro*. *J. Immunol.*, **136**, 2478–82

35. Bertolini, D., Nedwin, G., Brigman, T., Smith, D. and Mundy, G. (1986). Stimulation of bone resorption and inhibition of bone formation *in vitro* by human tumor necrosis factors. *Nature (London)*, **319**, 516–18

36. Girasole, G., Jilka, R. L., Passeri, G., Boswell, C., Boder, G., Williams, D. C. and Manolagas, S. C. (1992). 17β-Estradiol inhibits interleukin-6 production by bone marrow-derived stromal cells and osteoblasts *in vitro*: a potential mechanism for the antiosteoporotic effect of estrogens. *J. Clin. Invest.*, **89**, 883–91

37. Kassem, M., Harris, S. A., Spelsberg, T. C. and Riggs, B. L. (1996). Estrogen inhibits interleukin-6 production and gene expression in a human osteoblastic cell line with high levels of estrogen receptors. *J. Bone Min. Res.*, **11**, 193–9

38. Passeri, G., Girasole, G., Jilka, R. L. and Manolagas, S. C. (1993). Increased interleukin-6 production by murine bone marrow and bone cells after estrogen withdrawal. *Endocrinology*, **133**, 822–8

39. Jilka, R. L., Hangoc, G., Girasole, G., Passeri, G., Williams, D. C., Abrams, J. S., Boyce, B., Broxmeyer, H. and Manolagas, S. C. (1992). Increased osteoclast development after estrogen loss: mediation by interleukin-6. *Science*, **257**, 88–91

40. Poli, V., Balena, R., Fattori, E., Markatos, A., Yamamoto, M., Tanaka, H., Ciliberto, G., Rodan, G. A. and Costantini, F. (1994). Interleukin-6 deficient mice are protected from bone loss caused by estrogen depletion. *EMBO J.*, **13**, 1189–96

41. Lakatos, P., Foldes, J., Horvath, C., Kiss, L., Tatrai, A., Takacs, I., Tarjan, G. and Stern, P. H. (1997). Serum IL-6 and bone metabolism in patients with thyroid function disorders. *J. Clin. Endocrinol. Metab.*, **82**, 78–81

42. Tarjan, G. and Stern, P. H. (1995). Triiodothyronine potentiates the stimulatory effect of interleukin-1β on bone resorption and medium interleukin-6 content in fetal rat limb bone cultures. *J. Bone Min. Res.*, **10**, 1321–6

43. Sanders, J. L., Tarjan, G., Strieleman, P. J. and Stern, P. H. (1995). Protein kinase C mediates interleukin-6 production by parathyroid hormone in UMR-106 cells. *J. Bone Min. Res.*, **10** (Suppl. 1), S385

44. Joyce, M. E., Roberts, A. B., Sporn, M. B. and Bolander, M. E. (1990). Transforming growth factor-β and the initiation of chondrogenesis and osteogenesis in the rat femur. *J. Cell Biol.*, **110**, 2195–207

45. Pfeilschifter, J., Seyedin, S. M. and Mundy, G. R. (1988). Transforming growth factor beta inhibits bone resorption in fetal rat long bone cultures. *J. Clin. Invest.*, **82**, 680–5

46. Finkelman, R. D., Bell, N. H., Strong, D. D., Demers, L. M. and Baylink, D. J. (1992). Ovariectomy selectively reduces the concentration of transforming growth factor β in rat bone: implications for estrogen deficiency-associated bone loss. *Proc. Natl. Acad. Sci. USA*, **89**, 12190–3

47. Oursler, M. J. (1994). Osteoclast synthesis and secretion and activation of latent transforming growth factor β. *J. Bone Min. Res.*, **9**, 443–52

48. Robinson, J. A., Riggs, B. L., Spelsberg, T. C. and Oursler, M. J. (1996). Osteoclasts and transforming growth factor-β: estrogen-mediated isoform-specific regulation of production. *Endocrinology*, **137**, 615–21

49. Huo, B., Dossing, D. A., and DiMuzio, M. T. (1995). Generation and characterization of a human osteosarcoma cell line stably transfected with the human estrogen receptor gene. *J. Bone Min. Res.*, **10**, 769–81

50. Yang, N. N., Bryant, H. U., Hardikar, S., Sato, M., Galvin, R. J. S., Glasebrook, A. L. and Termine, J. D. (1996). Estrogen and raloxifene stimulate transforming growth factor-β3 gene expression in rat bone: a potential mechanism for estrogen- or raloxifene-mediated bone maintenance. *Endocrinology*, **137**, 2075–84

51. Sanders, J. L. and Stern, P. H. (1996). 17β-Estradiol and tamoxifen modulate protein kinase C isozyme expression in UMR-106 osteoblastic cells. *Pharmacologist*, in press

52. Williams, J. P., Blair, H. C., McKenna, M. A., Jordan, S. E. and McDonald, J. M. (1996). Regulation of avian osteoclastic H+-ATPase and bone resorption by tamoxifen and calmodulin antagonists. Effects independent of steroid receptors. *J. Biol. Chem.*, **271**, 12488–95

53. Stewart, P. J. and Stern, P. H. (1986). Effects of the antiestrogens tamoxifen and clomiphene on bone resorption *in vitro*. *Endocrinology*, **118**, 125–31

54. Gibson, M. K., Nemmers, L. A., Beckman, W. C., Davis, V. L., Curtis, S. W. and Korach, K. S. (1991). The mechanism of ICI 164,384 antiestrogenicity involves rapid loss of estrogen receptor in uterine tissue. *Endocrinology*, **129**, 2000–10

Bone structure and function in relation to aging and the menopause 19

Li. Mosekilde and J. S. Thomsen

Introduction

In Europe, vertebral fracture incidence has increased three- to four-fold for women and more than four-fold for men during the last 30 years[1]. In Scandinavia the other fragility fracture, the femoral neck fracture, has shown a similar pattern, with a two- to three-fold increase in incidence for both men and women. The data are age-adjusted and therefore highlight the fact that there is a decrease in bone mass or bone quality from generation to generation[2]. Recently it has been shown that the incidence of femoral neck fractures in Europe varies more between countries than between sexes, which suggests important genetic or environmental factors in the causation of hip fracture[3]. To arrest or reverse the increases in osteoporotic fractures, effective general preventive regimens must be established. However, as the described changes in the incidence of vertebral and femoral neck fracture cannot be related to the menopause alone, other etiological factors must be investigated. In order to do this, basic knowledge of normal age-related changes in bone structure and function is crucial. Also, a description of the work pattern of the remodeling process in the load-bearing trabecular network is essential for understanding the age-related changes, and for choosing the most appropriate therapeutic and preventive regimens.

In the following sections, normal age-related and menopause-related changes in human vertebral bodies will be described. As no data exist concerning menopause-related changes in vertebral trabecular bone structure, these changes have been deduced by applying a computer simulation model, based on dynamic data from human iliac crest bone biopsies[4], to trabecular thicknesses from the human vertebral network. In the following text, particular attention has been paid to the vertebral bodies, as vertebral fractures are the foremost and also the most common osteoporotic fractures.

Human bone – vertebrae

Peak bone mass and strength

The vertebral body is the load-bearing part of the vertebra. When peak bone mass has been attained (at the age of 25–30 years), the vertebral body consists of a central trabecular network demarcated by a bony shell approximately 400–500 µm thick. The central trabecular network is isotropic in the horizontal plane but anisotropic in all other directions (Figure 1). This special architecture provides great strength with minimum bone mass. The trabecular bone volume in relation to total tissue volume is 15–20% and ash-density 0.200–0.250 g/cm³. In young individuals the load-bearing capacity of a lumbar vertebral body is 1000 kg or more[5] (Table 1).

Peak bone mass is 25–30% higher in men than in women, mainly because the cross-sectional area is greater in men than in women, but the peak bone density is the same. Peak bone mass is determined by genetic factors and also by physical activity (loading) during childhood and adulthood[6].

Table 1 *In vitro* data concerning human vertebral body characteristics in relation to age

	Age (years)		
	20–40	70–80	Osteoporotic
Trabecular bone volume (%)	15–20	8–12	4–8
Ash-density (g/cm³)	0.200–0.250	0.100–0.150	0.060–0.090
Cortical thickness (μm)	400–500	200–300	120–150
Load-bearing capacity (kg)	1000–1200	150–250	60–150
Load-bearing capacity of cortical rim (% of total)	25–30	70–80	80–90

Normal age-related changes

With age, internal trabecular bone mass and architecture change due to a negative balance within the remodeling process (1–3 μm is lost during completion of each process). There is, therefore, a continuous loss of bone mass from the age of 25–30 years. These changes start in the center of the vertebral body (the vascular region) and progress both upwards and downwards from there. Furthermore, there is also an age-related thinning of the endplates and of the 'cortical' shell due to endosteal bone resorption. Concomitantly, cross-sectional area will change, partly due to periosteal bone formation (modeling)[5] and partly due to osteophyte formation[7]. This changes the strong vertebral body of a young individual to one with a load-bearing capacity of only 150–250 kg in an elderly individual[5] (Table 1). These are all normal, age-related changes but will, if they become pronounced, cause fragility fractures of the vertebral bodies (Figure 2).

Structural determinants of vertebral strength and mechanisms for loss of strength

The strength of the vertebral body is determined by several key factors, the most important being: (1) vertebral body cross-sectional area; (2) thickness of the 'cortical rim'; (3) thickness of the endplates; and (4) density, combined with the architecture of the central trabecular network. The exact roles of each of these factors have never been determined. This is partly because of the complexity of the structure and partly because each factor changes independently with age, menopause, immobilization, metabolic bone diseases and other conditions such as disc degeneration or osteophyte formation.

Cross-sectional area The cross-sectional area of the vertebral body is directly correlated with the load-bearing capacity of the vertebral body both during pure compression and during bending loads, which are the two dominating forces on the vertebral body during normal, daily activity[8,9]. The cross-sectional area of the vertebral bodies is 20–30% greater in young men than in women of corresponding ages[5]. Vigorous exercise exerts a direct effect on the vertebral body cross-sectional area[10], an effect that might be caused by direct periosteal stimulation, as shown by Pead and colleagues[11]. The 20–30% greater cross-sectional area of the male vertebral bodies (being genetic, hormonal or mechanically induced) will itself result in a 20–30% higher load-bearing capacity than that seen in female vertebral bodies. However, in many *in vivo* bone density measurements, this important size factor has been neglected.

The cross-sectional area of vertebral bodies seems to increase with age in men but not in women[5]. This age-related increase, seen solely in male vertebral bodies, can partly offset the concomitant decline in material properties (that is seen in both sexes), and it is therefore an important compensatory mechanism for the age-related decline in bone density. Also, at other skeletal sites, for example the long bones,

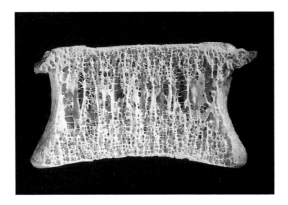

Figure 1 Photograph of vertebral body from young individual; central trabecular network is dense, with 'perfect' architecture

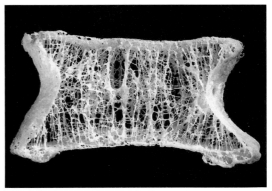

Figure 2 Photograph of vertebral body from elderly individual; trabecular bone density has decreased, and many perforations are seen

an age-related increase in cross-sectional area has been demonstrated for men, but not for women, and a direct stimulatory effect of loading on periosteal expansion has been suggested[12,13].

Thickness of the cortical shell The thickness of the cortical shell and the importance of this for the load-bearing capacity of the vertebral body is a matter of debate. The normally held view has been that the vertebral body consists of approximately 70% trabecular bone and 30% cortical bone[14]. However, Nottestad and co-workers[15] showed the opposite: 30–40% trabecular bone and 60–70% cortical bone. Both viewpoints could be correct, as with age the trabecular bone mass in the central part of the vertebral body declines much faster than cortical bone[16]. Therefore, a shift in trabecular/cortical bone mass ratio with age should be expected. While the central trabecular bone mass dominates in vertebral bodies in younger individuals, cortical bone seems to dominate in the very old. The relative importance of the cortical shell therefore increases with age – also in biomechanical terms[17,18]. In young individuals, the load-bearing capacity of the cortical rim is only 20–25 % of the total capacity of the vertebral body. With age, the cortical ring becomes thinner in both men and women, and at the age of 70–80 years has a thickness of only

200–300 μm. Despite the thinness of the cortical shell in elderly individuals, it might at this age contribute some 70–80% of the load-bearing capacity of the vertebral body, as the trabecular network has degraded (Table 1).

Thinning of the cortical shell is caused by endosteal resorption in both men and women, but in men there is also a significant modeling[5,18,19] of the cortical shell caused by slow periosteal apposition, as mentioned above. The thickness of the cortical ring has been directly measured in only a very few human studies[20]. However, even in young persons the cortical ring is very thin, and merely consists of condensed trabecular bone rather than real cortical bone with Haversian systems.

Endplates The endplates have a thickness of 200–400 μm. They are thin, perforated structures (perforated by vessels entering the fibrocartilage of the discs from the vertebral bodies). The endplates too can be described as condensed trabecular bone. Direct measurements of age-related changes have never been performed. No data exist concerning gender-related differences. On their external side the endplates have fibrocartilaginous tissue and discs, but on the internal face they are supported directly by the trabecular network. In young individuals the discs can absorb and distribute stresses and

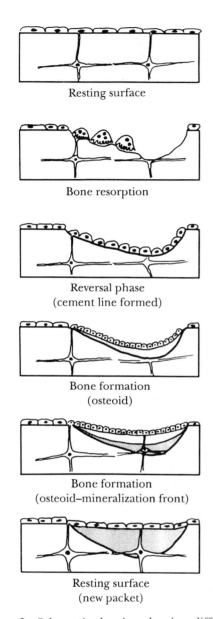

Resting surface

Bone resorption

Reversal phase
(cement line formed)

Bone formation
(osteoid)

Bone formation
(osteoid–mineralization front)

Resting surface
(new packet)

Figure 3 Schematic drawing showing different phases of bone remodeling process and negative balance on completion

depressions or biconcave vertebrae. This is further facilitated in elderly individuals, where the endplate lacks support because of little remaining trabecular connectivity. It also pinpoints that disc status (intact/some degeneration) is a very important factor concerning prevalent as well as incident vertebral deformities.

Vertebral trabecular network The vertebral trabecular network in younger individuals is dense and well connected. The volumetric density of the whole trabecular network is identical for young men and young women: the ash-density is approximately 0.2 g/cm³ and the trabecular bone volume 15–20%[22] (Table 1).

Hemopoietic marrow fills the space between the trabeculae, and has an internal hydraulic effect[23]. The marrow remains hemopoietic throughout life, although with age there is a slight increase in fat cells. Several of the bone cells involved in the remodeling process are directly recruited from the hemopoietic bone marrow or from the abundant sinusoidal capillaries in the marrow. Therefore, the close connection between red marrow and bone tissue in the vertebral bodies seems to be responsible for the high turnover (remodeling) at this site. At other skeletal sites where there has been a shift from hemopoietic to fat marrow in young adulthood (e.g. the diaphyses of the long bones), the bone turnover (remodeling activity) is much lower.

The remodeling process, having a slightly negative balance of 1–3 μm (Figure 3), primarily causes thinning of the horizontal struts in the load-bearing vertebral trabecular network (Figure 4), and secondarily, osteoclastic perforations. As resorption lacunae normally reach a depth of 45–50 μm[24], one resorption cavity covering more than half the circumference of a thin trabecula, or two resorption cavities, one on each side of a trabecular structure, would easily perforate a 90–110 μm thick horizontal trabecula[5,25] (Figure 5).

The decline in trabecular bone mass, the decline in trabecular thickness and the perforations in the network are all caused by

strains applied to the vertebrae[21], but with age the intervertebral discs lose elasticity and height, and thereby their capacity to absorb and distribute loads[21]. Even trivial forces therefore tend to reach extremely high values at small, localized areas, and can thereby cause endplate

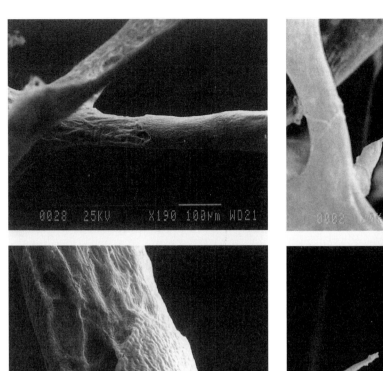

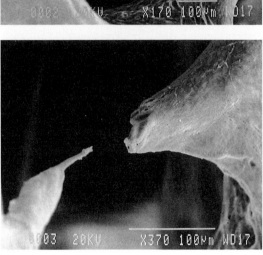

Figure 4 SEM micrographs demonstrating work-pattern of remodeling process on horizontal strut in network; such a remodeling process covering more than half of thin trabecula or a process on each side of trabecula would be able to cause perforation

Figure 5 SEM micrographs with focus on perforated trabecular strut; osteoclastic footprints are seen at end of horizontal strut

the remodeling process, and are therefore normal, age-related changes. The described pattern with selective thinning and perforation of horizontal struts, is seen in both men and women during normal aging[22,26].

Around the menopause the activation frequency increases[27], and at the same time resorption depth might increase[24]. These two factors accelerate the age-related changes and increase the number of trabecular perforations in the network[4]. Furthermore, once trabecular structures have been perforated they are no longer loaded, and they will therefore be resorbed rapidly by osteoclasts[25] (Figure 6).

The biomechanical consequences of the disruption of the load-bearing vertebral network are far-reaching. As the strength of a trabecular structure is proportional to its radius squared, thinning of the vertical structures has a tremendous influence on their strength. The situation is similar concerning the length between supporting, horizontal struts: the compressive strength of the network is proportional to the square of the distance between the supporting struts[28].

It should be recognized that not only is bone strength highly dependent on bone architecture and on connectivity, but also that loss of

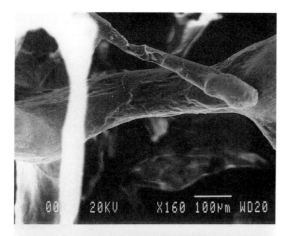

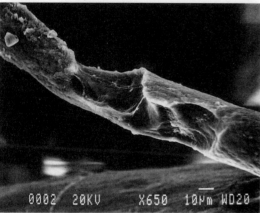

Figure 6 SEM micrographs of perforated and unloaded horizontal strut in vertebral trabecular network; structure is being removed by osteoclastic resorption

connectivity in the load-bearing network seems irreversible. Remodeling sites on disconnected, unloaded structures show no sign of bone formation (uncoupling)[25]. Strain or stress applied to bone seems essential to enable osteoblasts to form new bone on existing surfaces[29-31]. The osteoblasts will therefore be unable to refill the gaps in the network under normal circumstances. Most therapeutic regimens, being primarily antiresorptive, cannot facilitate this process either – but whether powerful anabolic agents like parathyroid hormone will be able to do so still remains unresolved.

Sex-related differences

Cross-sectional studies on human autopsy cases have clearly shown that age itself is the major determinant of vertebral bone mass, strength and structure[5] (Figure 7). When sex-related differences were investigated, three different factors were disclosed:

(1) Men at the age of 20–30 years had a higher peak bone mass and strength than women (20–30% higher).

(2) Men showed an age-related compensatory increase in bone size (cross-sectional area of the vertebral bodies) that could not be found in women. Furthermore, women with osteoporosis have been shown in clinical studies to have very small vertebral bodies and thereby low load-bearing capacity[32].

(3) After the age of 50 years (menopause), women showed a higher tendency than men to disconnection of the horizontal trabecular struts. This led to a more pronounced deterioration of the network in women, and thereby to an increased loss of strength.

However, to date very little attention has been paid to the first two points mentioned above: peak bone mass and changes in cross-sectional area. These are two factors closely related to physical activity (loading). On the other hand, the specific menopause-related changes have attracted almost all the attention and research effort.

Menopause

Research effort has been focused on measuring changes in bone mass (dual energy X-ray absorptiometry (DEXA), quantitative computed tomography (QCT)) or measuring changes in biochemical markers in relation to the menopause. Of the menopause-related studies, only very few have looked at changes in bone structure in relation to estrogen depletion (or estrogen treatment). However, recently two

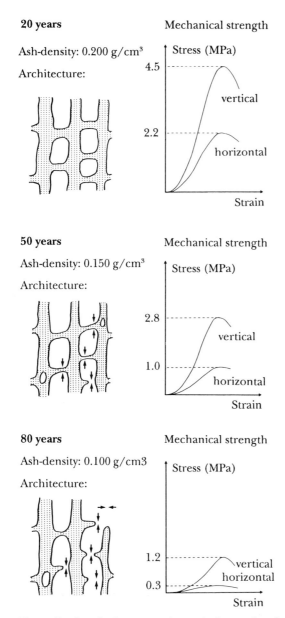

Figure 7 Graphs demonstrating typical age-related changes in vertebral trabecular network: density, architecture and biomechanical competence

structural changes in relation to estrogen therapy. The two studies were both longitudinal and thereby very valuable. The lack of detected changes could be caused by: (1) the material (small sample size, heterogeneity of individuals); (2) the sample site (the iliac crest, which is not load-bearing and has a very different structure to the vertebral bodies); or (3) the time span of the studies (2 years, which is possibly too short).

However, another way of analyzing the effect of the menopause on bone structure is the use of computer simulation models. This avenue will be briefly described in the following section.

Computer simulation models concerning menopause-related changes in bone mass and structure

A 'non-invasive', quick method for elucidating the importance of the architecture and the regularity of a load-bearing trabecular network is by use of computer models for simulation of different, normally-occurring events[35,36]. Realistic models based on human, biological material might also provide some insight into the capability of therapeutic agents to delay disruption of the network or eventually to restore connectivity. Such a model of bone dynamics has recently been developed[4,37].

There are advantages in using computer models based upon human data: (1) the method is 'non-invasive'; (2) the long-term effects of menopause-related changes in remodeling activity can be assessed very easily; (3) the effect of changes can be assessed on different types of trabecular network; and (4) the effect of changes in various remodeling parameters can be assessed independently.

The computer simulation model created by Thomsen and colleagues was based on structural data from human vertebral bodies and dynamic histomorphometry data from human iliac crest bone biopsies[4]. In the computer model, the menopause was simulated in accordance with two different theories, either: (1) the menopause causes an increase in activation frequency alone, or (2) the

such studies have been published[33,34]. Very importantly, both these studies failed to show any changes in bone structure (assessed by node–strut analysis, trabecular bone pattern factor, or marrow space star volume) around the menopause. They also failed to show any

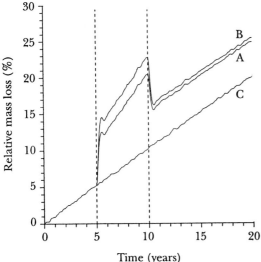

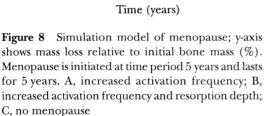

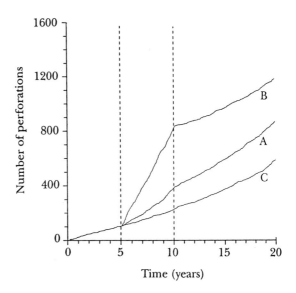

Figure 8 Simulation model of menopause; y-axis shows mass loss relative to initial bone mass (%). Menopause is initiated at time period 5 years and lasts for 5 years. A, increased activation frequency; B, increased activation frequency and resorption depth; C, no menopause

Figure 9 Simulation of menopause; y-axis shows number of perforations. Menopause is initiated at time period 5 years and lasts for 5 years. A, increased activation frequency; B, increased activation frequency and resorption depth; C, no menopause

menopause causes an increase in activation frequency accompanied by an increase in resorption depth. The endpoints of the model were bone mass loss, trabecular thinning and trabecular perforations.

The model clearly showed that during the menopause there is an increased mass loss relative to the initial mass (Figure 8), an increased thinning of trabecular structures and an increase in the number of perforations. However, most of the changes in bone mass and trabecular thickness are reversible and are caused by increased remodeling space. A small fraction of the loss of bone mass is, though, irreversible and is due to the increased number of perforations (Figure 9). In accordance with the second theory – that both activation frequency and resorption depth are increased during the menopause[34] – there is a more pronounced increase in number of perforations and therefore a slightly more pronounced irreversible loss of bone mass. The described changes appear large when presented on a very narrow y-axis (Figure 10a), but they are much

less 'dramatic' when a larger scale is used (Figure 10b). Precisely the same phenomenon is true in clinical assessments of changes in bone mass during the menopause. The 'seriousness' of the changes depends on the y-axis scale used!

Although the simulation model and clinical studies could be interpreted as showing a 20% bone loss during the 5 years of menopause, this is not actually the case as some of the bone mass loss is reversible, and some of it is related to the aging process *per se* and not to estrogen depletion. Furthermore, it is clear from inspecting Figure 10 that when the simulations with the menopause are compared with simulation without the menopause, the loss of trabecular thickness during menopause roughly corresponds to a 'normal' aging over a period of 5 years. It should still be kept in mind that the age-related bone loss is 40–50% when considering trabecular bone – and that this is seen in both men and women!

In summary, the simulation model has clearly shown the increased bone loss during the menopause (reversible and irreversible) and

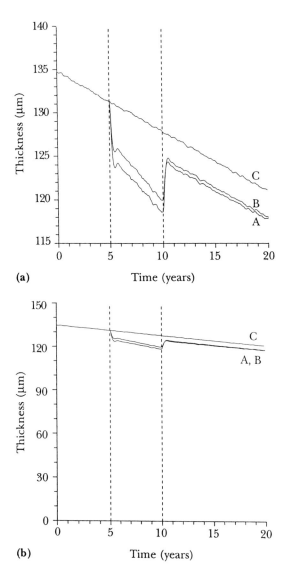

(a)

(b)

Figure 10 Simulation of menopause; (a) y-axis is horizontal trabecular thickness (μm), (b) shows the same as (a) but a larger scale is used. Menopause is initiated at time period 5 years and last for 5 years. A, increased activation frequency; B, increased activation frequency and resorption depth; C, no menopause

also that an increased resorption depth, as indicated by the study of Eriksen and colleagues[34], causes a further increase in bone loss. However, if the menopausal changes are followed for only a few years, they become heavily overestimated in relation to the age-related bone loss.

Conclusions

Vertebral bone strength is determined by several factors: cortical thickness, bone size, trabecular bone density and architecture. All these factors change with age as a result of the remodeling process. When the changes become pronounced, osteoporotic fractures occur. There is a different aging pattern for men and women: men achieve a higher peak bone mass than women (mainly because of a larger cross-sectional area of their bones), they have no accelerated bone loss in middle age, and they seem to be able to compensate for their loss of bone material strength by increasing their vertebral cross-sectional area with age.

The general pattern though for both men and women, is that of an extreme (70–80%) decline in vertebral bone strength during normal aging. The accompanying decline in bone density is much less pronounced (35–45%), and especially in men may be partly offset by osteophyte formation.

Focusing very closely on the menopause, the changes in bone mass and turnover seem very impressive. However, in a larger perspective they are minor, and the age-related changes become much more important, and half of the mass loss around the menopause is reversed without any intervention.

Only very recently has effort been devoted to studying the age-related changes as such, and only very recently has it been acknowledged that men have a high incidence of fragility fractures and that this incidence is increasing at a faster rate than it is in women.

Loading plays an important role in achieving peak bone mass, in the maintenance of trabecular architecture (through the remodeling process), and in the orientation of the trabeculae and the periosteal apposition (through the modeling process). Loading is therefore important throughout life for the maintenance of bone mass and strength during normal aging – for women as for men.

134

It is therefore very promising that the causes of osteoporotic fractures and of the increase in incidence of fragility fractures are now being investigated intensively – not only with regard to the menopause but also with regard to genetic and environmental factors.

References

1. Bengnér, U., Johnell, O. and Redlund-Johnell, I. (1988). Changes in incidence and prevalence of vertebral fractures during 30 years. *Calcif. Tissue Int.*, **42**, 293–6
2. Obrant, K. J., Bengnér, U., Johnell, O., Nilsson, B. E. and Sernbo, I. (1989). Increasing age-adjusted risk of fragility fractures: a sign of increasing osteoporosis in successive generations? *Calcif. Tissue Int.*, **44**, 157–67
3. Johnell, O., Gullberg, B., Allander, E. and Kanis, J. A. (1992). The apparent incidence of hip fracture in Europe: a study of national register sources. *Osteoporosis Int.*, **2**, 298–302
4. Thomsen, J. S., Mosekilde, L., Boyce, R. W. and Mosekilde, E. (1994). Stochastic simulation of vertebral trabecular bone remodeling. *Bone*, **15**, 655–66
5. Mosekilde L. (1993). Normal age-related changes in bone mass, structure and strength – consequences of the remodeling process. *Dan. Med. Bull.*, **1**, 65–84
6. Gilsanz, V., Gibbens, D. T., Carlson, M., Boechat, M. I., Cann, C. E. and Schulz, E. E. (1988). Peak trabecular vertebral density: a comparison of adolescent and adult females. *Calcif. Tissue Int.*, **43**, 260–2
7. Schmorl, G. and Junghanns, H. (1971). Development, growth, anatomy and function of the spine. In Besemann, E. F. (ed.) *The Human Spine in Health and Disease II*, pp. 6–9. (New York and London: Grune and Stratton)
8. Biggemann, M., Hilweg, D. and Brinckmann, P. (1988). Prediction of the compressive strength of vertebral bodies of the lumbar spine by quantitative computed tomography. *Skeletal Radiol.*, **17**, 264–9
9. Brinkmann, P., Biggemann, M. and Hilweg, D. (1989). Prediction of the compressive strength of human lumbar vertebrae. *Spine*, **14**, 606–10
10. Block, J. E., Genant, H. K. and Black, D. (1986). Greater vertebral bone mineral mass in exercising young men. *West. J. Med.*, **145**, 39–42
11. Pead, M. J., Skerry, T. M. and Lanyon, L. E. (1988). Direct transformation from quiescence to bone formation in the adult periosteum following a single brief period of bone loading. *J. Bone Min. Res.*, **3**, 647–56
12. Ruff, C. B. and Hayes, W. C. (1983). Cross-sectional geometry of Pecos Pueblo femora and tibiae – a biomechanical investigation: II. Sex, age and side differences. *Am. J. Phys. Anthropol.*, **60**, 383–400
13. Ruff, C. B. and Hayes, W. C. (1988). Sex differences in age-related remodeling of the femur and tibia. *J. Orthop. Res.*, **6**, 886–96
14. Eastell, R., Mosekilde, L., Hodgson, S. F. and Riggs, B. L. (1990). Proportion of human vertebral body bone that is cancellous. *J. Bone Min. Res.*, **5**, 1237–41
15. Nottestad, S. Y., Baumel, J. J., Kimmel, D. B., Recker, R. R. and Heaney, R. P. (1987). The properties of trabecular bone in human vertebrae. *J. Bone Min. Res.*, **2**, 221–9
16. Cann, C. E. (1988). Quantitative CT for determination of bone mineral density: a review. *Radiology*, **166**, 509–22
17. Rockoff, S. D., Sweet, E. and Bleustein, J. (1969). The relative contribution of trabecular and cortical bone to the strength of human lumbar vertebrae. *Calcif. Tissue Res.*, **3**, 163–75
18. Mosekilde, L. and Mosekilde, L. (1986). Normal vertebral body size and compressive strength: relations to age and to vertebral and iliac trabecular bone compressive strength. *Bone*, **7**, 207–12
19. Mosekilde, L. and Mosekilde, L., (1990). Sex differences in age-related changes in vertebral body size, density and biomechanical competence in normal individuals. *Bone*, **11**, 67–73
20. Vesterby, A., Mosekilde, L., Gundersen, H. J. G., Melsen, F., Mosekilde, L., Holme, K. and Sørensen, L. (1991). Biologically meaningful determinants of the *in vitro* strength of lumbar vertebra. *Bone*, **12**, 219–24
21. Hansson, T. and Roos, B. (1981). The relation between bone mineral content, experimental compression fractures, and disc degeneration in lumbar vertebrae. *Spine*, **6**, 147–53
22. Mosekilde, L., (1989). Sex differences in age-related loss of vertebral trabecular bone mass and structure – biomechanical consequences. *Bone*, **10**, 425–32
23. Kazarian, L. and Graves, G. A. (1977). Compressive strength characteristics of the human vertebral centrum. *Spine*, **2**, 1–14

24. Eriksen, E. F. (1986). Normal and pathological remodeling of human trabecular bone: three dimensional reconstruction of the remodeling sequence in normals and in metabolic bone disease. *Endocr. Rev.*, **7**, 379–408

25. Mosekilde, L. (1990). Consequences of the remodelling process for vertebral trabecular bone structure – a scanning electron microscopy study (uncoupling of unloaded structures). *Bone Miner.*, **10**, 13–35

26. Mosekilde, L. (1988). Age related changes in vertebral trabecular bone architecture – assessed by a new method. *Bone*, **9**, 247–50

27. Brockstedt, H., Kassem, M., Eriksen, E. F., Mosekilde, L. and Melsen, F. (1993). Age- and sex-related changes in iliac crest cortical bone mass and remodeling. *Bone*, **14**, 681–91

28. Mosekilde, L., Mosekilde, L. and Danielsen, C. C. (1987). Biomechanical competence of vertebral trabecular bone in relation to ash density and age in normal individuals. *Bone*, **8**, 79–85

29. Parfitt, A. M. (1984). Age-related structural changes in trabecular and cortical bone: cellular mechanisms and biomechanical consequences. *Calcif. Tissue Int.*, **36**, 37–45

30. Parfitt, A. M. (1987). Trabecular bone architecture in the pathogenesis and prevention of fracture. *Am. J. Med.*, **82**, 68–72

31. Parfitt, A. M. (1988). Bone remodeling: relationship to the amount and structure of bone, and the pathogenesis and prevention of

fractures. In Riggs, B. L. and Melton, L. J. III (eds.) *Osteoporosis: Etiology, Diagnosis and Management*, pp. 45–93. (New York: Raven Press)

32. Gilsanz, V., Loro, M. L., Roe, T. F., Sayre, J., Gilsanz, R. and Schulz, E. E. (1995). Vertebral size in elderly women with osteoporosis: mechanical implications and relationship to fractures. *J. Clin. Invest.*, **95**, 2332–7

33. Vedi, S., Croucher, P. I., Garrahan, N. J. and Compston, J. E. (1996). Effects of hormone replacement therapy on cancellous bone microstructure in postmenopausal women. *Bone*, **19**, 69–72

34. Eriksen, E. F., Landahl, B., Glerup, H., Vesterby, A., Rungby, J. and Kassem, M. (1996). Hormone replacement therapy (HRT) preserves bone balance by preventing osteoclastic hyperactivity in postmenopausal women: a randomized, prospective, histomorphometric study. *J. Bone. Miner. Res.*, S449, abstr.

35. Reeve, J. (1986). A stochastic analysis of iliac trabecular bone dynamics. *Clin. Orthop. Rel. Res.*, **213**, 264–78

36. Jensen, K. S., Mosekilde, L. and Mosekilde, L. (1990). A model of vertebral trabecular bone architecture and its mechanical properties. *Bone*, **11**, 417–23

37. Thomsen, J. S., Mosekilde, L. and Mosekilde, E. (1996). Factors influencing perforations and mass loss in the vertebral trabecular network – assessed by a computer simulation model. *Bone*, **19**, 505–11

Clinical aspects of estrogens and osteoporosis

20

E. F. Eriksen

Introduction

Hormone replacement therapy (HRT) has been the most widely used agent for treatment of and prophylaxis against osteoporosis over the past 25 years. This short review aims at summarizing current knowledge in this area.

Treatment regimens

Estrogen is still mainly given in oral formulations, but dermal patches are gaining increased recognition. In non-hysterectomized women progestogens have to be added to protect against endometrial cancer, while hysterectomized women can be treated with estrogen alone. Traditionally the United States has used estrogens (equinolones) derived from the urine of pregnant mares, while Europe has used synthetic estradiol preparations.

In recent years transdermal preparations have emerged that permit lower dosing of hormone, because these formulations bypass hepatic first-pass metabolism. Initially, only estradiol could be supplied transdermally, but recent formulations permit simultaneous administration of progestogens. Since the transdermal route of administration bypasses hepatic first-pass metabolism, changes in hepatic protein synthesis commonly associated with the oral route are avoided. Whether these changes are reflected in differences pertaining to side-effects remains to be established. Weissberger and colleagues[1] demonstrated that transdermal estrogen administration led to increases in circulating IGF-I levels and suppression of circulating levels of growth hormone (GH), while oral administration caused opposite changes in the two peptides. Although both peptides exert pronounced effects on skeletal remodeling, there is no evidence to date that the differences demonstrated are reflected in different skeletal responses to transdermal and oral estrogen/progestogen formulations. Stevenson and co-workers compared Premarin® and transdermal estrogen, and found similar increases in bone mass after 18 months of treatment[2], but long-term studies are lacking. Some studies indicate that especially female smokers lose the protective effect of oral estrogens[3], and might benefit more from the transdermal route of administration, but the evidence is still disputed[4].

Effects of hormone replacement therapy on bone mass

A vast number of studies have demonstrated similar increases in bone mass after 2-3 years of estrogen/progestogen treatment. The response seen in these studies is similar in both immediate postmenopausal and older women. Generally a 5–7% increase in bone mass occurs within 12–18 months, followed by a plateau[5–9]. The subsequent changes in bone mass have been controversial: some studies have described a decrease in bone mass, while others have described constant bone mass. Once estrogen treatment is stopped, bone loss ensues, but the rate of loss seems to be similar to that of untreated postmenopausal women[10].

The response to estrogen of areas rich in cortical bone differs from the response in areas of the skeleton rich in cancellous bone. The most pronounced increases in bone mass are seen in cancellous bone, while data obtained from areas rich in cortical bone, such as the forearm, just indicate preservation of bone mass (Figure 1)[11]. In a long-term study by Lindsay and Tohme where oophorectomized women were studied over a period of 10 years, the metacarpal index, which mainly reflects changes in cortical bone mass, also remained constant, while the values in controls decreased[8].

Recent data, however, suggest that a pronounced continuous increase in cancellous bone mass can be achieved with long-term HRT. Eiken and colleagues[12] recently presented data based on a randomized, prospective study of postmenopausal women treated with either cyclic or continuous combined estrogen/progestogen for 10 years. Estrogen-treated women exhibited 14.5% higher bone mass in the spine than controls. The most surprising finding was a continued increase in bone mass, even between years 5 and 8 of the study, suggesting slight anabolic properties of the treatment regimen. Bone mass in the forearm was preserved, but was 18% higher than in untreated women, who displayed a continuous decrease.

The role of progestogen in bone response is still unknown. One study by Lindsay and associates reported that two progestogens, gestronol and mestranol, also preserved bone mass[13]. Over a period of 1 year the women treated with the two progestogens increased their metacarpal bone mineral density by 0.1–0.6%, which is less than most responses recorded in estrogen users. The placebo group lost 1.7% bone mineral density (BMD). No firm evidence for synergistic action of estrogens and progestogens however has been provided to date. The vast majority of studies suggest no difference in BMD response between estrogen alone and combined estrogen/progestogen therapy[5–9]. In the study by Eiken and colleagues[12] no significant difference between cyclic and continuous combined treatment was demonstrable, albeit that BMD increased 15.9%

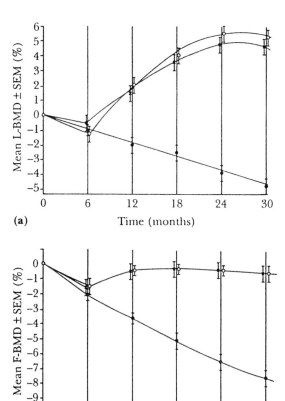

Figure 1 Changes in postmenopausal bone mineral density of (a) the spine (L-BMD) and (b) forearm (F-BMD) after 3 years of HRT with either cyclic or continuous estradiol/norethisterone. ○, Continuous group; ×, sequential group; ●, placebo group. Adapted from reference 11, with permission

in the continuous combined group compared with 11.1% in the sequential group. However, we still lack much knowledge concerning the action of progestogens on bone.

Effects of hormone replacement therapy on fracture

Numerous retrospective studies have demonstrated antifracture efficacy of HRT with a compound reduction in relative risk for hip fracture ranging between 0.5 and 0.75[4–7]. Only one randomized prospective study on the antifracture efficacy of estrogen exists, namely the study by Lufkin and co-workers[18], showing significant reduction in vertebral fracture rates in women receiving transdermal estrogen plus oral progestogen for 1 year.

The mean duration of estrogen treatment in many patients participating in most retrospective studies (3–5 years) is far below the time considered necessary to achieve significant effects on the skeleton (10 years or more). One of the few long-term studies was published by Ettinger and associates[19], who studied the antifracture efficacy of estrogen in women treated for a mean period of 17.6 years. They reported a 50% reduction in spinal fracture rate (Figure 2). Thus in the few studies on women subjected to prolonged exposure to estrogen, pronounced reductions in fracture rate have been recorded. Therefore, the current large randomized investigations under way in different countries using longer treatment periods, will be of significant interest.

Effects of estrogen on bone remodeling

Histologically, the main action of estrogen treatment is a reduction of bone turnover[20]. Women in menopause develop increased bone turnover, and a lowering of turnover reduces bone loss. Estrogen reduces the risk of disintegration of trabecular bone structure due to perforative resorption of trabeculae[20]. This is thought to be the main mechanism of action, and is also corroborated by the different responses seen in areas of the skeleton rich in cancellous bone versus areas dominated by cortical bone. The recent data by Eiken and colleagues[12], however, suggest some anabolic action of long-term HRT, otherwise no continuous increase in bone mass would be demonstrable.

The histological studies published to date have mainly investigated women around the age of 65 years with osteoporosis[20]. No evidence for a reversal of bone balance from negative to positive was demonstrable[20]. The only significant effect demonstrable was a 50% reduction of

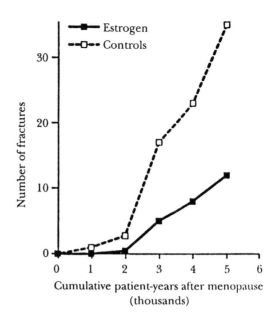

Figure 2 Cumulative fractures of spine in women receiving estrogen compared with untreated age-matched controls. Adapted from reference 19, with permission

activation frequency (i.e. birth-rate of new remodeling cycles)[20]. We recently studied bone biopsies obtained in early postmenopausal women before and after 2 years of treatment with either sequential estrogen/progestogen or placebo. In this study we found that the untreated women displayed an increase in resorptive activity and a progressively more negative bone balance at the level of individual remodeling units[21]. In the women treated with HRT, however, no such increase was observed, and bone balance was preserved, actually becoming slightly positive[21]. Osteoclastic resorption rate was more than halved in the women treated with HRT.

The reduced resorption activity leads to a reduction in turnover, which has been demonstrated with almost all of the biochemical markers of bone remodeling available (e.g. osteocalcin, alkaline phosphatase, procollagen peptides, hydroxyproline and collagen cross-links). Generally a 50% reduction of turnover is seen (Figure 3)[22,23].

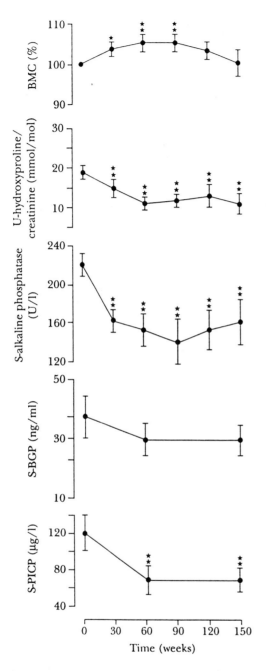

Figure 3 Changes in bone mineral content (BMC), biochemical markers of bone resorption (urinary hydroxyproline/creatinine excretion) and bone formation (serum alkaline phosphatase, serum osteocalcin (S-BGP) and serum human type I procollagen propeptide (S-PICP)) after 3 years of sequential estrogen/progestogen treatment. $*p < 0.05$; $**p < 0.01$. Adapted from reference 23, with permission

Monitoring estrogen therapy

Various biochemical markers of bone turnover have been suggested for monitoring responses to therapy. In numerous clinical studies formative markers like osteocalcin, bone alkaline phosphatase and resorption markers like hydroxyproline and collagen cross-links in urine have been found to decrease within a few months after institution of estrogen therapy[22,23]. The use in single patients, however, is hampered by the large intraindividual variation of these markers. When repeated measurements are performed in the same individual, the day-to-day variation ranges between 25 and 40%[24]. This means that quite pronounced changes in bone turnover have to take place before a reduction can be demonstrated with certainty in a single individual. Therefore, useful as these markers may be for monitoring bone remodeling in groups, it is still premature to use them for monitoring therapy in individual patients. More specific and/or less variable markers have to be characterized, before this strategy can be said to be cost-effective. Repeated measurements of biochemical markers would of course reduce the variation, but are unrealistic to perform in the large populations currently treated with HRT.

Repeated BMD measurements in the spine and hip currently constitute the best way to monitor the response to estrogen therapy. However, with the error for BMD measurements ranging between 1% in the spine and 1–3% in the hip, and changes in bone mass after HRT varying between 1 and 3% per year, the interval between measurements should be at least 2 years to detect a significant response. Bone mineral density values obtained at shorter intervals will be difficult to interpret with certainty. Furthermore, very few women do not respond to estrogen therapy, so certain researchers have advocated to omit monitoring altogether. With bad compliance being one of the main problems facing doctors treating women with estrogen, however, regular controls have to be instituted.

Future prospects

After initial animal experiments showed preservation of bone mass in ovariectomized rats treated with antiestrogens like tamoxifen, this field has expanded widely in recent years. Currently, a large multicenter phase 3 study is under way with the antiestrogens raloxifene and droloxifene. The hope is that these compounds will be able to exert positive effects on bone, cardiovascular system and brain, without causing serious estrogen-related side-effects like endometrial cancer and breast cancer, eliminating the need for concomitant progestogen administration. These regimens may also permit the treatment of women with previous breast cancer, who are currently faced with very different messages depending on whether they see a gynecologist or an oncologist.

The place for these new regimens in the future treatment of osteoporosis remains to be established. Until then, traditional estrogen/progestogen therapy remains the drug of choice for the treatment of postmenopausal osteoporosis. The estrogen effects on bone are similar to those of other antiresorptive regimens like bisphosphonates and vitamin D. However, these drugs lack the positive effects on hot flushes, vagina, cardiovascular system, brain and skin.

The biggest clinical problem in relation to HRT is still the pronounced lack of compliance due to bleeding disturbances, breast tenderness, weight gain and last but not least fear of breast cancer. It is therefore important to take time with every woman to discuss side-effects and their time course thoroughly. The putative risk for breast cancer has to be put in perspective in relation to the risk for other diseases, especially cardiovascular disease. Finally, it is important to discuss the duration of therapy, which has to be prolonged (exceeding 10 years) in order to achieve optimal bone protection. The message will probably be much clearer and more specific in years to come, when the results of several long-term randomized studies on estrogen effects should be on hand.

References

1. Weissberger, A. J., Ho, K. K. and Lazarus, L. (1991). Contrasting effects of oral and transdermal routes of oestrogen replacement therapy on 24-hour growth hormone (GH) secretion, insulin-like growth factor I and GH-binding protein in postmenopausal women. *J. Clin. Endocrinol. Metab.*, **72**, 374–81

2. Stevenson, J. C., Cust, M. P., Gangar, K. F., Hillard, T. C., Lees, B. and Whitehead, M. I. (1990). Effects of transdermal versus oral hormone replacement therapy on bone density in spine and proximal femur in postmenopausal women. *Lancet*, **336**, 265–9

3. Kiel, D. P., Baron, J. A., Anderson, J. J., Hannan, M. and Felson, D. T. (1992). Smoking eliminates the protective effect of oral oestrogens on the rlsk for hip fracture among women. *Ann. Int. Med.*, **116**, 716–21

4. Naessén, T., Persson, I., Thor, L., Mallmin, H., Ljughall, S. and Bergström, R. (1993). Maintained bone density at advanced ages after long term treatment with low dose oestradiol implants. *Br. J. Obstet. Gynaecol.*, **100**, 454–9

5. Ettinger, B., Genant, H. K. and Cann, C. E. (1987). Postmenopausal bone loss is prevented by treatment with low-dose oestrogen with calcium. *Ann. Intern. Med.*, **106**, 40–3

6. Christiansen, C., Christensen, M. S. and Transbøl, I. (1981). Bone mass in post-menopausal women after withdrawal of oestrogen/progestogen replacement therapy. *Lancet*, **1**, 459–61

7. Christiansen, C. and Riis, B. J. (1990). 17β-estradiol and continuous norethisterone: a unique treatment for established osteoporosis in elderly women. *J. Clin. Endocrinol. Metab.*, **71**, 836–41

8. Lindsay, R. and Tohme, J. F. (1990). Oestrogen treatment of patients with established post-menopausal osteoporosis. *Obstet. Gynecol.*, **76**, 290–5

9. Prince, R. L., Smith, M. and Dick, I. M. (1991). Prevention of postmenopausal osteoporosis. A comparative study of exercise, calcium supplementation, and hormone-replacement therapy. *N. Engl. J. Med.*, **325**, 1189–95

10. Christiansen, C., Christensen, M. S., McNair, P.,

Hagen, C., Stocklund, K. E. and Transbøl, I. (1980). Prevention of early postmenopausal bone loss: controlled 2-year study in 315 normal females. *Eur. J. Clin. Invest.*, **10**, 273–9

11. Munk Jensen, N., Nielsen, S. P., Obel, E. B. and Eriksen, P. B. (1988). Reversal of postmenopausal vertebral bone loss by oestrogen and progestogen: a double blind placebo controlled study. *Br. Med. J.*, **296**, 1150–2

12. Eiken, P., Kolthoff, N. and Nielsen, S. P. (1996). Effect of 10 years hormone replacement therapy on bone mineral content in postemenopausal women, in press

13. Lindsay, R., Hart, D. M., Purdie, D., Ferguson, M. M., Clark, A. S. and Krazewski, A. (1978). Comparative effects of oestrogen and a progestogen on bone loss in postmenopausal women. *Clin. Sci. Mol. Med.*, **54**, 193–5

14. Hutchinson, T. A., Polansky, S. M. and Feinstein, A. R. (1979). Postmenopausal oestrogens protect against fractures of hip and distal radius. *Lancet*, **2**, 705–7

15. Johnson, R. E. and Specht, E. E. (1981). The risk of hip fracture in postmenopausal females with and without estrogen exposure. *Am. J. Publ. Health*, **71**, 139–44

16. Paganini-Hill, A., Ross, R. K., Gerkins, V. R., Henderson, B. E., Arthur, M. and Mack, T. M. (1981). Menopausal oestrogen therapy and hip fractures. *Ann. Intern. Med.*, **95**, 28–31

17. Khoyi, A. A. and Middleton, R. K. (1992). Oral contraceptives in osteoporosis. *Ann. Pharmacother.*, **26**, 1094–5

18. Lufkin, E. G., Wahner, H. W., O'Fallon, W. M.,

Hodgson S. F., Kotowisz, M. A., Lane, A. W., Judd, H. L., Caplan, R. H. and Riggs, B. L. (1992). Treatment of postmenopausal osteoporosis with transdermal oestrogen. *Ann. Intern. Med.*, **117**, 1–9

19. Ettinger, B., Genant, H. K. and Cann, C. E. (1985). Long term oestrogen replacement therapy prevents bone loss and fractures. *Ann. Intern. Med.*, **102**, 319–24

20. Steiniche, T., Hasling, C., Charles, P., Eriksen, E. F., Mosekilde, L. and Melsen, F. (1989). A randomized study on the effects of estrogen–progestogen or high dose oral calcium on trabecular bone remodeling in postmenopausal osteoporosis. *Bone*, **10**, 313–20

21. Eriksen, E. F., Langdahl, B. L., Glerup, H., Vesterby, A., Rungby, J. and Kassem, M. (1996). HRT preserves bone balance by preventing osteoclastic hyperactivity in postmenopausal women: a randomized prospective, histo-morphometric study. *J. Bone Miner. Res.*, **1S** (abstr.)

22. Riis, B. J., Johanson, J. and Christiansen, C. (1988). Continuous oestrogen-progestogen treatment and bone metabolism in postmenopausal women. *Maturitas*, **10**, 51–8

23. Hasling, C., Eriksen, E. F., Melkko, J. and Ristelli, J. (1992). Effects of a combined estrogen–progestogen regimen on serum levels of the carboxy-terminal propeptide of human type I procollagen in osteoporosis. *J. Bone Miner. Res.*, **6**, 1295–9

24. Blumsohn, A. and Eastell, R. (1992). Prediction of bone loss in postmenopausal women. *Eur. J. Clin. Invest.*, **22**, 764–6

Prevention of osteoporosis with estrogen and its analogs: what is new?

21

D. W. Purdie

Introduction

There is general acceptance in the clinical field that estrogens are the treatment of choice for the arrest of bone resorption in postmenopausal, or otherwise estrogen-deficient women. The mechanism of estrogen action in relation to the skeleton is still imperfectly understood but is clearly intimately involved with the critical balance between bone formation and bone resorption[1]. This balance, in the absence of estrogen, tilts towards resorption,with a consequent progressive fall in bone mineral density (BMD), the principal variant in describing an individual's risk of fracture. The skeletal effect of estrogens appears to operate at all ages and continues for as long as the treatment is taken. Bone loss begins again on withdrawal of estrogen therapy, and the extent to which the preceding protection is lost is still a matter of considerable controversy. The use of a concomitant progestogen, necessary in women who have not undergone hysterectomy, does not detract from the skeletal benefits of estrogen[2].

Despite the unquestionable benefits for the skeleton, the use of estrogen replacement therapy is associated with numerous drawbacks and difficulties which are progressively being addressed by the medical profession and the pharmaceutical industry. There is little doubt that all concerned, not least the patient with osteoporosis, would welcome the advent of an estrogen-replacement regimen which would deliver symptom control and bone protection with long-term freedom from bleeding and from the fear of breast malignancy. This paper will cover some recent developments in the field, with particular reference to osteoporosis and its prevention.

Continuation

Compliance with prescribed estrogen has always been a severe problem. Patients sometimes fail to fill their prescriptions and, if incompletely briefed about the start-up syndrome, they may adversely react to the occurrence of such symptoms and terminate treatment (Table 1).

Our own data on patient acceptance and continuation, in a population aware that it was at risk of osteoporosis, are as shown in Tables 2 and 3[3]. Clearly, if it were possible to eliminate those side-effects consequent on breast and uterine stimulation, it is likely that

Table 1 Estrogen start-up syndrome

Symptoms
Breast tenderness
Calf cramps
Headaches
Appetite rise
Libido shift

Table 2 Patient rejection of offered HRT in screening feasibility trial ($n = 298$). Adapted from reference 3, with permission

Reason for rejection	n	%
Return to cycle	117	40
Fear of side-effects	90	30
breast cancer	34	11
Acceptance of risk	20	7
Rejection of medication	16	5
Conceptual rejection of HRT	9	3
Other	46	15

Table 3 Duration of HRT in prospective bone mineral density study (DXA) ($n = 434$). Adapted from reference 3, with permission

Reason for discontinuation	n	%
Return to cycle	110	25.3
Headaches	40	9.2
Weight gain	28	6.5
Unspecified side-effects	28	4.8
Depression	21	4.8
Breast pain	19	4.4
Dyspepsia	10	2.3
Initial effects	10	2.3
Other	168	38.7

acceptance and continuation results would be greatly improved.

Continuous combined therapy

One measure which has received much attention in the prevention of bleeding problems with hormone replacement therapy (HRT) is the replacement of cyclic (10–12 days/month) progestogens with a continuous regimen. This has the effect of inhibiting estrogen receptor production and hence maintains a flat unresponsive endometrium. Most clinical studies have indicated that, when such agents are correctly restricted to patients who are more than 1 year postmenopausal, then about 80% of patients will be amenorrheic following 6 months' treatment. Some initial spotting is experienced by many women in the first 6 months of therapy, but this is usually self-limiting. The continuous, combined regimens have been available for a relatively short time and hence long-term safety data in respect of the breast and cardiovascular systems are awaited. All such regimens hitherto have been oral, and a continuous, combined patch is awaited with interest.

With regard to bone, there have been several randomized studies addressing the effectiveness of continued combined therapy in bone protection, particularly at the spine[4,5]. In general, it would seem that bone loss at the distal radius and the lumbar spine is successfully arrested by this regimen, both in women with low bone mass and in those with established osteoporosis. Long-term data on hip bone density and a fracture risk are awaited.

Quarterly cycling regimens

Another maneuver designed to reduce the patient burden of withdrawal bleeding is the use of estrogen for 3 months, followed by progestogen delivery and withdrawal. This regimen has not been reported to be associated with excess endometrial hyperplasia. The precise minimum number of HRT cycles per year which will safely effect shedding is not known with certainty. There has been a recent report indicating that the use of cyclic progestogen is not attended by an absolute protection of the endometrium from hyperplasia or neoplasia. The rise in the incidence of endometrial cancer observed when estrogen is given alone[6] is substantially reduced, but perhaps not abolished, by the addition of a progestogen[7]. Clearly, the engagement of both estrogen and progestogen receptors by the components of HRT regimens constitutes a continuing problem.

Tibolone

Tibolone remains unique as a 'designer' agent which has estrogenic progestogenic and androgenic properties. As with the continuous, combined regimens it is recommended only to be used at least 1 year after menopause, when the circulating estradiol level is presumed to be low. The percentage of patients reporting amenorrhea at 6 months is in the order of 80%. This product has recently been licensed in the UK for the prevention of bone loss and should be a useful addition to the antiresorptive armamenterium.

Matrix patches

The use of transdermal systems has evolved rapidly in recent years and is of considerable value in the delivery of estrogen, since the active hormone is released into the systemic, not the portal circulation, and hence, like ovarian estrogen, it is distributed directly to the target organs. The advent of the matrix patch has seen a great improvement in patient acceptance with this useful and highly physiological mode of estrogen delivery. The absence of an alcohol carrier is believed to be largely responsible for the improved skin tolerance. Patches in general have to be changed at 3- or 4-day intervals, an eccentric regimen in which patients may find difficulty in remembering precisely when a change is due.

The advent of a new 7-day patch is therefore a significant advance. This agent is well tolerated and achieves a delivery 50 μg of estradiol throughout its week of activity (Figure 1)[8]. Despite being in skin contact for double the time of previous patches, the 7-day (FemSeven) patch is equally well tolerated.

Selective estrogen receptor modulation

As noted above, the principal problems encountered with HRT regimens center on the reproductive organs of the breast and uterus, the two prime sites of the estrogens' central action in modulating female fertility. However, it is now clear that evolution has also bestowed upon the estrogens essential functions in the skeletal cardiovascular and central nervous systems. When the advent of the menopause causes the plasma estrogen concentration to fall by an order of magnitude, pathological dysfunction in these organ systems may be provoked.

It has thus been a long-held ambition of pharmacologists and clinicians to have available an estrogen which would act as an agonist at the desired sites of bone, blood vessel and brain, while remaining neutral or antagonistic a the breast and uterus. Our rapidly evolving knowledge of the heterogeneity of the estrogen response in different tissues has indeed opened the door to selective response, and the clinical advent of selective estrogen receptor modulation is close.

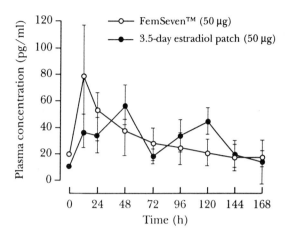

Figure 1 Pharmacokinetics of FemSeven™ (50 μg) vs. the 3.5-day estradiol atch (50 μg). Adapted from reference 8, with permission

It has been reported by Yang[9] that raloxifene, a triphenylethylene related to tamoxifen, appears to engage the estrogen receptor and then bind a response element without the participation of the DNA binding domain of the receptor. This new pathway of estrogen receptor-controlled gene activation is involved in the differential tissue response wherein raloxifene behaves as a true antagonist to estrogen action at the uterus and breast. The ability of raloxifene to inhibit proliferation of the MCF-7 breast cancer cell line as reported by Short and colleagues[10], holds out the, as yet untested, clinical possibility that these agents may confer protection against breast cancer. At present, there is a general consensus that conventional HRT is associated with a loading of the patients' underlying risk at a point between 5 and 10 years' therapy, and hence the advent of a breast cancer-neutral or even -protective agent is appealing. Draper and colleagues[11] reported recently that uterine biopsies taken from raloxifene-treated patients showed no evidence of endometrial stimulation when compared to control subjects given estrogen in a short-term 2-month study.

Caution should be applied to all the above data, however, since, to date, there has been no medium- or long-term data on the safety and efficacy of raloxifene, and since its failure to prevent vasomotor symptoms suggests that its central nervous system action may be, at best, patchy. The latter is an important point, since it was recently reported by Tang and colleagues[12] that the incidence of Alzheimer's disease and related dementias in conventionally HRT-treated US women was substantially reduced when such patients were compared to untreated age-matched controls. The ability of estrogen to modify or prevent the clinical course of these distressing conditions will, if confirmed, constitute another powerful indication for their use. Hence, it will be necessary to establish if any new selective estrogen receptor modulator (SERM) agent also delivers estrogen agonist effects in those key areas of the central nervous system, such as the hippocampus, which are believed to be involved in the development of Alzheimer's disease and related dementias.

Conclusion

Much has been done in recent years to render HRT regimens more acceptable to their users. The advent of the continuous, combined regimens, the 7-day matrix patch (FemSeven)

and the 'designer' estrogen/progestogens have contributed to the development of a therapy which is generally safe and is attended by relief of significant cessation of bone loss, inhibition of atherogenesis and, perhaps, protection of the central nervous system.

However, the acceptance and continuation of HRT regimens remain poor and will do so until a way is found to avoid engagement of the mammary and endometrial estrogen receptor. Although the advent of SERMs may provide part of the answer by selectively engaging skeletal, clinical and cardiovascular estrogen receptors, there will remain a major requirement for traditional hormone replacement therapy in perimenopausal women. All women should be seen at the time of menopause by their primary care physician, in order that a careful history and examination may determine those women in whom the use of HRT regimens is likely to be attended by a significant improvement in their health or in the prevention of disease. All such women should then be offered HRT so that the woman herself may exercise her central right to accept or not accept such a treatment.

References

1. Lindsay, R., Bush, T., Grady, D. *et al.* (1996). Oetrogen replacement in the menopause. *J. Clin. Endocrinol. Metab.*, **81**, 3829–38

2. Marcus, R. (1995). Effects of hormone replacement therapies on bone mineral density (BMD) results from the postmenopausal estrogen and progestin interventions trial (PEPI). *J. Bone Min. Res.*, **10**, S197

3. Purdie, D. W., Steel, S. A., Howey, S. and Doherty, S. M. (1996). The technical and logistical feasibility of population densitometry using DXA and directed HRT interventions: A 2-year prospective study. *Osteoporosis Int.*, **3**, S31–6

4. Riis, B. J., Johansen, J. and Christiansen, C. (1988). Continuous oestrogen–progestogen treatment and bone metabolism in post-menopausal women. *Maturitas*, **10**, 51–8

5. Grey, A. B., Candy, T. F. and Reid, I. R. (1994). Continuous combined oestrogen/progestin

therapy is well tolerated and increases bone density at the hip and spine in postmenopausal osteoporosis. *Clin. Endocrinol.*, **40**, 671–7

6. Voigt, L. F., Weiss, N. S., Chu, J. *et al.* (1991). Progestogen supplementation of exogenous oestrogens and risk of endometrial cancer. *Lancet*, **338**, 274–7

7. Jick, S. S., Walker, A. M. and Jick, H. (1993). Estrogens, progesterone, and endometrial cancer. *Epidemiology*, **4**, 20–4

8. Hughes, D. E., Lutkie, A. W. H. M. and Hackel, S. (1997). Efficacy, tolerability and compliance of FemSeven®, a once weekly transdermal system compared with Estraderm TTS 50®. *Eur. J. Clin. Res.*, **9**, 111–22

9. Yang, N. N, Venugopalan, M., Hardikar, S. and Glasebrook, A. (1996). Identification of an estrogen response element activated by metabolites and 17β-estradiol and raloxifene. *Science*, **273**, 1222–4

10. Short, L., Glasebrook, A., Adrian, M. *et al.* (1996). Distinct effects of SERMs on estrogen dependent and estrogen independent human breast cancer cell proliferation. Presented at the *American Society for Bone & Mineral Research,* 18th Annual Meeting, Abstract T731

11. Draper, M. W., Flowers, D. E., Huster, W. J. *et al.* (1996). A controlled trial of raloxifene (LY139481) Hcl: impact on bone turnover and serum lipid profile in healthy postmenopausal women. *J. Bone Min. Res.,* **11**, 835–42

12. Tang, M. X., Jacobs, D., Stern, Y., *et al.* (1996). Effect of oestrogen during menopause on risk and age at onset of Alzheimer's disease. *Lancet,* **348**, 429–32

Osteoporosis: treatment options

22

E. Seeman

Introduction

The aim of treatment of osteoporosis is to maintain, and ideally to restore, bone strength safely. Anti-vertebral fracture efficacy has been reported using bisphosphonates[1-4], estrogen[5,6], calcitonin[7], 1,25-dihydroxyvitamin D[8,9], 1α-hydroxyvitamin D[10], calcium supplements[11,12] and fluoride in some, but not all, studies[13-16]. Anti-hip fracture efficacy was reported using calcium plus vitamin D in elderly women in nursing homes[17], but not in elderly women living independently[18]. Annual parenteral vitamin D has been reported to reduce hip fractures in elderly persons in the community[19]. Hip protectors prevent hip fractures in women and men in nursing homes[20]. Alendronate has been reported to reduce the incidence of hip fractures in women with osteoporosis[4].

Remodeling transients, reduced bone turnover and balance at the basic multicellular unit – the meaning of increased bone mineral density

For bone loss to occur there must be a negative bone balance at the level of the basic multicellular unit (BMU): the amount of bone resorbed must be greater than the amount replaced. Given this, the rate of bone loss will be determined by the size of the imbalance at each BMU and by the turnover rate – the rate at which new remodeling sites are created[21,22]. When an antiresorptive agent such as hormone replacement therapy (HRT), bisphosphonate or calcitonin is given, bone turnover is reduced. The initial rise in bone mineral density (BMD) is about 4–7% in the first 1–2 years and occurs because bone formation initiated in the preceding remodeling cycle fills the remodeling space created during that cycle[22-24].

After this initial increase in BMD, bone loss resumes from the higher BMD at a rate determined by the effect of the drug on bone turnover and on bone resorption, and formation balance at the BMU. If bone loss is 1% per year and a drug reduces turnover by 50% but has no effect on bone balance at the BMU, bone loss will be 0.5% per year. If the imbalance at the BMU is also reduced by 50% (by the drug reducing the depth of resorption and/or increasing bone formation) then the rate of bone loss will be 0.25% per year. If the BMU imbalance is abolished, bone loss will cease irrespective of the rate of bone turnover (Figure 1).

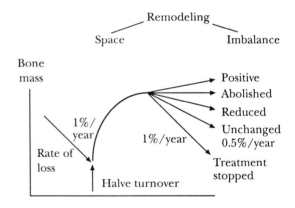

Figure 1 Initial increase in bone mineral density (BMD) following administration of resorption inhibitor is due to filling of remodeling space. If bone loss is 1% per year and resorption inhibitor halves bone turnover, rate of loss will be 0.5% per year; if drug also halves imbalance in basic multicellular unit (BMU), bone loss will be 0.25% per year; if imbalance is abolished no bone loss will occur; if drug increases bone balance at BMU then BMD would be expected to increase

Histomorphometry is needed to establish whether resorption depth is reduced and bone formation (mean wall thickness) is increased. Using beagles, Boyce and colleagues showed that risedronate reduced activation frequency, bone resorption and tissue-level bone formation but not bone formation at the cellular level[25]. Bone formation increased resulting in increasing mean wall thickness. In women with osteoporosis, Storm and co-workers showed that etidronate decreased activation frequency and decreased resorption depth[26]. Increased mean wall thickness using alendronate has been reported (unpublished data).

Thus, the antiresorptive drugs increase BMD initially by filling of the remodeling space and reducing the rate of bone turnover, and then perhaps by reducing the imbalance at the level of the BMU (by reducing resorption depth and increasing formation). The average increase in BMD over 2–3 years with bisphosphonates, estrogens and perhaps calcitonin is about 4–7%. As the starting BMD in these patients with osteoporosis is already low, this increase in BMD is small in absolute terms. Can fracture rates be expected to decline as a consequence of such small changes in BMD?

It is never too late

There is a need to consider treatment because bone loss continues throughout life[27–31]. Prospective studies suggest that bone loss actually accelerates with advancing age. Ensrud and associates showed that rates of decline in BMD at the proximal femur in 5698 white women increased four-fold from 2.5 mg/cm^2 per year in women aged 67–69 years to 10.4 mg/cm^2 per year in women over 85 years[31].

Contrary to the perception held by patients, it is not 'too late' for treatment. The breaking strength of bone is proportional to BMD squared. This power function suggests that continued bone loss should disproportionately increase fracture risk as BMD falls. A treatment that stops the accelerated bone loss in the elderly should prevent the rise in fracture rate

predicted by the falling BMD. There is evidence to support this notion. Tilyard and colleagues showed that the number of women sustaining fractures increased in the control group receiving calcium while the number of women having vertebral fractures while taking 1,25-dihydroxyvitamin D remained unchanged[8]. Storm and co-workers showed that the spinal deformity index increased in the placebo and remained unchanged in the treated group and differed between groups at week 150[1].

Whether the converse holds true is less certain. Do fracture rates decrease as BMD increases with treatment? There are cross-sectional data showing that higher BMD is associated with lower fracture rates. These cross-sectional data have led to the view that the greater the increase in BMD, the greater will be the reduction in fracture rates. The increase in BMD discussed above associated with treatment and the decrease in fracture rates (to be discussed below) are assumed to be causally related. However, the concomitant changes in bone turnover may contribute. The test of this hypothesis is to demonstrate an association betweeen the change in BMD and the change in fracture rates. There is no evidence of this relationship. We still do not know whether increasing BMD equates with reduced fracture rates. The effect of fluoride on BMD is evidence to the contrary[13,14].

Resorption inhibitors

Hormone replacement therapy

Elderly patients often believe it is 'too late' for HRT. HRT can reduce markers of bone resorption in the elderly, reduce the rate of bone loss and the incidence of fractures[5]. Lufkin and colleagues reported that transdermal estrogen resulted in an increase in BMD of about 5% at the spine and 7.6% at the trochanter. This was a double-blind placebo controlled trial, but the duration of the study was 1 year. Eight fractures occurred in 7 of 34 women in the HRT group, while 20 fractures occurred in 12 of 34 women given placebo. The reduction in fracture events was significant but the reduction in numbers of patients having fractures did not achieve statistical significance[5]. Lindsay and associates showed that vertebral deformities were less in the HRT (mestranol)-treated patients than controls in the double-blind placebo-controlled study[6]: 16 of 42 placebo- and 2 of 58 estrogen-treated women reviewed after 6–12 years. Both of these randomized studies support the view that HRT reduces vertebral fracture rates.

Observational studies suggest a reduction in fracture risk by 40–60% in women receiving HRT. An effect of sampling cannot be excluded; healthier individuals may have sought, and taken, HRT. Among 9704 women aged 65 years or older, current HRT use was associated with a 60% reduction in risk for wrist fracture and 34% reduction in risk for all non-spinal fractures[29]. Results were similar for women under and over 75 years of age. Current use reduced hip fracture risk by 40%. In users starting HRT within 5 years of menopause, relative risk (RR) was 0.29 for hip fracture, 0.29 for wrist fracture, and 0.50 for all non-spinal fractures. Maxim and co-workers followed up 245 postmenopausal women using 0.9 mg conjugated estrogen daily for a mean of 17 years[30]. Relative to 245 untreated women, age-adjusted incidence ratios were 0.55 for wrist fracture, 0.57 for vertebral fracture and 0.85 (NS) for hip fracture.

There are reasons to question the role of HRT in the prevention of hip fractures. Anti-hip fracture efficacy of HRT has not been assessed in randomized controlled studies. The confidence intervals around the reduced risk estimated included unity in several of the observational studies cited above. There was no detectable increase in BMD at the femoral neck in the study by Lufkin and colleagues[5]. Ensrud and associates reported that annual rates of bone loss in current estrogen users was 33% less at total hip and 35% less at calcaneus. Thus, bone loss at the proximal femur was slowed but not abolished. Higher (and less well-tolerated) doses of HRT may be needed to prevent bone loss at the proximal femur[32]. Long-term compliance with HRT is poor. These are important considerations given that hip fractures occur late in life, and HRT exposure to large numbers will be needed for many years to prevent hip fractures.

Felson and colleagues addressed the issue of whether HRT taken after the menopause provides residual benefit many years after it has been ceased[33]. In women aged under 75 years, with more than seven years' HRT exposure, BMD was about 11% higher than in untreated women. In women more than 75 years of age with comparable duration of treatment, BMD was only 3.2% higher. The authors suggested that any benefit of HRT was lost after stopping HRT. The observation is likely to be correct. Bone loss does resume after stopping HRT, so it is likely that HRT should be given long term.

Estrogens must be given with a progestin to protect against the estrogen-induced increased risk of endometrial cancer. Whether the 19-nor progestins have an independent anabolic effect on bone as well as protecting the endometrium remains to be established[34]. If there is no independent effect on the skeleton, it would be preferable to have an estrogen that has no effect on the endometrium.

Tissue-selective estrogen agonists may prevent bone loss while having no proliferative effect on the breast or endometrium. Raloxifene prevents bone loss following oophorectomy in animals and maintains the breaking strength of bone. Uterine weight increases with ethinyl estradiol administration but remains no different from ovariectomized animals treated with raloxifene[35]. Thus progestin therapy may not be required if this new agent is efficacious and safe.

Bisphosphonates

Two randomized trials reported in 1990[1,2] support the notion that etidronate may, or is likely to, reduce fracture rates, but problems in the study design such as the small sample sizes, the short duration of follow-up and the unblinding with loss of controls may have limited the power of the studies to detect a true beneficial effect if there was one.

Storm and co-workers studied 66 patients of mean age 68 years (range 57–75 years) with one or more spine fractures. Twenty patients in each group completed the study[1]. Mean spine BMD increased by 5.3% and decreased in placebo by 2.7%. The rate of new fractures (expressed per 100 patient-years) during 150 weeks was 18 in the treated group and 43 in controls (NS). Unplanned subgroup analyses revealed that the respective fracture rates were 38 versus 35 from 0–60 weeks (NS), and 6 versus 54 for weeks 60 to 150 ($p < 0.03$).

Watts and associates randomized 423 patients with one or more vertebral compression fractures to eight cycles of phosphate or placebo for 3 days, then etidronate or placebo for 14 days, then calcium for 72 days[2]. Mean spine BMD increased by 4.2% and 5.2% in the etidronate groups receiving placebo or phosphate respectively, among 363 patients completing 24 months. Fractures occurred in 17 non-etidronate-treated patients while eight patients had fractures in the etidronate groups ($p < 0.05$). The two etidronate groups were combined because of the small numbers of fracture cases in the individual groups. The new vertebral fracture rate (per 1000 patient-years) in the etidronate groups combined was 29.5 versus 62.9 in the combined non-etidronate groups ($p < 0.05$). In the group with BMD below the 50th percentile, fracture rates were 42.3 versus 132.7 per 1000 patient-years ($p = 0.004$).

In the extension of the study by Watts and colleagues, 357 continued in year 3 (305 agreed to blinded therapy, 52 received calcium) and 277 continued in year 4 (all receiving etidronate)[36]. Spine BMD increased to about 5% from baseline by year 4, and increased by 1.4 to 2.6% at the proximal femur depending on the region and group. There were no controls in the 4th year because all the remaining participants were given etidronate. Although fracture rates decreased in those with low BMD with three or more fractures: 228 versus 412 fractures per 1000 patient-years ($p < 0.05$), the numbers of patients sustaining vertebral fractures did not differ in the etidronate and non-etidronate groups during the 4-year period.

During years 0–3, 14% of the non-etidronate-treated patients had 86 fractures per 1000 patient-years while 17% of the etidronate-treated patients had 117 fractures per 1000 patient-years (NS).

Two multicenter double-blind studies provide compelling evidence of the antifracture efficacy of alendronate (ALN). The first, published by Liberman and co-workers, involved 994 postmenopausal women aged 64 years (range 45–80 years) with osteoporosis defined as a spine BMD 2.5 standard deviations below the young normal mean[3]. The presence of a fracture was not a requirement for inclusion. Placebo was given for 3 years, ALN as 5 mg per day for 3 years, 10 mg per day for 3 years or 20 mg per day for 2 years then 5 mg in the 3rd year. All received 500 mg elemental calcium. Bone mineral density increased using all dose regimens and decreased in the patients receiving placebo. At the end of 3 years, BMD was higher in the patients treated with 10 mg/day ALN than in patients receiving placebo by a mean of 8.8% at the lumbar spine, by 5.9% at the femoral neck and by 7.8% at the trochanter. The 10-mg dose was more effective than the 5-mg dose but no less effective than the 20/5-mg regimen. Urinary deoxypyridinoline and total alkaline phosphatase decreased with all doses.

The proportion of patients having vertebral fractures was 6.2% receiving placebo and 3.2% receiving ALN: a 48% reduction in numbers of women having fractures ($p < 0.04$). Of the patients having new vertebral fractures, two or more fractures occurred in 15 of 22 (68%) receiving placebo and 3 of 17 (18%) ALN-treated patients. That is, two or more vertebral fractures occurred in 4.2% (15 of 355) receiving placebo and 0.6% (3 of 526) of patients receiving ALN, a risk reduction of 87% (odds ratio (OR) 0.13, 95% confidence interval (CI) 0.05–0.38). The patients receiving placebo with new fractures lost 23.3 mm in height; ALN-treated patients who sustained one or more fractures lost 5.9 mm in height, consistent with less severe fractures. Non-vertebral fracture rates were based on preplanned pooling of these two studies with three similar but smaller studies of at least 2 years' duration. Non-vertebral fractures occurred in 73 of 1012 ALN-treated women and 60 of 590 patients receiving placebo. After 3 years, the cumulative incidences (ALN versus placebo) were 9% and 12.6%; a 29% reduction in risk compared to placebo ($p < 0.05$).

In the fracture intervention trial (FIT), 2027 women aged 71 years (range 55–81 years) with one or more vertebral fractures at baseline and reduced BMD were randomized at 11 centers in the USA to receive either placebo ($n = 1005$) or ALN ($n = 1022$, 5 mg for 2 years, 10 mg year 3)[4]. Calcium and vitamin D were supplemented if the diet was less than 1000 mg per day. Bone mineral density increased by 6.2% above placebo at the spine and by 4.7% above placebo at the total hip region.

The percentages of women with new vertebral fractures in placebo versus ALN respectively were as follows: those with one or more fractures, 15% versus 8%, RR = 0.53 (95% CI 0.41–0.72); those with two or more fractures, 4.9% versus 0.5%, RR = 0.10 (95% CI 0.05–0.29); and those with clinically apparent fractures 5.0% versus 2.3%, RR = 0.45, (95% CI 0.25–0.71). The cumulative proportion of women with any clinically apparent vertebral or non-vertebral fracture after 3 years was 18.3% versus 13.7%, RR = 0.72 (95% CI 0.57–0.90). The incidence of all non-spine fractures was 14.2% versus 11.4%, RR = 0.78 (95% CI 0.61–0.99), hip fractures was 2.2% versus 1.1%, RR = 0.49 (95% CI 0.23–0.98) and wrist fractures 4.1% versus 2.2%, RR = 0.52 (95% CI 0.33–0.94).

Bisphosphonates combined with other agents

The studies comparing effects of bisphosphonates and HRT suggest that both prevent bone loss relative to controls. Cyclic intravenous clodronate (200 mg per month during 2 years, $n = 31$) and HRT ($n = 33$) prevented bone loss with equal efficacy relative to 28 controls[37]. The spine BMD was unchanged in the treated groups and declined

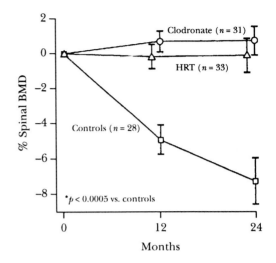

Figure 2 Cyclic intravenous clodronate (200 mg per month during 2 years) and hormone replacement therapy (HRT) prevented bone loss with equal efficacy relative to controls[37]

by 7.3% in the untreated group (Figure 2). In a 4-year study comparing etidronate with and without HRT, lumbar spine BMD increased 6.8% (estrogen), 6.8% (etidronate) and 10.9% (both), and decreased by 3.8% in placebo (Figure 3). Femoral neck BMD increased by 4.0% (estrogen), 1.2% (etidronate) and 7.3% (both) and decreased by 5.0% in placebo. This study suggested that the combination may be better than either alone in terms of BMD[38]. Antifracture efficacy studies comparing HRT, bisphosphonate, neither and both are needed to establish whether fracture rates will be lower with combined therapy than with either drug alone.

Calcium and vitamin D metabolites

Calcium supplementation may reduce the rate of bone loss and fracture rates[11,12]. In a double-blind placebo controlled trial, Recker and colleagues showed that 4 years of treatment with 1200 g calcium supplementation reduced vertebral fracture rates by about 45% in women with vertebral fractures at entry. Fracture rates were not reduced in calcium-treated women without fractures at entry to the study[11]. The

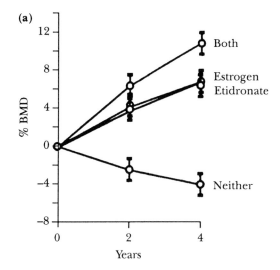

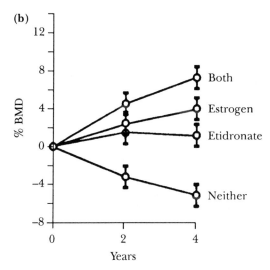

Figure 3 Lumbar spine (a) bone mineral density (BMD) increased similarly in estrogen- and etidronate-treated patients and by greater amount using both[38]. Femoral neck (b) BMD also increased more with combined therapy

significance of the differing efficacy in women with and without a fracture at entry to the study is unclear.

In a double-blind placebo-controlled study of nursing home residents, Chapuy and co-workers found that 800 units vitamin D plus 1.2 g calcium was associated with a reduction in fracture rates by about 25% relative to placebo-treated controls[17]. Lips and associates conducted a double-blind placebo-controlled trial of 1916 women and 662 men of mean age 80 years[18]. Fracture rates were no lower in subjects given 400 units vitamin D plus 1.2 g total dietary intake of calcium relative to placebo-treated controls in this community-based study. The incidence of fractures in the nursing home study was three times higher than in the community-based study, in part perhaps because nursing home residents often have illnesses, vitamin D or vitamin K deficiency or protein malnutrition (Figure 4).

The use of 1,25-dihydroxyvitamin D and 1 α-hydroxyvitamin D show promise as drugs that may reduce fracture rates, but inconsistencies in the literature leave uncertainty[8-10]. For example, in several prospective randomized blinded trials, BMD remained unchanged, decreased or increased by 1–4%[39-44]. Loss of vertebral height in the calcitriol treated group has been reported[42]. Gallagher and colleagues reported a decline in fracture rates at the end of 1 year relative to controls in patients treated at Creighton University but not Mayo Clinic in this combined study[9]. As all patients received treatment after 12 months, the lower fracture rates in the 2nd and 3rd years relative to the fracture rates in the placebo in year 1 are difficult to interpret.

Tilyard and co-workers conducted a randomized but unblinded study of 622 women with one or more fractures given 0.5 μg per day of calcitriol or calcium gluconate 1g/day[8]. Four hundred and thirty-two women (70%) completed the 3-year study. The numbers of patients with fractures did not change in the calcitriol group and increased three-fold in the control group. As 25-hydroxyvitamin D levels were 4–32 μg/l, many subjects may have been vitamin D deficient. BMD was not measured.

Calcitonin

There has been only one study of the antifracture efficacy of calcitonin. Overgaard and associates studied the effects of intranasal

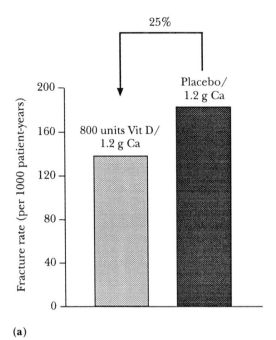

(a)

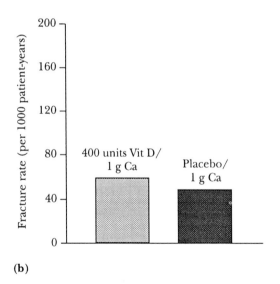

(b)

Figure 4 Chapuy and colleagues (a) found that 800 units vitamin D plus 1.2 g calcium was associated with 25% reduction in hip fracture rates in 3270 nursing home residents over 3 years[17]; Lips and associates (b) found no reduction in fracture rates over 3.5 years in 2578 subjects aged 80 years living in the community, given 400 units vitamin D plus 1 g total dietary intake of calcium[18]; incidence of fractures in nursing home study was three times that of community-based study.

salmon calcitonin in a 2-year double-blind placebo-controlled trial of women aged 68–72 years randomized to 50, 100, or 200 iu or placebo[7]. All patients received a 500 mg calcium supplement. Among the 162 completing the study, spine BMD increased by 1% (95% CI 0.1–1.5) in the placebo, 3% (95% CI 1.8–4.2) in the 200 iu-treated group. The numbers of fractures varied according to the method of assessment of vertebral morphometry. By one method, fractures occurred in seven patients receiving placebo and five patients treated with calcitonin, and in six patients receiving placebo and 4 patients treated with calcitonin using the second method. Pooling was not preplanned. Peripheral fractures occurred in two placebo and two treated patients. Incidence of new patients having vertebral fractures per 1000 patient-years was (pooled treated groups versus placebo group) 23 versus 92 by one method of assessing fractures and 19 versus 83 by the other (p = 0.006 and 0.008, respectively). Expressing the numbers of fractures per 1000 patient-years obscures the small absolute numbers of fractures that may be present. An extra fracture or misclassification under these circumstances can change the result and inferences made. The small numbers of fractures leave uncertainty.

Anabolic agents

The resorption inhibitors increase bone density by 4–8% over 2–3 years. Formation-stimulating agents may restore a greater amount of bone lost. Agents such as fluoride, anabolic steroids, intermittent parathyroid hormone, growth and local factors such as insulin-like growth factor-I (IGF-I), transforming growth factor-β (TGF-β), and prostaglandins are being studied, but there is no convincing evidence of a satisfactory anabolic agent that can be used in humans.

Fluoride increases BMD by about 10% per year so that after 4 years the BMD is restored to premenopausal levels. The rigorously conducted studies by Riggs and colleagues and Kleerekoper and associates showed that this increase in BMD could not be assumed to reflect an increase in bone strength[13,14]. Fracture rates did not differ from controls in either study. Positive results have been reported in two other studies but the loss of bone from the appendicular skeleton and the increased rates of peripheral fractures remain concerns[15,16].

In another study by Riggs and co-workers, fracture rates (per 100 person-years) in the treated versus control groups were 47 versus 52 (NS). There were 13 hip fractures in the sodium fluoride group (rate = 4.2%) and four in the controls (rate = 1.2%) in the first 4 years. There were two additional hip fractures in the 50 patients in the 2-year extension study (rate = 2.2%). Non-vertebral fractures decreased during the 2-year extension, but remained higher in the sodium fluoride than in the placebo group[45].

The study has been criticized because of the high doses used. Six-year follow-up in 50 women from the sodium fluoride group showed that higher fracture rates were associated with low initial BMD, bone loss, high BMD with rapid increases in BMD, or large increases in serum fluoride. Reduced fracture rates were associated with high BMD associated with slow increases in BMD (less than 17% per year) or increases in fluoride of less than 8 μmol/l above baseline. These associations must be tested prospectively.

The negative results of the Fluoride and Vertebral Osteoporosis Study (FAVOS) suggest that lower doses may not be efficacious[46]. No reduction in the proportion of patients having new vertebral fractures was found in this 2-year study of 354 women aged 65.7 years with 1–4 vertebral fractures at baseline. Treatments were 1 g calcium and 800 units vitamin D in addition to placebo ($n = 146$), or 50 mg per day sodium fluoride (22.6 mg F ion, $n = 73$), or 150 mg monofluorophosphate (19.8 mg F ion, $n = 68$) or 200 mg monofluorophosphate (26.4 mg F ion, $n = 67$). Bone mineral density in the fluoride-treated patients increased by 10.8% and in controls by 2.4%. By intention to treat (F versus no F), spine fractures occurred in 33.3% versus 26.5% patients, symptomatic fractures in 14% versus 14% patients, hip fractures in 1.9% versus 1.4% patients, forearm fractures in 2.4% versus 2.7% patients, and

height loss was 11 mm versus 9 mm. Fluoride should remain a research tool but cannot be recommended as a treatment modality at this time.

Intermittent parathyroid hormone (PTH) increases periosteal bone formation and trabecular connectivity, reduces cortical porosity and increases bone strength in animal studies. Combined with estrogen, intermittent PTH has been shown to increase trabecular connectivity and number in oophorectomized rats[47]. Ejersted and colleagues showed that intermittent PTH increased cortical area by 20%, reduced medullary area by 26% and reduced cortical porosity by 71%[48]. Bone strength as assessed by ultimate load increased by 71% and ultimate stiffness by 51%.

Local factors such as IGF-I may act directly, or partly mediate the anabolic effects of systemic factors such as PTH. IGF-I combined with its binding protein IGF-IBP3 may increase periosteal, endosteal and endocortical bone formation and so increase cortical thickness and trabecular number and reduce trabecular separation[49]. Other local agents having anabolic effects include prostaglandin E2, TGF-β, and bone morphogenic protein 2[50–52]. Some of these local factors must be targeted to bone as they cannot be given systemically[53]. Further studies are needed to evaluate the effects of strontium salts and flavonoids[54].

Which women to treat?

According to a study group of the World Health Organization (WHO), a woman with BMD of 2.5 or more standard deviations (SD) below the mean of the young normal range has osteoporosis. Thus, ~30% of women over 50 years have osteoporosis (15% of 50–59 year-olds, 22% of 60–69 year-olds, 40% of 70–79 year-olds). Should all these women be treated? If so, for how long? Starting at what age? With what drug?

The relative risk (RR) for fracture may double for each SD decrease in BMD, but the numbers requiring treatment to prevent one fracture depend on the efficacy of the drug and the underlying fracture rate of the age group being studied. The absolute risk for fracture is ~1–2 per 1000 person-years in < 60-year-old women, increasing by an order of magnitude to ~1–2 per 100 person-years in > 65-year-old women, reaching a maximum of ~10–14 per 100 person-years in women in the highest-risk group (elderly, low BMD, with fractures). For example, among the patients with BMD more than 2.5 SD below the young normal mean reported by Liberman and co-workers[3], the fracture rate in those with BMD in the highest tertile (of all of these women with low bone density) was about 2%, so that about 200 women must be treated to prevent one fracture. Fracture rate in the lowest tertile of this group was about 13.9%, so that only about 20 women must be treated to prevent one fracture.

If the fracture rate is 4% per year, in 3 years, 12 patients will sustain a fracture (assuming these fractures occur in different individuals) and 88 will not. If a drug has a 50% efficacy, in 3 years, 6 patients will have a fracture despite treatment, and 6 fractures will be prevented at the price of treating and exposing all the patients to side-effects, including the 88 who would not have had a fracture had no treatment been given. Long-term safety is a critical issue in prevention.

Safety is more difficult to demonstrate than efficacy. Concerns about the risk of breast cancer remain with HRT. The bisphosphonates remain in bone permanently. Osteomalacia may occur if etidronate is taken incorrectly. Although alendronate was well tolerated in clinical trials, gastrointestinal side-effects may occur when the drug is taken incorrectly. Few data are available for drugs of any kind beyond 3 years so that close monitoring will be needed when HRT, the bisphosphonates and vitamin D metabolites are in widespread use in the prevention and treatment of osteoporosis.

Conclusion

Effective treatments for osteoporosis are available. HRT and the bisphosphonates, particularly alendronate, appear to be first-line treatments for osteoporosis. The long-term effects of all drugs are unknown so that caution in the use of these agents is needed, particularly when preventive treatment is directed at individuals at high relative risk but low annual absolute risk because the treatment will have to be long-term.

Whether one treatment is 'better' than another, or whether both are better than either alone is uncertain as there have been no trials directly comparing their antifracture efficacy. Based on studies comparing HRT with etidronate and clodronate, HRT and the bisphosphonates are probably equally efficacious in preventing bone loss and increasing BMD. The choice of bisphosphonate or HRT may relate more to differences in tolerability and safety than efficacy, yet data concerning long-term safety are unavailable. A leaning towards HRT in younger and bisphosphonates in older persons seems to be a reasonable approach given the available information.

References

1. Storm, T., Thamsborg, G., Steiniche, T., Genant, H. K. and Sorensen, O. H. (1990). Effect of cyclical etidronate therapy on bone mass and fracture rate in women with postmenopausal osteoporosis. N. Engl. J. Med., **322**, 1265–71

2. Watts, N. B., Harris, S. T., Genant, H. K., Wasnich, R. D., Miller, P. D., et al. (1990). Intermittent cyclical etidronate therapy of post-menopausal osteoporosis. N. Engl. J. Med., **323**, 73–9

3. Liberman, U. A., Weiss, S. R., Broll, J., Minne, H. W., Quan Hui, Bell, N. H., Rodriguez-Portales, J., Downs, R. W., Dequecker, J., Favus, M. and Seeman, E. (1995). Effects of three years treatment with oral alendronate on fracture incidence in women with post-menopausal osteoporosis. N. Engl. J. Med., **333**, 1437–43

4. Black, D. M., Cummings, S. R. and Thompson, D. for the FIT research group (1996).

Alendronate reduces risk of vertebral and clinical fractures in women with existing vertebral fractures: results of the fracture intervention trial. *J. Bone. Min. Res.*, **11**, pS151, abstr. P242

5. Lufkin, E. G., Wahner, H. W., O'Fallon, W. M., Hodgson, S. F., Kotowicz, M. A., Lane, A. W., Judd, H. L., Caplan, R. H. and Riggs, B. L. (1992).Treatment of postmenopausal osteoporosis with transdermal estrogen. *Ann. Int. Med.*, **117**, 1–9

6. Lindsay, R., Hart, D. M., Forrest, C. and Baird C. (1980). Prevention of spinal osteoporosis in oophorectomised women. *Lancet*, **2**, 1151–4

7. Overgaard, K., Hansen, M. A., Jensen, S. B. and Christiansen, C. (1992). Effect of salcatonin given intra nasally on bone mass and fracture rates in established osteoporosis: a dose-response study. *Br. Med J.*, **305**, 556–61

8. Tilyard, M. W., Spears, G. F. S., Thomson, J. and Dovey, S. (1992). Treatment of postmenopausal osteoporosis with calcitriol or calcium. *N. Engl. J. Med.*, **326**, 357–62

9. Gallagher, J. C., Riggs, B. L., Recker, R. R. and Goldgar, D. (1989). The effect of calcitriol on patients with postmenopausal osteoporosis with special reference to fracture frequency. *Proc. Soc. Exp. Biol. Med.*, **191**, 287–92

10. Orimo, H., Shiraki, M., Hayashi, T. and Nakamura, T. (1987). Reduced occurrence of vertebral crush fractures in senile osteoporosis treated with 1a(OH)-vitamin D_3. *Bone Min.*, **3**, 47–52

11. Recker, R., Kimmel, D. B., Hinders, S. and Davies, K. M. (1994). Antifracture efficacy of calcium in elderly women. *J. Bone Min. Res.*, **9** (Suppl. 1) S154

12. Reid, I. R., Ames, R. W., Evans, M. C., Gamble, G. D. and Sharpe, S. J. (1996). Long-term effects of calcium supplementation on bone loss and fractures in postmenopausal women – a randomised controlled trial. *Am. J. Med.*, in press.

13. Riggs, B. L., Hodgson, S. F., O'Fallon, W. M., Chao, E. Y. S., Wahner, H. W., Muhs, J. M., *et al.* (1990). Effect of fluoride treatment on fracture rate in post-menopausal women with osteoporosis. *N. Engl. J. Med.*, **322**, 802–9

14. Kleerekoper, M., Peterson, E. L., Nelson, D. A., Phillips, E., Schork, M. A., Tilley, B. C. and Parfitt, A. M. (1991). A randomized trial of sodium fluoride as a treatment for postmenopausal osteoporosis. *Osteoporosis Int.*, **1**, 155–61

15. Mamelle, N., Meunier, P. J., Dusan, R., *et al.* (1988). Risk–benefit ratio of sodium fluoride treatment in primary vertebral osteoporosis. *Lancet*, **2**, 3651–5

16. Pak, C. Y. C., Sakhaee, K., Piziak, V., Peterson, R. D., Breslau, N. A., Boyd, P., Poindexter, J. R., Herzog, J., Heard-Sakhaee, Haynes S, Adams-

Huet, B., Reisch, J. S. (1994). Slow-release sodium fluoride in the management of postmenopausal osteoporosis. *Ann. Int. Med.*, **120**, 625–32

17. Chapuy, M. C., Arlot, M. E., Duboeuf, F., Brun, J., Crouzet, B., Arnaud, S., Delmas, P. D. and Meunier, P. J. (1992). Vitamin D_3 and calcium to prevent hip fractures in elderly women. *N. Engl. J. Med.*, **327**, 1637–42

18. Lips, P., Graafmans, W. C., Ooms, M. E., Bezemer, P. D. and Bouter, L. M. (1996). Vitamin D supplemention and fracture incidence in elderly people. *Ann. Int. Med.*, **124**, 400–6

19. Heikinheimo, R. J., Inkovaara, J. A., Harju, E. J., Haavisto, M. J., Kaarela, R. H., Kataja, J. M., Kokko, A. M., Kolho, L. A. and Rajala, S. A. (1992). Annual injection of vitamin D and fractures of aged bones. *Calcif. Tissue Int.*, **51**, 105–10

20. Lauritzen, J. B., Petersen, M. M. and Lund, B. (1993). Effect of external hip protectors on hip fractures. *Lancet*, **341**, 11–13

21. Parfitt, A. M. (1980). Morphologic basis of bone mineral measurements: transient and steady state effects of treatment in osteoporosis. *Min. Electrolyte Metab.*, **4**, 273–87

22. Heaney, R. P. (1994). The bone-remodelling transient: implications for the interpretation of clinical studies of bone mass change. *J. Bone Min. Res.*, **9**, 1515–23

23. Kraenzlin, C. A., Haas, H. G. and Kraenzlin, M. E. (1994). The effectiveness of estrogen-therapy to increase bone mineral density is dependent on the basal bone resorption rate. *J. Bone Min. Res.*, **9** (Suppl. 1), abstr.

24. Civitelli, R., Gopnelli, S., Zacchei, F., Bigazzi, S., Vattimo, A. and Avioli, L. V. (1988). Bone turnover in postmenopausal osteoporosis: effect of calcitonin treatment. *J. Clin. Invest.*, **82**, 1268–74

25. Boyce, R. W., Paddock, C. L., Gleason, J. R., Sletsema, W. K. and Ericksen, E. F. (1995). The effect of risedronate on canine cancellous bone remodelling: three dimensional kinetic reconstruction of the remodelling site. *J. Bone Min. Res.*, **10**, 211–21

26. Storm, T., Steiniche, T., Thamsborg, G. and Melsen, F. (1993). Changes in bone histomorphometry after long-term treatment with intermittent, cyclic etidronate for postmenopausal osteoporosis. *J. Bone Min. Res.*, **8**, 199–208

27. Jones, G., Nguyen, T., Sambrook, P., Kelly, P. J. and Eisman, J. A. (1994). Progessive loss of bone in the femoral neck in elderly people: longitudinal findings from the Dubbo osteoporosis epidemiology study. *Br. Med. J.*, **309**, 691–5

28. Foldes, J., Parfitt, A. M., Shin, M.-S., Rao, D. S.

and Kleerekoper, M. (1991). Structural and geometric changes in iliac bone: relationship to normal aging and osteoporosis. *J. Bone Min. Res.*, **6**, 759–66

29. Cauley, J. A., Seeley, D. G., Ensrud, K., Ettinger, B., Black, D. and Cummings, S. R. (1995). Estrogen replacement therapy and fractures in older women. *Ann. Int. Med.*, **122**, 9–16

30. Maxim, P., Ettinger, B. and Spitalny, G. M. (1995). Fracture protection provided by long-term estrogen treatment. *Osteoporosis Int.*, **5**, 23–9

31. Ensrud, K. E., Palermo, L., Black, D. M., Cauley, J., Jergas, M., Orwoll, E. S., Nevitt, M. C., Fox, K. M. and Cummings, S. R. (1995). Hip and calcaneal bone loss increase with advancing age: longitudinal results from the study of osteoporotic fractures. *J. Bone Min. Res.*, **10**, 1778–87

32. Gallagher, J. C. and Baylink, D. (1990). Effect of estrone sulphate on bone mineral density of the femoral neck and spine *J. Bone Min. Res.*, **5** (Suppl. 2), S275

33. Felson, D. T., Zhang, Y., Hannan, M. T., Kiel, D. P., Wilson, P. W. F. and Anderson J. J. (1993). The effect of postmenopausal estrogen therapy on bone density in elderly women. *N. Engl. J. Med.*, **329**, 1141–6

34. Christiansen, C. and Riis, B. J. (1990). 17β-estradiol and continuous norethisterone: a unique treatment for established osteoporosis in elderly women. *J. Clin. Endocrinol. Metab.*, **71**, 836–84

35. Turner, C. H., Sto, M. and Bryant, H. U. (1994). Raloxifene preserves bone strength and bone mass in ovarectomized rats. *Endocrinology*, **135**, 2001–5

36. Harris, S. T., Watts, N. B., Jackson, R. D., Genant, H. K., Wasnich, R. D., Miller, P. D., Licata, A. A. and Chesnut C. H. III (1993). Four-year study of intermittent cyclic etidronate treatment of postmenopausal osteoporosis: three years of blinded therapy followed by one year of open therapy. *Am. J. Med.*, **95**, 557–67

37. Filipponi, P., Pedetti, M., Fedeli, L., Cini, L., Palumbo, R., Boldrini, S., Massoni, C. and Cristallini, S. (1995). Cyclical clodronate is effective in preventing postmenopausal bone loss: a comparative study with transcutaneous hormone replacement therapy. *J. Bone Min. Res.*, **10**, 697–703

38. Wimalawansa, S. J. (1995). Combined therapy with estrogen and etidronate has an additive effect on bone mineral density in the hip and vertebrae: four-year randomized study. *Am. J. Med.*, **99**, 36–42

39. Falch, J. A., Odegaard, O. R., Finnanger, M. and Matheson, I. (1987). Postmenopausal osteo-porosis: no effect of three years treatment with 1,25-dihydroxycholecalciferol. *Proc. Soc. Exp. Biol. Med.*, **191**, 199–204

40. Gallagher, J. C. and Goldgar, D. (1989). Treatment of postmenopausal osteoporosis with high doses of synthetic calcitriol. A randomized controlled study. *Ann. Int. Med.*, **113**, 649–55

41. Christiansen, C., Christensen, M. S., Rodbro, P., Hagen, C. and Transbol, I. (1981). Effect of 1,25-dihydroxy-vitamin D$_3$ in itself or combined with hormone treatment in preventing post-menopausal osteoporosis. *Eur. J. Clin. Invest.*, **11**, 305–9

42. Jensen, G. F., Christiansen, C. and Transbol, I. (1982). Treatment of post-menopausal osteoporosis. A controlled therapeutic trial comparing oestrogen/gestagen, 1,25-dihydroxy-vitamin D$_3$ and calcium. *Clin. Endocrinol.*, **16**, 515–24

43. Ott, S. M. and Chesnut, C. (1989). Calcitriol treatment is not effective in post-menopausal osteoporosis. *Ann. Int. Med.*, **84**, 267–74

44. Alioa, J. F., Vaswani, A., Yeh, J. K., Ellis, K., Yasumaura, S. and Cohn, S. H. (1988). Calcitriol in the treatment of postmenopausal osteoporosis. *Am. J. Med.*, **84**, 401–8

45. Riggs, B. L., O'Fallon, W. M., Lane, A., Hodgson, S. F., Wahner, H. W., Muhs, J., Chao, E. and Melton, L. J. III (1994). Clinical trial of fluoride therapy in postmenopausal osteoporotic women: extended observations and additional analysis. *J. Bone Min. Res.*, 9, 265–75

46. Meunier, P. J. (1996). Bone forming agents. *Osteoporosis Int.*, **6** (Suppl. 1), 94

47. Shen, V., Dempster, D. W., Birchman, R., Xu, R. and Lindsay, R. (1993). Loss of cancellous bone mass and connectivity in ovariectomized rats can be restored by combined treatment with parathyroid hormone and estradiol. *J. Clin. Invest.*, **91**, 2479–87

48. Ejersted, C., Andreassen, T. T., Nilsson, M. H. L. and Oxlund, H. (1994). Human parathyroid hormone(1–34) increases bone formation and strength of cortical bone in aged rats. *Eur. J. Endocrinol.*, **130**, 201–7

49. Bagi, C. M., van der Meulen, M. C., Adams, S. and Rosen, D. (1994). Treatment with rhIGF-1/IGFBP-3 complex improves cortical bone structure and strength in ovariectomized rats. *J. Bone Min. Res.*, **9** (Suppl. 1), S392

50. Jee, W. S. S., Ueno, K., Deng, Y. P. and Woodbury, D. M. (1985). The effects of prostaglandin E2 in growing rats: increased metaphyseal hard tissue and cortico-endosteal bone formation. *Calcif. Tissue Int.*, **37**, 148–57

51. Centrella, M., McCarthy, T. L. and Canalis, E. (1988). Skeletal tissue and transforming growth factor β. *FASEB J.*, **2**, 3066–73

52. Yasko, A. W., Lane, J. M., Fellinger, E. J., Rosen, V., Wozney, J. M. and Wang, E. A. (1992). The healing of segmental bone defects, induced by recombinant human bone morphogenetic protein (rhBMP-2). *J. Bone Joint Surg.*, **74A**, 659–70

53. Mundy, G. R. (1994). Peptides and growth regulatory factors in bone. *Osteoporosis*, **20**, 577–88

54. Riggs, B. L. (1993). Formation-stimulating regimens other than sodium fluoride. *Am. J. Med.*, **95** (Suppl. 5A), 62S–8S

Alternatives to hormone replacement therapy: what is the role of calcium and vitamin D?

J. D. Ringe

Introduction

One of the challenging public health issues today is the maintenance of skeletal health into old age. Given the worldwide demographic trends towards increasing life-expectancy, there is an urgent need for different concepts of preventing osteoporosis with the aim to reduce health care costs related to vertebral and hip fractures.

Bone is a sex steroid-dependent tissue as proved by a rapid increase of bone mass around the time of puberty and a corresponding loss of bone substance around menopause. Hormone replacement therapy (HRT) is therefore generally regarded as the most physiological and effective prevention of early postmenopausal bone loss. Since there are women with contraindications for HRT and an even larger number primarily non-accepting, or briefly after initiation stopping replacement for various reasons, alternatives are needed to prevent osteoporosis.

Furthermore, the major benefit of HRT is related to the prevention of spinal bone loss, while at the proximal femur a proportion of females may lose bone despite correct hormone replacement[1]. Table 1 gives a listing of hormones and drugs that have been adopted as alternatives for prevention, or early treatment, of postmenopausal osteoporosis. For all these substances more or less positive effects on bone mineral content have been documented[2,3].

The decision for a preventive regimen for an individual patient has to consider age, degree of initial osteopenia, contributing risk factors

Table 1 Alternatives to hormone replacement therapy (HRT) for prevention of postmenopausal osteoporosis

Calcium substitution
Calcium plus vitamin D supplementation
Selective estrogen receptor modulators (SERMs, e.g. tamoxifen, raloxifen)
Synthetic sex steroids (e.g. tibolone)
Salmon calcitonin nasal spray
Bisphosphonates (e.g. etidronate, tiludronate, alendronate)
Low-dose fluoride plus calcium
Vitamin D-metabolites (e.g. alfacalcidol, calcitriol)

and possible comorbidity, and depends furthermore on the personal experience of the prescribing physician. As an important additive to each single or combined treatment selected from Table 1 increased physical activity and exercise can be recommended.

Besides exercise, calcium substitution or calcium plus vitamin D supplementation is of course the most harmless and the cheapest intervention to prevent bone loss. Below, existing data and specific circumstances will be discussed where a positive effect of this simple supplementation can be expected.

Calcium supplementation

Calcium intake is one of many environmental or life-style factors that influence bone loss and risk of osteoporosis. Since calcium is a threshold nutrient, the effect of supplementation above the threshold is a very different issue from the effect of a chronically inadequate calcium intake. The latter may contribute to low bone mass either because calcium intake during growth limits achievement of genetically programmed peak skeletal mass, or because low consumption later in life aggravates involutional loss, or both[4,5].

There is accumulated evidence today that in perimenopausal and early postmenopausal years calcium supplementation alone is not able to prevent progressive bone loss in most women[6,7]. Obviously the rather mild anti-resorptive effect of calcium is not sufficient to stop high bone turnover in this phase of female life. It was shown, however, that in early postmenopausal years calcium has an additive effect to HRT, or may allow a dose reduction of estrogen[8]. This effect can be achieved with both increasing dietary calcium content, mainly by a high intake of dairy products, or by oral calcium supplementation.

The efficacy of pure dietary supplementation has not been studied extensively to date. In one trial with an increased dairy intake corresponding to an average calcium supply of 500 mg/day there was no impact on vertebral bone mass until month 18. After 36 months, however, there was a significant treatment effect that resulted mainly from an acute decline in bone density in the control group[9].

The daily oral calcium intake should amount to 1000 or even better 1500 mg[10]. Since this is in general not feasible with diet alone and may be accompanied by a too high calorie and cholesterol supply for individual cases, we recommend that the basal dietary calcium intake should be roughly assessed and the remainder given by oral supplements.

Eight to 10 years after menopause, calcium alone may become a realistic alternative to HRT in the prevention of osteoporosis[11]. In two different studies comparing HRT with calcium and/or exercise or placebo, HRT increased bone mineral density (BMD) slightly and calcium kept BMD in its initial range while the groups with placebo or exercise showed significant losses[12,13]. In a 2-year study on 236

postmenopausal women, supplementation with 800 mg calcium per day had no effect on bone density in a subgroup of younger women (mean age 54.5 years), but a bone-sparing potency in older women (mean age 59.9 years)[6]. This effect was only statistically significant in women with a dietary calcium intake below 400 mg and not in cases with a daily consumption between 400 and 650 mg. Another result from this study was that supplementation with calcium citrate–maleate was more effective than with calcium carbonate[6]. It may be concluded from this study that the chance of a benefit from calcium supplements is inversely related to the basal dietary intake.

In a placebo-controlled study from New Zealand on 122 normal postmenopausal women with an average dietary intake of 750 mg calcium per day, the addition of 1000 mg calcium per day significantly slowed down axial and appendicular bone loss[14]. The mean age of the women was 58 years and the average time since menopause was 9.5 years. The course of lumbar BMD expressed as per cent change from base-line during the 2 years of this important study is shown in Figure 1.

More important than modest benefits in BMD is the impact of supplemented calcium on fracture rate. Information on the antifracture efficacy of added calcium from prospective studies is limited. There is one report of a randomized calcium intervention trial with a mean follow-up of over 4 years[15]. In

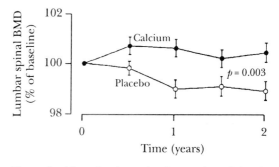

Figure 1 Mean lumbar spine bone mineral density (BMD) ($\pm$ SE) in postmenopausal women given calcium supplementation or placebo for 2 years. Based on a reanalysis from reference 14

this study postmenopausal women with a mean dietary calcium intake of 433 mg per day were supplemented with 1200 mg elemental calcium or placebo (Table 2). Spine X-rays were performed at the beginning and end of the study. Use of calcium reduced the vertebral fracture rate in a high-risk subset with pre-existing vertebral fractures but not in subjects without previous fracture events[15].

During another 4-year study, nine fractures occurred in seven women in the placebo group (two proximal femur, three forearm, one vertebral, three phalanges metatarsal) and only two were observed in the calcium group (one forearm, one metatarsal)[16]. Although the total number of fractures was small, the difference in fracture incidence between the two groups was significant (Figure 2).

Calcium alone is not considered adequate treatment for patients with established osteoporosis but as an essential adjunct to therapy with antiresorptive or osteoanabolic agents. For prevention, however, in healthy women or patients with preclinical osteoporosis (T-score between –1.0 and –2.5 SD), it has additive effects to HRT and stops bone loss by itself in women 8 or more years after menopause.

Vitamin D plus calcium

Cholecalciferol given as a monotherapy in physiological doses has no significant effect on postmenopausal bone loss. In a controlled 2-year study on healthy postmenopausal women there was no significant difference in the radial bone mineral content between the vitamin D or placebo group[17].

No further acceptable studies were performed to assess the efficacy of native vitamin D alone for prevention of postmenopausal osteoporosis. For treatment with pharmacological doses, however, two studies had already been carried out in the 1970s[18,19]. The conclusion from both studies using doses between 10 000 and 50 000 iu per day was nearly the same, i.e. that calciferol alone was no promising therapy for established

Table 2 Incidence of vertebral fractures in calcium-treated postmenopausal women, with and without pre-existing fractures. From reference 15, with permission

	No. treated with	
Fracture status and outcome	Placebo	Calcium
With pre-existing fractures ($n = 94$)		
new fractures	21	15*
no new fractures	20	38*
Without pre-existing fractures ($n = 103$)		
new fractures	13	12
no new fractures	48	30

*Differs from placebo, $p = 0.023$

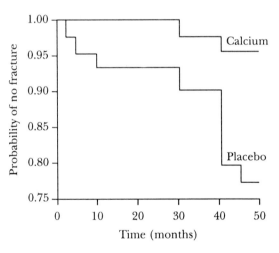

Figure 2 Probability of no fracture in calcium and placebo group. The difference in fracture rates between the two groups was significant ($p = 0.037$). Modified from reference 16

postmenopausal osteoporosis. In a third study including several treatment arms with different combinations of HRT, calcium, vitamin D and sodium fluoride, there was also no evidence to support the use of pharmacological doses of vitamin D (50 000 iu twice weekly) for established postmenopausal osteoporosis except than as cotherapy with fluoride[20].

More recently interest has centered on the correction of subclinical vitamin D deficiency in later life with small, physiological doses of vitamin D. Several studies had revealed that vitamin D deficiency is a frequent metabolic disorder in the elderly. Up to 60% of elderly persons and 70–100% of residents of homes for elderly people have an inadequate vitamin D status often combined with increased parathyroid hormone values[2].

This secondary hyperparathyroidism causes increased bone turnover with a negative bone balance[21]. There is a correlation between decreased levels of 25-hydroxy-cholecalciferol and clinical manifestation of senile osteoporosis, especially occurrence of hip fractures. Women with hip fractures have lower serum levels of vitamin D than age-matched controls. Another independent risk factor is little protein intake or even undernutrition in the elderly. Correspondingly in a study performed on 172 patients with hip fracture in Lausanne, low albumin was a strong biochemical predictor of increased risk[22]. Further important risk factors for hip fracture include low BMD, living in nursing homes and sedentariness.

Today it is generally accepted, however, that in the complex pathogenesis of senile osteoporosis, the secondary hyperparathyroidism due to vitamin D deficiency and low calcium intake is a very important contributing factor. In a study from Lyon it was shown in 1987 that vitamin D in a dose range from only 400 to 800 iu per day was able to increase 25-hydroxy-vitamin D levels in blood, and to normalize parathyroid hormone[23]. Recently it has again been shown that a supplementation with calcium and vitamin D in elderly women is very effective in suppressing parathyroid hormone levels and reducing bone turnover[24].

Three large trials have been conducted to date assessing the effect of calciferol administration with or without calcium on fractures in the elderly. In the study from Finland almost 800 elderly persons were randomized to receive 150 000 iu vitamin D_2 annually (in 1 of 5 years 300 000 iu were given) or to act as controls[25]. Circulating levels of 25-hydroxy-vitamin D were normalized in patients receiving the ergocalciferol injections, but a significant fall in

alkaline phosphatase was only observed during the year with 300 000 iu injection (corresponding approximately to 800 iu per day). The total number of symptomatic fractures was reduced by 25% in the vitamin D-treated subjects ($p = 0.03$).

In the French 3-year study 3270 women aged 69–106 years living in institutions for the elderly were included[26]. One-half received after random allocation 800 iu vitamin D and tricalcium phosphate corresponding to 1.2 g elemental calcium per day. At the end of 3 years the probabilities of nonvertebral fractures and hip fractures were reduced by 24 and 29% respectively (Figure 3) in the active intervention group ($p < 0.001$).

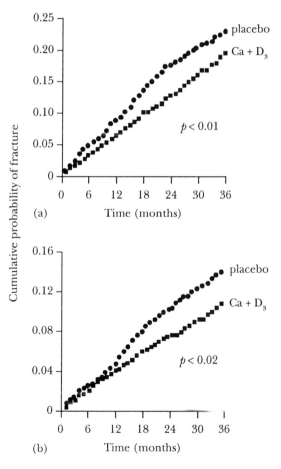

(a)

(b)

Figure 3 Cumulative probability for hip fractures (a) or all non-vertebral fractures (b) in placebo or vitamin D plus calcium group. From reference 2

Table 3 Features of three major studies assessing efficacy of vitamin D supplements with or without calcium for prevention of fractures in the elderly

	Heikinheimo et al. 1992[25]	Chapuy et al. 1994[26]	Ooms et al. 1995[27]
Patients included (*n*)	800	3270	2578
Mean age (years)	86	84	80
Follow-up (years)	5.0	3.0	3.5
Dietary calcium (mg/day)	ND	500	600–1000
Intervention			
vitamin D (iu)	150–300th./year	800/day	400/day
calcium (mg)	—	1200/day	—
Outcome: reduction of			
hip fractures	—	29%	NS
non-vertebral fractures	—	24%	—
total fractures	25%	—	—

ND, not determined; NS, not significant

In the Dutch study on 2578 subjects over age 70 years only 400 iu vitamin D per day were given[27]. Since the average calcium intake of the participants by diet had been estimated rather highly at 600–1000 mg per day, no additional calcium was supplemented. A significant effect on hip fracture incidence could not be proved in this study although BMD at the proximal femur improved in the vitamin D group.

Table 3 gives an overview of these three controlled intervention trials. Obviously a supplementation of 400 iu is too low and additional calcium substitution is essential to improve not only biochemical indices and BMD but also to reduce fracture rates.

Conclusions

Hormone replacement therapy is the first choice for prevention of postmenopausal spinal bone loss but there are data suggesting that it is not always effective in reducing bone loss at the proximal femur.

From the different alternatives for prevention of postmenopausal osteoporosis, supplementation with calcium and physiological doses of vitamin D is an inexpensive and effective approach under suitable circumstances.

Calcium substitution *per se* has an additive effect to HRT. However, calcium alone is not sufficient to stop increased early postmenopausal bone loss and only becomes effective 6–8 years post menopause.

Cholecalciferol has no significant preventive or therapeutic effect in vitamin D-replete postmenopausal women. Since vitamin D deficiency increases with advancing age, cholecalciferol supplements in combination with calcium are very effective, however, in later life, in reducing secondary hyperparathyroidism, bone loss and fracture incidence.

References

1. Hillard, T. C., Whitcroft, S. J., Marsh, M. S., Ellerington, M. C., Lees, B., Whitehead, M. I. and Stevenson, J. C. (1994). Long-term effects of transdermal and oral hormone replacement therapy on postmenopausal bone loss. *Osteoporosis Int.*, **4**, 341–8
2. Ringe, J. D. and Meunier, P. J. (1996). *Osteoporotic Fractures in the Elderly. Clinical*

Management and Prevention. (Stuttgart and New York: Georg Thieme)

3. Marcus, R., Feldman, D. and Kelsey, J. (eds.) (1996). *Osteoporosis*, pp. 1159–87. (San Diego, New York, London: Academic Press)

4. Nelson, D. A. (1996). An anthropological perspective on optimizing calcium consumption for the prevention of osteoporosis. *Osteoporosis Int.*, **6**, 325–8

5. Heaney, R. P. (1992). Calcium in the prevention and treatment of osteoporosis. *J. Intern. Med.*, **231**, 169–80

6. Dawson-Hughes, B., Dallal, G. E., Krall, E. A., Sadowski, L., Sahyoun, N. and Tannenbaum, S. (1990). A controlled trial of the effect of calcium supplementation on bone density in postmenopausal women. *N. Engl. J. Med.*, **323**, 878–83

7. Riis, B., Thomsen, K. and Christiansen, C. (1987). Does calcium supplementation prevent postmenopausal bone loss? *N. Engl. J. Med.*, **316**, 173–7

8. Ettinger, B., Genant H. K. and Cann, C. E. (1987). Postmenopausal bone loss is prevented by treatment with low-dosage estrogen with calcium. *Ann. Intern. Med.*, **106**, 40–5

9. Baran, D., Sorensen, A., Grimes, J., Lew, R., Karellas, A., Johnson, B. and Roche, J. (1989). Dietary modification with dairy products for preventing vertebral bone loss in postmenopausal women: a three-year prospective study. *J. Clin. Endocrinol. Metab.*, **70**, 264–70

10. National Institutes of Health consensus development panel on optimal calcium intake (1994). Optimal calcium intake. *J. Am. Med. Assoc.*, **4**, 469–75

11. Ettinger, B. (1992). Role of calcium in preserving the skeletal health of aging women. *South. Med. J.*, **85** (Suppl. 2), 22–30

12. Aloia, J. F., Vaswani, A., Yeh, J. K., Ross, P. L., Flaster, E. and Dilmanian, F. A. (1994). Calcium supplementation with and without hormone replacement therapy to prevent postmenopausal bone loss. *Ann. Intern. Med.*, **120**, 57–103

13. Prince, R. L., Smith, M., Dick, I. M., Price, R. I., Webb, P. G., Henderson, N. K. and Harris, M. M. (1991). Prevention of postmenopausal osteoporosis. A comparative study of exercise, calcium supplementation, and hormone-replacement therapy. *N. Engl. J. Med.*, **325**, 1189–95

14. Reid, I. R., Ames, R. W., Evans, M. C., Gamble, G. D. and Sharpe, S. J. (1993). Effect of calcium supplementation on bone loss in post-menopausal women. *N. Engl. J. Med.*, **328**, 460–4

15. Recker, R. R., Kimmel, D. B., Hinders, S. and Davies, K. M. (1994). Antifracture efficacy of calcium in elderly women. *J. Bone Min. Res.*, **9** (Suppl. 1), 135

16. Reid, I. R., Ames, R. W., Evans, M. C., Gamble, G. D. and Sharpe, S. J. (1995). Long-term effects of calcium supplementation on bone loss and fractures in postmenopausal women: a randomized controlled study. *Am. J. Med.*, **98**, 331–5

17. Christiansen, C., Christensen, M. S. and McNair, P. (1980). Prevention of early postmenopausal bone loss: controlled 2-year study in normal postmenopausal females. *Eur. J. Clin. Invest.*, **10**, 273–9

18. Buring, K., Hulth, A. G., Nilsson, B. E., Westlin, N. E. and Wiklund, P. E. (1974). Treatment of osteoporosis with vitamin D. *Acta Med. Scand.*, **195**, 471–2

19. Nordin, B. E. C., Horsman, A., Crilly R. G., Marshall, D. H. and Simpson, M. (1980). Treatment of spinal osteoporosis in postmenopausal women. *Br. Med. J.*, **1**, 451–4

20. Riggs, B. L., Seeman, E., Hodgson, S. F., Taves, D. R. and O'Fallon, W. M. (1982). Effect of fluoride/calcium regimen on vertebral fracture occurrence in postmenopausal osteoporosis. *N. Engl. J. Med.*, **306**, 444–50

21. Ashby, J. P., Newman, D. J. and Rinsler, M. G. (1989). Is intact PTH a sensitive biochemical indicator of deranged calcium homeostasis in vitamin D deficiency? *Ann. Clin. Biochem.*, **26**, 324

22. Burckhardt, P., Burnand, B., Thiebaud, D., Constanza, M., Sloutskis, D., Giliard, D., Quinodoz, F., Landry, M. and Paacaud, F. (1995). Low albumin is a major risk factor for hip fracture. *Bone*, **16** (Suppl. 189), Abstr. 416

23. Chapuy, M. C., Chapuy, P. and Meunier, P. J. (1987). Calcium and vitamin D supplements: effects on calcium metabolism in the elderly. *Am. J. Clin. Nutr.*, **46**, 324

24. Prestwood, K. M., Pannullo, A. M., Kenny, A. M., Pilbeam, C. C. and Raisz, L. G. (1996). The effect of a short course of calcium and vitamin D on bone turnover in older women. *Osteoporosis Int.*, **6**, 314–9

25. Heikinheimo, R. J., Inhkovaara, J. A., Harju, E. J., Haavisto, M. V., Kaarela, R. H., Kataja, J. M., Kokko, A. M., Kolho, L. A. and Rajala, S. A. (1992). Annual injection of vitamin D and fractures of aged bones. *Calcif. Tissue Int.*, **51**, 105–10

26. Chapuy, M. C., Arlot, M. E., Delmas, P. D. and Meunier, P. J. (1994). Effect of calcium and cholecalciferol treatment for three years on hip fractures in elderly women. *Br. Med. J.*, **308**, 1081–2

27. Ooms, M. E., Lips, P., Roos, J. C., Bezemer, P. D. and Bouter, L. M. (1994). Prevention of bone loss by vitamin D supplementation in elderly women: a randomized double blind trial. *Endocrinol. Metab.*, **80**, 1052

A new estrogen gel: clinical benefits 24

A. Viitanen

Introduction

Today, estrogen treatment is still most frequently used to relieve the symptoms related to estrogen deficiency during the perimenopause. With increasing age, the relative number of users decreases. It is widely accepted, however, that estrogen replacement therapy also has long-term benefits such as prevention of osteoporosis[1] and prevention of cardiovascular diseases[2,3]. Recent evidence even suggests that prevention of dementia and maintenance of cognitive functions could be achieved with estrogen treatment[4]. For long-term benefit treatment compliance is of critical importance. One determinant of compliance is the mode of treatment. Therefore, treatment alternatives with new features are welcomed; a gel formulation, Divigel®/Sandrena®, represents such an alternative.

Pharmacokinetic studies

The pharmacokinetics of the gel have been studied in postmenopausal women (Nykänen, unpublished data, 1996). After administration of the gel, estradiol is rapidly absorbed through the skin. In this study with a 1.0 mg estradiol dose corresponding to 1.0 g of the gel, the average maximum estradiol concentration was around 400 pmol/l (397 ± 80 pmol/l); the maximum concentration was achieved 3–4 h after administration. The estradiol level remained around 200 pmol/l until the next dose.

The effect of the size of the application area on the bioavailability of the gel was studied in the same randomized crossover trial with postmenopausal women. One gram of the gel was applied on an area of 200 cm² or 400 cm², or an undefined area that was as large as possible on one or both thighs. Bioavailability decreased with increasing application area: area under the curve (AUC) values were (mean ± SEM) 5827 ± 788, 4934 ± 1232 and 2748 ± 222 pmol/l) × h, respectively. Based on our experience from clinical trials, 1.0 g of the gel (1.0 mg estradiol) is most conveniently applied on an area of approximately 200–400 cm², which corresponds to the size of an area of one to two hands.

It is unlikely that patients would wash the area of application soon after applying the gel. However, the effect on bioavailability of washing the application area has also been studied (Nykänen, unpublished data, 1996). A 1.0 g dose of the gel was applied on the 14th study day to an area of 400 cm², and blood samples for determining the concentration–time curve were obtained. On the 15th study day the same amount of gel was applied to the same area, but the area was washed with water and soap 30 min after the application. Blood samples for determining the concentration–time curve were obtained as for day 14. After washing, the bioavailability was lower but the effect of washing did not appear to be clinically significant, as the mean concentration maxima and minima and the concentration–time curve profiles were quite similar.

It can be concluded from the pharmacokinetic studies that estradiol is well absorbed from the gel, and that sufficient estradiol levels are reached with administration of 1.0 g of the gel on an area corresponding to that of one or two hands.

Clinical studies

The clinical effects of the gel have been evaluated in several clinical trials. In these

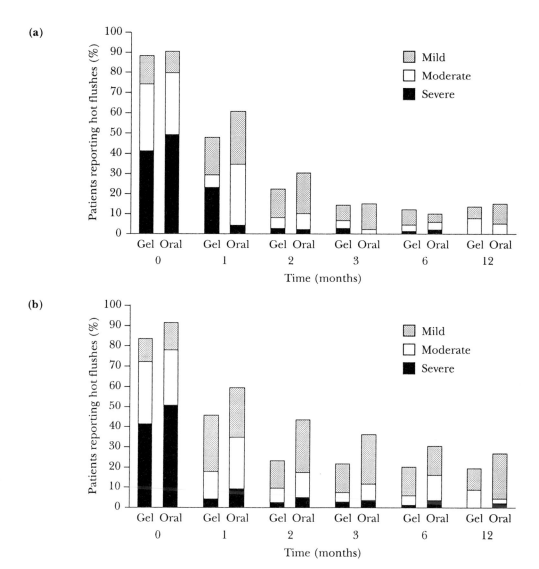

Figure 1 Effect of estrogen gel (1.0 mg estradiol) and oral estradiol valerate (2 mg) on (a) hot flushes and (b) sweating

studies, the effective dose range has been 0.5–1.5 mg of estradiol (corresponding to 0.5–1.5 g of the gel).

Although the aim is often towards the long-term benefits of estrogen treatment, most patients seek alleviation of their menopausal symptoms. The effect of 1.0 mg of estradiol as the gel on menopausal symptoms was compared with that of 2 mg of oral estradiol valerate in a parallel-group controlled study (Hirvonen,

unpublished data, 1990). Both treatments highly significantly and equally effectively reduced the frequency of occurrence of hot flushes and sweating (Figure 1a and b).

In another parallel-group controlled study, the gel (0.5–1.5 g dose) was compared with a patch (25–100 µg estradiol dose). Similar statistically significant and equal effects on alleviation of hot flushes (Figure 2a) and sweating (Figure 2b) were seen (Hirvonen, unpublished data, 1993).

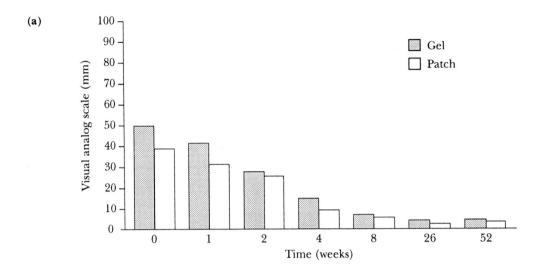

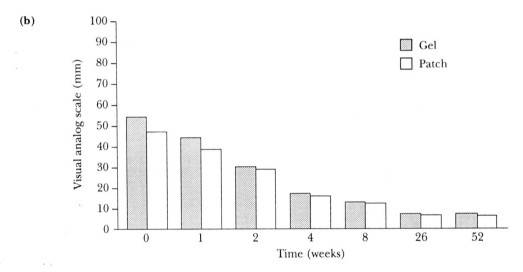

Figure 2 Effect of estrogen gel (0.5–1.5 mg estradiol) and patch (25–100 µg estradiol/24 h) on (a) hot flushes and (b) sweating

In an early study, bone mineral density was measured with single photon absorptiometry (Hirvonen, unpublished data, 1990). Although the number of patients followed up for 24 months was small, the effect on bone density seemed to be equal with the 1.0 mg estradiol dose of gel and 2 mg of oral estradiol valerate. A more recent study compared a patch delivering 25–100 µg of estradiol in 24 h with a 0.5–1.5 mg estradiol dose as the gel (Hirvonen, unpublished data, 1993). After 12 months of follow-up, the effects of the treatments on bone mineral density were comparable.

One important factor that has an influence on compliance is the occurrence of adverse events. Breast tension is one of the most common adverse drug reactions to estrogen replacement therapy. In the study of Kesäniemi and colleagues, breast tension was reported by 20% of the patients treated with the 1.0 g dose of the gel, but by 35% of those treated with 2 mg of oral estradiol valerate (Kesäniemi, unpublished data, 1996). In the study comparing the gel and a patch, the reported incidence of breast tension was lower, 7% and 3%, respectively (Hirvonen, unpublished data, 1993).

Skin irritation, which has been a frequent adverse event with a patch, has been mild and transient with the gel treatment. Out of approximately 600 patients treated with the gel in the clinical study series, only one patient discontinued the study because of skin irritation related to the formulation. About 5% of patients reported skin irritation; the vast majority of cases were of mild to moderate intensity and transient. This is in clear contrast with the reported rate (20–40%) of skin irritation with patches[5]. In a study where the gel and a patch were compared, the incidence of skin irritation was 47% with the patch compared to 3% with the gel (Hirvonen, unpublished data, 1993).

In conclusion, this new gel provides an effective and well-tolerated transdermal treatment mode for estrogen replacement therapy with a low incidence of skin irritation. It has a further advantage of being invisible.

References

1. Conference report (1993). Consensus Development Conference: diagnosis, prophylaxis and treatment of osteoporosis. *Am. J. Med.*, **94**, 646–50
2. Grodstein, F., Stampfer, M. J., Manson, J. E., Colditz, G. A., Willett, W. C., Rosner, B., Speizer, F. E. and Hennekens, C. H. (1996). Postmenopausal estrogen and progestin use and the risk of cardiovascular disease. *N. Engl. J. Med.*, **335**, 453–61
3. Bush, T. C., Barret-Connor, E. and Cowan, L. D. (1987). Cardiovascular mortality and non-contraceptive use of estrogen in women: results from the Lipid Research Clinics Program Follow-up Study. *Circulation*, **75**, 1102–9
4. Tang, M., Jacobs, D., Stern, Y., Marder, M., Schofield, P., Gurland, B., Andrews, II. and Mayeux, R. (1996). Effect of oestrogen during menopause on risk and age at onset of Alzheimer's disease. *Lancet*, **348**, 429–32
5. Balfour, J. A. and Heel, R. C. (1990). Transdermal estradiol. A review of its pharmacodynamic and pharmacokinetic properties, and therapeutic efficacy in the treatment of menopausal complaints. *Drugs*, **40**, 561–82

The health economics of osteoporosis and estrogen replacement therapy

25

R. L. Prince

Introduction

In this review various assumptions commonly made about the role of estrogen in health care are challenged. The first is that health economics is irrelevant to patient care. The second, based on a health–economic analysis, is that estrogen treatment is best started at the menopause.

Health economics as a tool has a variety of uses in the maintenance and improvement of the health of individuals and societies. In essence it is a comparative evaluation of costs and outcomes of different methods of preventing and treating disease. As such it may be used by a variety of professional groups, all of whom presumably want the best health outcomes for the least cost. To date economic analysis has been the preserve of the academic health economist and governments. However, there are benefits to the clinician in terms of medical decision-making which may be assisted by an understanding of the health–economic approach. For the clinician advising the individual with a disease, the question is 'which intervention is going to provide the best control of the disease impact with the fewest side-effects for the least cost?' In this situation a comparative evaluation of outcomes, for example fractures saved or life-years gained, using different therapies would be extremely valuable in deciding which therapy should be used. If the patient has a brief self-limiting disease with one causative factor, such as pneumonia, the answer to this question may be clear. However, for many chronic diseases, for example osteoporosis, the answer is by no means as clear. This is because the connection between the development of disability due to the disease and interventions to prevent this progression are not intuitively obvious, due to the longer duration of time over which the disabilities develop and the multifactorial nature of the disease process. In these circumstances a comparative mathematical evaluation of interventions and outcomes is often required, to allow a decision to be made on which intervention actually is the best under the particular circumstances of the case.

In considering inputs to prevention of disability due to disease it is necessary to consider cost. The question of cost that the patient can afford depends on the social and economic structure, present in an individual country, set up to pay for disease management. In countries where private or public insurance underwrites the cost of disease management, the decision on what treatment is available to the patient may be determined by a central organization rather than the patient and clinician. It is imperative that, under these circumstances, decisions having cost implications are taken with improved patient care in mind. Furthermore it is important that these decisions are understood and supported by clinicians and patients. Thus the remainder of this review will be written to highlight some of these issues primarily with the clinician in mind.

Types of health–economic evaluation

The methodology used in health–economic evaluation is clearly critically important for understanding its effects. The major problem relates to assessment of outcomes, as the cost of the intervention itself is usually clear-cut. There are three types of outcome evaluation commonly used: cost effectiveness, cost utility and cost benefit. The first, cost effectiveness, is the closest to clinical end-points as it uses these as the denominator, for example in cost per fracture saved. To get a broader view, cost per life-year gained may be the end-point. If so, it is necessary to estimate not only the number of fractures saved but the effect these will have on longevity. Furthermore the monetary cost of the fracture saved must be evaluated as this will reduce the numerator. The monetary cost of particular interventions varies from one country to another, and depends not only on the monetary cost of fracture management but also on the cost of the consequent disability.

A further level of complexity is to consider a cost–utility analysis which involves an assessment of the quality of life with the aim of maximizing it; the units are cost per quality-adjusted life-year gained. The advantage of this approach is that health care is directed towards the maximization of quality as well as quantity of life. The disadvantage of this approach is that quality of life is, according to its very nature, subjective so that few people agree on the factors constituting quality of life. This becomes a particular problem when quality comes to be measured. A variety of approaches have been developed, all of which are dependent on questionnaires designed to determine the value that individuals put on a particular disease state. This may be done by asking how many years of life an individual would forgo to avoid the disease state in question (time trade-off). Alternatively, questionnaires have been developed, for example the Short Form 36 (SF 36), which include evaluation of a variety of quality-of-life 'domains'. Other questionnaires include the Nottingham Health Profile and Euroquol. Although comprehensive, these questionnaires are often not sensitive or specific enough to detect the impact of a specific disease. Thus disease-specific questionnaires have been developed.

Finally, cost-benefit analyses are purely economic analyses which simply consider costs of the treatment versus the monetary costs of disability saved in terms of the actual cost of health care supplied to the individual and in terms of wages lost. This form of analysis would, for example, discriminate against patients who were not in the work-force.

Having decided the outcome measure to be used, it is then necessary to decide the magnitude of the treatment effect. The reliability with which this can be determined depends on the time frame over which the analysis is to occur. In analysis of effects lasting 3–5 years it is likely that data will be available from randomized trials. If analyses are directed to longer time frames, treatment effects have to be derived from epidemiological studies which have a lower validity. The data for these analyses are usually derived from meta-analyses of large numbers of studies. Furthermore, over long time frames and with agents having effects on various diseases, it is necessary to use conditional probability models to allow for interactions between disease processes.

Effects of estrogen on competing risks of disease

Evaluating the effects of estrogen must be one of the most complex of health–economic analyses to be undertaken. This is because it has effects on so many organ systems in the body (Figure 1). The critical issue is that if the patient survives one disease as a result of the treatment, she is available to die of another disease. Since the diseases that estrogen affects cause mortality

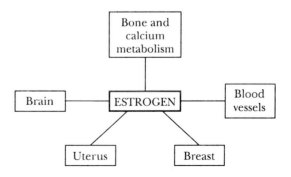

Figure 1 Sites of estrogen action

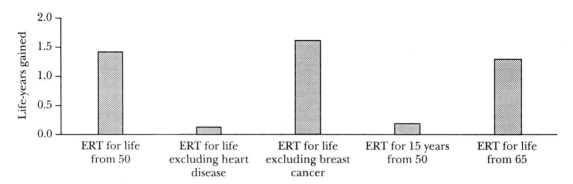

Figure 2 Quality-adjusted life-years gained from estrogen replacement therapy (ERT). With no intervention, average life expectancy is 82 years

in old age, any saving of life-years at this time is likely to be small, because if the patient survives one disease she is available to die of another.

We have examined these interactions in a conditional probability model using current data on long-term effects of estrogen derived from meta-analysis[1,2]. We utilized relative risks of 0.5 for heart disease, 0.96 for stroke, 1.3 for breast cancer and 0.1 for hip fracture[3]. This optimistic evaluation of lifetime risk of hip fracture with estrogen treatment is derived from a model which relates hip fracture to bone density and age. We concluded that, with these assumptions, the overall benefit of estrogen for life is limited to about 1.4 extra life-years in addition to the average life expectancy of 82 years, a relatively small gain that many would consider insignificant when the decision to commence treatment is being made at the age of 50 (Figure 2). In view of the long time frame between commencing estrogen at the menopause and prevention of disease such as hip fracture or heart disease, we have examined the concept of introducing estrogen at age 50 or 65 for life, or from age 50 for 15 years. In this last scenario we assumed that the benefits of estrogen disappear after 5 years. The results of the analysis are shown in Figure 2. Treatment for just 15 years from age 50 to 65 increased longevity by only 0.2 years. However treating with estrogen from the age of 65 for the rest of life produced results very similar to treating from age 50 for life, at 1.3 life-years gained. This

is because most preventable events are occurring after age 65.

More recently we have recalculated the overall survival benefit following estrogen using relative risks of 0.65 for heart disease, 0.96 for stroke, 1.45 for breast cancer and 0.75 for hip fracture. Under this scenario there is an increase in longevity of 1.2 years following lifetime estrogen treatment from age 50. Furthermore the excess mortality from breast cancer is only slightly less than the reduced mortality from heart disease for the first 10 years of treatment (Figure 3).

Costs

We next examined the costs of the three interventions (Figure 4). Not unexpectedly it showed that estrogen treatment for 15 years was much cheaper than treating for the whole of life from age 50 or 65. Somewhat more surprising is the fact that a large part of the incremental cost was due to extra nursing-home costs after estrogen treatment. The reason for this is that if the subject does not die of a myocardial infarct, she is then available to enter a nursing home as a result of other disease processes. As the risk of entry into a nursing home is very age-dependent, any increased longevity will increase the probability that the subject will enter a nursing home with its consequent costs.

Finally, to get an overall picture it is usual to calculate the cost per life-year gained (Figure

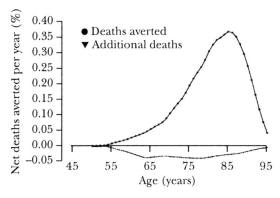

Figure 3 Net deaths averted, and caused, in cohort per year with estrogen intervention from age 50. Most deaths averted were due to the reduction in heart disease. All deaths caused were due to breast cancer

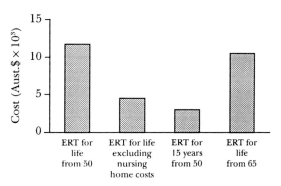

Figure 4 Extra costs for estrogen replacement therapy (ERT), including those for drugs, hip fracture treatment, endometrial monitoring, endometrial and breast cancer treatment, heart disease treatment and nursing home fees. Cost of no intervention is Aust.$74 000

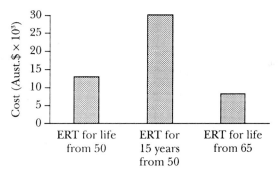

Figure 5 Discounted cost for estrogen replacement therapy (ERT) per quality-adjusted life-year gained

5). It is clear that estrogen treatment for 15 years is much less cost-effective than either of the other two interventions, because although costs of therapy are reduced, the benefits of intervention are also reduced. These data are in contrast to a study of Tosteson and colleagues[4] which suggested a much more optimistic scenario for 15 years' treatment. The differences arise because their analysis assumed that the benefits of treatment were maintained over a longer time frame than the 5 years we assumed.

It is also clear from Figure 5 that estrogen treatment from age 65 is slightly more cost-effective if discounting for future events at 5% per year is included in the analysis. Discounting has the effect of favoring the later intervention simply because costs (and benefits) are occurring further into the future and therefore cost less. Without discounting, the two interventions are more comparable.

Conclusions

As a result of these analyses it is apparent that, if the aim of estrogen replacement is to prevent heart disease and hip fracture, there is little point in commencing treatment at age 50 when the events to be prevented will not occur for 20–30 years. Furthermore these women are still at a relatively high risk of breast cancer which may be increased by estrogen therapy. After the age of 65 breast cancer becomes a less likely way to die when compared with heart disease.

It is clear that economic analyses have significant limitations. For example there are problems in evaluating quality of life and extrapolation over 30–50 years may not be valid. However, the modeling approach does allow one to make explicit assumptions and to examine their effects. Currently many women are prescribed estrogen to prevent events that are not expected to occur for many years. The approach presented in this paper allows a more precise evaluation of the likely effects of estrogen treatment.

References

1. Grady, D., Rubin, S. M., Pettiti, D. B., Fox, C. S., Black, D., Ettinger, B. *et al.* (1992). Hormone therapy to prevent disease and prolong life in postmenopausal women. *Ann. Intern. Med.*, **117**, 1016–37

2. Stampfer, M. J. and Colditz, G. A. (1991). Estrogen replacement therapy and coronary heart disease: a quantitative assessment of the epidemiologic evidence. *Prevent. Med.*, **20**, 47–63

3. Geelhoed, E., Harris, A. and Prince, R. (1994). Cost-effectiveness analysis of hormone replacement therapy and lifestyle intervention for hip fracture. *Aust. J. Public Health*, **18**, 153–60

4. Tosteson, A. N. A., Rosenthal, D. I., Melton, J. M. III and Weinstein, M. C. (1990). Cost effectiveness of screening perimenopausal white women for osteoporosis: bone densitometry and hormone replacement therapy. *Ann. Intern. Med.*, **113**, 594–603

A screening model for osteoporosis using dermal skin thickness and bone densitometry

26

M. P. Brincat, R. Galea and Y. Muscat Baron

Introduction

Increasingly, the postmenopausal phase of a woman's life is being viewed as a time during which the whole body experiences an accelerated aging process. Acute symptoms of menopause such as hot flushes and sweats herald the beginning of this new phase in a woman's life. Unlike these acute symptoms, more serious sequelae such as postmenopausal osteoporosis and cardiovascular disease are more difficult to extricate from the effects of aging[1].

The quality of bone is not easy to assess, although it can be reliably quantified by measurement of bone density. The diagnosis of osteoporosis and its response to hormone replacement therapy is therefore rather difficult[2]. Postmenopausal osteoporosis is increasingly considered to be due to accelerated collagen loss[3–5], similarly to the effect of the menopause on organs of mesodermal origin (skin dermis, cardiovascular system and bladder trigone). Collagen loss from the skin has been shown to correlate with bone mass[6–8]. Brincat and co-workers have shown that hormone replacement therapy increases the collagen content in both bone and skin in postmenopausal women, compared with age-matched controls[6]. Skin thickness, similarly to bone mass and skin collagen, has been shown to increase in postmenopausal women treated with estrogen[6,9]. The mode of action of hormone replacement therapy in increasing bone mass has not been clearly defined, and the pathology of postmenopausal osteoporotic fracture requires further investigation. Any additional information relating to the quality of bone, rather than simply its quantity, would thereby aid in determining who is likely to have strong bones and therefore less likely to incur fracture.

By the age of 75 years, more than 25% of women develop osteoporotic fractures[10]. The three classic osteoporotic fractures are: fractures of the vertebrae, distal end of the radius and neck of the femur. Fractures of the femoral neck lead to considerable morbidity and mortality.

Albright and colleagues noted that postmenopausal women with osteoporotic fractures had thin skin. They suggested that these women had a general diminution of connective tissue[11]. Skin and bone parameters have been investigated, and their potential in the screening of menopausal osteoporosis by using combined indices has been assessed. It is possible that both osteoblastic and osteoclastic activity might be responsible in the etiology of bone loss and its response to estrogens, with the entire bone remodeling unit functioning at a different level.

Bone densitometry alone, however, is not effective for the screening of osteoporotic fracture[12], and screening methods continue to be inaccurate. In an attempt to improve accuracy, a connective-tissue parameter, dermal skin thickness, was combined with bone mineral density measurement in our study. The aims of the study were: (1) to determine the efficacy of skin thickness as a screening test for osteoporotic fracture, either alone or (2) in combination with other bone-density parameters.

Patients and methods

Women were recruited sequentially from the gynecology out-patients' department and the bone density unit at the Department of Obstetrics and Gynecology, University of Malta Medical School. Women who had sustained osteoporotic fractures were referred by the Department of Orthopedics. A total of 540 postmenopausal women were recruited. Patient data are given in Table 1.

All women had their bone density and skin thickness measured. Bone density measurements were carried out using a Norland dual energy X-ray absorptiometry (DEXA) 386 machine, and were taken from the lumbar spine (L2–L4), femoral neck and Ward's triangle. Skin thickness was measured at the medial side of the left arm using an Osteoson 22-MHz ultrasound probe (Minhorst, Germany). An average of five measurements was taken in order to minimize any error. The bone densitometer was specified as having a coefficient of variation of 1.5%, while the ultrasound probe was specified as having a coefficient of variation of 1.7%.

Statistical analysis

The following formulae were used in order to calculate the various risk factors.

Specificity was calculated using the formula

$$\frac{\text{false positives}}{\text{false positives} + \text{true negatives}}$$

Sensitivity was calculated using the formula

$$\frac{\text{true positives}}{\text{true positives} + \text{false negatives}}$$

Accuracy was calculated using the formula

$$\frac{\text{true positives} + \text{true negatives}}{\text{true positives} + \text{false positives} + \text{false negatives} + \text{true negatives}}$$

This method compares true positives and negatives with the total tested; results were expressed as percentages.

Table 1 Study patient data

	Controls	Fractures
Patients (*n*)	411	129
Mean age (SD) (years)	54 (9.0)	68 (11)
Mean duration of menopause (SD) (years)	8 (8.0)	21 (11)

Results

Scattergrams of bone densities at L2–L4 and at Ward's triangle in relation to skin thickness are shown in Figure 1(a) and (b). At a cut-off point of 0.9 mm skin thickness, the highest accuracy as defined above of 58% for measurement of skin thickness alone was obtained. This was, however, at the expense of sensitivity and specificity which were decreased to 59% and 42% respectively. At a cut-off point of 1 mm skin

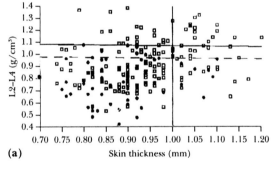

(a)

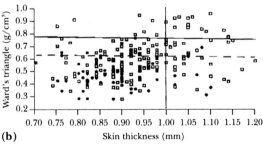

(b)

Figure 1 Scattergrams of bone densities at (a) lumbar spine (L2–L4) and (b) Ward's triangle vs. skin thickness. Open squares, controls (*n* = 411); solid circles, fractures (*n* = 129)

thickness, the accuracy of the method decreased to 39% but the sensitivity increased to about 91% (Table 2). In order to attain a balance between accuracy and sensitivity, a combination of skin thickness and bone density measurement was used.

The combination of skin thickness to bone density measurements showed that a very high sensitivity could be maintained (91.7 and 91.8%). Accuracy was in the range 39.6–50.9% with the various bone density measurements on their own, but using the combination model (represented in Figure 1 as the measurements enclosed in a box) the accuracy was increased to a range 50.1–59.1%. This represents a useful increase in accuracy.

Conclusions

This study indicates that skin thickness is as effective a screening test for the likelihood of osteoporotic fracture as bone density measurement. When skin thickness measure-

Table 2 Calculated sensitivities and accuracies of skin thickness and bone density measurements

	Sensitivity (%)	Accuracy (%)
Skin thickness	91.7	39.2
Ward's triangle	100.0	50.9
Lumbar spine (L2–L4)	100.0	39.6
*Box Ward's triangle	91.7	59.1
*Box lumbar spine (L2–L4)	91.8	50.1

*'Box' values refer to the combination model

ments are combined with bone density measurements the accuracy of this screening method increases.

Skin thickness measurement alone achieved sensitivity of 91.7% but an accuracy of 39.2%; however, this measurement has the advantage of being very rapid and cheap to perform. Furthermore, the equipment used is small and mobile, unlike the usual bone densitometer.

References

1. Brincat, M., Studd, J. W. W., O'Dowd, T., Magos, A. L., Cardozo, L., Wardle, P. J. and Cooper, D. (1984). Subcutaneous hormone implants for the control of climacteric symptoms: a prospective study. *Lancet*, **1**, 16–18

2. Lindsay, R. (1988). Pathogenesis, detection and prevention of postmenopausal osteoporosis. In Studd, J. W. W. and Whitehead, M. I. (eds.) *The Menopause*, pp. 156–67. (Oxford, London, Edinburgh: Blackwell Scientific Publications)

3. Brincat, M., Moniz, C. J., Kabalan, S., Versi, E., O'Dowd, T., Magos, A. L., Montgomery, J. and Studd, J. W. W. (1987). Decline in skin collagen content and metacarpal index after the menopause and its prevention with sex hormone replacement. *Br. J. Obstet. Gynaecol.*, **94**, 126–9

4. Sarrell, P. M. (1990). Ovarian hormones and circulation. *Maturitas*, **12**, 287–98

5. Versi, E., Cardozo, L. D., Brincat, M., Cooper, D., Montgomery, J. C. and Studd, J. W. W. (1988). Correlation of urethral physiology and skin collagen in postmenopausal women. *Br. J. Obstet. Gynaecol.*, **95**, 147–52

6. Brincat, M., Moniz, C. J., Studd, J. W. W., Darby, A., Magos, A., Emburey, G. and Versi, E. (1985). Long term effects of the menopause and sex hormones on skin thickness. *Br. J. Obstet. Gynaecol.*, **92**, 256–9

7. Brincat, M., Moniz, C. F., Studd, J. W. W., Darby, A. J., Magos, A. L. and Cooper, D. (1983). Sex hormones and skin collagen content in postmenopausal women. *Br. Med. J.*, **287**, 1337–8

8. Castelo-Branco, C., Pons, F., Gratacós, E., Fortuny, A., Vanrell, J. A. and González-Merlo, J. (1994). Relationship between skin collagen and bone changes during aging. *Maturitas*, **18**, 199–206

9. Meschia, M., Bruschi, F., Amicarelli, F. and Barbacini, P. (1994). Transdermal hormone replacement therapy and skin in post-menopausal women: a placebo controlled study. *Menopause*, **1**(2), 79–82

10. Jensen, G. F., Christiansen, C., Boesen, J., Hegedus, V. and Transbol, I. (1982). Epidemiology of postmenopausal spine and longbone fractures: a unifying approach to

postmenopausal osteoporosis. *Clin. Orthopaed. Rel. Res.*, **166**, 75–81

11. Albright, F., Smith, P. H. and Richardson, A. M. (1941). Postmenopausal osteoporosis – its clinical features. *J. Am. Med. Assoc.*, **116**, 2465–74

12. Johnston, C. C., Slemenda, C. W. and Milton, L. J. III (1991). Clinical use of bone densitometry. *N. Engl. J. Med.*, **324**, 1105–9

Bone density and skin thickness changes in postmenopausal women on long-term corticosteroid therapy

27

Y. Muscat Baron, M. Brincat and R. Galea

Introduction

In his original series of studies on hypercortilism due to basophil adenomas, Cushing noted certain dermatological changes, and some patients had also sustained osteoporotic fractures[1]. Since the widespread application of long-term steroid therapy in clinical practice, skin- and bone-related complications in addition to many others are more frequently being encountered. This study was carried out to measure skin thickness and bone density changes in postmenopausal women taking long-term corticosteroids. Measurements were compared with those from a number of controls (postmenopausal females), patients who had sustained osteoporotic fractures and post-menopausal women on hormone replacement therapy.

Methods

The study was carried out in the bone density unit at St Luke's Hospital in Malta, between the years 1993 and 1995. Skin thickness was measured by a high-resolution 22.5-MHz ultrasound probe (Minhorst D III). Bone density measurements were carried out on a dual X-ray absorptiometry unit (Norland DEXA 386).

The skin thickness of the medial aspect of the left mid-arm was measured. Five readings were taken from each patient and the average was then determined. Bone density measurements of the lumbar spine (L2–L4) and the left hip were performed.

Sixty-four postmenopausal females who had been on long-term corticosteroids for more than 2 years were recruited. These were compared with three groups of women: (1) control population; (2) patients who had sustained osteoporotic fractures; (3) women on hormone replacement therapy for more than 2 years (Table 1).

A smaller prospective study was carried out whereby 29 postmenopausal women on steroid therapy had been followed up for 1 year at 6-monthly intervals. Of these women, nine were on hormone replacement therapy, 14 were not having any treatment and six were taking either etidronate, calcitonin or progesterone.

Results

Significant differences were found in the skin thickness and bone density of the post-menopausal women on long-term steroid

Table 1 Patient data. HRT, hormone replacement therapy

	Controls	Osteoporotic fractures	HRT	Steroid therapy
Patients (*n*)	557	180	399	64
Age (years)	53	67	53	56
Menopausal age (years)	45.4	47.3	46.2	47.9

therapy. The lowest (0.83 mm) skin thickness measurements were obtained with women taking corticosteroids (Figure 1). Patients who had sustained osteoporotic fractures had a mean skin thickness of 0.88 mm. Statistical significance was found when comparing the skin thickness of the steroid and fracture groups with the control population and the group of women on hormone replacement therapy. The mean skin thickness of both the control group and the women on hormone replacement therapy was found to be 0.93 mm.

Bone density measurements of the lumbar spine and left hip showed very similar patterns to those of the skin thickness. The mean bone density of the lumbar spine for both the fracture group and the women on steroid therapy was 0.81 g/cm³. This was significantly lower than the readings obtained for the control population and the women on hormone replacement therapy, who were found to have a mean bone density of 0.93 g/cm³ (Figure 2).

A similar pattern of bone density measurements was obtained for the left femoral neck. The bone densities of the steroid and fracture groups were again very similar, the mean being 0.71 g/cm³ (Figure 3). This was found to be significantly lower than that of the control population (0.80 g/cm³, and the group of women on hormone replacement therapy (0.82 g/cm³).

The small prospective study showed significant increases in both bone density and skin thickness in the women given hormone replacement therapy (Figures 4, 5 and 6).

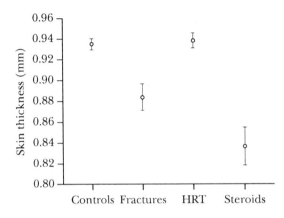

Figure 1 Skin thickness measurements of four study groups. HRT, hormone replacement therapy. Significant differences: controls vs. fractures, fractures vs. HRT, $p < 0.001$; controls vs. steroids, HRT vs. steroids, $p < 0.0001$

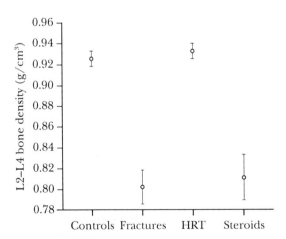

Figure 2 Lumbar spine (L2–L4) bone density measurements of four study groups. HRT, hormone replacement therapy. Significant differences: controls vs. fractures, fractures vs. HRT, HRT vs. steroids, $p < 0.0001$; controls vs. steroids, $p < 0.0002$

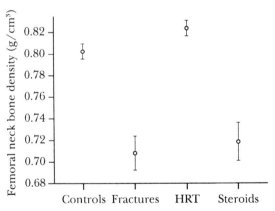

Figure 3 Femoral neck bone density measurements of four study groups. HRT, hormone replacement therapy. Significant differences: controls vs. fractures, controls vs. steroids, fractures vs. HRT, HRT vs. steroids, $p < 0.0001$

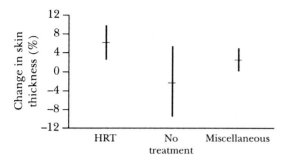

Figure 4 Average annual percentage change in skin thickness for three study groups. HRT, hormone replacement therapy. Significant difference: controls vs. HRT, $p < 0.001$

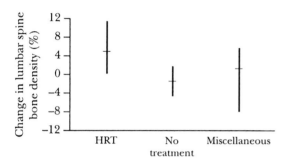

Figure 5 Average annual percentage change in lumbar spine bone density for three study groups. HRT, hormone replacement therapy. Significant difference: controls vs. HRT, $p < 0.0001$

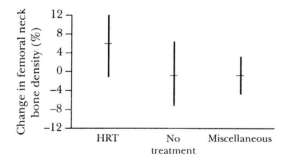

Figure 6 Average annual percentage change in femoral neck bone density for three study groups. HRT, hormone replacement therapy. Significant differences: controls vs. HRT, $p < 0.001$; HRT vs. miscellaneous, $p < 0.01$

Discussion

The therapeutic effect of glucocorticoids as anti-inflammatory agents was first recognized by Hirsch and colleagues in 1949[2]. This effect was inferred from the relief pregnancy induced in women who suffered from rheumatoid arthritis. This relief is due to the high serum levels of corticosteroids during pregnancy.

Since the 1950s the indications for the use of glucocorticoids have expanded considerably. Concomitantly it became evident that serious side-effects accompanied prolonged exposure to these anti-inflammatory agents.

Osteoporosis is one serious side-effect of long-term steroid therapy, leading to severe morbidity and mortality. Since the initial use of these anti-inflammatory agents, a large number of patients have reached an age whereby the combination of the aging process, the menopause and long-term steroid therapy has dealt a severe blow to the skeleton. This is reflected in significantly reduced bone density measurements, reaching critical fracture levels. The effect can be easily appreciated from our study whereby the bone density readings of patients on long-term steroids were very low, on a par with those patients who had sustained osteoporotic fractures.

At the cellular level, steroid-induced osteoporosis appears to occur as a result of the reversal of bone formation[2]. The reduction of osteoblastic matrix formation has been recognized after corticosteroid therapy[3]. Simultaneously it appears that osteoclastic activity is accelerated, encouraging osseous breakdown[4].

Calcium metabolism appears to be adversely affected by prolonged glucocorticoid therapy. Diminished gut sensitivity to vitamin D reduces calcium absorption[5]. Secondary hyperparathyroidism may occur leading to loss of renal and intestinal calcium[6]. Prolonged glucocorticoid use may also significantly decrease serum levels of sex hormones such as estradiol, estrone and androstenedione[7].

Throughout the cross-sectional study reported here, the patterns of both bone density and skin thickness closely mirrored each other for all four categories of postmenopausal women. This suggests a close relationship of skin and bone in the response to long-term steroid therapy.

Albright and co-workers[8] recognized the frequency of thin skin of patients who had sustained osteoporotic fractures. It was suggested that the loss of connective tissue in the skin may be more generalized and may also occur in bone. Connective tissue is found throughout the body to such an extent that collagen, its main component, constitutes one-third of the body mass[9].

Significant loss in human and animal skin has been noted after long-term corticosteroid therapy[9]. Purpuras and skin thickness loss of 28–39% have been recorded following oral glucocorticoid treatment. This loss still persisted albeit to a smaller degree (15–19%) when high-dose inhaled steroids were used[10].

The small prospective study showed that the women treated with hormone replacement therapy had significant increases in bone density and skin thickness. Optimum levels of estrogen given to postmenopausal women appear to increase the skin collagen content, increasing the skin thickness[11]. This may also contribute to the increased bone density and skin thickness observed in our study.

In conclusion, this study showed that significantly low skin thickness and bone density measurements were obtained for patients on long-term steroid therapy. These results were very similar to those obtained in patients who had sustained osteoporotic fractures. The small prospective study suggests that hormone replacement therapy may be a useful adjunct for women on long-term glucocorticoids.

References

1. Cushing, H. (1932). Basophil adenomas. *J. Neur. Ment. Dis.*, **76**, 50
2. Avern, H. and Clellingworth, M. (1994). Prevention and management of steroid induced osteoporosis. *Br. J. Hosp. Med.*, **52**, 86–92
3. Canalis, E. M. (1983). Effect of glucocorticoids on type I collagen synthesis, alkaline phosphatase activity and deoxyribonucleic acid content in cultured rat calvariae. *Endocrinology*, **112**, 931
4. Reid, I. R., Katz, J. R. *et al.* (1986). The effects of hydrocortisone, parathyroid hormone and the biphosphonate APD on bone resorption in neonatal mouse calvariae. *Calcif. Tiss. Int.*, **38**, 38
5. Hahn, T. J., Halstead, L. R. and Teiralbaun, S. L. (1988). Altered mineral metabolism in glucocorticoid induced osteopaenia: effect of 25-hydroxyvitamin D administration. *J. Clin. Invest.*, **64**, 655–65
6. Suzuki, Y., Ichiwana, Y., Saito, E. and Homm, A. M. (1983). Importance of increased urinary calcium excretion in the development of secondary hyperparathyroidism of patients under glucocorticoid therapy. *Metabolism*, **32**, 151–6
7. Crilly, R. G., Francis, R. M. and Nordin, B. E. C. (1981). Steroid hormones, ageing and bone. *Clin. Endocrinol. Metab.*, **10**, 115–39
8. Albright, F., Bloomberg, E. C. and Smith, P. H. (1940). Postmenopausal osteoporosis. *Trans. Assoc. Am. Phys.*, **55**, 298–305
9. Hall, D. (1981). Gerontology and collagen diseases. *Clin. Endocrinol. Metab.*, **2**, 23
10. Finlay, A., Capewell, S., Reynolds, S., Shuttleworth, D. and Edwards, D. (1990). Purpura and dermal thinning associated with high dose inhaled corticosteroids. *Br. Med. J.*, **300**, 1548–51
11. Brincat, M., Versi, E., Moniz, C., Magos, A, de Trafford, J. and Studd, J. W. W. (1987). Skin collagen changes in postmenopasusal women receiving different regimens of oestrogen therapy. *Obstet. Gynaecol.*, **70**, 123

5

Hormones and breast cancer

Role of hormones in human breast development: the menopausal breast

28

J. Russo and I. H. Russo

Introduction

The human breast, which at birth is a rudimentary bilateral organ, develops as the result of a combination of external and internal factors, all of which are intimately linked to the female reproductive system[1]. These factors, in turn, are modified by cultural, socioeconomic and environmental influences. Thus, in modern industrialized societies the fundamental role of the breast, nourishment of the offspring, becomes progressively less relevant, but at the same time this organ acquires new relevance because it constitutes the source of the most frequent malignancy in women. The higher risk of developing breast cancer has been associated with lengthened ovarian function, such as that occurring with early menarche and late menopause[2-8]. The increased risk associated with nulliparity or late first full-term pregnancy, or the protection afforded by early first full-term pregnancy are an indication that reproductive events, mainly through the hormonal influences of the new endocrine organ represented by the placenta, play important roles in modulating the susceptibility of the breast to undergo malignant transformation[1].

In order to clarify the complexity of these interactions the development of the breast has to be viewed as an integral component of a four-tiered system, which is comprised of the central nervous system, with the hypothalamus and the anterior pituitary gland as major directors, exerting their influence on the reproductive system, mainly the ovaries, which in turn act on the ductal structures, the uterus, the Fallopian tubes and the breast[9-12].

Hypothalamic–pituitary influences on breast development

The hallmark of childhood is body growth which is in great part regulated by growth hormone (GH), produced by cells of the anterior pituitary gland. This hormone belongs, together with prolactin (PRL) and the placental lactogen (PL), to a family of polypeptide hormones that have arisen by duplication of an ancestral gene. Two major effects are mediated by GH: stimulation of skeletal and soft tissue growth, mediated by insulin-like growth factor I (IGF-I) or somatomedin, and a receptor-mediated direct effect on carbohydrate and lipid metabolism. Fetal GH appears in the first trimester of pregnancy, reaching a maximum level at the 20th week, its concentration falling thereafter. During childhood the secretion of GH peaks approximately 1 h after the onset of deep sleep, with smaller peaks occurring at later periods in the sleep cycle. Breast development during these periods parallels body growth. Specific changes in breast morphology occur with the initiation of ovarian function. The driving signal of female gonadal function is the hypothalamic decapeptides gonadotropin-releasing hormone (GnRH) or luteinizing hormone-releasing hormone (LHRH)[9-11]. Gonadotropin secretion in childhood is minimal. The pubertal awakening of gonadotropic secretion is thought to be of central origin; it is genetically controlled and linked to the attainment of a critical body weight. Gonadotropin secretion is first related to sleep periods, but later occurs throughout the 24 h of the day, increasing for 3–4 years before a cyclic pattern begins and regular menstrual periods are established. Gonadotropin-releasing hormone is secreted in a pulsatile manner by hypophysiotropic neurons in the arcuate nucleus of the hypothalamus. Its release is modified by the opposing influences of at least two catecholamines: dopamine, acting as an inhibitor, and norepinephrine, acting as a facilitator. GnRH is transported to the gonadotropic cells of the anterior pituitary via the pituitary portal system. After binding to specific membrane receptors, GnRH stimulates the production of two gonadotropins, follicle-stimulating hormone (FSH) and luteinizing hormone (LH). Luteinizing hormone secretion is pulsatile; each pulse reflects a prior pulse of GnRH, with sequential changes in both the amplitude and the frequency of LH pulses throughout the menstrual cycle. When a regular cycle is established, FSH secretion begins to rise during the last few days of the prior menstrual period; this secretion stimulates the ripening of a cohort of ovarian follicles, of which one soon dominates. Increasing estradiol secretion by this follicle potentiates the local action of FSH and also exerts positive feedback at the pituitary, contributing to a sudden midcycle rise in FSH and LH. This midcycle surge, crucial to ovulation, appears to require ovarian steroids, an increase in GnRH pulse frequency and probably other factors. The peak of LH contributes to ovulation, manifested as the rupture of the leading follicle, and to the formation of the corpus luteum. During the luteal phase LH pulses are of greater amplitude than in the follicular phase, but the frequency is sometimes reduced to one pulse per day, with an abrupt decline in the serum levels.

The anterior pituitary synthesizes and releases PRL, an activity that is negatively controlled by the hypothalamus via production of prolactin-inhibiting factor (PIF). This inhibition in turn is controlled by the amount of catecholamines released from nerve endings in the hypothalamus. Estrogen acts on the pituitary gland to increase PRL release and on the hypothalamus to decrease PIF, thus increasing prolactin secretion by dual mechanisms. In addition the thyroid hormones, acting directly on the pituitary, increase prolactin secretion[1]. Data seem to substantiate the theory that estrogens are mammary carcinogens in rodents because of their stimulatory effects on prolactin secretion. However, the role of prolactin in the development of breast cancer in women is uncertain[13].

Ovarian influences on breast development

The ovary secretes estrogens, inhibins, progesterone and androgens. The principal estrogen, 17β-estradiol, has dramatic stimulatory effects on the breast, uterus, vagina and distal urethra. In the first half of each menstrual cycle, estrogen stimulates endometrial proliferation and induces production of estrogen and progesterone receptors in endometrial cells. Progesterone is the primary product of the corpus luteum; its level rises progressively after ovulation, accompanied by a second peak of estradiol. In the first 1 to 2 years after menarche, only about 10% of cycles are ovulatory. In these cycles, the amount of progesterone secreted is lower than in adults, and the length of the luteal phase is shorter. In the course of the 2 to 3-year period after menarche, the proportion of ovulatory cycles increases, the peak levels and total secretion of progesterone rise, and the luteal phase reaches its normal duration of 14 days. During the luteal phase, FSH and LH levels are presumably suppressed by the rise in estrogen and progesterone. Towards the end of the 2-week life-span of the corpus luteum, estrogen and progesterone levels fall, endometrial shedding begins, and a menstrual period results. A new cycle begins immediately, as FSH levels start to rise and several follicles mature. The ovary also synthesizes inhibins and activins that affect the FSH level. Inhibins suppress pituitary secretion of FSH. The serum level of inhibin rises late in the follicular phase of each cycle and reaches a peak on the day of ovulation. Thereafter, inhibin is produced in the corpus luteum, and rising levels of this hormone during the early luteal phase may contribute to the falling levels of FSH that occur during the luteal phase. Activins, on the other hand, increase FSH secretion. Both compounds have other endocrine, paracrine, and probably autocrine influences, but their exact roles in the menstrual cycle have yet to be defined[14,15]. Testosterone and androstenedione are secreted directly by the ovary. They contribute to the anabolic state in females, and secreted androstenedione serves as a prohormone for peripheral conversion to testosterone or estrone. In excess they inhibit the normal menstrual cycle[11].

Influence of placental hormones and growth factors on breast development

The reproductive process from initiation is deeply dependent on hormonal and neural factors. The maternal corpus luteum that is instrumental in the preparation of the endometrium for implantation, is in turn rescued by the luteotropic hormone chorionic gonadotropin (CG) secreted by the primitive trophoblast of the blastocyst within hours of implantation. In women, human CG (hCG) stimulates the corpus luteum to synthesize progesterone, 17-hydroxyprogesterone, estradiol, inhibin and relaxin[1]. The corpus luteum constitutes the major source of progestational steroids until the 9th week of gestation, when the placenta becomes the sole source of these hormones, as demonstrated by the lack of effect of ovariectomy after the 9th week on the progression of pregnancy. The placenta has evolved in mammals as an efficient mechanism for transporting nutrients to the fetus, excreting waste products into the maternal blood stream, and for influencing maternal physiology through the newly secreted placental and fetal hormones. In humans, the placenta becomes fully developed by the end of the first trimester of pregnancy. The syncytiotrophoblast of the chorionic villus, the functional unit of the placenta, synthesizes progesterone, hCG and human placental lactogen (hPL). The cytotrophoblast is the

source of several neuropeptides first discovered in the brain, such as gonadotropin-releasing hormone (GnRH), thyrotropin-releasing hormone (TRH), somatostatin, corticotropin-releasing factor (CRF), and propiomelano-cortin, and the gonadal peptide inhibin[16]. Chorionic gonadotropin (CG) is a polypeptide hormone composed of an α and a β subunit. The α subunit is identical to that of pituitary gonadotropins, whereas the β subunit differs in aminoacid sequence[17]. The most widely known action of CG is the maintenance of the corpus luteum during pregnancy, an action that is identical to that of the pituitary gonadotropin LH, with a small degree of FSH activity[18,19]. The breast has been traditionally considered to be a passive target of sex steroid hormones. This concept, however, is being challenged by modern day research reporting the discovery of a direct inhibitory effect of hCG on human breast epithelial cell proliferation, and the induction of inhibin synthesis[1]. New hormones and growth factors are being discovered to be locally synthesized in the breast, suggesting that this organ might self-regulate its development through autocrine or paracrine effects. This promising area of research remains to be developed.

Human breast as a developing organ

The human breast is one of the few organs of the body that is not completely developed at birth; it reaches its fully differentiated condition only after a full term pregnancy, under the stimulus of new endocrine organs, the placenta and the developing fetus. These new hormonal influences induce a profuse branching of the mammary parenchyma leading to the formation of fully secretory lobular structures[20]. The study of the branching pattern of the breast requires a three-dimensional analysis of the organ in order to evaluate the relationship of terminal and lateral branches to the main lactiferous ducts. A more limited vision is provided by the classical two-dimensional histological sections in which the topographic arrangement of ducts, ductules and alveoli or acini allows reconstruction and categorization of specific lobular units. Each lobular structure has been morphologically characterized by its size, number of ductules per unit and the number of cells per ductule, reflecting different stages of development. The earliest or more undifferentiated structure identified in the breast of postpubertal nulliparous women is the lobule type 1 (Lob 1), also called terminal ductal lobular unit (TDLU); it is composed of clusters of 6 to 11 ductules per lobule. These progress to lobules type 2 (Lob 2), which have a more complex morphology, being composed of a higher number of ductular structures per lobule. During pregnancy, Lob 1 and Lob 2 rapidly progress to lobules type 3 (Lob 3), and secretory lobules type 4 (Lob 4). Lob 3 are characterized by having an average of 80 small alveoli per lobule. When active milk secretion supervenes, the alveoli become distended, a characteristic of the Lob 4 present during the lactational period. After weaning, all the secretory units of the breast regress, reverting to Lob 3 and Lob 2.

Influence of menopause on breast structure

Menopause supervenes as the consequence of the atresia of more than 99% of the 7 million follicles that are present in the ovaries of a female fetus at a gestational age of 5 months[21]. Gonadotropin-releasing hormone secretion is also implicated in this phenomenon, indicating that a hypothalamic process is involved in the development of menopause. The most characteristic sign of menopause is amenorrhea, which is the result of the almost complete cessation of ovarian estrogen and progesterone production. The years leading up to the final menstrual period, until menopause sets in generally at around age 51 years, constitute the perimenopause. During this time, many women ovulate irregularly, either because the rise in estrogen during the follicular phase is insufficient for triggering an LH surge, or because the remaining follicles are resistant to the ovulatory stimulus. The increase in human

longevity occurring in our society has caused a considerable increment in the number of women who will live one-third or more of their lives in the menopausal period, namely without natural estrogen and progesterone[22]. After menopause the breast undergoes a regressive phenomenon both in nulliparous and parous women. This regression is manifested as an increase in the number of Lob 1, and a concomitant decline in the number of Lob 2 and Lob 3[23,24]. At the end of the fifth decade of life the breast of both nulliparous and parous women contains Lob 1 (Figure 1). These observations led us to conclude that the understanding of breast development requires a horizontal study in which all the different phases of growth are taken into consideration. For example, the analysis of breast structures at a single given point, i.e. age 50 years, would lead us to conclude that the breast of both nulliparous and parous women appears identical. However, the phenomena occurring in prior years might have imprinted permanent changes in breast biology that affect the

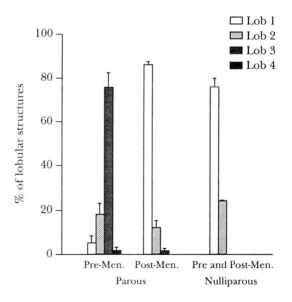

Figure 1 Percentage of lobular structures in breast of pre- (Pre-Men.) and postmenopausal (Post-Men.) parous and nulliparous women. Lob 1, lobules type 1; Lob 2, lobules type 2; Lob 3, lobules type 3; Lob 4, lobules type 4

potential of the breast for neoplasia, but are no longer morphologically observable. Thus, from a quantitative point of view the regressive phenomenon occurring in the breast at menopause differs in nulliparous and parous women. In the breast of nulliparous women the predominant structure is the Lob 1, which comprises 65–80% of the total lobular component, and their relative percentage is independent of age. Second in frequency is the Lob 2, which represents 20–35% of the total. The least frequent is the Lob 3, which represents only 0–5% of the total lobular population. In the breast of premenopausal parous women, on the other hand, the predominant lobular structure is the Lob 3, which comprises 70–90% of the total lobular component[23]. Only after menopause do they decline in number, and the relative proportion of the three lobular types present approaches that observed in nulliparous women. These observations led us to conclude that early parous women truly underwent lobular differentiation, which was evident at a younger age, whereas nulliparous women seldom reached the Lob 3, and never the Lob 4 stages.

The epidemiological observation that nulliparous women exhibit a higher incidence of breast cancer than early parous women[2], and the fact that the most frequent breast malignancy is the ductal carcinoma that originates in Lob 1, or TDLU[25], suggest that the lobules type 1 present in the breast of these two groups of women might be biologically different, or exhibit different susceptibility to carcinogenesis[23,24,26]. The morphological differences however are subtle. Lob 1 of the nulliparous woman's breast have a very active intralobular stroma, composed of loose connective tissue. In the parous woman's breast, Lob 1 have a stroma with a hyalinized appearance. Similar differences indicative of a regressive phenomenon have been observed in the breast tissue of women treated with hormones. Another important difference is that the Lob 1 have higher proliferative activity in the nulliparous than in the parous woman's breast, as determined by the use of the Ki67

marker. More significant is the fact that in the nulliparous breast there is a low proportion of cells in the G_0 phase of the cycle, being the opposite in the parous woman's breast, even if Lob 1 are present. These observations indicate that the lobules type 1 of the nulliparous breast are active centers of proliferation. These characteristics might explain the higher susceptibility of these structures to develop carcinomas. We concluded that the lobules type 1 found in the breast of nulliparous women never went through the process of differentiation, whereas the lobules type 1 of parous women did.

Cell proliferation and hormone receptors in relation to breast structure

Although ductal breast cancer originates in Lob 1, or TDLU[25], the epidemiological observation that nulliparous women exhibit a higher incidence of breast cancer than early parous women[2] suggests that Lob 1 in these two groups of women might be biologically different, or exhibit different susceptibility to carcinogenesis[27–30]. At the present time it is not known whether specific genes are responsible for or control these differences. What is known is that the branching of the mammary ducts proceeds under the influence of circulating hormones for stimulation of and synchronization with reproductive events. The branching is also influenced by local factors which provide signals that influence glandular growth, differentiation and morphogenesis.

Cell proliferation is a cell function essential for normal growth. It also plays a crucial role in the development of malignancies[23,24,31]. Normal growth requires a net increase of cycling cells over two other cell populations, resting cells (arrested in G_0) and dying cells (cells lost through programmed cell death or apoptosis). The proliferative activity of the mammary epithelium varies as a function of the degree of lobular differentiation. Lob 1 have a higher proliferative index than Lob 2, 3 and 4 (Table 1). These differences are not abrogated when

Table 1 Cell proliferation in lobular structures of nulliparous and parous women's breast, determined immunocytochemically using monoclonal antibody against Ki67 antigen. Results are expressed as mean ± SD

Group	Age (years)	Lob 1 (% labeled cells)	Lob 2 (% labeled cells)	Lob 3 (% labeled cells)	Lob 4 (% labeled cells)	Ducts (% labeled cells)	Total (% labeled cells)
Nulliparous	42 ± 10	5.53 ± 2.68*	0.77 ± 0.31*	—	—	3.23 ± 1.31**	3.68 ± 2.27***
Parous	48 ± 11	0.89 ± 0.20*	0.18 ± 0.07*	0.11 ± 0.06*	0.0*	1.36 ± 0.23**	1.05 ± 0.15***

* $p < 0.01$, nulliparous Lob 1 vs. Lob 2, parous Lob 1 vs. Lob 2, Lob 3 and Lob 4, nulliparous Lob 1 vs. parous Lob 1, nulliparous Lob 2 vs. parous Lob 2; **$p < 0.02$, nulliparous Ducts vs. parous Ducts; ***$p < 0.03$, nulliparous Total vs. parous Total

the phases of the menstrual cycle are taken into consideration[32]. In addition to exerting an important influence in the lobular composition of the breast as described above, parity profoundly influences the proliferative activity of the mammary epithelium. Lob 1 and Lob 2 present in the breast of premenopausal nulliparous women exhibit a significantly higher proliferative activity than those lobules found in the breast of parous women (Table 1). After menopause sets in the proliferative activity of the mammary epithelium decreases, but although less pronounced, the differences between the nulliparous woman and parous woman's cell proliferation in breast structures are maintained.

Estrogens and progesterone are known to promote proliferation and differentiation in the normal breast epithelium. Both steroids act intracellularly through a receptor which, when activated by its binding with the hormone, regulates the expression of specific genes[33,34]. However, the mechanism by which these molecules exert their mitogenic and differentiation effect has not been clearly established[35–43]. One of the accepted mechanisms of action of steroid hormones postulates that the proliferation of cells is the response to direct stimulation, as the result of the interaction of the estradiol bound to the estrogen receptor (ER) with the DNA[34]. Measurement of the levels of ER and progesterone receptor (PgR) in normal breast in the cytosol fraction, using standard biochemical techniques, is inaccurate because

of the low cellularity of the tissue. The use of monoclonal antibodies which specifically recognize ER and PgR makes it possible to identify and to quantitate the cells expressing these receptors[32]. Both ER and PgR are present in the nucleus of epithelial cells. However, the percentage of cells expressing these receptors varies as a function of the degree of lobular development of the breast, and therefore of the type of lobular structure analyzed. Lob 1 are the structures more consistently containing a higher percentage of ER- and PgR-positive cells than Lob 2, 3 and 4, an observation that indicates that a progressive decrease in the percentage of cells exhibiting an immunocytochemically positive reaction for these markers occurs as the structures become more differentiated (Tables 2 and 3). These data allowed us to conclude that degree of differentiation of the breast is an important determinant in the expression of both ER and PgR, in addition to modulating the proliferative activity of the breast epithelium. Neither age (Figures 2 and 3) nor parity history affect the percentage of cells reacting for both receptors (Tables 2 and 3).

Lob 1 as the site of origin of breast cancer

An important concept that emerged from our study of breast development is that the TDLU, which had been originally identified by Wellings and colleagues as the site of origin of the most common breast malignancy, the ductal

Table 2 Distribution of estrogen receptors in lobular structures of nulliparous and parous women's breast, immunocytochemically detected as described in reference 32. Results are expressed as percentage of cells exhibiting positive nuclear reaction, mean ± SD

Group	Lob 1 (% positive cells)	Lob 2 (% positive cells)	Lob 3 (% positive cells)	Lob 4 (% positive cells)	Ducts (% positive cells)
Nulliparous	10.45 ± 1.42*	4.27 ± 1.09*	—	—	0.85 ± 9.47*†
Parous	14.25 ± 6.04**	4.24 ± 1.00**	0.31 ± 0.28**	0.01 ± 0.01**	14.25 ± 6.04†

*$p < 0.01$, nulliparous Lob 1 vs. Lob 2 and Ducts; ** $p < 0.006$, parous Lob 1 vs. Lob 2, Lob 3 and Lob 4; †$p < 0.05$, percentage of estrogen receptor positive cells significantly lower in ducts of nulliparous than parous women

Table 3 Distribution of progesterone receptors in lobular structures of nulliparous and parous women's breast, immunocytochemically detected as described in reference 32. Results are expressed as percentage of cells exhibiting positive nuclear reaction, mean ± SD

Group	Lob 1 (% positive cells)	Lob 2 (% positive cells)	Lob 3 (% positive cells)	Lob 4 (% positive cells)	Ducts (% positive cells)
Nulliparous	12.19 ± 2.54*	1.98 ± 0.21*	—	—	16.11 ± 5.72*†
Parous	12.92 ± 1.67**	7.00 ± 1.91**	1.50 ± 0.50**	0.24 ± 0.12**	7.66 ± 2.70†

*$p < 0.01$, nulliparous Lob 1 vs. Lob 2 and Ducts; ** $p < 0.003$, parous Lob 1 vs. Lob 2, Lob 3 and Lob 4; †$p < 0.05$, percentage of progesterone receptor positive cells significantly higher in ducts of nulliparous than parous women

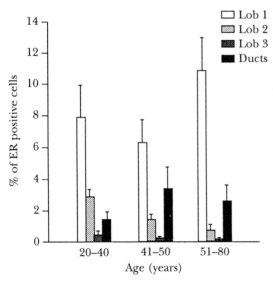
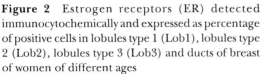
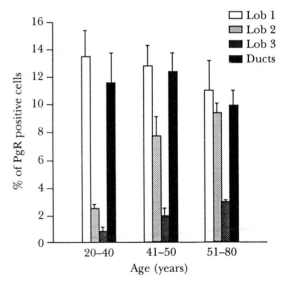

Figure 2 Estrogen receptors (ER) detected immunocytochemically and expressed as percentage of positive cells in lobules type 1 (Lob1), lobules type 2 (Lob2), lobules type 3 (Lob3) and ducts of breast of women of different ages

Figure 3 Progesterone receptors (PgR) detected immunocytochemically and expressed as percentage of positive cells in lobules type 1 (Lob1), lobules type 2 (Lob2), lobules type 3 (Lob3) and ducts of breast of women of different ages

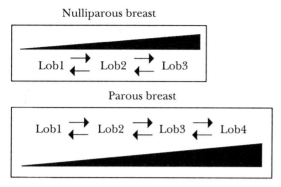

Nulliparous breast

Parous breast

Figure 4 Schematic representation of evolution of lobular structures in breast of nulliparous and parous women

carcinoma[44,45], corresponds to a specific stage of development of the mammary parenchyma, the lobules type 1. This observation is supported by comparative studies of normal and cancer-bearing breasts obtained at autopsy. It was found that the non-tumoral parenchyma in cancer-associated breasts contained a significantly higher number of hyperplastic terminal ducts, atypical Lob 1 and ductal carcinomas *in situ* originating in Lob 1 than those breasts of women free of breast cancer. These observations indicate that Lob 1 are affected by preneoplastic as well as by neoplastic processes[23,24]. The finding that the most undifferentiated structures originate the most undifferentiated and aggressive neoplasm acquires relevance to the understanding that these structures are more numerous in the breast of nulliparous women, who are in turn at a higher risk of developing breast cancer. We concluded that the Lob 1 found in the breast of nulliparous women never went through the process of differentiation, whereas the same structures, when found in the breast of postmenopausal parous women, did (Figure 4)[23].

Conclusions

Our studies have allowed us to determine that mammary cancer originates in undifferentiated terminal structures of the mammary gland. The terminal ducts of the Lob 1 or TDLU of the human female breast are the site of origin of ductal carcinomas. Cell replication in Lob 1 is

at its peak during early adulthood, at a time during which the breast is more susceptible to carcinogenesis, decreasing considerably with aging. *In vitro* studies have demonstrated that the Lob 1 express phenotypes indicative of neoplastic transformation when treated with chemical carcinogens. These studies indicate that in the human breast the epithelium of Lob 1 represents a target of carcinogens. These target cells will become the 'stem cells' of the neoplastic event, depending upon: (1) topographic location within the mammary gland tree; (2) age at exposure to a known or putative genotoxic agent; and (3) reproductive history of the host. This concept is supported by epidemiological findings that indicate a higher incidence of breast cancer occurs in nulliparous women and in women having an early menarche. Thus, the protection afforded by early full-term pregnancy in women could be explained by the higher degree of differentiation of the mammary gland at the time in which a given etiologic agent or agents might act. Even though differentiation significantly reduces cell proliferation in the mammary gland, the mammary epithelium remains capable of responding with proliferation to specific stimuli, such as a new pregnancy. Under these circumstances, however, the cells that are stimulated to proliferate are from structures that have already been primed by the first cycle of differentiation, thus creating a second type of 'stem cells'. These cells should be able to metabolize a carcinogen and to repair any induced DNA damage more efficiently than those cells of the virginal gland, thus becoming less susceptible to trans-formation. The findings that cell proliferation is of importance for cancer initiation, whereas differentiation is a powerful inhibitor, provide novel tools for developing rational strategies for breast cancer prevention.

Acknowledgements

This work was supported by National Cancer Institute grants CA64896 and CA67238, and National Institute of Environmental Health Science grant ESO7280.

References

1. Russo, I. H. and Russo, J. (1996). Mammary gland neoplasia in long-term rodent studies. *Environ. Health Perspect.*, **104**, 938–67

2. MacMahon, B., Cole, P., Liu, M., Lowe, C. R., Mirra, A. P., Ravinihar, B., Salber, E. J., Valaoras, V. G. and Yuasa, S. (1970). Age at first birth and breast cancer risk. *Bull. WHO*, **34**, 209–21

3. McGregor, D. H., Land, C. E., Choi, K., Tokuoka, S., Liu, P. I., Wakabayashi, I. and Beebe, G. W. (1977). Breast cancer incidence among atomic bomb survivors, Hiroshima and Nagasaki 1950–1989. *J. Natl. Cancer Inst.*, **59**, 799–811

4. De Waard, F. and Trichopoulos, D. (1988). A unifying concept of the etiology of breast cancer. *Int. J. Cancer*, **41**, 666–9

5. Henderson, B. E., Ross, R. K. and Pike, M. C. (1993). Hormonal chemoprevention of cancer in women. *Science*, **259**, 633–8

6. Boring, C.C., Squires, T. S. and Tang, T. (1993). Cancer statistics. *CA-Cancer J. Clin.*, **43**, 72–6

7. Rosner, B., Colditz, G. A. and Willett, W. C. (1994). Reproductive risk factors in a prospective study of breast cancer: the nurses' health study. *Am. J. Epidemiol.*, **139**, 819–35

8. Parker, S. L., Tong, T., Bolden, S. and Wingo, P. A. (1996). Cancer statistics. *CA-Cancer J. Clin.*, **65**, 5–27

9. South, S. A., Yankov, V. I. and Evans, W. S. (1993); Normal reproductive neuroendocrinology in the female. *Endocrinol. Metab. Clin. N. Am.*, **22**, 1–22

10. Marshall, J. C. and Griffin, M. L. (1993). The role of changing pulse frequency in the regulation of ovulation. *Hum. Reprod.*, **8** (Suppl. 2), 57–68

11. Carr, B. R. (1992). Disorders of the ovary and female reproductive tract. In Wilson, J. D. and Foster, D. W. (eds.) *Williams Textbook of Endocrinology*, pp. 733–57. (Philadelphia: W. B. Saunders)

12. Espey, L. L. and Ben Halim, I. A. (1990). Characteristics and control of the normal menstrual cycle. *Obstet. Gynecol. Clin. N. Am.*, **17**, 275–8

13. MacLeod, R. M. (1976). Regulation of prolactin secretion. In Martini, L. and Ganong, W. F. (eds.) *Frontiers in Neuroendocrinology*, pp. 164–94. (New York: Raven Press)

14. Roseff, S. J., Banagh, M. L., Kettel, L. M., *et al.* (1989). Dynamic changes in circulating inhibin levels during the luteal–follicular transition of the human menstrual cycle. *J. Clin. Endocrinol. Metab.*, **69**, 1033–8

15. Dye, R. B., Rabinovici, J. and Jaffe, R. B. (1992). Inhibin and activin in reproductive biology. *Obstet. Gynecol. Surv.*, **47**, 173–6

16. Yen, S. C. C. (1990). Clinical endocrinology of reproduction. In Balieu, E. E. and Kelly, P. A. (eds.) *Hormones: from Molecules to Disease*, pp. 445–82. (New York: Chapman and Hall)

17. Russo, I. H. and Russo, J. (1993). Chorionic gonadotropin: a tumoristatic and preventive agent in breast cancer. In Teicher, B. A. (ed.) *Drug Resistance in Oncology*, pp. 537–60. (New York, Basel, Hong Kong: Marcel Dekker, Inc.)

18. Russo, I. H. and Russo, J. (1994). Role of hCG and inhibin in breast cancer. *Int. J. Oncol.*, **4**, 297–306

19. Nisula, B. C., Taliadouros, G. S. and Carayon, P. (1980). Primary and secondary biologic activities intrinsic to the human chorionic gonadotropin molecule. In Segal, S. J. (ed.) *Chorionic Gonadotropin*, pp. 17–35. (New York: Plenum Press)

20. Russo, J. and Russo, I. H. (1987). Biological and molecular bases of mammary carcinogenesis. *Lab. Invest.*, **57**, 112–37

21. Schwartzman, R. A. and Cidlowski, J. A. (1993). Apoptosis: the biochemistry and molecular biology of programmed cell death. *Endocr. Rev.*, **14**, 133–53

22. Grady, D., Rubin, S. M., Petitti, D. B., *et al.* (1992). Hormone therapy to prevent disease and prolong life in postmenopausal women. *Ann. Intern. Med.*, **7**, 1016–132

23. Russo, J., Rivera, R. and Russo, I. H. (1992). Influence of age and parity on the development of the human breast. *Breast Cancer Res. Treat.*, **23**, 211–18

24. Russo, J., Romero, A. L. and Russo, I. H. (1994). Architectural pattern of the normal and cancerous breast under the influence of parity. *J. Cancer Epidemiol. Biomark. Prevent.* **3**, 219–24

25. Russo, J., Gusterson, B. A., Rogers, A. E., Russo, I. H., Wellings, S. R. and Van Zwieten, M. J. (1990). Comparative study of human and rat mammary tumorigenesis. *Lab. Invest.*, **62**, 1–32

26. Russo, J., Mills, M. J, Moussalli, M. J. and Russo, I. H. (1989). Influence of breast development and growth properties *in vitro*. *In Vitro Cell Dev. Biol.*, **25**, 643–9

27. Russo, J., Reina, D., Frederick, J. and Russo, I. H. (1988). Expression of phenotypical changes by human breast epithelial cells treated with carcinogens *in vitro*. *Cancer Res.*, **48**, 2837–57

28. Russo, J., Calaf, G. and Russo, I. H. (1993). A critical approach to the malignant trans-

formation of human breast epithelial cells. *CRC Crit. Rev. Oncogen.*, **4**, 403–17

29. Russo, J. and Russo, I. H. (1994). Toward a physiological approach to breast cancer prevention. *Cancer Epidemiol. Biomark. Prevent.*, **3**, 353–64

30. Russo, J. and Russo, I. H. (1995). Hormonally induced differentiation: a novel approach to breast cancer prevention. *J. Cell Biochem.*, **22**, 58–64

31. Russo, J. and Russo, I. H (1987). Development of the human mammary gland. In Neville, M. C. and Daniel, C. W. (eds.) *The Mammary Gland. Development, Regulation, and Function*, pp. 67–93. (New York: Plenum Publ. Corp.)

32. Russo, J. and Russo, I. H. (1996). Role of differentiation in the pathogenesis and prevention of breast cancer. *Curr. Top. Breast Cancer Res.* in press

33. Kumar, V., Stack, G. S., Berry, M., Jin, J. R. and Chambon, P. (1987). Functional domains of the human estrogen receptor. *Cell*, **51**, 941–51

34. King, R. J. B. (1992). Effects of steroid hormones and related compounds on gene transcription. *Clin. Endocrinol.*, **36**, 1–14

35. Soto, A. M. and Sonnenschein, C. (1987). Cell proliferation of estrogen-sensitive cells: the case for negative control. *Endocr. Rev.*, **48**, 52–8

36. Huseby, R. A., Maloney, T. M. and McGrath, C. M. (1987). Evidence for a direct growth-stimulating effect of estradiol on human MCF-7 cells *in vitro*. *Cancer Res.*, **144**, 2654–9

37. Huff, K. K., Knabbe, C., Lindsey, R., Kaufman, D., Bronzert, D., Lippman, M. E and Dickson, R. B. (1988). Multihormonal regulation of insulin-like growth factor-1-related protein in MCF-7 human breast cancer cells. *Mol. Endocrinol.*, **2**, 200–8

38. Dickson, R. B., Huff, K. K., Spencer, E. M. and Lippman, M. E. (1986). Introduction of epidermal growth factor related polypeptides by 17β-estradiol in MCF-7 human breast cancer cells. *Endocrinology* **118**, 138–42

39. Page, M. J., Field, J. K., Everett, P and Green, C. D. (1983). Serum regulation of the estrogen responsiveness of the human breast cancer cell line MCF-7. *Cancer Res.*, **43**, 1244–50

40. Katzenellenbogen, B. S., Kendra, K. L., Norman, M. J. and Berthois, Y. (1987). Proliferation, hormonal responsiveness, and estrogen receptor content of MCF-7 human breast cancer cells grown in the short-term and long-term absence of estrogens. *Cancer Res.*, **47**, 4355–60

41. Aakvaag, A., Utaacker, E., Thorsen, T., Lea, O. A. and Lahooti, H. (1990). Growth control of human mammary cancer cells (MCF-7 cells) in culture: effect of estradiol and growth factors in serum containing medium. *Cancer Res.*, **50**, 7806–10

42. Dell'aquilla, M. L., Pigott, D. A., Bonaquist, D. L. and Gaffney, E. V. (1984). A factor from plasma derived human serum that inhibits the growth of the mammary cell line MCF-7: characterization and purification. *J. Natl. Cancer Inst.*, **72**, 291–8

43. Markaverich, B. M., Gregory, R. R., Alejandro, M. A., Clark, J. H., Johnson, G. A. and Middleditch, B. S. (1988). Methyl p-hydroxyphenyl lactate. An inhibitor of cell growth and proliferation and an endogenous ligand for nuclear type-II binding sites. *J. Biol. Chem.*, **263**, 7203–10

44. Wellings, S. R. (1980). Development of human breast cancer. *Adv. Cancer Res.*, **31**, 287–99

45. Wellings, S. R., Jensen, H. M. and Marcum, R. G. (1975). An atlas of subgross pathology of 16 human breasts with special reference to possible precancerous lesions. *J. Natl. Cancer Inst.*, **55**, 231–75

Steroidal control of cell proliferation in the breast and breast cancer

29

E. A. Musgrove and R. L. Sutherland

Introduction

The control of normal cellular proliferation involves a delicate balance between different influences in the extracellular environment, including signaling molecules and cell–cell interactions. The two major female sex-steroid hormones, estradiol and progesterone, are key elements in the regulation of growth and development of female sex organs. Estrogen, acting in concert with other hormones and growth factors, appears to be the main drive to proliferation in these tissues. In contrast with the 'proliferative' effects of estrogen, progesterone can be seen as the 'differentiating' female sex steroid. In this role it can either stimulate or inhibit proliferation. For example, progesterone causes the glandular elements of the mammary gland to grow and develop into secretory epithelium with the ultimate effect of acting in concert with other hormones, particularly prolactin, to facilitate milk production. While the biology of these processes is well documented, it is only recently that progress has been made towards understanding the molecular basis of steroidal control of cell cycle progression. Despite this progress, much remains to be learnt.

Steroid-responsive breast cancer cells are a widely used model for studying steroid hormone action *in vitro*, and some of the most detailed mechanistic studies have been performed using such cells. These studies provide insights relevant to some of the processes of normal development in the mammary gland. In addition, they have application to questions raised by the pharmacological use of steroids in oral contraceptives and hormone replacement therapies, for example the possibility that increased cell proliferation may increase the risk of developing breast cancer or accelerate its progression. Furthermore, the majority of breast cancers retain some degree of steroid responsiveness, a fact that has been exploited therapeutically by the use of agents that interfere with the production or action of estrogens. Synthetic progestins also have an established role as first- and second-line therapy for the treatment of breast and endometrial cancer. Research in this laboratory in recent years, reviewed in this chapter, has centered on control of cell cycle progression by steroids in breast cancer cell lines, with the aim of identifying cell cycle phase-specific effects and ultimately the genes which might mediate these effects.

Steroid effects on cell cycle progression

The effects of steroids on cell proliferation have been examined in a variety of models *in vivo* and *in vitro*. While it is clear that there is both cell and tissue specificity in the response to steroid treatment, some clear patterns emerge. Studies of cell proliferation in the rodent uterus and mammary gland *in vivo* indicated that estrogen increases the proportion of cells engaged in DNA synthesis predominantly by recruiting non-cycling cells into the cell cycle and reducing the duration of G_1 phase in cells which are already cycling[1] (Figure 1). The roles of estrogen in mediating breast epithelial cell proliferation in humans are more difficult to examine directly, but the consensus to emerge from studies using a variety of techniques including organ culture and primary cell culture is that estrogen is capable of stimulating breast epithelial cell growth *in vitro*. Breast

Estrogen

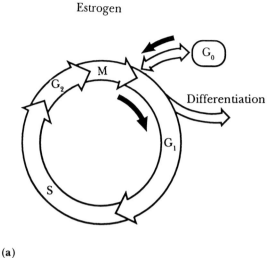

(a)

Progestins

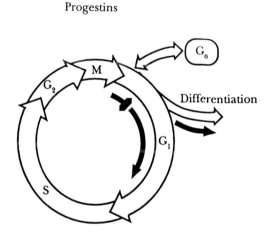

(b)

Figure 1 Cell cycle phase specific effects of estrogen and progestins in mammary epithelial cells. Four phases of the cell cycle: G_1, DNA synthesis or S phase, G_2 and mitosis (M) are illustrated. Cells can leave the cell cycle and enter resting or G_0 phase which allows re-entry into the cell cycle. Alternatively, cells can exit the cell cycle to enter irreversible program of differentiation. Examples of effects of estrogen and progestins on mammary epithelium, illustrated using solid arrows, include mitogenic effects of estrogen in early G_1 phase, progestin inhibition of cell cycle progression in early G_1 phase and progestin acceleration later in G_1 phase

cancer cells have been a more widely used model and some of the earliest studies using these cells documented a mitogenic effect of estrogen[2]. Using breast cancer cells synchronised at G_2/M by treatment with the microtubule inhibitor nocodazole, Leung and Potter[3] concluded that the sensitive cells were in early G_1 phase, immediately following mitosis. These data supported observations that antiestrogens arrest estrogen receptor-positive breast cancer cells in G_1 phase and that the sensitive cells are in early-to-mid G_1 phase[4-6]. Overall, the data clearly indicate that estrogen is mitogenic via an early G_1 phase site of action in human breast cancer cells, consistent with the limited data from normal breast epithelial cells.

Progestin effects on breast epithelial cell cycle progression have been less readily dissected than those of estrogen. A wave of breast epithelial cell proliferation in the late secretory phase of the menstrual cycle coincides with, or immediately follows, a rise in the serum concentrations of both estrogen and progesterone. Since an earlier rise in estrogen alone is not accompanied by a similar wave of proliferation, several authors have proposed that progestins have a primary mitogenic role in the human breast[7]. However, direct evidence for this is lacking from studies of human breast epithelium both *in vitro* and *in vivo*[8,9], and synthetic progestins are effective agents in the treatment of metastatic breast carcinoma.

Studies *in vitro* show a predominantly inhibitory effect of progestins on breast cancer cells stimulated to proliferate by a range of hormonal and growth factor mitogens[7]. A detailed analysis of the effects of progestins in T-47D human breast cancer cells growing at suboptimal rates under defined conditions[10] revealed both stimulation and inhibition, providing evidence for two distinct effects of progestins on cell cycle progression within the one cell type. Together these effects resulted in a biphasic change in the rate of cell cycle progression, consisting of an initial transient acceleration through G_1 phase and subsequent increase in the S phase fraction, followed by cell cycle arrest and growth inhibition accompanied by a decrease in the S phase fraction. The decreased S phase fraction is maintained so that the predominant effect is long-term growth inhibition.

Progestins increase the rate at which cells enter S phase, implying that progestins target a rate-limiting process within G_1 phase[10]. This stimulatory effect of progestins is temporally distinct from that of other breast cancer cell mitogens: progestin-stimulated cells began to enter S phase approximately 4–6 h before estrogen-, growth factor- or serum-stimulated cells[10]. The inhibitory effect also occurs in G_1 phase[10,11], but the two effects of progestins apparently target distinct processes within G_1 phase (Figure 1). One possibility is that these effects are mediated by two independent mechanisms. However, since in a number of tissues progestins can be viewed as inducers of differentiation[7], the transient increase in cell cycle progression might arise from a necessity for DNA replication before full expression of a differentiated phenotype after growth arrest. This interpretation is consistent with progesterone stimulation of proliferation in the mammary gland, where the development of alveoli is a requirement for subsequent lactation, the ultimate differentiated function of this organ.

Mechanisms for control of cell cycle progression

The demonstration of steroidal control of cell cycle progression at defined points within G_1 phase suggests that these agents act via their respective receptors to directly or indirectly regulate the expression of genes which control cell cycle progression through G_1 phase. The identification of these molecular targets has been a focus of recent research.

Transient accumulation of cyclins, consequent assembly and activation of cyclin/ cyclin-dependent kinase (CDK) complexes leading to phosphorylation of specific substrates regulates passage through the eukaryotic cell cycle. The best characterized mammalian cyclins comprise four classes: A, B, D and E. Of these, cyclins D and E have G_1 specific roles, as illustrated in Figure 2. The expression of cyclin D1 is strongly mitogen-inducible but does not oscillate throughout the cell cycle as dramatically as other cyclins[12,13]. Following mitogenic stimulation, cyclin D/Cdk4 or cyclin D/Cdk6 are the first active CDKs detected[12,13]. This is followed by cyclin E/Cdk2 activation near the G_1/S phase boundary. Microinjection of cyclin D1 antibodies or antisense plasmids leads to cell cycle arrest when performed in early G_1 phase cells but not in cells past the G_1/ S phase boundary, indicating that cyclin D1 is essential during G_1 phase[14]. Conversely, increased expression of cyclin D1 shortens G_1[13,15–17]. In breast cancer cells cyclin D1 is also sufficient for G_1 progression: induction of ectopic cyclin D1 in cells arrested by serum deprivation leads to re-entry into the cell cycle with subsequent DNA synthesis and mitosis[17]. The substrates for the CDKs which associate preferentially with cyclin D1, Cdk4 and Cdk6, have yet to be defined, but include the retinoblastoma tumor suppressor protein, pRB[13]. The protein is hypophosphorylated during early G_1 and in this form is growth-inhibitory[18]. Phosphorylation of pRB by cyclin/ CDK complexes during G_1 phase relieves this inhibition and allows S phase entry[18]. It is likely that cyclin E/Cdk2 also phosphorylates pRB *in vivo*, perhaps contributing to the further phosphorylation of pRB as cells progress into S phase[18] (Figure 2).

While changes in cyclin abundance govern much of the regulation of CDK activity as cells progress through the cell cycle, the catalytic activity of CDKs depends not only on cyclin association but also on appropriate phosphorylation of the CDK subunit[19]. A further means of regulating cyclin/CDK function is provided by endogenous low molecular weight proteins which physically associate with the cyclins, CDKs or their complexes and inhibit CDK activity[20]. A growing family of such inhibitors, for which p16[INK4] is the prototype, selectively targets cyclin D-associated kinases. A second, structurally unrelated family of inhibitors includes p21 (WAF1, Cip1, Sdi1) and p27 (Kip1).

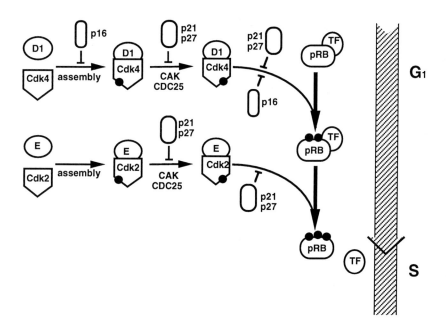

Figure 2 Control of G_1 phase progression in breast cancer cells. Sequential activation of cyclin D1 (D1)/ Cdk4 and cyclin E (E)/Cdk2 leads to phosphorylation (filled circles) of the retinoblastoma tumor suppressor gene product pRB with consequent release of transcription factors (TF) and entry into S phase. Kinase activity depends on several steps including assembly of the cyclin/cyclin-dependent kinase (CDK) complex and appropriate phosphorylation of CDK subunit, mediated in part by action of CDK-activating kinases (CAK) and CDK-activating phosphatases (CDC25). A variety of CDK inhibitors (p16, p21, p27) can inhibit kinase activity by mechanisms including competition with cyclins for CDK binding (p16) and inhibition of CAK activation, probably mediated by occlusion of the target residue (p21, p27)

Figure 2 presents a simplified model of interactions between some of the molecules involved in G_1 phase progression. Activation of cyclin D-associated kinases, cyclin E/Cdk2 activation and phosphorylation of pRB are necessary for transit from G_1 into S phase. Although it is clear that there are many additional complexities associated with G_1 control, this model provides a framework for investigation of mechanisms underlying steroidal regulation of cell cycle progression in breast cancer cells.

Effects of steroids on cell cycle regulatory genes

Estrogen

A number of different experimental paradigms tailored to specific responses have been used to focus on various aspects of the steroidal control of cell proliferation. For example, inhibition of cell proliferation following antiestrogen treatment can be 'rescued' by addition of estrogen, leading to synchronous progression of a substantial fraction of the cell population through G_1 phase, S phase and subsequent cell division[21,22]. Some selective magnification of estrogen-regulated gene expression might be expected from this strategy and would compound the additional sensitivity afforded by the use of synchronized cells. Thus, this model provides a sensitive experimental system for the study of specific estrogen-regulated events associated with cell cycle progression.

Estrogen rescue of MCF-7 breast cancer cells inhibited using the pure estrogen antagonist ICI 182780 was accompanied by induction of cyclin

D1 mRNA and protein[21]. This change in gene expression occurred prior to any change in the proportion of cells entering S phase, which was first apparent after ~12 h. The activity of Cdk4, the major catalytic partner for cyclin D1 in these cells, was likewise significantly elevated within 3 h of estradiol treatment, maximally elevated at 6–8 h (> six-fold) and thereafter declined[21]. The initial changes in Cdk4 activity were temporally similar to the changes in expression for cyclin D1 protein and consequent cyclin D1/Cdk4 association. Although there was no significant change in the expression of cyclin E as estrogen-stimulated cells progressed through G_1 phase, cyclin E-associated kinase activity increased within 4 h and reached a maximum at 16 h, approximately seven-fold relative to control levels[21]. The substantial and early changes in both Cdk4 activity and cyclin E-associated kinase activity preceding entry into S phase indicated that both kinases were likely to contribute to increased cell cycle progression following estradiol treatment. While an important activating mechanism for Cdk4 was likely to be increased cyclin D1 expression, activation of cyclin E/Cdk2 complexes was not associated with changes in the level of cyclin E, Cdk2 or the CDK inhibitors p21 or p27, pointing to another level of regulation by estrogen that has yet to be defined.

Progestins: mitogenesis

Our first studies investigating the possible effects of progestins on CDK function focused on the stimulatory component of the response[23]. The entry of progestin-stimulated cells into S phase was preceded by increases in cyclin D1 mRNA abundance (Figure 3). The increase in cyclin D1 mRNA expression was inhibited by simultaneous treatment with actinomycin D, consistent with a transcriptional effect. Addition of the progestin antagonist RU 486 either at the same time as, or 3 h subsequent to progestin treatment rapidly reversed the increase in cyclin D1 mRNA abundance, although by 3 h a substantial increase had already occurred[23] (Figure 3). In either circumstance, i.e.

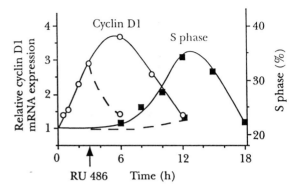

Figure 3 Effect of progestin stimulation on cyclin D1 mRNA expression and S phase fraction. T-47D cells proliferating at suboptimal rates in serum-free medium containing insulin were treated with progestin (ORG 2058) and harvested for Northern blot analysis at intervals thereafter. Some progestin-treated flasks were additionally treated with antiprogestin (RU 486) added 3 h after progestin; effects of such RU 486 treatment on cyclin D1 and S phase fraction are shown by dashed lines. Redrawn from reference 23

simultaneous or delayed progestin antagonist addition, progestin antagonist addition was sufficient to prevent progestin-induced entry into S phase[10] (Figure 3).

The increase in cyclin D1 mRNA following progestin treatment was accompanied by an increase in cyclin D1 protein abundance (Figure 4). Little effect was apparent within 3 h but by 6 h cyclin D1 levels had increased by three- to four-fold (Musgrove and colleagues, in preparation). This response preceded entry into S phase, which began after > 9 h treatment. The induction of cyclin D1 protein was accompanied by a corresponding increase in the abundance of cyclin D1/Cdk4 complexes and an increase in the relative amount of pRB in the hyperphosphorylated form (Figure 5). In contrast with the marked increase in cyclin D1 abundance, cyclin E abundance and kinase activity increased by at most two-fold (Figure 4). Overall, the data indicate substantial induction of cyclin D1 but more modest effects on cyclin E, consistent with induction of cyclin D1 being a critical component of the mitogenic response to progestins.

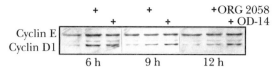

Figure 4 Cyclin expression following progestin stimulation. T-47D human breast cancer cells proliferating at suboptimal rates in medium containing 5% charcoal-treated fetal calf serum were treated with progestins ORG 2058 or ORG OD-14 or vehicle (ethanol). Whole-cell lysates were immunoblotted using antibodies specific for cyclin D1 and cyclin E. Redrawn from Musgrove and colleagues (in preparation)

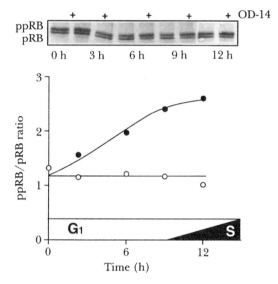

Figure 5 Retinoblastoma tumor suppressor protein (pRB) phosphorylation following progestin stimulation. T-47D human breast cancer cells proliferating at suboptimal rates in medium containing 5% charcoal-treated fetal calf serum (FCS) were treated with progestin ORG OD-14 or vehicle (ethanol). Whole-cell lysates were immunoblotted using antibodies specific for pRB. Ratio between intensity of hyperphosphorylated pRB (lower band) and hypophosphorylated pRB (ppRB, upper band) was calculated following densitometric analysis of same blot. (o), control; (●), ORG OD-14. Redrawn from Musgrove and colleagues (in preparation)

Experiments using T-47D breast cancer cells expressing cyclin D1 under the control of a metal-inducible metallothionein promoter[17,24] demonstrated that induction of cyclin D1 alone mimicked the effects of progestins. Zinc treatment of these cells resulted in rapid induction of cyclin D1 mRNA, beginning within 1 h, and consequent induction of cyclin D1 protein, typically reaching ~five-fold between 6 and 12 h. These responses were followed by increased cyclin E abundance (~two-fold) and pRB phosphorylation, and ultimately by an increase in the proportion of cells reaching S phase between 12 and 24 h after zinc treatment[17,24]. Cell kinetic experiments indicated that cyclin D1 induction led to both an increase in the rate of G_1 transit and an increase in the proportion of the cell population engaged in active transit through G_1[17]. Thus, induction of cyclin D1 could account for progestin-mediated acceleration of G_1 phase progression.

The conclusion that cyclin D1 induction is a critical component of the mitogenic response to progestins is supported by studies in transgenic and knockout mice. Overexpression of cyclin D1 in the mammary gland of transgenic mice led to increased lobuloalveolar development, reminiscent of the changes associated with pregnancy, while conversely, development of the lobular alveoli did not occur in pregnant cyclin D1-null mice[25-27]. This indicates a very specific impairment in alveolar proliferation; ductal proliferation apparently occurs normally, allowing both pubertal development of the gland and some side-branching during pregnancy[26]. These phases of mammary development involve complex interactions between different hormones including estrogen and prolactin or growth hormone. However, a major difference between the hormonal requirements of alveolar and ductal epithelial cells is a necessity for progesterone for alveolar but not ductal proliferation[7]. This conclusion is further supported by the similarities in phenotype between cyclin D1-null and progesterone receptor-null mice[28]. Thus while cyclin D1 action is apparently dispensable for proliferation in many tissues, it appears to be essential for progesterone-driven mammary epithelial proliferation.

Progestins: inhibition

The effects of progestin-induced inhibition of cell proliferation on CDK function are less clear than the mitogenic effects of either estradiol or progestins. Under optimal growth conditions for T-47D cells the predominant effect of progestin treatment is inhibition of entry into S phase[11]. S phase begins to decline after 12 h or more treatment and reaches a minimum by 24 h. These changes were associated with decreased phosphorylation of pRB. At 18 h both the hypo- and hyper-phosphorylated forms were clearly present although the proportion of hyperphosphorylated pRB decreased (Figure 6). However, by 24 h essentially no hyper-phosphorylated pRB was evident, consistent with the low proportion of S phase cells associated with almost total inhibition of cell proliferation. Both cyclin D1-associated and cyclin E-associated kinase activity began to decrease after 12 h and by 24 h had declined to < 20% of control (Figure 6), accompanying or slightly preceding the decrease in %S phase cells. Changes in the abundance of cyclin D1 and cyclin E accompany the decreases in kinase activity (Musgrove and associates, in preparation) but these data do not exclude the possibility that other factors might also contribute to the marked loss of CDK activity. Furthermore, while clear effects on CDK activity are associated with progestin inhibition of proliferation, extended progestin treatment is required before these responses are manifest, and whether they are a cause or a consequence of the changes in the rate of cell proliferation remains to be defined.

Conclusions

The hypothesis that estradiol and progesterone could contribute to breast cancer development because stimulation of cell division may increase the possibility of accumulation of oncogenic mutations, is based on the association of increased breast epithelial mitosis with increased steroid hormone levels in the luteal phase of the menstrual cycle[29]. However,

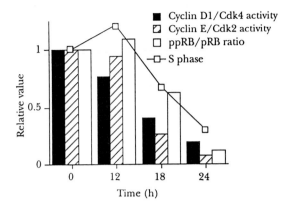

Figure 6 Inhibition of cyclin/cyclin-dependent kinase (CDK) activity and retinoblastoma tumor suppressor protein (pRB) phosphorylation following progestin treatment. T-47D human breast cancer cells proliferating at maximal rates in medium containing 5% fetal calf serum were treated with progestin (ORG 2058) or vehicle (ethanol). Antibodies to cyclin D1 or cyclin E were used to immunoprecipitate cyclin/CDK complexes and kinase activity of immunoprecipitates determined by phosphorylation of GST-pRB$^{773-923}$ (cyclin D1/Cdk4 activity) or histone H1 (cyclin E/Cdk2). Changes in kinase activity and S phase fraction relative to that in cultures treated with ethanol vehicle instead of progestin are shown. Ratio between intensity of the hyperphosphorylated pRB and hypophosphorylated pRB (ppRB/pRB) is also presented relative to that in control cultures. Redrawn from Musgrove and colleagues (in preparation)

increased proliferation as measured by thymidine labeling index identifies cells synthesizing DNA, but does not provide evidence for a sustained proliferative effect. Thus cells which undergo mitosis may do so on their path to terminal differentiation and exit from the cell cycle. The experimental data discussed above suggest that this might be the case in breast epithelium following exposure to progestins, providing a potential resolution of the apparent paradox between progestin inhibition of breast cancer cell proliferation and the postulated proliferative role in the normal breast. This interpretation implies that progestin administration would be expected to have little effect on breast cancer risk, consistent with the limited epidemiologic data[30]. Although some support for this interpretation is thus available, breast epithelium *in vivo* is composed of a number of phenotypically distinct cell types which may display differential responses to the same stimuli, and there is in addition the potential for indirect effects mediated by the stroma. Thus several issues remain to be addressed before the *in vitro* studies can be extrapolated with any confidence to the human breast *in vivo*.

The studies summarized above identified the induction of cyclin D1 gene expression as an early response to mitogenic steroids in breast cancer cells. It is clear that cyclin D1 has a critical regulatory role in steroidal control of progression through G_1 phase, but it is important to note, however, that the induction of cyclin D1 by estrogen or progestin is preceded by the induction of other genes, and that the effect on cyclin D1 expression may not be direct, but rather result from prior induction of another gene or genes. Furthermore, there are additional complexities in steroidal control of breast epithelial cell proliferation which have yet to be addressed. These include, for example, the suggestion that cyclin D1 function is essential for progesterone-dependent but not estrogen-dependent proliferation in the normal mammary gland.

Acknowledgements

This research has been supported by grants from the National Health and Medical Research Council of Australia and the New South Wales State Cancer Council. The authors thank Dr Colin Watts, Dr Owen Prall, Dr Boris Sarcevic, Christine Lee, Ann Cornish and Alex Swarbrick for their invaluable contributions to these studies.

References

1. Sutherland, R. L., Reddel, R. R. and Green, M. D. (1983). Effects of oestrogens on cell proliferation and cell cycle kinetics. A hypothesis on the cell cycle effects of antioestrogens. *Eur. J. Cancer Clin. Oncol.*, **19**, 307–18

2. Lippman, M. E. and Bolan, G. (1975). Oestrogen-responsive human breast cancer in long term tissue culture. *Nature (London)*, **256**, 592–3

3. Leung, B. S. and Potter, A. H. (1987). Mode of estrogen action on cell proliferation in CAMA-1 cells: II. Sensitivity of G1 phase population. *J. Cell. Biochem.*, **34**, 213–25

4. Sutherland, R. L., Green, M. D., Hall, R. E., Reddel, R. R. and Taylor, I. W. (1983). Tamoxifen induces accumulation of MCF-7 human mammary carcinoma cells in the G_0/G_1 phase of the cell cycle. *Eur. J. Cancer Clin. Oncol.*, **19**, 615–21

5. Sutherland, R. L., Hall, R. E. and Taylor, I. W. (1983). Cell proliferation kinetics of MCF-7 human mammary carcinoma cells in culture and effects of tamoxifen on exponentially growing and plateau-phase cells. *Cancer Res.*, **43**, 3998–4006

6. Taylor, I. W., Hodson, P. J., Green, M. D. and Sutherland, R. L. (1983). Effects of tamoxifen on cell cycle progression of synchronous MCF-7 human mammary carcinoma cells. *Cancer Res.*, **43**, 4007–10

7. Clarke, C. L. and Sutherland, R. L. (1990). Progestin regulation of cellular proliferation. *Endocr. Rev.*, **11**, 266–302

8. Gompel, A., Malet, C., Spritzer, P., Lalardrie, J. P., Kuttenn, F. and Mauvais Jarvis, P. (1986). Progestin effect on cell proliferation and 17β-hydroxysteroid dehydrogenase activity in normal human breast cells in culture. *J. Clin. Endocrinol. Metab.*, **63**, 1174–80

9. Laidlaw, I. J., Clarke, R. B., Howell, A., Owen, A. W. M. C., Potten, C. S. and Anderson, E. (1995). The proliferation of normal human breast tissue implanted into athymic nude mice is stimulated by oestrogen but not progesterone. *Endocrinology*, **136**, 164–71

10. Musgrove, E. A., Lee, C. S. L. and Sutherland, R. L. (1991). Progestins both stimulate and inhibit breast cancer cell cycle progression while increasing expression of transforming growth factor α, epidermal growth factor receptor, c-*fos* and c-*myc* genes. *Mol. Cell. Biol.*, **11**, 5032–43

11. Sutherland, R. L., Hall, R. E., Pang, G. Y. N.,

Musgrove, E. A. and Clarke, C. L. (1988). Effect of medroxyprogesterone acetate on proliferation and cell cycle kinetics of human mammary carcinoma cells. *Cancer Res.*, **48**, 5084–91

12. Hunter, T. and Pines, J. (1994). Cyclins and cancer II: cyclin D and CDK inhibitors come of age. *Cell*, **79**, 573–82

13. Sherr, C. J. (1994). G1 phase progression: cycling on cue. *Cell*, **79**, 551–5

14. Baldin, V., Lukas, J., Marcote, M. J., Pagano, M. and Draetta, G. (1993). Cyclin D1 is a nuclear protein required for cell cycle progression in G_1. *Genes Dev.*, **7**, 812–21

15. Quelle, D. E., Ashmun, R. A., Shurtleff, S. A., Kato, J.-Y., Bar-Sagi, D., Roussel, M. F. and Sherr, C. J. (1993). Overexpression of mouse D-type cyclins accelerates G_1 phase in rodent fibroblasts. *Genes Dev.*, **7**,1559–71

16. Resnitzky, D., Gossen, M., Bujard, H. and Reed, S. I. (1994). Acceleration of the G_1/S phase transition by expression of cyclins D1 and E with an inducible system. *Mol. Cell. Biol.*, **14**, 1669–79

17. Musgrove, E. A., Lee, C. S. L., Buckley, M. F. and Sutherland, R. L. (1994). Cyclin D1 induction in breast cancer cells shortens G_1 and is sufficient for cells arrested in G_1 to complete the cell cycle. *Proc. Natl. Acad. Sci. USA*, **91**, 8022–6

18. Weinberg, R. A. (1995). The retinoblastoma protein and cell cycle control. *Cell*, **81**, 323–30

19. Morgan, D. O. (1995). Principles of CDK regulation. *Nature (London)*, **374**, 131–4

20. Sherr, C. J. and Roberts, J. M. (1995). Inhibitors of mammalian G1 cyclin-dependent kinases. *Genes Dev.*, **9**, 1149–63

21. Prall, O. W. J., Sarcevic, B., Musgrove, E. A., Watts, C. K. W. and Sutherland, R. L. (1996). Estrogen-induced activation of Cdk4 and Cdk2 during G_1-S phase progression is accompanied by increased cyclin D1 expression and decreased CDK inhibitor association with cyclin E/Cdk2. Submitted for publication

22. Osborne, C. K., Boldt, D. H. and Estrada, P. (1984). Human breast cancer cell cycle synchronization by estrogens and antiestrogens in culture. *Cancer Res.*, **44**, 1433–9

23. Musgrove, E. A., Hamilton, J. A., Lee, C. S. L., Sweeney, K. J. E., Watts, C. K. W. and Sutherland, R. L. (1993). Growth factor, steroid and steroid antagonist regulation of cyclin gene expression associated with changes in T-47D human breast cancer cell cycle progression. *Mol. Cell. Biol.*, **13**, 3577–87

24. Musgrove, E. A., Sarcevic, B. and Sutherland, R. L. (1996). Inducible expression of cyclin D1 in T-47D human breast cancer cells is sufficient for CDK2 activation and pRB hyperphosphorylation. *J. Cell Biochem.*, **60**, 362–77

25. Wang, T. C., Cardiff, R. D., Zukerberg, L., Lees, E., Arnold, A. and Schmidt, E. V. (1994). Mammary hyperplasia and carcinoma in MMTV-cyclin D1 transgenic mice. *Nature (London)*, **369**, 669–71

26. Sicinski, P., Liu Donaher, J., Parker, S. B., Li, T., Fazeli, A., Gardner, H., Haslam, S. Z., Bronson, R. B., Elledge, S. J. and Weinberg, R. A. (1995). Cyclin D1 provides a link between development and oncogenesis in the retina and breast. *Cell*, **82**, 621–30

27. Fantl, V., Stamp, G., Andrews, A., Rosewell, I. and Dickson, C. (1995). Mice lacking cyclin D1 are small and show defects in eye and mammaru gland development. *Genes Dev.*, **9**, 2364–72

28. Lyndon, J. P., DeMayo, F. J., Funk, C. R., Mani, S. K., Hughes, A. R., Montgomery, C. A., Shyamala, G., Conneely, O. M. and O'Malley, B. W. (1995). Mice lacking progesterone receptor exhibit pleiotrophic reproductive abnormalities. *Genes Dev.*, **9**, 2266–78

29. Henderson, B. E., Ross, R. K. and Pike, M. C. (1991). Toward the primary prevention of cancer. *Science*, **254**,1131–8

30. Staffa, J. A., Newschaffer, C. J., Jones, J. K. and Miller, V. (1992). Progestins and breast cancer: an epidemiologic review. *Fertil. Steril.*, **57**, 473–91

Progestogen use and breast cancer 30

R. Sitruk-Ware and G. Plu-Bureau

Introduction

Breast cancer is the most commonly diagnosed cancer and the second leading cause of cancer death among women in most developed countries[1]. The annual incidence of female breast cancer increased by approximately 52% during the second half of this century from 1950 to 1990[2] especially in the United States. The lifetime risk has also risen from an estimate of 1 : 10 in the mid 1970s to 1 : 8 in the early 1990s[3].

However, the lifetime risk of dying from breast cancer has not changed, and the mortality curves have remained level over the same period. It is recognized that the increased use of mammographic screening, helping to detect breast cancer earlier, would account for the apparent sharp increase of breast cancer cases in the late 1980s.

The relationship between female sex hormones and breast cancer incidence has been evaluated in a considerable number of epidemiological studies. Controversy arises time and again, each time a new publication appears in the literature. Estrogen replacement therapy (ERT) where used for more than 10–15 years, may increase the risk of breast cancer by 30% according to meta-analysis of epidemiological studies[4-6]. However a causal relationship cannot be established, and only large long-term randomized placebo-controlled prospective trials could definitely be conclusive. The results of the Women's Health Initiative study designed in such a direction may bring the answer, but not before the next decade.

Although most studies concur about the role of estrogens, contradictory results have been published about the risks associated with the use of progestins alone or estrogens combined with progestins. Also, opposite results have been found in experimental studies about the role of progesterone and various progestins on the breast cells. The discrepancies may be explained in both cases by the variety in study designs, populations studied, progestins used and also in the interpretation of observed results.

Epidemiologic data and controversies about role of progestins on breast-cancer risk

Although many epidemiological studies have been conducted to assess the relationship between ERT and breast-cancer risk, only a few of them specifically address the role of the progestins. This relates to the rather recent coprescription of progestins with estrogens for menopausal therapy, especially in the United States where most of the large epidemiological surveys were conducted. Also, one must bear in mind that the progestins prescribed for hormone replacement therapy (HRT) differ from country to country, and their effects also differ according to the category to which they belong. In the United States, most of the prescriptions of progestins relate to medroxyprogesterone acetate (MPA), while in Europe derivatives of progesterone are preferred for HRT, such as micronized progesterone (MP), dydrogesterone (DDG), chlormadinone acetate (CLA) derived from 17OH-progesterone, or nomegestrol acetate (NOM Ac) derived from 19-norprogesterone.

Therefore several compounds are used and the population of HRT users would not be homogeneous as it appears in the United States. In addition, 17β-estradiol and estradiol valerate are more often prescribed in Europe than conjugated estrogens, which have been mostly prescribed in the United States for several decades.

Controversy started with the publication of Pike and colleagues[7] who evaluated breast cancer risk in young women using oral contraceptives (OCs). These researchers showed an increased risk of breast cancer in those women who used high doses of OCs, especially those containing high doses of progestins. Their classification of progestational potency was criticized, as indeed the OCs containing a high progestin dose also contained a high estrogen dose. That study was never repeated and had the merit to generate a huge number of other studies both epidemiologic and experimental, examining the specific role of progestins on the mammary gland.

Among the epidemiological studies specifically examining the role of progestins and breast cancer, the first one published in the United States by Gambrell and co-workers[8] pointed out that progestins would reduce the risk of breast cancer. However, their study was criticized as the authors did not adjust for the other known risk factors for breast cancer. The longest study of experimental design, randomized and placebo-controlled, was published by Nachtigall and associates[9] and again showed a lower number of breast cancer cases in combined HRT users than in the placebo group. This study followed 84 matched pairs of women for more than 22 years. However, the number of patients is too small to draw definite conclusions.

In Scandinavian countries, two major studies appeared in the late 1980s. The study from Bergkvist and colleagues[10] raised the controversy and a public alarm as the results indicated that long-term users of estrogens for 9 years and above would have a relative risk (RR) of 1.7 as compared to non-users, and those who used combined therapy would have a RR which was interpreted by the media as a four-fold increase in risk. Unfortunately, although the scientists very wisely indicated that the RR at 4.4 was not at all statistically significant, as the confidence interval (CI) was

large at 0.9–22.4 including the value 1, the lay press spread an alarming message.

Later on, with further follow-up, the same Swedish group indicated that the combined HRT users had a RR of 1.6, which was statistically significant, but not much different from the risk observed in estrogen-only users[11]. Ewertz[12] in Denmark also published results specific to progestin users, and in her study the sequential use of progestins added to ERT led to a RR of 1.4 (CI 0.9–2.1), not statistically significant. The only subgroup with a significant increase in risk was the one where androgens were added to estrogens: RR, 2.3 (CI 1.4–3.8). In that group the HRT was given as implants combining high doses of both estrogens and androgens.

More recently the large Nurses Health Cohort study appeared, where around 70 000 women were followed up to 16 years[13]. In that study, which also raised public concern, the relative risk of breast cancer was significantly increased among women who were current users of estrogens (RR 1.32; CI 1.14–1.54) or of combined estrogens and progestins (RR 1.41; CI 1.15–1.74). No difference was obvious between the two groups using either estrogens alone or combined HRT. The main concern was related to an earlier appearance of risk, after only 5 years of use of ERT or HRT, than that found in previous studies[4,10].

Shortly after the Colditz and associates[13] report, two population-based North American studies appeared[14,15], indicating no increase in risk in any group of ERT or HRT users with long-term use, up to 15 years or above in the Newcomb and co-workers[15] report. Stanford and colleagues[14] also reported a significant reduction in risk for long-term users of combination HRT.

In another population of premenopausal French women suffering from benign breast diseases, we followed 1150 patients for 10 years and longer comparing women who received high doses of 19-norsteroids for 15 days per cycle, to those who did not. The relative risk of breast cancer in the progestin users was 0.48 (CI 0.26–0.93) with a significant linear trend for a decrease in the RR of breast cancer with duration of use[16]. Although the population was not of postmenopausal but younger women, these results suggest at least that high doses of 19-norsteroid progestins did not increase the risk of breast cancer.

The above-mentioned conflicting results have resulted in an active controversy as to whether progestins should be added to estrogens in HRT and especially whether hysterectomized women would need the progestins.

Laboratory data on progestin action on breast cells

Experimental studies on human breast cells have also generated conflicting results but tend to shed some light on the true effects of progestins on the breast.

Histological findings and controversy

The first wave of controversies linked to the study of Pike and colleagues[7] followed the publication of Ferguson and Anderson[17] to whom Pike referred. This study was designed to examine the mitosis rate in histological sections of breast tissue collected in young women who underwent surgery for non-cancerous lesions. The tissues were collected at various stages of their menstrual cycle and the authors concluded that an increased rate of mitosis was present during the luteal phase as well as a peak in apoptosis.

Although Vogel and co-workers[18] in similar experiments found a different pattern with increased mitosis activity during the follicular phase, the histological data were diversely interpreted and opposing hypotheses arose as to the effect of sex steroids on breast-cell activity.

It was correctly argued that breast cells would react to the cumulative effect of estrogens and progesterone secreted over several cycles rather than to the daily change in hormonal production[19], and also that, breast cells being much slower to respond to estrogen than are endometrial cells, the observed mitosis increase

in the early luteal phase might rather reflect the rising level of estrogen over the late follicular phase[20].

Biological studies

Several experiments have helped to understand a number of mechanisms through which progesterone and some progestins regulate the estrogenic action on the breast tissue.

Enzyme and receptor in vitro studies It has been shown that progesterone, and some progestins, stimulate the 17β-estradiol dehydrogenase which converts estradiol into estrone, a less active metabolite. Also, progestins decrease the content of epithelial cells in estradiol (E_2) receptors thus decreasing the estrogen-induced effects, and also, under certain conditions, decrease breast-cell proliferation[21-23].

Musgrove and colleagues[24] have performed elegant *in vitro* studies demonstrating that breast cells in the late phase of cell cycle activity are initially driven to the S phase of DNA synthesis by progestins. This effect is transient and further application of progestins suppresses the cyclins, then halting the breast cell division in early G_1 phase.

These experiments underline a dual effect of progestins according to the duration of their application, and may reconcile both hypotheses for the role of progestins: stimulator or suppressor of breast cell mitoses[20].

Animal studies Progesterone (P) induces a secretory transformation of the breast buds into acini which are then insensitive to chemical carcinogens[25,26]. In *in vivo* studies performed in surgically postmenopausal female monkeys, it was suggested by Cline and associates[27] that MPA administered orally, at doses equivalent to those used in women for HRT, would increase the tissue proliferation. These authors indeed showed from morphometric studies that the mammary gland thickness was increased under therapy, and also the percentage of mammary gland occupied by glandular tissue was increased more markedly in the group of animals receiving HRT. This finding has been interpreted as a marker of a mitogenic role of the progestin. However it was clearly stated by the authors that there was no statistical difference in the proliferative index measured in animals receiving estrogen alone from that measured in those receiving combined therapy.

In addition, it is well known that progestins act synergistically with estrogens to promote cell differentiation and acini formation. Therefore the glandular volume increases under combined E_2 and P action and this may account for the findings of Cline and colleagues[27] reflecting merely a physiological phenomenon.

Earlier, McManus and Welsch[28] grafting normal human breast tissue to athymic nude mice showed that estrogen increased the growth of the ductal epithelium within the transplants while progesterone alone did not have any influence. When added to estrogens, progesterone did not enhance their effect.

Human studies and ex vivo studies In premenopausal women undergoing surgery for benign mammary lesions, Chang and coworkers[29] applied either estradiol gel or progesterone gel or a placebo on the breast for 11–13 days before surgery. The treatments were applied during the first phase of their cycle as surgery was scheduled between days 11 and 13 of the menstrual cycle, before presumed ovulation. Samples of glandular tissue were collected and the mitotic activity measured. They found a striking difference between groups: those women receiving estradiol exhibited a high rate of mitosis (0.83/1000 cells) while those with progesterone had a low mitotic activity in their glandular tissue (0.17/1000 cells) as compared to placebo (0.5/1000 cells). The authors concluded that *in vivo*, high intra-tissular concentrations of progesterone were able to decrease the mitotic activity of the normal lobular epithelial cells.

In an *in vivo* study, Maudelonde and colleagues[30] used a 19-nortestosterone derivative in premenopausal women with benign breast disease (BBD) and showed a significant decrease in estrogen receptor-stained breast cells. The authors suggested that the drug may decrease the stimulatory effects of estrogens on breast tissue by decreasing the number of functional receptors.

Finally the phenomenon of apoptosis or 'programmed cell death', already evidenced in human breast biopsies at the end of the luteal phase[17], is now believed to be one of the regulatory mechanisms by which the breast cells shed at the end of each cycle[31]. It was indeed shown by Foidart and associates[31] that in *ex vivo* experiments using human breast tissue grafted to nude mice, some progestins would trigger apoptosis, the maximum effect appearing after the progestin application was stopped. One interpretation, close to the physiological situation, would be that at the end of each cycle, the drop in progesterone levels would trigger the apoptosis of some breast cells allowing for a regulation of the breast tissue[32]. This hypothesis would fit with the observations of Ferguson and Anderson in the human breast of menstrually cycling women[17].

Role of different progestins on human breast cells As mentioned above, the progestins prescribed for HRT vary between Europe and the USA, and it is not possible to assume a 'class-effect' of these different molecules on the breast cells, given their varying properties.

Using human breast-cancer cell lines in culture, Catherino and co-workers[33] described the estrogenic activity of some 19-nortestosterone derivatives such as norgestrel and gestodene, which were shown to stimulate breast-cancer cell growth through an estrogen-receptor mechanism. Later, Catherino and Jordan[34] tested 19-norprogesterone derivatives using the same model. They showed that nomegestrol acetate, a 19-norprogesterone derivative, inhibited T47D-cell growth and did not exhibit any estrogenic effect. They found that only estradiol, norgestrel and RU486 stimulate cell proliferation while R5020, MPA and nomegestrol acetate were unable to provide a proliferative stimulus. They also demonstrated that this effect of the former molecules on proliferation was an estrogen receptor-mediated effect.

These experiments may partly explain the contradictory results of some epidemiological studies. It must be stressed that the study of Bergkvist and colleagues[10] mostly included users of estradiol valerate in combination with norgestrel or norethisterone acetate, while the studies from the United States were mostly referring to MPA as the main progestin used for combined HRT.

Trends in world progestin consumption over recent years

As already mentioned above, the progestins prescribed for HRT vary from country to country, and the coprescription of progestins together with estrogens is only a recent phenomenon in most countries. The progestin molecule most often prescribed in the United States remains medroxyprogesterone acetate (MPA), a 17OH-progesterone derivative exhibiting some glucocorticoid activity and a partial androgenic effect[35,36]. In Europe, several combinations of estrogens and progestins have been developed and the progestational molecules are often derivatives of 19-nortestosterone which have lost their main androgenic effect, but still bind to the androgen receptor. These well-known 19-nortestosterone compounds include both the estrane derivatives such as norethisterone, and the gonane category such as norgestrel. Progesterone itself, and its derivatives such as dydrogesterone and the 19-norprogesterone compounds, are also largely prescribed in Europe.

France is a particular country where several progestins have been registered and the coprescription of progestins with estrogens has been recommended since the late 1970s. In addition, several progestins have been widely used in France to treat various gynecological disorders whenever a transitory suppression of the ovarian function was necessary. The most common prescriptions for HRT include natural progesterone in a micronized form (MP), the 19-norprogesterones such as nomegestrol acetate (NOM Ac) and promegestone (R5020), dydrogesterone (DDG) and also chlormadinone acetate (CLA), another 17OH-progesterone derivative differing from MPA as it does not exert glucocorticoid or androgenic effects. All of these compounds are devoid of androgenic properties and also devoid of estrogenic effect, an important factor in view of breast cell cycle regulation[33,34].

Examining the prescription curves for progestins in all related indications including HRT as well, a striking difference exists between the USA and the European countries. In 1985 when adjusted to the number of women, the number of progestin tablets sold in France was 12 times as high as the number sold in the USA. In 1995, the ratio France/USA was 3. The volume for Europe is represented essentially by the French market (Information Medical and Statistics data).

The increase in prescriptions rose steadily in Europe but strikingly in the USA since 1991. Indeed, the Food and Drug Administration (FDA) recommended the coprescription of progestins with estrogens for HRT in non-hysterectomized women in 1991[37]. In 1995 the number of prescriptions was about 800 million tablets per year in the USA and 600 million in France, a very small difference if we consider the population numbers of the two countries. Although it would be inaccurate to draw any parallel between progestin sales and breast-cancer incidence as so many other factors are involved in breast-cancer risk, it is however interesting also to note striking differences over the years in breast cancer incidence between the USA and Europe. According to Surveillance, Epidemiology, End Result (SEER) information[2,3] the annual incidence of breast cancer among American women increased by approximately 52% during the years 1940–90. During the same period prescriptions of progestins for HRT were minimal, and it is unlikely that progestins could be considered as one of the factors involved in that trend. In France, where progestins were largely prescribed since the late 1970s it is not obvious that any relationship could be established between the incidence of breast cancer and progestin sales. When examining progestin consumption and breast-cancer incidence, the trends are those of a higher consumption of progestins for a lower breast-cancer incidence, in France as compared to the USA. Hence, data from the International Agency for Research on Cancer established a breast-cancer incidence for the period 1983–87 at 64.4 and 89.2 per 100 000 women for five French registries and United States SEER white women, respectively[38]. For the same period, the consumption of progestins was about ten times greater in France than in the USA.

Given the magnitude of progestin consumption in France, should these molecules increase breast-cancer risk, it would affect the trend for breast-cancer incidence in France as compared to other countries. Obviously, curve analysis does not permit the establishment of any causal relationship between progestin consumption and breast-cancer incidence.

The lifetime odds ratio for breast cancer in North America was 1 : 10.6 in the late 1970s and is at present 1 : 8 while in Europe the trends are less intense. In France the lifetime odds were about 1 : 11 and have remained close to 1 : 11, or 1 : 14 when adjusted for death occurring before age 90 years[39].

Obviously, the improvement in mammographic screening which explained the peak of cancers observed in the mid 1980s in the USA has also occurred in France. Also, it has become mandatory to perform a breast X-ray before any prescription of estrogens and HRT since the mid 1980s. Therefore the screening effect alone could not account for the difference in breast-cancer incidence curves observed between the countries.

Conclusion

Although the relationship between progestin use and breast-cancer risk is still the subject of debate and controversy, the data reported to date do not allow any conclusion in favor of a harmful effect. Therefore there should be no change in the currently accepted coprescription of progestins with ERT. Further studies are still needed, randomized long-term prospective studies as well as from the laboratory, especially to determine whether a sequential or continuous regimen would be preferable as far as breast-cell response and apoptosis are concerned, and what are the effects of the various molecules used for HRT.

From a practical viewpoint and until these trials give us a clear answer, it would be wise to prescribe long-term HRT to postmenopausal women with a low risk of breast cancer, when a first X-ray excludes the diagnosis. The lowest effective dose of estrogens is the rule, and the progestin to be added should be devoid of androgenic and estrogenic effects. The avoidance of androgenic side-effects would prevent any negative effect on the estrogen-related cardiovascular benefit, and the avoidance of estrogenic effects would prevent potential breast-cell stimulation.

For women at risk or with a previous diagnosis of breast cancer, risks must be weighed against benefits according to the patient's symptoms and other risks, bearing in mind that the median age at diagnosis of breast cancer is 64, of myocardial infarction is 74 and of hip fracture is 79 years[40].

Acknowledgements

The authors wish to express their thanks to Ms M. J. Goldfrad for her technical assistance and to Professor J. C. Thalabard for his scientific advice.

References

1. McPherson, K., Steel, C. M. and Dixon, J.M. (1994). Breast cancer – epidemiology, risk factors, and genetics. *Br. Med. J.*, **309**, 1003–6
2. Cancer Surveillance Section, CDC (1994). Deaths from breast cancer – United States, 1991. *J. Am. Med. Assoc.*, **271** (18), 1395–7
3. Feuer, E. J., Wum, L. M., Boring, C. C., Flanders, W. D., Timmel, M. J. and Tong, T. (1993). The lifetime risk of developing breast cancer. *J. Natl. Cancer Inst.*, **85**, 892–7
4. Steinberg, K. K., Thacker, S. B., Smith, S. J., Stroup, D. F., Zack, M. M., Flanders, D. and Berkelman, R. L. (1991). A meta-analysis of the effects of oestrogen replacement therapy and the risk of breast cancer. *J. Am. Med. Assoc.*, **265**, 1985–90
5. Grady, D., Rubin, S. M., Petitti, D. B., Fox, C. S., Black, D., Ettinger, B., Ernster, V. L. and Cummings, S. R. (1992). Hormone therapy to prevent disease and prolong life in postmenopausal women. *Ann. Intern. Med.*, **117**, 1016–37
6. Daly, E., Roche, M., Barlow, D., Gray, A., McPherson, K. and Vessey, M. (1992). HRT: an analysis of benefits, risks and costs. *Br. Med. Bull.*, **48**, 368–400
7. Pike, M. C., Henderson, B. E., Krailo, M. D., Duke, A. and Roy, S. (1983). Breast cancer in young women and use of oral contraceptive: possible modifying effect of formulation and age at use. *Lancet*, **2**, 926–30
8. Gambrell, R. D. Jr, Maier, R. and Sanders, B. (1983). Decreased incidence of breast cancer in postmenopausal oestrogen and progestogen? *Obstet. Gynecol.*, **62**, 435–43
9. Nachtigall, M. J., Smiler, S. W., Nachtigall, R. D., Nachtigall, R. H. and Nachtigall, L. E. (1992). Incidence of breast cancer in a 22 year study of women receiving estrogen-progestin replacement therapy. *Obstet. Gynecol.*, **80**, 827–30
10. Bergkvist, L., Adami, H. O., Persson, I., Hoover, R. and Schairer, C. (1989). The risk of breast cancer after oestrogen and oestrogen/progestogen replacement. *N. Engl. J. Med.*, **321**, 293–7
11. Persson, I., Yuen, J., Bergkvist, L., Adami, H. O., Hoover, R. and Schairer, C. (1992). Combined oestrogen-progestogen and breast cancer risk. *Lancet*, **340**, 1044
12. Ewertz, M. (1988). Influence of non-contraceptive exogenous and endogenous sex hormones on breast cancer risk in Denmark. *Int. J. Cancer*, **42**, 832–8
13. Colditz, G. A., Hankinson, S. E., Hunter, D. J., Willett, W. C., Manson, J. E., Stampfer, M. J., Hennekens, C., Rosner, B. and Speizer, F. E. (1995). The use of oestrogens and progestins and the risk of breast cancer in postmenopausal women. *N. Engl. J. Med.*, **332**, 1589–93
14. Stanford, J. K., Weiss, N. S., Voigt, L. F., Daling, J. R., Habel, L. A. and Rossing, M. A. (1995). Combined estrogen and progestin hormone replacement therapy in relation to risk of breast cancer in middle-aged women. *J. Am. Med. Assoc.*, **274**, 137–42
15. Newcomb, P. A., Longnecker, M. P., Storer, B. E., Mittendorf, R., Baron, J., Clapp, R. W., Bogdan, G. and Willet, W. C. (1995). Long-term hormone replacement therapy and risk of breast cancer in postmenopausal women. *Am. J. Epidemiol.*, **142**, 788–95
16. Plu-Bureau, G., Lê, M., Sitruk-Ware, R., Thalabard, J. C. and Mauvais-Jarvis, P. (1994). Progestogen use and the decreased risk of breast cancer in a cohort of premenopausal women with benign breast disease. *Br. J. Cancer*, **70**, 270–7
17. Ferguson, D. J. P. and Anderson, T. J. (1981). Morphological evaluation of cell turnover in relation to the menstrual cycle in the resting human breast. *Br. J. Cancer*, **44**, 177–81
18. Vogel, P. M., Geogiade, N. G., Fetter, B. E., Vogel, F.S. and McCarty, K.S. (1981). The correlation of histologic changes in the human breast with the menstrual cycle. *Am. J. Pathol.*, **104**, 23–34
19. Sitruk-Ware, R. (1992). Estrogens, progestins and breast cancer risk in postmenopausal women: state of the ongoing controversy in 1992. *Maturitas*, **15**, 129–39
20. Wren, B. G. (1995). Hormonal replacement therapy and breast cancer. *Eur. Menopause J.*, **2**, 13–19
21. Fournier, S., Kuttenn, F., De Cicco, F., Baudot, N., Malet, C. and Mauvais-Jarvis P. (1982). Estradiol 17β hydroxysteroid dehydrogenase activity in human breast fibro adenomas. *J. Clin. Endocrinol. Metab.*, **55**, 428–33
22. Botella, J., Duranti, E., Duc, I., Cognet, A. M., Delansorne, R. and Paris, J. (1994). Inhibition by nomegestrol acetate and other synthetic progestins on proliferation and progesterone receptor content of T47-D human breast cancer cells. *J. Steroid Biochem. Mol. Biol.*, **50**, 41–7
23. Clarke, C. L. and Sutherland, R. L. (1990). Progestin regulation of cellular proliferation. *Endocr. Rev.*, **11**, 266–301
24. Musgrove, E. A., Lee, C. S. L. and Sutherland, R. L. (1991). Progestins both stimulate and inhibit

breast cancer cell cycle progression while increasing expression of transforming growth factor, epidermal growth factor receptor, c-fos and c-myc genes. *Mol. Cell Biol.*, 11, 5032–43

25. Russo, J., Tay, L. K. and Russo, I. H. (1982). Differentiation of the mammary gland and susceptibility to carcinogenesis. *Breast Cancer Res. Treat.*, 2, 5–73

26. Labrie., F., Li, S., Bélanger, A., Côté, J., Mérand, Y. and Lepage, M. (1993). Controlled release low dose medroxyprogesterone acetate (MPA) inhibits the development of mammary tumors induced by dimethyl-benz(a) anthracene in the rat. *Breast Cancer Res. Treat.*, 26, 253–65

27. Cline, J. M., Soderqvist, G., Von Schoultz, E., Skoog, L. and Von Schoultz, B. (1996). Effects of hormone replacement therapy on the mammary gland of surgically postmenopausal cynomolgus macaques. *Am. J. Obstet. Gynecol.*, 174, 93–100

28. McManus, M. J. and Welsch, C. W. (1984). The effect of estrogen, progesterone, thyroxine, and human placental lactogen on DNA synthesis of human breast ductal epithelium maintained in athymic nude mice. *Cancer*, 54, 1920–7

29. Chang, K. J., Lee, T. T. Y., Linares-Cruz, G., Fournier, S. and de Lignières, B. (1995). Influence of percutaneous administration of estradiol and progesterone on human breast epithelial cell cycle *in vivo*. *Fertil. Steril.*, 63, 785–91

30. Maudelonde, T., Lavaud, P., Salazar, G., Laffargue, F. and Rochefort, H. (1991). Progestin treatment depresses oestrogen receptor but not cathepsin D levels in needle aspirates of benign breast disease. *Breast Cancer Res. Treat.*, 19, 95–102

31. Foidart, J. M., Colin, C., Denoo, X., Desreux, J., Fournier, S. and de Lignières, B. (1996). Influence of percutaneous administration of estradiol and progesterone on the proliferation of human breast epithelial cells. In Calvo, F., Crépin, M. and Magdelenat, H. (eds.) *Breast Cancer, Advances in Biology and Therapeutics*, pp. 329–34. (London: John Libbey Eurotext)

32. Wren, B. G. and Eden, J. A. (1996). Do progestogens reduce the risk of breast cancer? A review of the evidence. *Menopause*, 3, 4–12

33. Catherino, W. H., Jeng, M. H. and Jordan, V.C. (1993). Norgestrel and gestodene stimulate breast cancer cell growth through an oestrogen receptor mediated mechanism. *Br. J. Cancer*, 67, 945–52

34. Catherino, W. H. and Jordan, V. C. (1995). Nomegestrol acetate, a clinically useful 19-norprogesterone derivative which lacks estrogenic activity. *J. Steroid Biochem. Mol. Biol.*, 55(2), 239–46

35. Hellman, I., Yoshida, K., Zumoff, B., Levin, J., Kream, J. and Fukushima D. K. (1976). The effect of medroxyprogesterone acetate on the pituitary-adrenal axis. *J. Clin. Endocrinol. Metab.*, 42, 912–17

36. Bullock, L. P. and Bardin, C. W. (1977). Androgenic, synandrogenic and anti-androgenic actions of progestins. *Ann. NY Acad. Sci.*, 286, 321-30

37. Food and Drug Administration (1991). FDA Committee recommends approval of estrogen/progestogen use. SCRIP 24, 1632

38. Menegoz, F., Black, R. J., Arveux, P., Magne, F., Ferlay, J., Buemi, A., Carli, P. M., Chapelain, G., Faivre, J., Guignoux, M., Grosclaude, P., Macelesec'h, J., Raverdy, N. and Schaffer, P. (1996). Cancer incidence and mortality in France in 1975–1995. Submitted for publication

39. Hill, C., Benhamou, E. and Auquier A. (1994). What is the risk of breast cancer in a given population? *Bull. Cancer (Paris)*, 81, 785–7

40. Hulka, B. S. and Stark, A. T. (1995). Breast cancer: cause and prevention. *Lancet*, 346, 883–7

6

Hormone activity in the endometrium

Hormonal activity in the endometrium: tissue remodeling and uterine bleeding   31

L. A. Salamonsen

Ovarian steroid hormones orchestrate the cyclical remodeling of the endometrium that occurs during reproductive life and after the menopause. When ovarian follicular activity ceases, endometrial remodeling also ceases and the endometrium enters a phase of quiescence which remains for the rest of a woman's life. As the menopause approaches, the hormonal milieu becomes unpredictable and liable to large fluctuations, and considerable disturbances in patterns of menstrual bleeding occur. Similar disturbances of uterine bleeding are also experienced by women using progestagenic steroids as contraceptives (particularly the long-acting progestins), or hormone replacement therapy: such disturbances occur predominantly during the first year of use.

Actions of estrogen and progesterone on the endometrium can be direct or indirect (Figure 1). The hormones either directly influence those cells containing receptors, resulting in direct actions, or stimulate production of paracrine factors, often growth factors or cytokines, which in turn modulate the actions of adjacent cells. Thirdly, steroid hormones can stimulate the entry, differentiation or activation of resident cells of hemopoietic origin within tissues (Miller and Hunt, 1996) and these also contribute an array of bioactive molecules. Estrogen and progesterone receptors (ER and PR respectively), which have been localized by immunohistochemistry in the endometrium across the menstrual cycle[1], appear in both epithelial and stromal cells during the

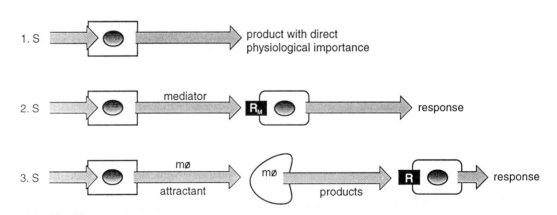

Figure 1 Possible mechanisms by which steroid hormones may exert effects in tissue. (1) Steroid hormone (S) acts directly on target cell bearing specific receptor, resulting in production of molecule of direct physiological importance. (2) Target cell produces mediator which then acts on adjacent cell through specific receptor, generally on cell membrane (R_M), second cell producing response. (3) Steroid hormone acts to induce production of chemokine, which attracts cell of hematopoietic origin into tissue: products of this cell elicit physiological response.

Table 1 Potential paracrine regulators of matrix metalloproteinases and tissue inhibitors (MMPs/TIMPs) in human endometrium. Reprinted from reference 3, with permission

Regulator	Cellular source	Phase of peak production
TGFβ[21]	epithelial, stromal	secretory (M,L)
TNFα[22]	epithelial, stromal	secretory (M,L)
LIF[23]	epithelial	secretory (M,L)
RLX[24]	decidual, epithelial	secretory (M,L)
PRL[24]	decidual,epithelial	secretory (M,L)
ET[25]	epithelial	secretory, menstrual
PGE/PGF$_{2\alpha}$[26]	stromal/epithelial	menstrual
IL-1[27]	stromal/epithelial	secretory (M,L)

TGFβ, transforming growth factor-β; TNFα, tumor necrosis factor-α; LIF, leukemia inhibiting factor; RLX, relaxin; PRL, prolactin; ET, endothelin; PGE/PGF, prostaglandin E/F; IL-1, interleukin-1; M, mid; L, late

proliferative phase reaching a peak around mid-cycle. Subsequently, the ER decline, being more rapidly lost from stromal than epithelial cells, with PR being retained on stroma in the functionalis layer throughout the secretory phase, while they decline in the epithelium after about day 20. Some factors produced by different endometrial cell types, which exert paracrine effects, and whose production undergoes cyclical variability, are detailed in Table 1.

Menstruation can be defined as the partial breakdown and loss of the functionalis layer of the endometrium that occurs following the fall of progesterone and estrogen at the end of a normal ovulatory cycle. This process can be mimicked by withdrawal of exogenous hormones or administration of progesterone antagonists such as mifipristone (RU486) at the appropriate time of the cycle. Until recently, little has been known of the mechanisms of normal menstruation, most of our understanding being derived from morphological studies using intraocular autotransplants of endometrium in rhesus monkeys[2]. Recently, a paradigm shift in this understanding has occurred, with combined data from a number of laboratories demonstrating a clear and central role for a

family of matrix-degrading enzymes, the matrix metalloproteinases (MMPs), in menstruation (for review see reference 3). These enzymes[4] degrade extracellular matrix components, including both interstitial matrix and basement membranes. While individual MMPs have different substrate specificities, there is considerable overlap and a number of enzymes acting in concert are able to fully degrade most matrices. Matrix metalloproteinases have a number of specific properties: all are Zn^{2+}-dependent ectoenzymes, which are secreted in latent forms requiring activation by cleavage of the propeptide; this can be achieved by a number of proteases with specificity for different MMPs and also some pro-MMPs can be activated by others or autoactivated. In this respect, MMP-3 probably has a central role as once activated, it can further activate other family members, thus setting up a cascade of enzyme activities. MMPs are also specifically inhibited by members of a family of specific tissue inhibitors (TIMPs) and it is the balance between the MMPs and TIMPs that is probably ultimately of most importance in determining whether degradation will occur at any focal point in a tissue.

A number of MMPs are produced within the endometrium at menstruation. MMP-1 (interstitial collagenase), MMP-2 (gelatinase A) and MMP-3 (stromelysin 1) are produced by endometrial stromal cells[5] while MMP-7 (matrilysin) is produced by endometrial epithelial cells[6] and another gelatinase (MMP-9, gelatinase B) is a product of neutrophils and other migratory cells within menstrual endometrium[7]. The location of the enzymes coincides exactly with sites of tissue degradation[3] and in tissue explants, such degradation can be inhibited by specific inhibitors of MMPs[8]. An area of current active research is into the mechanisms by which these enzymes are regulated. Regulation can be at a number of levels: expression and translation of mRNA, activation of latent enzymes in the extracellular environment, and increase or decrease of TIMPs at focal points.

Progesterone has long been recognized as a regulator of collagenase (MMP-1) activity in the uterus[9,10]. Glucocorticoids and retinoids but not estrogen have also been identified as important steroids in regulation of MMP genes (reviewed in reference 11). In the human endometrium, progesterone is clearly an important player: withdrawal of progesterone increases the production of MMPs from both tissue explants[12] and decidualized stromal cells in culture[13–15], while not altering the expression of TIMPs[15]. However, the focal nature of MMP action at menstruation, and the occurrence of menstruation only in certain primates, including humans, while progesterone withdrawal at the end of the estrous cycle occurs in most mammalian species, suggests that while progesterone withdrawal may be obligatory for menstruation, it is not the essential causative factor of MMP production and activation.

Cytokine products of adjacent cell types can regulate MMP production by endometrial cells in culture. Both interleukin-1α and tumor necrosis factor-α stimulate the production of MMP-1, -3 and -9 but not MMP-2 from endometrial stromal cells[5], while transforming growth factor β has been identified as the stromal factor mediating progesterone effects on epithelial cell production of MMP-7[16]. Both mast cells and eosinophils are activated in perimenopausal endometrium[17] and these can also provide all the above cytokines as well as a myriad of other potential regulators[18,19]. Mast cell tryptase is of particular interest as it activates pro-MMP-3 *in vitro*[20] and thus could be responsible for setting up a cascade of MMP activity at focal points.

It is apparent from these summarized studies and others, that while progesterone withdrawal may be obligatory for the production and activation of MMPs at menstruation, its effects are largely indirect, being mediated by cytokines and other regulatory molecules produced by endometrial cells themselves, or by hemopoietic cells which migrate into, or are resident in the endometrium. A simplified scenario is presented in Figure 2. It is likely that the unstable estrogen and progesterone levels seen around the time of the menopause drive endometrial disturbances, particularly altering migration and activation of hemopoietic cells and production of bioactive molecules by stromal and epithelial cells, resulting in an alteration in the production of MMPs and hence tissue breakdown and bleeding. Studies are currently under way to examine such mechanisms.

Acknowledgements

Studies in the author's laboratory are funded by the National Health and Medical Research Council (NH&MRC, project grant 940538), the National Institutes of Health (NIH, grant D33233) and the Human Reproduction Program of the World Health Organization (WHO, grant 92909).

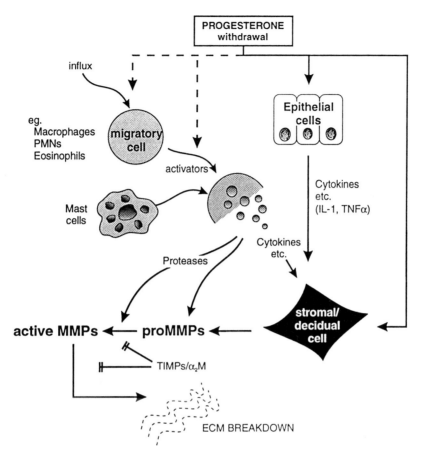

Figure 2 Schematic illustration of potential mechanisms for initiation of matirx metallo-proteinase (MMP) activity at menstruation. (1) Withdrawal of progesterone may induce entry or activation of migratory cells into endometrium, upregulation of cytokine production or other paracrine factors from epithelium, or directly promote MMP production from these cells and from endometrial stromal and/or decidual cells. (2) Mediators derived from epithelial or migratory cells may also stimulate stromal/decidual cell production of MMPs. (3) Proteases from migratory cells will activate latent MMPs and cascade of activation will be established with some active MMPs activating other members of this gene family. (4) Resultant MMP-mediated degradation of endometrial extracellular matrix (ECM) and basement membranes removes most of functionalis layer in preparation for next cycle. Reproduced from reference 3, with permission

References

1. Lessey, B. A., Killam, A. P., Metzger, D. A., Haney, A. F., Greene, G. I. and McCarty K. S. Jr (1988). Immunohistochemical analysis of human uterine estrogen and progesterone receptors throughout the menstrual cycle. *J. Clin Endocrinol. Metab.*, **67**, 334–40

2. Markee, J. E. (1940). Menstruation in intraocular endometrial transplants in the rhesus monkey. *Contrib. Embryol.*, **177**, 220–320

3. Salamonsen, L. A. and Woolley, D. E. (1996). Matrix metalloproteinases in normal menstruation. *Human Reprod.*, **11** (Suppl. 2), 124–33

4. Birkedal-Hansen, H., Moore, W. G. I., Bodden, M. K., Windsor, L. J., Birkedal-Hansen, B., De Carlo, A. and Engler, J. A. (1993). Matrix metalloproteinases: a review. *Crit. Rev. Oral Biol. Med.*, **4**, 199–250

5. Rawdanowicz, T. J., Hampton, A. L., Nagase, H.,

Woolley, D. E. and Salamonsen, L. A. (1994). Matrix metalloproteinase secretion by cultured human endometrial stromal cells: identification of interstitial collagenase, gelatinase A, gelatinase B and stromelysin 1. Differential regulation by interleukin-1α and tumor necrosis factor β. *J. Clin. Endocrinol. Metab.*, **79**, 530–6

6. Rodgers, W. H., Osteen, K. G., Matrisian, L. M., Navre, M., Guidice, L.C. and Gorstein, F. (1993). Expression and localisation of matrilysin, a matrix metalloproteinase, in human endometrium during the reproductive cycle. *Am. J. Obstet. Gynecol.*, **168**, 253–60

7. Jeziorska, M., Nagase, H., Salamonsen, L. A. and Woolley, D. E. (1996). Immunolocalization of the matrix metalloproteinases, gelatinase B and stromelysin-1 in human endometrium throughout the menstrual cycle. *J. Reprod. Fertil.*, **107**, 43–51

8. Marbaix, E., Kokorine, I., Moulin, P., Donnez, J., Eeckhout, Y. and Courtoy, P. J. (1996). Menstrual breakdown of human endometrium can be mimicked *in vitro* and is selectively and reversibly blocked by inhibitors of matrix metalloproteinases. *Proc. Natl. Acad. Sci. USA*, **93**, 9120–5

9. Jeffrey, J. J., Coffey, R. J. and Eisen, A. Z. (1971). Studies on uterine collagenase in tissue culture. II. Effect of steroid hormones on enzyme production. *Biochim. Biophys. Acta*, **252**, 143–50

10. Wilcox, B. D., Rydelek-Fitzgerald, L. and Jeffrey, J. J. (1992). Regulation of collagenase gene expression by serotonin and progesterone in rat uterine smooth muscle cells. *J. Biol. Chem.*, **267**, 20752–7

11. Salamonsen, L. A. (1996). Matrix metalloproteinases and their tissue inhibitors in endocrinology. *Trends Endocrinol.*, **7**, 28–34

12. Marbaix, E., Donnez, J., Courtoy, P. J. and Eeckhout, Y. (1992). Progesterone regulates the activity of collagenase and related gelatinases A and B in human endometrial explants. *Proc. Natl. Acad. Sci. USA*, **89**, 11789–93

13. Schatz, F., Papp, C., Toth-Pal, E. and Lockwood, C. J. (1994). Ovarian steroid-modulated stromelysin-1 expression in human endometrial stromal and decidual cells. *J. Clin. Endocrinol. Metab.*, **78**, 1467–72

14. Irwin, J. C., Kirk, D., Gwatkin, R. B. L., Navre, M., Cannon, P. and Guidice, L. C. (1996). Human endometrial matrix metalloproteinase-2, a putative menstrual proteinase. Hormonal regulation in cultured stromal cells and messenger RNA expression during the menstrual cycle. *J. Clin. Invest.*, **97**, 438–47

15. Salamonsen, L. A., Butt, A. R., Hammond, F. R., Garcia, S. and Zhang, J. (1997). Production of endometrial matrix metalloproteinases but not their tissue inhibitors is modulated by progesterone withdrawal in an *in vitro* model for menstruation. *J. Clin. Endocrinol. Metab.*, in press

16. Bruner, K. L., Rodgers, W. H., Gold, L. I., Korc, M., Hargrove, J. T., Matrisian, L. M. and Osteen, K. G. (1995). Transforming growth factor β mediates the progesterone suppression of an epithelial metalloproteinase by adjacent stroma in the human endometrium. *Proc. Natl. Acad. Sci. USA*, **92**, 7362–6

17. Jeziorska, M., Nagase, H., Salamonsen, L. A. and Woolley, D. E. (1996). Immunolocalization of the matrix metalloproteinases, gelatinase B and stromelysin-1 in human endometrium throughout the menstrual cycle. *J. Reprod. Fertil.*, **107**, 43–51

18. Galli, S. J. (1993). New concepts about the mast cell. *N. Engl. J. Med.*, **328**, 257–65

19. Kroegel, C., Virchow, J.-C., Luttmann, W., Walker, C. and Warner J. A. (1994). Pulmonary immune cells in health and disease: the eosinophil leukocyte (Part 1). *Eur. Resp. J.*, **7**, 519–43

20. Lees, M., Taylor, D. J. and Woolley, D. E. (1994). Mast cell proteinases activate precursor forms of collagenase and stromelysin 1, but not of gelatinases A and B. *Eur. J. Biochem.*, **223**, 171–7

21. Kauma, S., Matt, D., Strom, S., Eierman, D. and Turner, T. (1990). Interleukin-1β, human leukocyte antigen HLA-DRa, and transforming growth factor-β expression in endometrium, placenta and placental membranes. *Am. J. Obstet. Gynecol.*, **163**, 130–7

22. Hunt, J. S., Chen, H.-L., Hu, X.-L. and Tabibzadeh, S. (1992). Tumor necrosis factor-α messenger ribonucleic acid and protein in human endometrium. *Biol. Reprod.*, **47**, 141–7

23. Vogiagis, D., Marsh, M. M., Fry, R. C. and Salamonsen, L. A. (1996). Leukemia inhibitory factor in human endometrium throughout the menstrual cycle. *J. Endocrinol.*, **148**, 95–102

24. Bryant-Greenwood, G. D., Rutanen, E.-M., Partanen, S., Coelho, T. K. and Yamamoto, S. Y. (1993). Sequential appearance of relaxin, prolactin and IGFBP-1 during growth and differentiation of the human endometrium. *Mol. Cell. Endocrinol.*, **95**, 23–9

25. Salamonsen, L. A., Butt, A. R., Macpherson, A. M., Rogers, P. A. W. and Findlay, J. K. (1992). Immunolocalization of the vasoconstrictor endothelin in human endometrium during the menstrual cycle and in umbilical cord at birth. *Am. J. Obstet. Gynecol.*, **167**, 163–7

26. Abel, M. H. and Kelly, R.W. (1979). Differential production of prostaglandins within the human uterus. *Prostaglandins*, **18**, 821–8

27. Tabibzadeh, S. and Sun, X. Z. (1992). Cytokine expression in human endometrium throughout the menstrual cycle. *Human Reprod.*, **7**, 1214–21

Biology of the endometrium

32

E.-M. Rutanen

Endometrial components and cyclic changes

The basis for all understanding of endometrial biology is to realize that this tissue is composed of different cell types. The major cell types in the endometrium are epithelial cells, stromal cells and vascular endothelial cells. Epithelial cells in glands and the luminal epithelium are functionally quite different, and even within the same anatomical position epithelial cells may have different functions. Endometrial stroma is composed of a heterogeneous population of cells, the fibroblast-like cells being the major cell type. In addition, endometrial stroma contains various types of leukocytes, the number of which varies depending on the phase of the menstrual cycle. Some of the fibroblast-like stromal cells undergo decidual differentiation during the late luteal phase. Also, the extracellular matrix that underlies the epithelium as the basement membrane and surrounds the stromal cells as interstitial matrix is assumed to play an important role in endometrial biology.

Two morphologically different compartments can be distinguished in the endometrium, i.e. stratum basalis and stratum functionalis. The latter is further divided into compact and spongy layers. During the normal menstrual period the functionalis is lost, while the basal layer is preserved and gives rise to regeneration of the endometrium during the next cycle. The vessels of the functionalis of the endometrium differ from vessels of other organs and tissues by their unique structure and their ability to respond quickly to hormonal stimuli. In contrast, the vessels of the basalis are influenced little by hormonal changes of the cycle.

As the most sensitive target organ of ovarian steroid hormones, endometrium undergoes strictly regulated cyclic changes in morphology as well as in biochemical and functional characteristics during each ovulatory menstrual cycle. Estrogen is the major stimulator of endometrial cell proliferation, whereas progesterone counteracts the action of estrogen and induces endometrial differentiation with differentiated functions during the postovulatory phase of the menstrual cycle. In general, estrogen priming is a requirement of progesterone action in the endometrium. First responses in human endometrium to ovarian steroid hormones can be demonstrated at 20–21 weeks' gestation, and this response is maintained in late postmenopausal years if endometrium is exposed to estrogen. Steroids can act directly or indirectly through cell–cell interactions to regulate not only proliferation and differentiation but also several other functions in different endometrial cell types. Different endometrial cell types synthesize molecules, which are differentially regulated by steroids and which may have different cell-specific functions in the cells that produce them (autocrine action) or in the neighbour cells (paracrine action). Especially decidual transformation is associated with remarkable biochemical changes in the endometrium. Also, extracellular matrix shows cyclic changes, suggesting hormonal regulation. The major components of the extracellular matrix include fibronectin, vitronectin, laminin, and different types of collagen and fibronectin which bind to specific receptors, such as integrins, cadherins and selectins[1,2]. Matrix metalloproteinases are a group of locally produced enzymes that are involved in degradation of matrix and endometrial remodeling[3]. In addition, metalloproteinases are assumed to play a role in implantation and angiogenesis, and in activation of growth factors. At a woman's reproductive age, the goal of all endometrial changes is to prepare the intrauterine environment for blastocyst implantation. If conception occurs the pregnant endometrium, called decidua, exhibits new characteristics and functions to maintain pregnancy. Following the physiologic decline of ovarian function and withdrawal of both estrogen and progesterone after the menopause, the resting endometrium finally becomes an atrophic endometrium a few years later. Thereafter, all signs of endometrial proliferation should be regarded as pathological.

Tremendous progress has been made in elucidating factors important for endometrial biology after the role of sex steroids as endometrial regulators was discovered in the early 1900s. Identification of receptors as mediators of steroid hormone actions – as transcriptional activators – occurred much later. Yet characterization of several steroid receptor genes, their cloning, sequencing and elucidation of domains vital for receptor functions have added another dimension to the mechanism of steroid action during the past decade. Besides steroid hormones, many peptide hormones, such as prolactin, oxytocin, gonadotropin releasing hormone (GnRH) and luteinizing hormone (LH) have been shown to have binding sites in the human endometrium, but their biological significance is not yet known. During the past 10 years, the development of molecular biology has greatly increased our understanding of the molecular mechanisms of steroid hormone actions. Attention has been focused on growth factors and cytokines which are believed to mediate steroid hormone actions and maintain cell–cell interactions as well as cell–extracellular matrix interactions. The role and significance of local regulators after cessation of ovarian function are still unknown.

This chapter will briefly review molecular processes involved in steroid hormone action in the endometrium. More attention is focused on steroid regulation of growth factor production and the roles of growth factors in modulation of steroid-induced cell proliferation/differentiation. At this point the insulin-like growth factor system will be used as an example.

Steroid receptors and their functions

In addition to steroid hormones, their receptors play a key role in the regulation of cellular events in the endometrium. Estrogen and progesterone receptors are intracellularly located ligand-inducible transcription factors that interact with specific hormone-response elements in target genes[4,5]. The three different domains of the receptor molecule possess specific functions (e.g. steroid and DNA-binding domains). A revolution in receptor studies was the realization that steroid hormone receptors are associated with non-steroid binding proteins that play a role in regulation of receptor function. Some of those proteins, such as heat shock protein 90, are speculated to stabilize the unactivated form of the steroid receptor in the absence of hormone[6]. The steroid-controlled regulatory genes can further regulate the expression of a multitude of genes either via transcription or post-transcriptional pathways. Some of the final protein products may remain intracellular; others are secreted and capable of mediating the steroid action to other cells. Figure 1 schematically represents a simplified model of signal transduction by steroid receptors. Despite many significant advances in the field of molecular biology, our understanding of how steroid receptors regulate gene transcription is still at an early stage.

Estrogen receptor

The estrogen receptor (ER) is a strong hormone-regulated transcription factor that regulates the expression of many structural and functional genes. Estrogen receptor gene

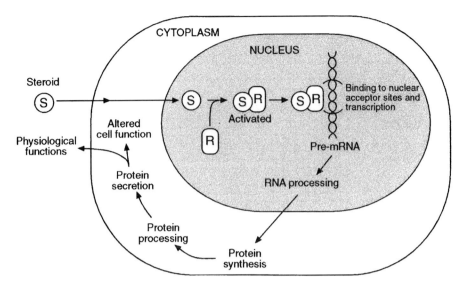

Figure 1 Schematic representation of steroid (S) hormone action. R, receptor

contains eight exons. Alternative splicing of mRNA generates ER variants, which may have different effects on the expression of endogenous estrogen-regulated genes and on growth, and response to the hormone and its antagonist in different tissues[7]. Estrogen is traditionally considered to be a predominant regulator of progesterone receptor gene expression in many systems, although this regulation is not well understood. It is thought that the progesterone receptor (PR) gene is transcriptionally activated by estrogen and inhibited by progesterone. However, it has been difficult definitely to demonstrate DNA sequences that the estrogen receptor recognizes within the progesterone receptor gene, in that the promoter does not contain consensus DNA sequences known to mediate the actions of estrogen receptor. This suggests that estrogen-induced transcription of PR gene is mediated by DNA sequences that are not classic estrogen-response elements but can interact with estrogen receptors.

Progesterone receptor

The complete structure of the human progesterone receptor (hPR) gene has been determined[5]. Progesterone receptor exists in two distinct isoforms, hPR-A and hPR-B, which differ only in that hPR-B contains an additional 164 amino acids at the amino terminus. Both isoforms bind progesterone using the same kinetics, but they exhibit quite different biological functions. The interaction between PR and progesterone induces a series of structural and functional changes in this protein, leading ultimately to an association of the receptor with specific DNA sequences in the regulatory regions of target genes in a cell-specific manner. The PR is down-regulated by its own ligand at the transcriptional level through inhibition of ER-mediated induction and through protein–protein interactions. In addition to estrogen, progesterone, transcription factor AP-1, growth factors such as insulin-like growth factor, and agents that increase intracellular cyclic adenosine monophosphate (cAMP) levels all modulate progesterone receptor or receptor mRNA levels.

In most contexts, PR-B functions as a transcriptional activator of progesterone-responsive genes, whereas PR-A functions as a transcriptional inhibitor of all steroid hormone receptors. For example, PR-A-mediated repression of human ER transcriptional activity seems to depend largely on the absolute expression level of PR-A. Progesterone receptor-

A appears to inhibit ER transcriptional activity as a consequence of a non-competitive interaction of PR-A with either distinct cellular targets or different contact sites on the same target. Thus, the alterations in the expression level of PR-A or its cellular target can have profound effects on the physiological and pharmacological responses to sex steroids. For example, the antiprogestin RU 486 inhibits estrogen action in the endometrium through a PR-A-mediated mechanism[8]. The dual role of PR-A provides a potential mechanism by which cells can generate dissimilar responses to a single hormone.

Post-translational modifications

Post-translational events such as glycosylation or phosphorylation, have turned out to be important in regulating the activity of steroid receptors[9]. Phosphorylation, for example, is essential for progesterone receptor function. There are also other proteins in steroid action cascade, the phosphorylation of which appears to be involved in modulation of steroid receptor-induced gene transcription. Phosphorylation may also be steroid dependent in such a way that, for example, it can inactivate the receptor when bound to estrogen, and the anti-estrogen effect is opposite. This may provide support for independent mechanisms of action for estrogen and anti-estrogen which bind to the same receptor. When a given steroid fails to stimulate its target tissues, it is usually because the tissues lack receptors for that hormone, or the function of the receptors is impaired.

The pattern of endometrial ER and PR during the menstrual cycle

Like ovarian estrogen and progesterone secretion, levels of receptors for estrogen and progesterone in the endometrium fluctuate markedly during the menstrual cycle. Both estrogen and progesterone receptor levels are higher in the proliferative phase and decline after ovulation[10]. Estrogen receptors are mainly located in epithelial cells, but occur also in stromal cells in proliferative phase endometrium. Progesterone receptors are most abundant around the time of ovulation, probably reflecting the ability of estrogen to increase progesterone receptors. Thereafter, they decrease in epithelial cells, but remain abundant in stromal cells also in the luteal phase of the menstrual cycle. The pattern of sex steroid receptors is maintained during the perimenopausal years. In addition, postmenopausal endometrium possesses ER and PR.

Growth factors in the endometrium

An increasing amount of evidence suggests that at least some of the actions of steroid hormones in the endometrium are mediated by growth factors and cytokines, which can act in a juxtacrine, paracrine or autocrine fashion (Figure 2)[11]. The list of growth factors and cytokines identified in human endometrium is growing all the time (Table 1)[12-21]. Each of the endometrial cell types may synthesize different growth factors/cytokines and each of them may mediate a specific steroid hormone-dependent function. Cytokines which modulate a variety of cellular functions in the endometrium have been comprehensively reviewed by Tabibzadeh[21]. Epidermal growth factor (EGF) is supposed to have a role in endometrial proliferation, differentiation and angiogenesis[13]. Glycodelin has immuno-suppressive and contraceptive activities[15]. Transforming growth factor (TGF) β has a variety of actions; for example, it enhances the production of extracellular matrix components and up-regulates a variety of receptors that are important in mediating cell–cell and cell–extracellular matrix interactions[19]. Endothelin (ET)-1 is a potent vasoconstrictor[12]. Vascular endothelial cell growth factor (VEGF) is an angiogenic factor[20]. The insulin-like growth factor (IGF) system, including IGF-I and IGF-II, their receptors and soluble IGF-binding proteins (IGFBP), is perhaps the best characterized growth factor system in the endometrium and will be presented here as an example[16].

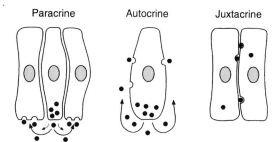

Figure 2 Schematic representation of autocrine, paracrine and juxtacrine cell regulation

Table 1 Growth factors and cytokines in the endometrium

Molecule	Cell type	Steroid-dependence
ET-1[12]	stromal/epithelial cells	?
EGF[13]	epithelial cells	+
bFGF[14]	?	+
Glycodelin[15]	epithelial cells	+
IGF-I[16]	stromal cells	+
IGF-II[16]	stromal cells	+
KGF[17]	stromal cells	?
PDGF[18]	macrophages	?
TGFα[13]	stromal/epithelial cells	+
TGFβ[19]	stromal/epithelial cells	+
VEGF[20]	vascular smooth muscle cells	—
	stromal/epithelial cells	—
CSF-1[21]	epithelial cells	+
IL-1[21]	stromal cells	+
INFγ[21]	lymphocytes	?
TNFα[21]	macrophages	+

ET-1, endothelin-1; EGF, epidermal growth factor; bFGF, basic fibroblast growth factor; IGF-I and II, insulin-like growth factor I and II; KGF, keratinocyte growth factor; PDGF, platelet-derived growth factor; TGFα and β, transforming growth factor α and β; VEGF, vascular endothelial cell growth factor; CSF-1, colony-stimulating factor-1; IL-1, interleukin-1; INFγ, interferon γ; TNFα,tumor necrosis factor α

The endometrial IGF system

Schematic representation of the endometrial IGF system is shown in Figure 3. IGF-I and IGF-II are polypeptides structurally and functionally related to insulin[22]. IGF-I stimulates

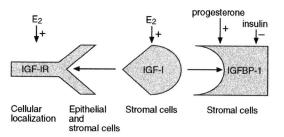

Figure 3 Major components of the endometrial insulin-like growth factor (IGF) system: regulation and cellular location. E_2, estradiol; IGF-IR, IGF-I receptor; IGFBP, IGF-binding protein

proliferation and differentiation of several cell types, and it also has insulin-like metabolic effects. The biological action of IGF-II is less clear, but it is assumed to be more important during fetal life. Either IGF-I or IGF-II, or both, as well as their cell membrane receptors have been identified in almost all tissues examined so far, including the endometrium. In human endometrium, IGF-I gene expression is elevated during the estrogen-dominated proliferative phase, whereas IGF-II gene expression is more abundant in late secretory phase endometrium, supporting the view that IGF-I mediates the mitogenic effects of estrogen, and that IGF-II is involved in the regulation of endometrial differentiation[16]. Boehm and colleagues[18] report in their studies high expression of IGF-II also in early proliferative endometrium. IGF acts through cell membrane receptors which are present in the endometrium throughout the menstrual cycle[23]. Estrogen has been shown to stimulate the gene expression of IGF-I receptor[16]. Both IGF-I and IGF-II are produced by endometrial stromal cells as shown by *in situ* hybridization experiments[24]. IGF receptors are abundant in surface and glandular epithelium and less abundant in stromal cells[24]. The cellular localization of IGFs and their receptors implies that these growth factors may have both auto- and paracrine functions. The stromal expression of IGFs and epithelial expression of IGF receptors are in keeping with the proposal that the proliferative response in epithelial cells is mediated through stromal factors. In animal studies, progesterone has been shown to inhibit the effects of estrogen on uterine IGF-I expression[25]. In agreement, preliminary studies in our laboratory have shown that an intrauterine device releasing levonorgestrel 20 µg per day suppresses IGF-I mRNA expression in human endometrium (to be published). Both this and the earlier studies by Boehm and co-workers[18] suggest that progesterone may attenuate IGF-I expression in the human endometrium as well. Regarding the lack of ovarian estrogen secretion in postmenopausal women, it is of interest to note that mRNAs encoding IGF-I and IGF-I receptor are expressed also in postmenopausal endometrium[26,27]. This suggests that estrogen may not be the only regulator of IGF-I expression in the endometrium. The expression of local factors which mediate estrogen effects during reproductive years, but which are stimulated by other factors as well, might provide an explanation why endometrial cancer, considered to be estrogen dependent, mostly occurs in postmenopausal women.

The biological actions of IGFs are regulated at the cellular level by soluble binding proteins. Six different IGFBPs, all products of different genes, have been cloned and sequenced[28]. IGFBPs can either inhibit or enhance IGF actions depending on the context. They are all expressed in the endometrium with variations in their levels and regulation[26]. The most strikingly regulated IGFBP in the endometrium is IGFBP-1, which is also the best characterized IGFBP. Besides being the major IGFBP in the endometrium, IGFBP-1 is also the major secretory protein of the human endometrium in late secretory phase and during pregnancy[29]. The pioneering work with regard to this protein was carried out in our laboratory in the early 1980s when the structure and function of the protein were not known, and the name of the protein was placental protein 12[29]. Progesterone is the major regulator of IGFBP-1 gene expression and protein secretion in human endometrium[30], whereas in the liver the major regulator of IGFBP-1 is insulin, which inhibits

IGFBP-1 production[31]. Insulin also suppresses IGFBP-1 mRNA expression in the endometrium[16]. IGFBP-1 mRNA is not expressed in proliferative phase endometrium, but is abundant in predecidualized endometrium at the end of the menstrual cycle[30]. The changes in endometrial IGFBP-1 production during the menstrual cycle are not reflected in serum IGFBP-1 levels which remain constant throughout the cycle[31]. When conception occurs, the IGFBP-1 mRNA expression in the endometrium increases and remains high throughout pregnancy[32]. IGFBP-1 inhibits the receptor binding and biological actions of IGF-I in endometrial tissues as well as in cultured trophoblastic cells in a dose-dependent manner, suggesting that the IGF-I-dependent functions in the endometrium as well as in endometrial–trophoblastic interaction during pregnancy are inhibited in the presence of IGFBP-1[23,33]. The IGF system thus provides an example in which growth factor expression is stimulated by estrogen and specifically inhibited by progesterone. Cellular localization of the IGF system supports the concept of stromal influence on epithelial cells. If IGFs mediate estrogen actions, the induction of IGFBP-1 expression may be one of the mechanisms by which progesterone counteracts estrogen effects at the molecular level. After cessation of ovarian function at the menopause, endometrial IGFBP-1 synthesis is inhibited and IGF-I, if expressed, is unopposed and may maintain cell proliferation. This might be one of the molecular mechanisms favoring the development of endometrial cancer at postmenopausal age[26]. Endometrial IGFBP-1 production can also be induced in postmenopausal women by progestin treatment, but not in all cases. Recently we have shown that an intrauterine system, releasing levonorgestrel 20 µg per day combined with various estradiol regimens is capable of inducing IGFBP-1 production in the endometrium in all postmenopausal women studied[34,35]. IGFBP-1 immunostaining was constant as long as intrauterine levonorgestrel was administered. Interestingly, the endometrial epithelium was atrophic in all these cases. In contrast, no IGFBP-1 could be detected in the endometrium of those women who were treated with either subdermal levonorgestrel implants or with micronized natural progesterone 100–200 mg orally or vaginally. In the latter groups no signs of progestin effect were detected by microscopic examination.

The striking hormonal regulation and the abundance of IGFBP-1 in predecidualized/decidualized endometrium strongly suggest that the IGF system has a biological function in the endometrium and in maternal–fetal interactions. However, we need to consider that the biological effects of ovarian steroids in the endometrium, whether stimulatory or inhibitory, are likely to be regulated by several mechanisms in parallel. It is well established that progesterone attenuates estrogen action by suppressing the expression of estrogen receptors as well as by increasing the activities of 17-β dehydrogenase and sulfotransferase, which are both important in converting estradiol to less active metabolites.

Conclusions

The heterogeneous population of endometrial cells and their functions are regulated at several levels including endocrine and auto/paracrine systems which can be stimulatory or inhibitory. The major hormonal regulators of endometrial function are estrogen and progesterone, which may act directly or indirectly through intercellular interactions mediated by growth factors and other local regulators. The IGF system is believed to be one of the growth factor systems that mediate estrogen and progesterone actions in the endometrium.

The complexity of the regulation of endometrial functions probably explains why normal blood levels of estrogen and progesterone which can be reached by external hormones, are unable to correct many endometrial disorders or diseases that we are trying to treat simply with steroid hormones. Efforts to increase our knowledge of the molecular basis of endometrial disorders should be a great challenge in all research dealing with women's reproductive health. Better understanding in this field might shed light on the mechanisms accounting for increased dysfunctional bleeding at perimenopausal years, as well as the increased risk of endometrial cancer at postmenopausal age. This knowledge might ultimately be used to improve diagnosis, and for developing new therapies, of women's reproductive diseases.

References

1. Aplin, J. D., Charlton, A. K. and Ayad, S. (1988). An immunohistochemical study of human endometrial extracellular matrix during the menstrual cycle and first trimester of pregnancy. *Cell Tissue Res.*, **253**, 231–40

2. Tabibzadeh, S. and Poubourides, D. (1990). Expression of leukocyte adhesion molecules in human endometrium. *Am. J. Clin. Pathol.*, **93**, 183–9

3. Salamonsen, L. A. and Nancarraw, C. D. (1994). Cell biology of the oviduct and endometrium. In Findlay, J. K. (ed.) *Molecular Biology of the Female Reproductive System*, pp. 289–328. (Sydney: Academic Press)

4. Evans, R. M. (1988). The steroid and thyroid hormone receptor superfamily. *Science*, **240**, 889–95

5. Misrahi, M., Venencie, P. Y., Saugier-Veber, P., Sar. S., Dessen, P. and Milgrom, E. (1993). Structure of the human progesterone receptor gene. *Biochim. Biophys. Acta*, **1216**, 289–92

6. Renoir, J. M., Radanyi, C., Faber, L. E. and Baulieu, E. E. (1990). The non-DNA-binding heterooligomeric form of mammalian steroid hormone receptors contains a hsp90-bound 59-kilodalton protein. *J. Biol. Chem.*, **265**, 10740–5

7. Truss, M. and Beato, M. (1993). Steroid hormone receptors: interaction with deoxyribonucleic acid and transcription factors. *Endocr. Rev.*, **14**, 459–79

8. McDonnell, D. P. and Goldman, M. E. (1994). RU486 exerts antiestrogenic activities through

a novel progesterone receptor A form-mediated mechanism. *J. Biol. Chem.*, **269**, 11945–9

9. Ali, S., Matzger, D., Bornet, J. M. and Chambon, P. (1993). Modulation of transcriptional activation by ligand-dependent phosphorylation of the human oestrogen receptor A/B region. *EMBO J.*, **12**, 1153–60

10. Lessey, B. A., Killam, A. P., Metzger, D. A., Haney A. F., Greene, G. L. and McCarty, K. S. Jr (1988). Immunohistochemical analysis of human uterine estrogen and progesterone receptors throughout the menstrual cycle. *J. Clin. Endocrinol. Metab.*, **67**, 334–40

11. Murphy, L. J. and Ballejo, G. (1994). Growth factor and cytokine expression in the endometrium. In Findlay, J. K. (ed.) *Molecular Biology of the Female Reproductive System*, pp. 345–77. (Sydney: Academic Press)

12. Economos, K., MacDonald, P. C. and Casey, M. L. (1992). Endothelin-1 gene expression and protein biosynthesis in human endometrium: potential modulator of endometrial blood flow. *J. Clin. Endocrinol. Metab.*, **74**, 14–19

13. Haining, R. E., Schofield, J. P., Jones, D. S., Rajput-Williams, J. and Smith, S. K. (1991). Identification of mRNA for epidermal growth factor and transforming growth factor-alpha present in low copy number in human endometrium using reverse transcriptase-polymerase chain reaction. *J. Mol. Endocrinol.*, **6**, 207–14

14. Brigstock, D. R., Heap, R. P. and Brown, K. D. (1989). Polypeptide growth factors in uterine tissues and secretions. *J. Reprod. Fertil.*, **85**, 747–58

15. Dell, A., Morris, H. R., Easton, R. L., Panico, M., Patankar, M., Oehninger, S., Koistinen, R., Koistinen, H., Seppälä, M. and Clark, G.F. (1995). Structural analysis of the oligosaccharides derived from glycodelin, a human glycoprotein with potent immunosuppressive and contraceptive activities. *J. Biol. Chem.*, **270**, 24116–26

16. Giudice, L. C. (1994). Growth factors and growth modulators in human uterine endometrium: their potential relevance to reproductive medicine. *Fertil. Steril.*, **61**, 1–17

17. Pekonen, F., Nyman, T. and Rutanen, E.-M. (1993). Differential expression of keratinocyte growth factor and its receptor in the human uterus. *Mol. Cell. Endocrinol.*, **95**, 43–9

18. Boehm, K. D., Daimon, M., Gorodeski, I. G., Sheean, L. A., Utian, W. H. and Ilan, J. (1990). Expression of the insulin-like and platelet-derived growth factor genes in human uterine tissues. *Mol. Reprod. Dev.*, **27**, 93–101

19. Kauma, S., Matt, D., Strom, S., Eierman, D. and Turner, T. (1990). Interleukin-1b, human leukocyte antigen HLA-DRa, and transforming growth factor-b expression in endometrium, placenta and placental membranes. *Am. J. Obstet. Gynecol.*, **163**, 130–7

20. Charnock-Jones, D. S., Sharkey, A. M., Rajput-Williams, J., Burch, D., Schofield, P. J., Fountain, S. A., Boocock, C. A. and Smith, S. K. (1993). Identification and localization of alternately spliced mRNAs for vascular endothelial growth factor in human uterus and estrogen regulation in endometrial carcinoma cell lines. *Biol. Reprod.*, **48**, 1120–8

21. Tabibzadeh, S. S. (1991). Human endometrium: an active site of cytokine production and action. *Endocr. Rev.*, **12**, 272–90

22. Rinderknecht, E. and Humbel, R. E. (1978). The amino acid sequence of human insulin-like growth factor-1 and its structural homology with proinsulin. *J. Biol. Chem.*, **253**, 2769–76

23. Rutanen, E.-M., Pekonen, F. and Mäkinen, T. (1988). Soluble 34K binding protein inhibits the binding of insulin-like growth factor I to its receptors in human secretory phase endometrium: evidence for autocrine/paracrine regulation of growth factor action. *J. Clin. Endocrinol. Metab.*, **66**, 173–80

24. Zhou, J., Dsupin, B. A., Giudice, L. C. and Bondy, C. A. (1994). Insulin-like growth factor system gene expression in human endometrium during the menstrual cycle. *J. Clin. Endocrinol. Metab.*, **79**, 1723–34

25. Croze, F., Kennedy, T., Schroedter, I. C., Friesen, H. G. and Murphy, L. J. (1990). Expression of insulin-like growth factor-I and insulin-like growth factor binding protein-1 in the rat uterus during decidualization. *Endocrinology*, **127**, 1995–2001

26. Rutanen, E.-M., Nyman, T., Lehtovirta, P., Ämmälä, M. and Pekonen, F. (1994). Suppressed expression of insulin-like growth factor binding protein-1 mRNA in the endometrium: a molecular mechanism associating endometrial cancer with its risk factors. *Int. J. Cancer*, **59**, 307–12

27. Laatikainen, T., Toma's, E. I. and Voutilainen, R. J. (1995). The expression of insulin-like growth factor and its binding protein mRNA in the endometrium of postmenopausal patients with breast cancer receiving tamoxifen. *Cancer*, **76**, 1406–10

28. Shimasaki, S. and Ling, N. (1991). Identification and molecular characterization of insulin-like growth factor binding proteins (IGFBP-1, -2, -3, -4, -5, and -6). *Prog. Growth Factor Res.*, **3**, 243–66

29. Koistinen, R., Kalkkinen, N., Huhtala, M.-L., Seppälä, M., Bohn, H. and Rutanen, E.-M. (1986). Placental protein 12 is a decidual protein that binds somatomedin and has an identical N-

terminal amino acid sequence with somatomedin-binding protein from human amniotic fluid. *Endocrinology*, **118**, 1375–8

30. Julkunen, M., Koistinen, R., Aalto-Setälä, K, Seppälä, M., Jänne, O. and Kontula, K. (1988). Primary structure of human insulin-like growth factor-binding protein/placental protein 12 and tissue-specific expression of its mRNA. *FEBS Lett.*, **236**, 295–302

31. Suikkari, A.-M., Koivisto, V., Rutanen, E.-M., Yki-Järvinen, H., Karonen, S.-L. and Seppälä, M. (1988). Insulin regulates the serum levels of low molecular weight insulin-like growth factor-binding protein. *J. Clin. Endocrinol. Metab.*, **66**, 266–72

32. Pekonen, F., Suikkari, A.-M., Mäkinen, T. and Rutanen, E.-M. (1988). Different insulin-like growth factor binding species in human placenta and decidua. *J. Clin. Endocrinol. Metab.*, **67**, 1250–7

33. Ritvos, O., Ranta, T., Jalkanen, J., Suikkari, A.-M., Voutilainen, R., Bohn, H. and Rutanen, E.-M. (1988). Insulin-like growth factor (IGF) binding protein from human decidua inhibits the binding and biological action of IGF-I in cultured choriocarcinoma cells. *Endocrinology*, **122**, 2150–7

34. Suvanto-Luukkonen, E., Sundström, H., Penttinen, J., Kauppila, A. and Rutanen, E.-M. (1996). Insulin-like growth factor-binding protein-1: a biochemical marker of endometrial response to progestin during hormone replacement therapy. *Maturitas*, **22**, 255–62

35. Suhonen, S., Haukkamaa, M., Holmström, T., Lähteenmäki, P. and Rutanen, E.-M. (1996). Endometrial response to hormone replacement therapy as assessed by expression of insulin-like growth factor-binding protein-1 in the endometrium. *Fertil. Steril.*, **65**, 776–82

Ultrasound and the endometrium in postmenopausal women

33

J. C. Grimwade, E. A. Farrell and A. L. Murkies

Introduction

Abnormal bleeding in menopausal patients is common, and may present as perimenopausal menstrual irregularity, breakthrough bleeding on hormone replacement therapy (HRT) or as a clearly defined episode of postmenopausal bleeding. The need exists to diagnose accurately endometrial pathology in such patients. Endometrial pathology is varied and mostly benign (Table 1). Endometrial carcinoma, however, is the most common of the reproductive malignancies with approximately 90% of endometrial cancers occurring in women of 50 years of age or more (Table 2). An easily applied and accurate diagnostic procedure for menopausal patients with abnormal bleeding would be a valuable guide for their management.

Transvaginal ultrasound is one of a number of diagnostic methods available to detect endometrial pathology and is the least invasive (Table 3). Ultrasound assessment includes measurement of the double endometrial width, display of the midline cavity echo, examination of the endometrial appearance and definition of the endometrial–myometrial interface.

This paper details the usefulness and limitations of transvaginal ultrasound in menopausal women with abnormal bleeding, and describes the technique of saline infusion sonohysterography (SIS) used to enhance diagnosis.

Subjects and methods

The double endometrial width was measured by a single observer (JCG) in 50 menopausal women who were a subgroup of 53 patients who

Table 1 Endometrial pathology in postmenopausal women

Endometrial polyp
Submucosal fibroid
Proliferative change
Tamoxifen-induced change
Hyperplasia
   simple, complex
   atypical
Carcinoma

Table 2 Incidence of female reproductive cancer in Victoria (Australia) in 1993, figures supplied by Anti-Cancer Council of Victoria. Female population 2.245 million, rate expressed per 100 000 females. Endometrial cancer: < 50 years of age, $n = 40$; ≥ 50 years of age, $n = 315$

Site	Incidence (n)	Rate
Endometrium	355	15.8
Ovary	283	12.6
Cervix	249	11.1
Other	59	2.6

Table 3 Methods of endometrial diagnosis

Transvaginal ultrasound
Saline infusion sonohysterography
Endometrial biopsy
Hysteroscopy
Hysteroscopy with directed biopsy
Hysteroscopy with curettage
Hysterectomy

had volunteered to participate in an HRT research trial organized by one of the authors (ALM) at the Monash Medical Centre Menopause Unit. Three women were excluded when found to have endometrial polyps. The mean age was 57 years (range 46–69 years). All women had ceased bleeding for at least 12 months and none were on HRT. The study used an ATL echoscope (HDI 3000) with a 5–9 MHz vaginal transducer.

In a second study, SIS was performed on 219 patients from November 1995 to September 1996 with the aim of establishing the technique and assessing the degree to which endometrial views could be enhanced. Patients were both pre- and postmenopausal and had presented with abnormal bleeding (age range 34–84 years: 65% of patients were 50 years of age or more). Patients were selected for SIS if transvaginal ultrasound showed the endometrium to be excessively thickened and intrauterine pathology suspected to be present, or if the endometrium could not be clearly displayed. The cervix was aseptically prepared with Betadine® 1% solution. In the first half of the study involving 109 patients, a chorion villus sample (CVS) cannula was inserted through the cervical canal and 5–10 ml of sterile saline was instilled into the uterine cavity. In the second half of the study (110 patients), three different instruments for saline instillation were used: a CVS cannula, one slightly modified to help retain saline in the uterus, or a soft 1.5 mm intrauterine insemination catheter. The latter became the preferred method and was used for 60 patients. No local anesthetic was needed. A transvaginal ultrasound was then performed and the endometrium assessed.

Results

The mean endometrial width in the 50 menopausal women was 2.5 mm, the 95% confidence interval 2.3–2.8 mm (Table 4, Figure 1). The endometrial width exceeded 4 mm in only four women and there was no measurement above 4.8 mm.

Table 4 Endometrial width (in mm) in 50 normal menopausal women, measurements are of double width. Age of patients: mean, 57 years; range, 46–69 years

Mean	2.5
95% confidence interval	2.3–2.8
Median	2.6
Range	0.8–4.8

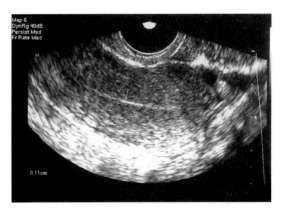

Figure 1 Longitudinal plane through menopausal uterus demonstrating atrophic endometrium (arrow) with double width of 1.1 mm

Endometrial assessment was enhanced by SIS in 181 of 219 patients (83%) (Table 5). In these patients, the endometrium and uterine cavity could be clearly displayed (Figure 2). In particular, pathology was seen to be either localized (focal) such as for an endometrial polyp

Table 5 Outcome of saline infusion sonohysterography in 219 patients, age range: 34–84 years. 143 patients (65%) were 50 years of age or more

Outcome	n	%
Endometrial view enhanced	181	83
first 109 patients	85	78
second 110 patients	96	87
Endometrial view unimproved	9	4
Procedure not possible		
vaginal atrophy/cervical stenosis	9	4
difficulty with cannula or catheter placement	20	9

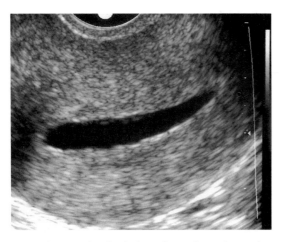

Figure 2 Longitudinal plane through uterine cavity after instillation of saline demonstrating empty cavity with atrophic endometrium

or submucosal fibroid (Figure 3), or more generalized (global) as for hyperplasia (Figure 4). There were 113 patients aged 50 years or more where SIS successfully enhanced the vaginal scan image. There was endometrial pathology in 50 of these patients (44%). Endometrial polyps were found in 29 patients, submucosal fibroids in 16, hyperplasia in four (one with atypia), and one patient had an endometrial carcinoma (endometrial width 10 mm).

The views were not improved in nine patients where either the saline was not retained in the cavity or fibroids obscured the display. The procedure was not possible in another nine patients because of vaginal atrophy or stenosis of the cervical external os. In a further 20 patients the catheter could not be easily passed through the cervical canal (16 of these patients were in the first half of the study). No patient experienced any vasovagal phenomenon and there was no incidence of infection. Of the six patients experiencing temporary discomfort, five were in the first half of the study, three requiring paracetamol.

Discussion

Saline infusion sonohysterography was found to be highly effective in defining endometrial pathology especially of a focal nature. The creation of a fluid–endometrial interface permits any lesion projecting into the cavity to be clearly outlined and accurately measured. Our study showed that with experience SIS enhanced endometrial diagnosis in almost 9 out of 10 patients. The increased success rate in the second half of the study was related to both improved technique and to an evolving preference for using the insemination catheter.

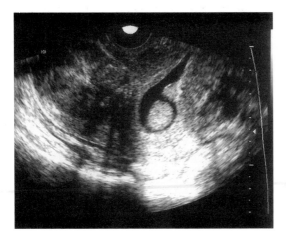

Figure 3 Longitudinal plane through uterine cavity after instillation of saline demonstrating two endometrial polyps and intramural fibroid

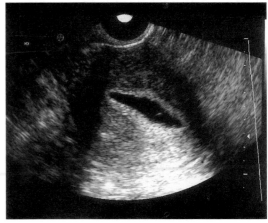

Figure 4 Longitudinal plane through uterine cavity after instillation of saline demonstrating hyperplasia

The procedure was virtually pain free in the second half, only one patient having temporary discomfort.

In our study of 50 normal menopausal women, the endometrial width was always less than 5 mm. A measurement of greater than 5 mm in patients not on HRT is therefore likely to be associated with pathology.

Pertinent to any discussion on endometrial diagnosis is the incidence of pathology when the measurement is less than 5 mm. The report by Karlsson and colleagues known as the Nordic study, has contributed significantly to this debate[1]. Karlsson and co-workers measured the endometrial width in 1138 patients with postmenopausal bleeding (PMB) prior to uterine curettage. Of the 518 patients with a measurement ≤ 4 mm, 14 had pathology (2.7%). They estimated that when the endometrium measured ≤ 4 mm, the 95% confidence limit for the probability of excluding an endometrial abnormality was 5.5%. They noted this estimate compared favorably with published false negative rates for curettage and endometrial biopsy by aspiration (2–6%).

There were 620 patients in the Nordic study with endometrium ≥ 5 mm and 394 (64%) had pathology. The 114 patients with endometrial cancer all had endometrial widths of 5 mm or more (mean 21 mm). The authors concluded that it would seem justifiable to refrain from curettage with an endometrial width of ≤ 4 mm. Using this cut-off limit, they would have reduced their number of curettages by 46%.

Bourne[2] in a review article noted a number of published papers in support of this view.

However, he sounded a note of caution since several recent papers have observed endometrial cancers in endometria of less than 5 mm[3–5] (Table 6).

When wishing to avoid hysteroscopy and biopsy or uterine curettage for PMB, it is tempting for clinicians to rely on the endometrial width as a guide to further management. When the endometrium measures ≤ 4 mm, it seems that only rarely will a small endometrial cancer be overlooked. This risk may well be lessened if other factors such as the degree to which the endometrium is clearly resolved and position of the midcavity echo are taken into account. Additionally, if the entire cavity can not be clearly visualized, SIS as well may help identify a small local lesion.

In any event, when abnormal bleeding persists in menopausal patients where the initial diagnostic test has been normal (as it would with pathology that has been overlooked), it is always sound clinical practice to pursue further investigation.

When the endometrial width is ≥ 5 mm in patients with PMB, there is a significant incidence of pathology as shown in the Nordic study (64%). The incidence of pathology in our patients with abnormal bleeding (44%), who were 50 years of age or more, is in agreement. In patients with PMB, SIS will both help define pathology and aid the clinician in planning the appropriate further management. The identification of a focal lesion, such as an endometrial polyp or submucosal fibroid, permits hysteroscopic resection to be considered. For extensive global endometrial

Table 6 Number of patients with endometrial cancer where endometrial width measured less than 5 mm; patients presented with postmenopausal bleeding (PMB). Endometrial width measured with transvaginal ultrasound

Study	n	Incidence of endometrial cancer (n)	Incidence of endometrial width < 5 mm (n)
Dorum (1993)[3]	100	15	3
Conoscenti (1995)[4]	149	16	1
Ferrazzi (1995)[5]	930	102	1

thickening, hysteroscopy and uterine curettage may be more suitable. Where global thickening is not so excessive (between 4 and 6 mm) and the patient is on HRT, a less invasive procedure, such as endometrial biopsy by aspiration, may initially be the treatment of choice.

There are a number of options available for the detection of endometrial pathology in patients with PMB. A view is now emerging that, following a thorough history and examination, transvaginal ultrasound should be considered as the first diagnostic investigation for many of these patients. In addition, SIS can be of considerable value both in defining focal lesions and displaying the endometrium when the transvaginal scan alone is poorly resolved. A more invasive diagnostic investigation would then be indicated either to establish the histology when the ultrasound examination showed an abnormality, or less commonly to follow up patients in whom symptoms were persisting when the ultrasound appeared normal.

References

1. Karlsson, B., Granberg, S., Wikland, M., Ylostalo, P., Torvid, K., Marsal, K. and Valentin, L. (1995). Transvaginal ultrasonography of the endometrium in women with postmenopausal bleeding – a Nordic multicenter study. *Am. J. Obstet. Gynecol.*, **172**, 1488–94

2. Bourne, T. H. (1995). Evaluating the endometrium of postmenopausal women with transvaginal ultrasonography. *Ultrasound Obstet. Gynecol.*, **6**, 75–80

3. Dorum, A., Kristensen, G. B., Langebrekke, A., Sornes, T. and Skaar, O. (1993). Evaluation of endometrial thickness measured by endovaginal ultrasound in women with menopausal bleeding. *Acta Obstet. Gynecol. Scand.*, **72**, 116–19

4. Conoscenti, G., Meir, Y. J., Fischer-Tomaro, L., Maieron, A., Natale, R., D'Ottavio, G., Rustico, M. and Mandruzzato, G. (1995). Endometrial assessment by transvaginal sonography and histological findings after D & C in women with postmenopausal bleeding. *Ultrasound Obstet. Gynecol.*, **6**, 108–15

5. Ferrazzi, E., Zannoni, E., Torri, N., Trio, D., Severi, F., Dordoni, D., Spagnolo, D. and Galbiati, G. (1995). Sonographic endometrial thickness: a useful test to predict atrophy in menopausal atypical bleeding. *Ultrasound Obstet. Gynecol.*, **5** (Suppl. 1), 42

Clinical implications for the endometrium 34
of hormone replacement therapy

J. H. Pickar

Introduction

The endometrium is a target tissue for both endogenous and exogenous hormones. Increasing our understanding of the effects of exogenous hormones on the endometrium may help both to avoid risks and to optimize patient satisfaction with hormone replacement therapy.

Risk of developing endometrial cancer

Grady and colleagues[1] performed a meta-analysis of 30 studies on the association of unopposed estrogen, or estrogen plus progestin, with the risk of developing endometrial cancer or dying from this disease. In women with a uterus, ever-use of unopposed estrogen therapy was associated with a relative risk (RR) of endometrial cancer of 2.3 (95% confidence interval (CI) 2.1–2.5). The RR increased to 9.5 (95% CI 7.4–12.3) with more than 10 years of use. The summary RR of endometrial cancer remained elevated (RR 2.3, 95% CI 1.8–3.1) five or more years after discontinuation of unopposed estrogen therapy. The risk for endometrial cancer death was elevated among unopposed estrogen users (RR 2.7, 95% CI 0.9–8.0). Among estrogen plus progestin users, cohort studies showed a decreased risk of endometrial cancer (RR 0.4, 95% CI 0.2–0.6) whereas case–control studies showed a small increase (RR 1.8, 95% CI 1.1–3.1)[1].

Continuous and interrupted estrogen-only regimens do not differ significantly in risk for endometrial hyperplasia or endometrial cancer. Twenty-five symptomatic postmenopausal women with an intact uterus were randomly assigned to receive 0.625 mg of conjugated estrogens (CE) on either a cyclic (3 weeks on, 1 week off) or continuous (daily) basis. The incidence of endometrial hyperplasia as demonstrated by screening biopsies at 6 and 12 months of therapy was 4.5 per 100 woman-months in the cyclic group, and 3.7 per 100 woman-months in the continuous group (difference not statistically significant)[2].

In a study by Kurman and associates[3], the diagnosis of endometrial cancer in women previously found to have endometrial hyperplasia varied from about 1% with simple hyperplasia to 29% with complex atypical hyperplasia. Two (1.6%) of 122 patients with hyperplasia without atypia progressed to carcinoma; this included one (1%) of 93 patients with simple hyperplasia and one (3%) of 29 patients with complex hyperplasia. Eleven (23%) of 48 women with atypical hyperplasia progressed to carcinoma, including one (8%) of 13 women with simple atypical hyperplasia and ten (29%) of 35 women with complex atypical hyperplasia. The difference in progression to carcinoma between women with and without atypia was significant ($p = 0.0001$)[3].

Effects of progestin addition to hormone replacement therapy on endometrial hyperplasia

The addition of a progestin to oral estrogen replacement, hormone replacement therapy (HRT), in cyclic or continuous combined regimens, has been shown to significantly decrease the incidence of endometrial hyperplasia. Endometrial hyperplasia occurs in about one-fifth of women with a uterus taking low-dose unopposed oral estrogen over a 1-year period. In the Menopause Study Group trial, women in each of five groups received conjugated estrogens (CE) 0.625 mg/day. Groups A and B also took continuous daily doses of medroxyprogesterone acetate (MPA) 2.5 and 5.0 mg, respectively. Groups C and D took MPA 5.0 and 10.0 mg, respectively, for the last 14 days of each 28-day cycle. Group E took continuous daily doses of placebo to match MPA. Endometrial hyperplasia developed after 12 months of treatment in 20% of 283 women with a uterus receiving oral unopposed conjugated estrogens (group E), yet in only about 1% or less of those in the continuous (553 women) or cyclic (549 women) combination treatment groups (Table 1)[4].

A recent report from the Postmenopausal Estrogen/Progestin Interventions (PEPI) Trial confirmed that cyclic or continuous oral progestin prevents the increased hyperplasia associated with unopposed estrogen therapy. A total of 596 postmenopausal women with a uterus were randomly assigned to receive: placebo; conjugated estrogen (CE) (0.625 mg/day) alone; CE (0.625 mg/day for 28 days) + MPA (10.0 mg/day for 12/28 days); CE (0.625 mg/day for 28 days) + MPA (2.5 mg/day for 28/28 days); or CE (0.625 mg/day for 28 days) + micronized progesterone (200 mg/day for 12/28 days). After 3 years, women receiving unopposed CE had a significantly higher rate of hyperplasia and more unscheduled biopsies and procedures than the placebo group ($p < 0.001$), while those receiving any of the estrogen plus progestin regimens had levels similar to the placebo group. With the continuous combined regimen, only one case of simple hyperplasia developed over 3 years; with placebo, there was one case each of simple hyperplasia complex hyperplasia and endometrial adenocarcinoma (Table 2)[5].

The addition of transdermal progestin to transdermal estrogen replacement also decreases the incidence of endometrial

Table 1 Incidence of endometrial hyperplasia at 12 months of treatment with conjugated estrogens, with or without medroxyprogesterone acetate. All groups received conjugated estrogens 0.625 mg every day of a 28-day cycle. The following medroxyprogesterone acetate dosages were taken: group A, 2.5 mg, days 1 to 28; group B, 5.0 mg, days 1 to 28; group C, 5.0 mg, days 15 to 28; group D, 10.0 mg, days 15 to 28; group E, no medroxyprogesterone acetate (placebo). Adapted from reference 4

Treatment group	No. of participants	% with hyperplasia
A	279	< 1*
B	274	0*
C	277	1*
D	272	0*
E	283	20

*Significantly different from conjugated estrogens alone

hyperplasia. This was investigated in a multicenter study of 136 postmenopausal women who received 12 cycles of 4 weeks each: 2 weeks transdermal estradiol 50 μg/day followed by 2 weeks of a combined patch delivering norethisterone acetate 0.25 mg/day and estradiol 50 μg/day. Of the 136 pretreatment biopsies, 89% provided no material, an inadequate sample, or an inactive (atrophic or non-secretory) endometrium. Of the post-treatment biopsies from 110 women who completed the study, 65% showed secretory endometrium, 3% proliferative endometrium, and 24% inadequate material or inactive endometrium. Hyperplasia was found in two biopsies (2%); in one case focal atypical hyperplasia was the diagnosis agreed upon by the two study pathologists, and in the other case, a hyperplastic endometrial polyp was diagnosed by one pathologist[6].

The role of long-cycle therapy (quarterly progestin) in reducing endometrial hyperplasia is, at this time, unclear. The Scandinavian Long Cycle Study, a randomized multicenter trial of a quarterly regimen (2 mg/day estradiol for 68 days; 2 mg estradiol + 1 mg norethindrone

Table 2 Distribution of endometrial procedures among participants and endometrial biopsy changes since normal baseline to most extreme abnormal results, by treatment regimen. Adapted from reference 5

Procedure or findings	Placebo (n =119)	CEE only (n = 119)	CEE + MPA (cyc) (n = 118)	CEE + MPA (con) (n = 120)	CEE + MP (cyc) (n = 120)
Unscheduled biopsy*	11/10	115/79	20/16	11/9	17/14
D&C	1	24/21*	2/2*	1	0
Hysterectomy	2	7	3	0	2
Normal findings	116	45	112	119	114
Simple hyperplasia	1	33	4	1	5
Complex hyperplasia	1	27	2	0	0
Atypia	0	14	0	0	1
Adenocarcinoma	1	0	0	0	0

*Total number of procedures/number of women; CEE, conjugated equine estrogens; MPA, medroxyprogesterone acetate; MP, micronized progesterone; cyc, cyclic; con, continuous; D&C, dilation and curettage

for 10 days; 1 mg estradiol for 6 days), was canceled after 3 years when 14 patients developed hyperplasia (one with atypia) and one developed endometrial cancer, a significantly ($p = 0.004$) higher rate than in the control group, who received a monthly regimen of 2 mg estradiol for 12 days; 2 mg estradiol + 1 mg norethindrone for 10 days; 1 mg estradiol for 6 days[7].

Evaluation of endometrial biopsies

The reporting of endometrial histology is both subjective and objective, and this fact may lead to differences in interpretation between pathologists. In one study, reported by Whitehead and Pickar[8], in postmenopausal women receiving an estrogen/progestogen combination, a single pathologist read all biopsy samples. All biopsies classified as abnormal, and a random sample of additional biopsies, were reviewed by two additional pathologists. The reported incidence of complex hyperplasia at month 6 ranged from 1.1% to 5.1%, and at month 12, from 1.1% to 7.1%. At month 6, each of the three pathologists reported one case of simple hyperplasia, but in three different patients; at month 12, two pathologists reported no simple hyperplasia and the third reported three cases. In addition to pathologists agreeing

on a standardized, common set of criteria for endometrial evaluation, procedures should be developed to reduce the degree of inter-observer variation, which may interfere with accurate assessment[8].

Vaginal administration of progesterone

In addition to oral and transdermal progestin administration, recent data indicate that selective endometrial concentration of progestin takes place following vaginal application and suggest possible utility of this route for HRT.

Studies with progesterone (P) in functionally agonadal women showed selective concentration of P in the endometrium after intravaginal administration, in contrast to intramuscular (i.m.) administration. All subjects received divided doses of oral micronized estradiol on a schedule designed for recipients of oocyte donation, with daily administration of 1 mg from day 1 to day 6, 2 mg from day 7 to day 10, 6 mg from day 11 to day 13, and 2 mg from day 14 to day 26. Starting with day 15, the subjects received either vaginally administered, micronized natural P capsules 200 mg every 6 h or i.m. P in oil 50 mg twice daily. Steady-state serum levels obtained by cycle day 21 (6 days of exogenous P) were significantly higher using i.m. P compared with vaginal P (69.80 ± 5.90 ng/ml versus 11.90 ± 1.20 ng/ml; $p < 0.05$). However, endometrial concentrations of P were greatest after vaginal P (vaginal P: 11.50 ± 2.60 ng/mg protein versus i.m. P: 1.40 ± 0.40 ng/mg protein, compared to P: 0.30 ± 0.10 ng/mg protein in normal ovulatory control women). No differences between control groups and either treatment regimen (vaginal or i.m.) in terms of endometrial factors were detected by histologic, ultrasonographic or immunocyto-chemical receptor analyses[9].

Effects of different doses of P administered transvaginally were tested in a physiological hormone replacement paradigm initially designed to prime endometrial receptivity in egg-donation recipients. Progesterone was administered via a vaginal gel with sustained-release properties at rates of 45, 90 and 180 mg every other day from cycle days 15 to 26. The lowest P dose raised plasma P to between (trough) 1 and (peak) 3 ng/ml, while levels were significantly higher with the higher doses. Despite the low plasma P levels achieved with the low P dose, endometrial changes observed in the mid (day 20) or late (day 24) luteal phase were indistinguishable from endometrial findings normally made in the menstrual cycle or when using higher vaginal P doses (300 mg/day) administered from soft gelatin capsules in previous studies[10].

Uterine route selectivity is believed to represent the practical reflection of a 'first uterine pass effect' linked to the vaginal route of administration. However, an anatomical support facilitating direct transport from the vagina to the uterus has not yet been identified. *Ex vivo* uterine perfusion studies showed significant accumulation of radiolabeled P in both the endometrium and myometrium; no gradient was observed between these two uterine components. Vaginal P administration may be particularly promising for women in whom oral progestins are contraindicated because of coexisting medical conditions or are not well tolerated[10].

Determining the adequacy of the progestin dose

As new data emerge from randomized clinical trials, it is becoming clear that markers used previously to demonstrate adequacy of progestational stimulus, such as proliferative[11] or secretory[12] endometrial response, or day of onset of withdrawal bleeding[13], may not be as reliable for indicating risk to the endometrium as hyperplasia, and may result in the use of excessive progestin doses.

Menopause Study Group data: bleeding with cyclic and continuous HRT

Cyclic HRT results in reasonably predictable withdrawal bleeding, while continuous combined regimens produce amenorrhea in a significant number of patients. Cyclic and continuous combined HRT regimens were compared in 1724 postmenopausal women by the Menopause Study Group[14]. This 1-year, double-blind, randomized study compared five treatment groups, as described previously in this paper. The two continuous combined regimens produced amenorrhea in 61.4 and 72.8% of the evaluable cycles in groups A and B respectively. Generally, the incidence of amenorrhea increased and irregular bleeding decreased with longer duration of treatment. More than one-half of those who took conjugated estrogens alone had amenorrhea[14].

According to an additional analysis of the Menopause Study Group bleeding data, approximately one-half of the women who took a continuous combined CE + MPA regimen or the CE-only regimen achieved amenorrhea halfway through the trial and remained amenorrheic for the 1-year study. The proportion of women receiving continuous combined therapy achieving amenorrheic status continued to rise as the trial progressed. Of the women who did not achieve amenorrheic status, a notable portion experienced only spotting at each cycle[15].

In the same study, the majority of women who received cyclic combination therapy experienced withdrawal bleeding that began, in the next cycle, within 3 days of the day of onset in the previous cycle throughout all 13 evaluable cycles (80% and 65.9% for women who took MPA at 5.0 and 10.0 mg, respectively,

for the last 14 days of each 28-day cycle along with the CE 0.625 mg/day in both cases)[15].

Forthcoming advances promise to expand our understanding of the mechanisms and consequences of HRT on the endometrium.

References

1. Grady, D., Gebretsadik, T., Kerlikowske,K., Ernster, V. and Petitti, D. (1995). Hormone replacement therapy and endometrial cancer risk: a meta-analysis. *Obstet. Gynecol.*, **85**, 304–13

2. Schiff, I., Sela, H. K., Cramer, D., Tulchinski, D. and Ryan, K. J. (1992). Endometrial hyperplasia in women on cyclic or continuous estrogen regimens. *Fertil. Steril.*, **37**, 79–82

3. Kurman,R. J., Kaminski, P. F. and Norris, H. J. (1985). The behavior of endometrial hyperplasia: a long-term study of 'untreated' hyperplasia in 170 patients. *Cancer*, **56**, 403–12

4. Woodruff, J. D. and Pickar, J. H. for the Menopause Study Group (1994). Incidence of endometrial hyperplasia in postmenopausal women taking conjugated estrogens (Premarin) with medroxyprogesterone acetate or conjugated estrogens alone. *Am. J. Obstet. Gynecol.*, **170**, 1213–23

5. The Writing Group for the PEPI Trial (1996). Effects of hormone replacement therapy on endometrial histology in postmenopausal women. The postmenopausal estrogen/progestin interventions (PEPI) trial. *J. Am. Med. Assoc.*, **275**, 370–5

6. Lindgren, R., Risberg, B., Hammar, M., Berg, G. and Pryse-Davies, J. (1992). Endometrial effects of transdermal estradiol/norethisterone acetate. *Maturitas*, **15**, 71–8

7. Cerin, A., Heldaas, K. and Moeller, B. for the Scandinavian Long Cycle Study Group (1996). Adverse endometrial effects of long-cycle estrogen and progestogen replacement therapy (Letter to the editor). *N. Engl. J. Med.*, **334**, 668–9

8. Whitehead, M. I. and Pickar, J. (1996). Variation between pathologists in the reportings of endometrial histology with combination oestrogen/progestogen therapies. British Medical Society meeting, Exeter, UK, July 4

9. Miles, R. A., Paulson, R. J., Lobo, R. A., Press, M. F., Dahmoush, L. and Sauer, M. V. (1994). Pharmacokinetics and endometrial tissue levels of progesterone after administration by intramuscular and vaginal routes: a comparative study. *Fertil. Steril.*, **62**, 485–90

10. de Ziegler, D., Scharer, E., Seidler, L., Fanchin, R. and Bergeron, C. (1995). Transvaginal administration of progesterone: the vaginal paradox and the first uterine pass effect hypothesis. *Ref. Gynecol. Obstet.*, **3**, 267–72

11. Fraser, D., Whitehead, M., Schenkel, L. and Pryse-Davies, J. (1993). Does low-dose, transdermal, norethisterone acetate reliably cause endometrial transformation in postmenopausal oestrogen-users? *Maturitas*, **16**, 23–30

12. Fraser, D. I., Parsons, A., Whitehead, M. I., Wordsworth, J., Stuart, G. and Pryse-Davies, J. (1990). The optimal dose of oral norethindrone acetate for addition to transdermal estradiol: a multicenter study. *Fertil. Steril.*, **53**, 460–8

13. Padwick, M. L., Pryse-Davies, J. and Whitehead, M. I. (1986). A simple method for determining the optimal dosage of progestin in postmenopausal women receiving estrogens. *N. Engl. J. Med.*, **315**, 930–4

14. Archer, D. F., Pickar, J. H. and Bottiglioni, F. for the Menopause Study Group (1994). Bleeding patterns in postmenopausal women taking continuous combined or sequential regimens of conjugated estrogens with medroxyprogesterone acetate. *Obstet. Gynecol.*, **83**, 686–92

15. Pickar, J. H., Bottiglioni, F. and Archer, D. F. for the Menopause Study Group. Continuous combined and cyclic hormone replacement therapies: frequency of amenorrhea and consistency of withdrawal bleeding. In preparation

Unresolved issues in endometrial cancer and postmenopausal hormone therapy

N. S. Weiss, S. A. A. Beresford, L. F. Voigt, P. K. Green and J. A. Shapiro

Introduction

Endometrial cancer is curable in most instances, particularly in a woman who is taking unopposed estrogens at the time the tumor is diagnosed. None the less, the concern over an increased incidence of endometrial cancer associated with the use of unopposed estrogen therapy has led to a decrease in the proportion of postmenopausal women who use unopposed estrogens, and also to changes in the way postmenopausal hormones are administered. Even though there are good reasons for many postmenopausal women to take estrogens for a very long period of time (to maximize benefits to their skeletal and cardiovascular systems), many women who have taken unopposed estrogens have now stopped taking hormones altogether. The data available to date are unclear regarding the incidence of endometrial cancer in these women in the years following their cessation of hormone-taking.

Other postmenopausal women have used a hormonal regimen that is believed not to be associated with much, if any, increased risk of endometrial cancer, namely daily estrogen plus a cyclic progestogen. However, data are limited regarding the duration each month that the progestogen must be taken in order for the incidence of endometrial cancer to be reduced. Also, the impact of long-term use of combined hormone therapy, irrespective of the monthly duration of progestogen, has not yet been evaluated. Finally, even if combined estrogen plus progestogen therapy does produce a decrease in the incidence of endometrial cancer relative to the use of estrogens alone, does it do so for all endometrial tumors, or only for those that have the least potential to spread and lead to a woman's death?

In our population-based case–control study of endometrial cancer in western Washington State (USA), we sought to provide information that addresses these questions.

Methods

Women eligible for this study were diagnosed with endometrial cancer between 1985 and 1991 and were residents of King, Pierce (1987–91 cases only) or Snohomish (1987–91 cases only) county. They were identified through the Cancer Surveillance System (CSS), a population-based cancer registry serving western Washington State. Cases were included if they were between the ages of 45 and 64 years (if diagnosed during 1985–86), 69 years (if diagnosed during 1991), or 74 years (if diagnosed during 1987–90). Of the 1154 eligible cases identified, 832 (72%) were interviewed in person regarding their use of hormones and other relevant aspects of their medical history.

Controls ($n = 1114$) were selected from female residents of these same three counties. They were chosen by means of random-digit telephone dialing using the Waksberg sampling method[1], and were given an in-person interview identical to that given to the women with cancer.

Menopausal hormone use was defined to be any non-contraceptive estrogen or progestogen use that was initiated within 12 months before a woman's natural menopause, any time after natural menopause, or after the age of 44 years. In addition, hormone use at any age was included if it was for menopausal symptoms or for osteoporosis.

Results

Incidence of endometrial cancer in relation to cessation of use of unopposed estrogens

In this analysis, women who had taken menopausal hormones for 6 months or less ($n = 192$) were categorized together with hormone non-users. Women who had used a progestogen for more than 6 months, either alone or together with estrogens ($n = 373$), and women who could not recall what type of hormone they had used ($n = 45$) were excluded. Details of this analysis and its results can be found elsewhere[2].

Women who were currently using unopposed estrogens, or had discontinued using them within the previous 2 years, were proportionately far more numerous among cases than controls (Table 1). The risk of endometrial cancer in women with such recent use was estimated to be nearly eight times that of non-hormone users. The relative risk declined in size with increasing time since last use of estrogens,

Table 1 Recency of unopposed estrogen use among cases and controls. Relative risk (RR) compared to non-users of menopausal estrogen, adjusted for age (< 55, 55–60, 60–65, > 65 years), body mass index (highest quartile vs. lowest three quartiles), cigarette smoking history (ever smoked vs. never smoked) and parity (parous vs. nulliparous)

Time since last use (years)	Cases	Controls	RR	95% CI
Non-user	337	685	1.0*	
< 2	213	68	7.9	5.7–10.9
2–8	27	21	2.7	1.4–5.0
> 8	77	89	1.7	1.1–2.4

*Reference category

but even beyond 8 years from the time of cessation a modest elevation in risk persisted (relative risk (RR) = 1.7, 95% confidence interval (CI) = 1.1–2.7). The elevated risk of endometrial cancer following cessation of estrogen use was present irrespective of the duration of use (beyond 6 months), but was particularly large for women with more than a decade of use (Table 2).

Table 2 Recency of unopposed menopausal estrogen use among cases of endometrial cancer and controls, by duration of use. Relative risk (RR) compared to non-users of unopposed estrogens, adjusted for age, body mass index (highest quartile vs. lowest three quartiles), cigarette smoking history (ever smoked vs. never smoked) and parity (parous vs. nulliparous)

Duration of use (years)	Recency (years)	Cases	Controls	RR	95% CI
6 months–3 years	< 2	26	25	2.5	1.4–4.4
	2–8	9	13	1.5	0.6–3.8
	> 8	46	56	1.7	1.1–2.7
4–7	< 2	25	13	4.9	2.4–10.0
	2–8	3	3	2.1	0.4–11.4
	> 8	14	23	1.3	0.6–2.7
8–12	< 2	36	11	8.8	4.3–17.8
	2–8	5	2	5.2	1.0–27.8
	> 8	7	7	1.7	0.5–5.0
> 12	< 2	126	19	16.5	9.8–27.9
	2–8	10	3	6.6	1.7–25.6
	> 8	10	3	5.6	1.5–21.3

Endometrial cancer in relation to combined hormone therapy

Excluded from this analysis are the very small number of women who had taken continuous combined therapy. Also, since we wanted to examine the effect of combined therapy in women whose risk of endometrial cancer was not already increased by unopposed estrogen, we excluded women who had previously taken estrogens alone. Finally, in the analysis of risk in relation to monthly duration of progestogen, we excluded women who had taken more than one regimen of combined hormones.

Using data from 45–64-year-old cases and controls in the early part of this study (1985–87), we previously observed that women who took cyclic combined therapy in which the progestogen was used for less than 10 days per cycle were at an increased risk of endometrial cancer[3]. Table 3 presents data that address the same hypothesis, excluding the women who had comprised our prior analysis. The same pattern of results was obtained. Compared to women who had never used hormones (or had done so for fewer than 6 months), those who used estrogen combined with progestogen for less than 10 days per month had a 3.1-fold increase in their risk of developing endometrial cancer (95% CI 1.7–5.7). In contrast, the relative risk associated with use of a progestogen for 10–21 days per month was only 1.3 (95% CI 0.8–2.2). The large majority of cases and controls had used medroxyprogesterone acetate as their progestational agent.

In the full dataset (394 cases and 788 controls), both in women who used a progestogen for less than 10 days per month and those who used it for 10 or more days, there was an increased risk of endometrial cancer associated with 5 or more years duration of use. The relative risks were 3.7 (95% CI 1.7–8.2) and 2.5 (95% CI 1.1–5.5), respectively.

For additional information regarding this phase of the study, see Beresford and colleagues[4].

Combined hormone therapy in relation to stage of endometrial cancer

The data suggest that women who took unopposed estrogen for 3 or more years had a large increase in risk of both endometrial cancers that had spread to the myometrium and cancers that had not. Use of combined therapy for 3 or more years was associated with about a two-fold increased risk of cancers confined to the endometrium (RR or odds ratio (OR) = 2.1, 95% CI = 1.2–3.7) and a smaller increase of more advanced cancers (RR or odds ratio (OR) = 1.3, 95% CI = 0.8–2.2). Relative to use of unopposed estrogen only (and adjusted for duration and recency of hormone use), use of combined therapy was associated with a substantially lower incidence of endometrial cancer irrespective of stage. The same pattern of results was present

Table 3 Endometrial cancer in relation to prior use of combined estrogen–progestogen therapy, by number of days per month progestogen was added. Table excludes women who used unopposed estrogen, users of more than one combined regimen, and continuous combined estrogen–progestin users. Analysis restricted to subjects not included in reference 3. Relative risk (RR) adjusted for age, body mass index and county of residence

	Cases		Controls			
Progestogen use	n	%	n	%	RR	95% CI
Never used hormones	270	84.4	593	86.8	1.0	
< 10 days/month	25	7.8	26	3.8	3.1	1.7–5.7
10–21 days/month	25	7.8	64	9.4	1.3	0.8–2.2

when we confined the analysis to the cases whose tumor had progressed to the outer half of the myometrium or to a more distant location. The results according to tumor grade were similar to those we found for tumor stage[5].

Discussion

As is true of nearly all interview-based case–control studies, the interpretation of our data is limited by not having information on all cases and controls, and by the likely inability of some of the participants to provide accurate information regarding the details of their hormone use. We sought to minimize the latter by providing visual displays of hormonal preparations to facilitate recall and, in our analyses, by restricting attention to hormone use that was maintained for at least 6 months (and therefore would be relatively less subject to being forgotten or recalled inaccurately).

Our results suggest that the increased risk of endometrial cancer present in users of unopposed estrogens declines after use of these hormones is discontinued. While this also has been true in all previous studies of this topic, there have been some differences across studies regarding how long after cessation of estrogen the incidence of endometrial cancer remains elevated. In our study there was an increased risk of endometrial cancer in prior users of unopposed estrogen, even among women who had discontinued taking this hormone more than 8 years earlier. The median duration of estrogen use among women in this category was 14.7 years. While four other studies also observed a persistent increase in endometrial cancer risk following cessation of unopposed estrogens[6–9], two relatively small studies[10,11] failed to do so. Also, in a relatively large study conducted among the female members of the Kaiser Foundation of Southern California[12], women who last used estrogens 4 or more years earlier had no increased risk of endometrial cancer. Reasons for the difference between these results and those of the majority of studies of endometrial cancer in relation to prior use of unopposed estrogen remain unknown.

Women who take estrogens with a cyclic progestogen for 10 or more days each month have a lower incidence of endometrial hyperplasia than the women who take a progestogen for a shorter duration. However, the incidence of endometrial *cancer* in relation to monthly duration of progestogen administration has been little studied. Apart from the research of Voigt and co-workers[3] cited earlier, there have only been two small studies. Brinton and colleagues[13], in a study that included only 11 cases and nine controls who had ever taken a progestogen, did not observe the risk of endometrial cancer to 'vary substantially' in relation to the number of days per month the progestogen was used. Jick and associates[14] obtained results more consistent with ours, in that a greater percentage of controls than cases had used more than 100 mg of medroxyprogesterone per month (presumably a larger total dose is indicative of a longer monthly duration of use). On the whole, the epidemiologic studies of endometrial cancer support the notion that, if a progestogen is to be given on a cyclic basis along with estrogens to postmenopausal women, protection against the development of endometrial cancer is best achieved with a duration of at least 10 days per month.

We observed that long-term use of estrogen with a cyclic progestogen is associated with an increased risk of endometrial cancer. Relative to non-users of hormones, the observed risk was increased some 2.5 times among women who took a progestogen for at least 10 days per month as part of a regimen of combined therapy that lasted 5 or more years. While this result is potentially worrisome, we recommend that it be interpreted cautiously, given that: (1) the confidence interval around the estimated relative risk is wide (1.1–5.5); (2) the study of Jick and colleagues[14] failed to find a difference between long- and short-term users of combined hormone therapy with regard to the risk of endometrial cancer.

While the addition of cyclic progestogen to postmenopausal estrogen therapy is associated with a greatly reduced risk of endometrial cancer in general, relative to the risk in users of unopposed estrogens, there have been no data regarding the influence of combined therapy on the occurrence of the relatively small percentage of endometrial cancers that are advanced, and therefore have the potential to be fatal. The data from our present study are encouraging in this regard: the reduced risk of endometrial cancer associated with cyclic progestogen (relative to the risk in users of unopposed estrogens) extends to the higher stage, higher grade, lesions. None the less, the number of cases in our study with these more advanced lesions was small, and it would be desirable for other large studies of endometrial cancer to confirm our finding.

Acknowledgements

This work was supported in part by two grants from the National Cancer Institute, R35 CA39779 and R01 CA47749.

References

1. Waksberg, J. (1978). Sampling methods for random digit dialing. *J. Am. Stat. Assoc.*, **73**, 40–6
2. Green, P. K., Weiss, N. S., McKnight, B., Voigt, L. F. and Beresford, S. A. A. (1996). Risk of endometrial cancer following cessation of menopausal hormone use. *Cancer Causes Control*, **7**, 575–80
3. Voigt, L. F., Weiss, N. S., Chu, J., Daling, J. R., McKnight, B. and van Belle, G. (1991). Progestogen supplementation of exogenous oestrogens and risk of endometrial cancer. *Lancet*, **338**, 274–7
4. Beresford, S. A. A., Weiss, N. S., Voigt, L. F. and McKnight, B. (1996). Endometrial cancer risk in relation to use of estrogen combined with cyclic progestin therapy in postmenopausal women. Submitted for publication
5. Shapiro, J. A., Weiss, N. S., Beresford, S. A. A. and Voigt, L. F. (1996). Menopausal hormone use and endometrial cancer, by tumor grade and invasion. Submitted for publication
6. Weiss, N. S., Szekeley, D. R., English, D. R. and Schweid, A. I. (1979). Endometrial cancer in relation to patterns of menopausal estrogen use. *J. Am. Med. Assoc.*, **242**, 261–4
7. Shapiro, S., Kelly, J. P., Rosenberg, L., Kaufman, D. W., Helmrich, S. P., Rosenhein, N. B., Lewis, J. L. Jr., Knapp, R. C., Stolley, P. D. and Schottenfeld, D. (1985). Risk of localized and widespread endometrial cancer in relation to recent and discontinued use of conjugated estrogens. *N. Engl. J. Med.*, **313**, 969–72
8. Paganini-Hill, A., Ross, R. K. and Henderson, B. E. (1989). Endometrial cancer and patterns of use of oestrogen replacement therapy: a cohort study. *Br. J. Cancer*, **59**, 445–7
9. Rubin, G. L., Peterson, H. B., Lee, N. C., Maes, E. F., Wingo, P. A. and Becker S. (1990). Estrogen replacement therapy and the risk of endometrial cancer: remaining controversies. *Am. J. Obstet. Gynecol.*, **162**, 148–54
10. Hulka, B. S., Fowler, W. C., Kaufman, D. G., Grimson, R. C., Greenberg, B. G., Hogue, C. J. R., Berger, G. S. and Pulliam, C. C. (1980). Estrogen and endometrial cancer: cases and two control groups from North Carolina. *Am. J. Obstet. Gynecol.*, **137**, 92–101
11. Pettersson, B., Adami, H. O., Persson, I., Bergstrom, R., Lindgren, A. and Johansson, E. D. B. (1986). Climacteric symptoms and estrogen replacement therapy in women with endometrial carcinoma. *Acta Obstet. Gynecol. Scand.*, **65**, 81–7
12. Finkle, W. D., Greenland, S., Miettinen, O. S. and Ziel, H. K. (1995). Endometrial cancer risk after discontinuing use of unopposed conjugated estrogens. *Cancer Causes Control*, **6**, 99–102
13. Brinton, L. A., Hoover, R. N. and The Endometrial Cancer Collaborative Group (1993). Estrogen replacement therapy and endometrial cancer risk: unresolved issues. *Obstet. Gynecol.*, **81**, 265–71
14. Jick, S. S., Walker, A. M. and Jick, H. (1993). Estrogens, progesterone, and endometrial cancer. *Epidemiology*, **4**, 20–4

Bleeding from an atrophic endometrium   36

S. K. Smith

Introduction

Hormone replacement therapy (HRT) provides considerable advantages to women with respect to prevention of osteoporosis and protection from ischemic heart disease and stroke[1]. Conversely, there is a slight increased risk of breast carcinoma[2] and thromboembolic phenomena[3]. However, many women are persuaded against using HRT because of the continuation of regular menstrual bleeding with sequential combined regimens. In order to minimize this inconvenience, continuous regimens have been developed in which either combined regimens (Kliofem®) or single agents (tibolone) are used in order to prevent regular steroid withdrawal bleeding. Unfortunately between 15 and 25% of patients on these regimens continue to have endometrial bleeding[4]. These episodes of bleeding are reduced if HRT is begun after 1 year of amenorrhea and declines over the 1st year of use. Why does this bleeding occur and why does it not occur in all patients?

Mechanisms of endometrial bleeding

Menstrual bleeding

Menstruation occurs in normal reproductive cycles when estrogen and progesterone are withdrawn from an estrogen-primed endometrium. This type of bleeding may also arise when exogenous steroids are withdrawn, as is the case with sequential combined HRT regimens. The mechanism is assumed to be similar to that observed by Markee[5] who transplanted endometrium of the rhesus macaque into the anterior chamber of the eye. On withdrawal of the steroid, the spiral arterioles undergo intense constriction resulting in distal hypoxia. For reasons which are unknown, these vessels then undergo dilatation and blood passes back into the distal endometrium. This results in the rupture of the blood vessel and the extravasation of blood into the stroma of the endometrium. The blood eventually reaches the surface epithelium which breaks down with release of the blood into the uterine cavity[6]. This mechanism occurs focally but eventually results in the loss of the superficial two-thirds of the endometrium.

However, tissue breakdown is not just mediated by the destructive effect of the extravasated blood. The matrix of the endometrium consists of collagens, fibronectin, laminin, gelatins, entactins, hyaluronic acid and proteoglycans. Cellular expression of the heterodimeric integrins in endometrium provides the link between the extracellular matrix and individual cells of the endometrium[7-10]. Degradation of the matrix is regulated by the matrix metalloproteins (MMPs). Three broad groups of enzymes have been described which include collagenases, gelatinases and stromelysins[11]. Endometrial stroma is known to express MMP-1, MMP-2 (type IV collagenase), MMP-3 (stromelysin-1) and MMP-10. The epithelium expresses MMP-7 (matrilysin). This expression is controlled by progesterone[12,13]. Interestingly, epithelial expression of MMP-7 is suppressed by transforming growth factor-β2 (TGF-β2) synthesized in the stromal compartment which is further regulated by progesterone. Removal of progesterone withdraws the suppressive action and releases metalloproteinase activity which results in the degradation of the extracellular matrix and the cleavage of the functionalis. With the loss of the stromal matrix, endometrial blood vessels would lose their support and their integrity which will lead to vessel rupture and bleeding.

Bleeding from atrophic endometrium

This carefully regulated mechanism of bleeding does not occur in patients with sustained systemic levels of steroid as is the case in bleeding from patients using continuous combined HRT. If atrophy is induced by these agents how is it that an 'inactive' endometrium can bleed? The mechanism of bleeding described above does not occur in these cases, so why do these women bleed? To answer this question a detailed understanding of the endometrial vasculature is required.

Endometrial vasculature Histological examination of the atrophic endometrium shows a profound reduction of mitotic indices in epithelial and stromal cells of the endometrium (Wells, personal communication). However, this is not matched by changes in the density of blood vessels in atrophic endometrium nor in their proliferative indices[14,15]. The endometrial vasculature consists of spiral arterioles which pass into the endometrium from the myometrium[16]. In the basal part of the endometrium, short non-branched basal arterioles supply the most proximal part of the endometrium. Remarkably, these transected vessels undergo repair during bleeding and growth in the proliferative phase of the cycle[17]. Arterioles are characterized by an intima and vascular smooth muscle coat. Approximately one-third of the way into the endometrium these vessels give off 'thinner' arterioles which continue towards the surface of the endometrium. Finally, a rich capillary plexus of microvessels supplies the superficial parts of the endometrium. These are collected into venules which pass back towards the myometrium[18]. In normal menstrual cycles, this profound angiogenesis does not result in significant

extravasation of blood despite the development of new vessels.

Factors which control endothelial integrity

Growth factors

A range of agents are known to control the complex process of angiogenesis in that they can stimulate proliferation of endothelial cells, induce their migration, promote proteolytic enzyme secretion resulting in degradation of the basement membrane, and promote the development of tubular structures (Table 1). Several of these, including vascular endothelial growth factor (VEGF) and fibroblast growth factors-1 and -2 (FGF-1 and -2), are expressed in human endometrium[19,20]. In the case of VEGF it is expressed by glandular and stromal cells in the proliferative phase of the cycle, but expression is more restricted to the glandular cells in the luteal phase (Figure 1). At menstruation arising from a natural cycle, high levels of mRNA are found in the glandular cells. Vascular endothelial growth factor expression in atrophic endometrium is unclear. In areas characterized by necrosis, bleeding and macrophage infiltration, high levels would be expected because macrophages produce large amounts of VEGF, and its expression in other

Table 1 Angiogenic growth factors and their receptors

Growth factor	Receptor
VEGF	flt, KDR
FGF-1	FGF-R+1
FGF-2	FGF-R+2
HGF	met
TGF-α	EGF-R
Angiotrophin	

VEGF, vascular endothelial growth factor; FGF, fibroblast growth factor; HGF, hybridoma growth factor; TGF, transforming growth factor; FGF-R, FGF-receptor; EGF-R, endothelial growth factor-receptor

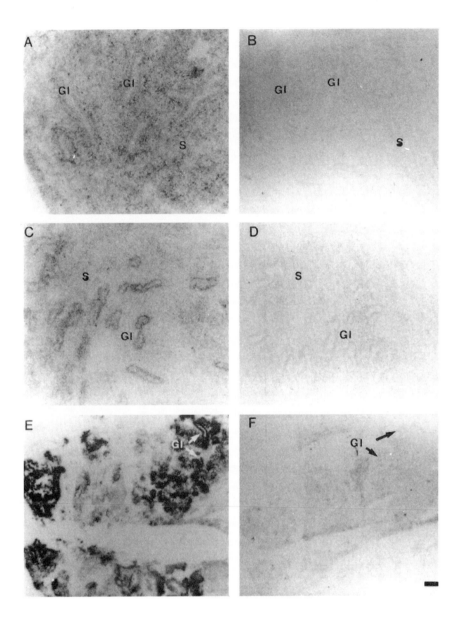

Figure 1 *In situ* localization of vascular endothelial growth factor (VEGF) mRNA in endometrial tissue. Bright-field photomicrographs of sections of endometrium after *in situ* hybridization with antisense VEGF RNA probe (A, C, E); equivalent sections hybridized with sense probe are shown for comparison (B, D, F). Sections are counterstained with hemalum. A, B, proliferative phase endometrium; C, D, secretory phase endometrium; E, F, menstrual tissue. Endometrial glands (GI) and stroma (S) are indicated. Scale bar: 250 μm

endometrial cells is induced by hypoxia[21]. In these circumstances increased wound repair would be expected. Of particular interest is the finding that atrophic endometrium has increased endometrial vascular density, further suggesting that enhanced VEGF presence arises in this tissue[15]. What is not known at this stage is whether significant disturbances of

VEGF expression cause abnormalities in endothelial cell integrity resulting in endometrial bleeding.

Endothelial cell biology

Endothelial cells have specific receptors for a range of angiogenic growth factors and these receptors are regulated by a range of agents including hypoxia itself. These cells lining blood vessels are highly specific for each organ in which they are found. Disorders in receptor expression or function could give rise to abnormal contact between the endothelial cells resulting in extravasation of blood cells into the endometrial stroma. Integrins, particularly the promiscuous $\alpha_v\beta_3$ are particularly expressed by growing endothelial cells and are regulated by a range of agents. They interact with VEGF through its capacity to promote extravasation and stimulate the extravascular coagulation system. Overexpression of VEGF could potentially result in endothelial cell disruption and bleeding[22,23].

Surrounding matrix

An alternative explanation for atrophic endometrial bleeding is that the surrounding matrix in which the vessel is situated becomes deranged when denied a continuing exposure to estrogens and progestogens, or at least a combination of both, which results histologically in a gross reduction in epithelial component and regression of the stroma. Progesterone stimulates degradation of urokinase plasminogen activator (u-PA) in endometrial stromal cells by increasing its inhibitor and surface expression of the u-PA receptor[24]. This diminishes its proteolytic activity. It also increases plasminogen activator inhibitor-1 (PAI-1) expression further reducing fibrinolytic activity in endometrium[25]. This is an example of a steroid regulating proteolytic enzyme activity but why and how this differs between patients and between different areas of the endometrium in the same uterus is not known.

Conclusion and avenues of new discovery

We do not know why women bleed from an atrophic endometrium; nor do we know why many women do not bleed from an atrophic endometrium. This is not surprising because the body of knowledge needed to understand these complex processes in the endometrium is not available. What is clear is that bleeding arises from blood vessels, and the understanding of their biology is the key to better control of bleeding from the atrophic endometrium.

The steroidal regulation of angiogenic growth factor expression is a critical part of the process, often being the conductor of the whole process of blood vessel growth and maintenance of the integrity of the endothelium. The specific means by which this is regulated in patients using replacement therapy needs to be determined. Particularly, the unusual changes that arise focally in the endometrium need to be studied by sight-directed biopsies of bleeding areas. The key to understanding endometrial bleeding is the endometrial vasculature.

References

1. Birkhauser, M. H. (1995). HRT and health: fact or fiction? *Eur. Menopause J.*, **2**, 2–3
2. Wren, B. (1995). Hormonal replacement therapy and breast cancer. *Eur. Menopause J.*, **2**, 13–19
3. Medicines Control Agency (1996). Risk of venous thromboembolism with hormone replacement therapy. *Medicines Control Agency*, **22**, 9–10
4. Archer, D. F. (1993). Hormone replacement therapy and uterine bleeding. *Menopausal Med.*, **1**, 1–12
5. Markee, J. E. (1940). Menstruation in intraocular endometrial transplants in the rhesus monkey. *Contrib. Embryol. Carnegie Inst.*, **28**, 219–308

6. Nogales-Ortiz, F., Puerta, J. and Nogales, F. F. (1978). Normal menstrual cycle. Chronology and mechanisms of endometrial desquamation. *Obstet. Gynecol.*, **51**, 259–64

7. Hynes, R. O. (1987). Integrins: a family of cell surface receptors. *Cell*, **40**, 549–54

8. Ruoslahti, E. and Yamaguchi, Y. (1991). Proteoglycans as modulators of growth factor activities. *Cell*, **6**, 867–9

9. Lessey, B. A., Damjanovich, L., Coutfaris, C., Castelbaum, A., Albelda, S. M. and Buck, C. A. (1992). Integrin adhesion molecules in the human endometrium. Correlation with the normal and abnormal menstrual cycle. *J. Clin. Invest.*, **90**, 188–95

10. Lessey, B. A., Castelbaum, A. J., Buck, C. A., Lei, Y., Yowell, C. W. and Sun, J. (1994). Further characterization of endometrial integrins during the menstrual cycle and in pregnancy. *Fertil. Steril.*, **62**, 497–506

11. Tabizzada, S. and Babaknia, A. (1995). The signals and molecular pathways involved in implantation, a symbiotic interaction between blastocyst and endometrium involving adhesion and tissue invasion. *Mol. Hum. Reprod.*, **1**, 1579–602

12. Osteen, K. G., Rodgers, W. H., Gaire, M., Hargrove, J. T., Gorstein, F. and Matrisian, L. M. (1994). Stromal–epithelial interaction mediates steroidal regulation of metalloproteinase expression in human endometrium. *Proc. Natl. Acad. Sci. USA*, **91**, 10129–33

13. Schatz, F., Papp, C., Toth Pal, E. and Lockwood, C. J. (1994). Ovarian steroid-modulated stromelysin-1 expression in human endometrial stromal and decidual cells. *J. Clin. Endocrinol. Metab.*, **78**, 1467–72

14. Rogers, P. A. W. (1996). Structure and function of endometrial blood vessels. *Hum. Reprod. Update*, **2**, 57–62

15. Hickey, M., Lau, T. M., Russell, P., Fraser, I. S. and Rogers, P. A. W. (1996). Microvascular density in conditions of endometrial atrophy. *Hum. Reprod.*, **11**, 2009–13

16. Ferenczy, A. (1976). Studies on the cytodynamics of human endometrial regeneration. I. Scanning electron microscopy. *Am. J. Obstet. Gynecol.*, **124**, 64–74

17. Ludwig, H., Metzger, H. and Frauli, M. (1990). Endometrium: tissue remodelling and regeneration. In D'Arcangues, C., Fraser, I. S., Newton, J. R. and Odlind, V. (eds.) WHO Symposium on Contraception and Mechanisms of Endometrial Bleeding, pp. 441–66. (Geneva: World Health Organization)

18. Roberts, D. K., Parmley, T. H., Walker, M. J. and Horbelt, D. V. (1992). Ultrastructure of the microvasculature in the human endometrium throughout the normal menstrual cycle. *Am. J. Obstet. Gynecol.*, **166**, 1393–406

19. Ferriani, R. A., Charnock-Jones, D. S., Prentice, A., Thomas, E. J. and Smith, S. K. (1993). Immunohistochemical localisation of acidic and basic fibroblast growth factors in normal human endometrium and endometriosis and the detection of their mRNA by PCR. *Hum. Reprod.*, **8**, 11–16

20. Charnock-Jones, D. S., Sharkey, A. M., Rajput-Williams, J., Burch, D., Schofield, J. P., Fountain, S. A., Boocock, C. A. and Smith, S. K. (1993). Identification and localization of alternately spliced mRNAs for vascular endothelial growth factor in human uterus and estrogen regulation in endometrial carcinoma cell lines. *Biol. Reprod.*, **48**, 1120–8

21. Song, J. Y., Russell, P., Markham, R., Manconi, F. and Fraser, I. S. (1996). Effect of high dose progestogens on white cells and necrosis in human endometrium. *Hum. Reprod.*, **11**, 1713–18

22. Cullinan-Bove, K. and Koos, R. D. (1993). Vascular endothelial growth factor/vascular permeability factor expression in the rat uterus: rapid stimulation by estrogen correlates with estrogen induced increases in uterine capillary permeability and growth. *Endocrinology*, **133**, 829–37

23. Senger, D. R., Ledbetter, S. R., Claffey, K. P., Papadopoulos-Sergiou, A., Perruzzi, C. A. and Detmar, M. (1996). Stimulation of endothelial cell migration by vascular permeability factor/vascular endothelial growth factor through cooperative mechanisms involving the alpha(v)beta3 integrin, osteopontin, and thrombin. *Am. J. Pathol.*, **149**, 293–305

24. Casslen, B., Nordengren, J., Gustavsson, B., Nilbert, M. and Lund, L. R. (1995). Progesterone stimulates degradation of urokinase plasminogen activator (u-PA) in endometrial stromal cells by increasing its inhibitor and surface expression of the u-PA receptor. *J. Clin. Endocrinol. Metab.*, **80**, 2776–84

25. Casslen, B., Tove, H. and Goran, S. (1996). Norethisterone and progesterone are potent comparable inducers of endometrial PAI-1 activity. Presented at the *8th International Congress on the Menopause*, Sydney, Australia, November, abstr. F223

7

Androgens and the menopause

Androgen production over the female life span

37

H. M. Buckler and W. R. Robertson

Introduction

Traditionally testosterone (T) and estrogen (E_2) have been regarded as the male and female hormones respectively, but this apparent mutual exclusivity no longer seems appropriate. Although most studies on androgens and women have focused on their role in various pathologies, e.g. polycystic ovarian syndrome, there is now good evidence emerging that demonstrates a role for testosterone (T) in both female embryologic development[1] as well as in normal female sexual function, mood, cognitive function and well-being[2-5]. There is also increasing awareness that androgens may be of therapeutic value in postmenopausal women, and low doses of androgens are being increasingly used in women for the treatment of sexual dysfunction[6].

Estrogens are formed in the ovary from androgen precursors which circulate at a higher concentration in the blood as well as having a greater production and secretion rate. Typically, estradiol production rate varies over the menstrual cycle from around 80 μg a day in the follicular phase with a peak of around 450–900 μg per day at mid-cycle[7], resulting in circulating levels of 130–500 and 500–1500 pmol/l for the follicular and mid-cycle phases respectively. In contrast, ovarian production rates of T are around 200–300 μg/day and circulating levels are about 2 nmol/l. Further, the production rates and circulating levels of the weaker androgens (dehydroepiandrosterone, DHEA and androstenedione, Adione) are even greater in women than in men, being 800 μg DHEA and about 3 mg/day Adione with one-half being derived from the ovary[8]. The remainder is secreted by the adrenal cortex or derived by extraglandular conversion. Clearly, the large quantities of androgen present in the healthy woman raises the question of what is their role in normal physiology.

Androgen production and secretion

Androstenedione, T and DHEA are produced by the ovary and the adrenals, with secretion from the latter being partially controlled by adrenocorticotropin hormone (ACTH); dehydroepiandrosterone sulfate (DHEAS) synthesis is entirely adrenal in origin. Androgen secretion from the ovary is under luteinizing hormone (LH) control and as it arises from the theca cells of the follicle, the corpus luteum and the stromal cells, it varies somewhat during the normal menstrual cycle. Examination of the androgen content of ovarian venous blood has shown that both T and Adione are secreted by the ovary with the dominant follicle[9] but the other ovary also contributes. Testosterone varies less than its major precursor Adione as at least 50% of circulating T is derived from the peripheral conversion of Adione and DHEA.

Although the plasma concentration of androgen determines the amount of hormone potentially available for action at target tissues, its rate of transport into cells is largely determined by a specific plasma binding protein (sex hormone-binding globulin, SHBG) which binds testosterone at such high affinity that only 1–2% of the hormone is free to act on the target cell. This free T level, which is usually expressed as the free T index (calculated from the levels of total T and SHBG) is a far better index of androgenicity than the total T. Under certain circumstances such as hyperthyroidism and pregnancy, SHBG is increased and this can have effects on the free level of plasma T. Moreover, estrogen administration, e.g. hormone replacement therapy (HRT) may increase SHBG levels and result in decreased free T levels which may have significance for the well-being of these patients, as it could be that T plays an important role in this process. Thus, the plasma level of free T is a variable fraction of the total hormone concentration and depends on the amount of binding protein present.

Androgen levels in childhood and puberty

There is a marked increase in plasma DHEA and DHEAS in prepubertal girls and boys which starts at around 8 years of age and continues through to ages 13–15 years[10,11]. This increase in the secretion of adrenal androgen, which contributes to the growth of pubic and axillary hair, is known as the adrenarche and its onset commences 2 years before the rise in gonadotropins and gonadal sex steroids that is the hallmark of puberty. In contrast, T levels remain low (< 1 nmol/l) in the prepubertal girl, but increase progressively between pubertal stages 1 and 4 to the normal adult levels of around 2 nmol/l. Prepubertally there are equal levels of SHBG in boys and girls, but at puberty there is a small decrease in levels in girls and a much larger decrease in boys. Adult males have one-half the SHBG concentrations of adult females, thus, although the plasma concentration of T is 20 times greater in men than in women the concentration of free T is 40 times greater[12].

Androgens and menstrual cycle

Ovarian androgen secretion varies considerably over the menstrual cycle with Adione and T being lowest (2600 and 200 µg/24 h respectively) in the early follicular phase before rising to the highest levels just prior to, or at the time of ovulation, by which time the production rates are 4700 and 240 µg/24 h respectively[13]. Testosterone levels then gradually fall in the luteal phase (170 µg/24 h) in contrast to Adione which peaks again during the luteal phase reflecting a production rate of 3400 µg/24 h[14,15]. Dihydrotestosterone (DHT) levels do not vary during the menstrual cycle and DHEA and DHEAS remain stable[15]. This mid-cycle androgen rise may serve two purposes. First, it may accelerate follicular atresia of the current cohort of follicles, with the exception of the single dominant follicle which will progress onto ovulation. Second, it may also play a role in stimulating libido as female sexual activity has been found to peak at mid-cycle[16].

Androgens and perimenopause

The menopausal transition, the perimenopause, is associated with characteristic endocrine changes, with a monotropic rise in follicle-stimulating hormone (FSH) and corresponding fall in inhibin levels being the first endocrine manifestation of ovarian aging[17]. However, the changes in circulating androgen levels during this process are less clear, although reproductive aging may be associated with a menstrual-cycle related decrease in androgen secretion, as a decline in T with increasing age has been reported in premenopausal women such that the levels in women in their 40s are about a one-third of those in their 20s[18]. Moreover, diminished free T and Adione levels are found at mid-cycle in older women[19]. No change was found in T, DHT or Adione levels over an 18-month period following the last menstrual period in one study[20], but more recently a small decline in T and Adione within a 6-month period encompassing the last menstrual period was described[21]. In their study, Longcope and colleagues[20] noted that the mean concentration of T in all their subjects was less than those of a group of young women. Taken together it is now becoming clear that a fall in circulating androgens is associated with aging and may in fact precede the menopause.

Androgens and menopause

The menopause is defined as the last menstrual period in a woman's life, and at the cessation of menstruation there is a steep decline in estradiol and estrone circulating concentrations (6 μg and 42 μg/24 h respectively[22]). Estrogen production in postmenopausal women is almost exclusively due to extraglandular aromatization of Adione, the levels of which are about 50% lower than in premenopausal women reflecting a production rate of about 1500 μg/24 h[22] primarily due to a fall in ovarian secretion. Although there is a concomitant decrease in adrenal production of Adione the relative contribution of the adrenal to circulating Adione increases to 80% following the menopause, as opposed to 50% premeno-pausally[22]. The other adrenal androgens, DHEA and DHEAS, also decrease with age, but this process appears to be independent of the menopausal transition[23].

The menopause is also associated with a decrease in overall T production (between 50 and 100 μg/24 h[22]) most of which is now secreted from the stroma. However, ovarian secretion of T is maintained at a level approaching that in younger women (50–70 μg/24 h premenopausally, 40–50 μg/24 h postmenopausally) although the marked fall in secretion of Adione, a major precursor of T, results in an overall decline in circulating T levels which is compounded by a decrease in non-ovarian production of T.

Thus the postmenopausal ovary remains an important source of T production, and the decline in total circulating androgens with age results from a combination of ovarian failure and decreasing adrenal and peripheral androgen synthesis. This relative androgen deficiency is compounded in women who have had bilateral oophorectomy, as this group has even lower levels of androgen with serum T falling by 50%; this may contribute to the increased morbidity in this group in comparison to the normal climacteric[24]. Overall, this deficiency state may be associated with a reduction in quality of life and increased sexual dysfunction as well as adverse effects on

bone mass[5]. In view of this there is an increasing belief that there may be a role for androgen replacement in addition to estrogen treatment in postmenopausal women. However, there are few studies on what doses of androgen may be needed, what is the best mode of delivery of the hormones and what are the relative benefits/disadvantages of such a therapy. There is an urgent need for good clinical trials as androgen replacement is becoming very topical because of mounting reports of the effects of these hormones ('the fountain of youth'[25]).

Androgen replacement therapy

As T cannot be administered orally owing to inactivation by the liver it has to be given by other routes. Subcutaneous T implants have been available for the treatment of male hypogonadism for many years and although their pharmacokinetics are not ideal they do not produce short-lived high T peaks, but result in more stable T levels over reasonable periods of time[26,27] (4–6 months). Compared to the available oral and injectable T esters they provide an effective form of androgen replacement for male hypogonadism[28].

The concept of adrenal androgen replacement in older women is now the subject of increasing investigation and a number of therapeutic strategies (oral medication, intramuscular injection, implants, transdermal patch-based delivery) are now available. For example, the fall in adrenal DHEA and DHEAS secretion has lead to the treatment of women of advancing age with DHEA, and this results in the restoration of circulating T and Adione to premenopausal levels[29] and is reported to be associated with an increased feeling of well-being. Further, the treatment of women with testosterone (100 or 50 mg) as well as estradiol implants has been shown to improve sexual function and have beneficial effects on bone density[6,30]. The long duration of subcutaneous implant therapy may not always be appropriate when initiating T treatment in women because of potential side-effects such as worsening of hirsutism or acne.

250

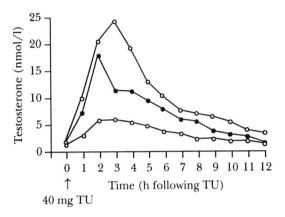

Figure 1 Testosterone undecanoate (TU) (40 mg) given to 10 healthy women at time zero 1 h after controlled fat meal. Median (closed circles) plus range (open circles) is shown for testosterone concentration hourly for 12 h

Testosterone undecanoate

An orally active preparation of T is available (testosterone undecanoate, TU) and this may be of value as a convenient method of administering T to women. It is widely used for androgen replacement in hypogonadal men but the circulating T levels can be unpredictable (peak concentrations with a dose of 80 mg twice daily, 11.5–60.1 nmol/l[31]). We have therefore examined the pharmacokinetics of various doses of TU in women (Buckler and Robertson, unpublished data). We found that using doses ranging from 10–40 mg produced inappropriate levels, and there was wide individual variation in T levels between subjects (Figures 1 and 2). It appears that TU may not be suitable for use in women.

Testosterone implants

Early work indicated that the use of T implants in women could lead to a controlled release of T. Thus, Thom and colleagues[32] showed a five-fold increase in plasma testosterone following a 100 mg testosterone implant, with peak levels occurring at 1–2 months followed by a return to pretreatment values at 5 months. Further studies showed that 100 and 50 mg

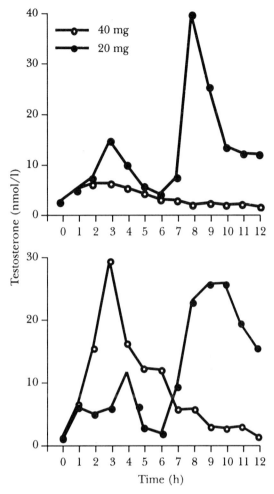

Figure 2 Two profiles from individual patients initally given testosterone undecanoate (TU) (40 mg; open circles) and then TU (2 × 20 mg; closed circles) at 6-h intervals a week later

implants produced peak T levels at 1 month of 6.7 and 3.5 nmol/l, respectively[6,33] (normal range up to 3 nmol/l), and our own data (Figure 3, Buckler and Robertson, unpublished data) with a 100 mg implant showed similar results with testosterone levels reaching 9.0 nmol/l 1 month after insertion followed by a rapid fall. Testosterone levels (2.9 nmol/l) were still above our normal range (up to 2.4 nmol/l) at 6 months.

Testosterone implants are usually used in conjunction with estradiol treatment when the

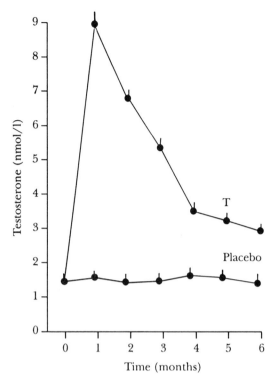

Figure 3 Serum testosterone (T) levels following subcutaneous T implant (100 mg; $n = 30$) or placebo ($n = 30$) measured monthly for 6 months. Data are mean + standard error

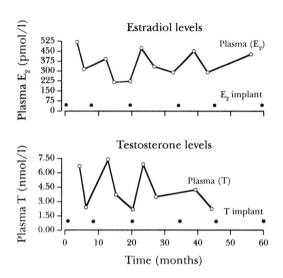

Figure 4 Estradiol (E_2) and testosterone (T) levels in a woman receiving combined E_2 + T implant therapy

latter alone does not improve sexual dysfunction. We have previously reported an audit of the long-term use of estradiol implant therapy in women[34]. More recently we have analyzed the additional use of T implants (100 mg) combined with E_2 implants in this group of patients. Two hundred and seventy-five women were included in this group receiving a total of 759 E_2 implants. One hundred and seven of these patients received a total of 242 T implants largely because they felt

that the symptoms of sexual dysfunction were not relieved. Interestingly, the patients opting for additional T implant treatment were younger than those receiving E_2 alone and 83% of them had had a bilateral oophorectomy (Table 1). Overall, the median frequency with which T implants were inserted was every 8 months, and based on the measurement of testosterone every 3 months during therapy T levels of around 3.5 nmol/l were achieved. An example of plasma estradiol and testosterone levels in relation to estradiol and testosterone implantation in a typical patient is shown in Figure 4.

Although subcutaneous testosterone treatment appears to be effective, the testosterone levels achieved are not physiological and the use of implants is

Table 1 Characteristics of patients receiving estradiol (E_2) (50 mg) alone or E_2 (50 mg) and testosterone (T) (100 mg) subcutaneous implants

	E_2 ($n = 275$)	$E_2 + T$ ($n = 107$)
Mean age at start of treatment (years)	46 (range 17–62)	42 (range 18–59)
Hysterectomy (n)	145 (53%)	91 (86%)
Oophorectomy (n)	91 (33%)	89 (83%)

characterized by rapid rises and falls of this potent steroid. On the other hand the pharmacokinetics of intramuscular injections of testosterone esters using existing preparations are unlikely to be entirely satisfactory in women either, as high levels of testosterone in the first 2–3 days after intramuscular injection are generally unavoidable even at low doses[35]. Further, as has been discussed, earlier oral testosterone also has its disadvantages and in view of this, alternative treatment strategies which give rise to a controlled and physiological pattern of testosterone release are clearly desirable.

Transdermal testosterone

We have therefore investigated a matrix transdermal delivery system in an attempt to achieve more physiological and stable levels in women. Transdermal delivery of drugs offers several advantages including rapid perfusion through the skin, painless delivery, increased compliance and avoidance of the first-pass hepatic metabolism. We have examined (Buckler, Robertson and Wu, unpublished data) the pharmacokinetics of a matrix transdermal system (TDS) for testosterone using various estimated daily T delivery rates aiming to produce stable physiological levels in women. As can be seen (Figures 5 and 6) this delivery system produced T levels which may be appropriate for use in women. The TDS was well tolerated by all subjects with no evidence of any local skin reaction even with repeated applications.

We conclude that this novel matrix TDS for T can produce and maintain stable T levels within the physiological range, with little within- and between-subject variation. The patches have the further advantage of being easy to use and remove without the need for

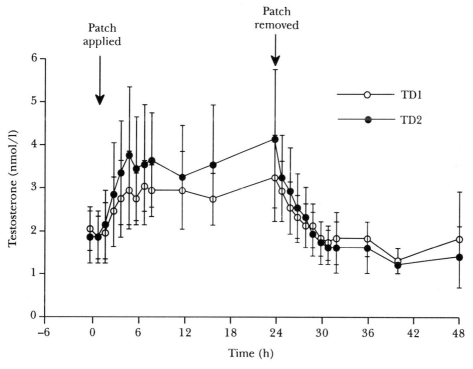

Figure 5 Testosterone (T) levels following application of two transdermal (TD) patches for delivery of T. Each patch was worn for 24 h and then removed; data are mean ± standard deviation. Two delivery rates were examined: TD1, 840 μg per 24 h; TD2, 1100 μg per 24 h

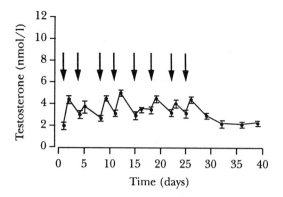

Figure 6 Testosterone (T) levels following administration of transdermal T (TD2) twice weekly (indicated by arrows) for 4 weeks

nursing or medical staff, and represent a major advance in patch technology. Although further studies are clearly required to establish the best therapeutic range, this new technology should allow for women to be treated with T in a far more physiological manner than is possible with existing methods.

Summary

Androgens are present in women in large quantities relative to estrogens but their function in women is not fully understood. They have an important role as precursors to estrogens, but it also appears that in addition they may play a part in well-being and sexual function. Therefore the decreased androgens associated with the postmenopausal state, particularly following oophorectomy, may result in a decreased quality of life in these women. The strategy of androgen replacement therefore merits further consideration.

References

1. McEwen, B. S. (1991). Sex differences in the brain, what are they and how do they arise? In Notman, M. T. and Nadelson, C. C. (eds.) *Women and Men, New Perspectives on Gender Differences*, pp. 35–41. (Washington DC: American Psychiatric Press)
2. Sherwin, B. B. and Gelfand, M. M. (1985). Sex steroids and affect in the surgical menopause. A double blind cross over study. *Psychoneuro-endocrinology*, **10**, 325–35
3. Sherwin, B. B. (1988). Affective changes with oestrogen and androgen replacement therapy in surgically menopausal women. *J. Affect. Disord.*, **14**, 177–87
4. Kaplan, H. S. and Owett, T. (1993). The female androgen deficiency syndrome. *Sex. Marital Ther.*, **19**, 3–24
5. Sands, R. and Studd, J. (1995). Exogenous androgens in post-menopausal women. *Am. J. Med.*, **98** (Suppl. 1A), 76S–9S
6. Burger, H. G., Hailes, J., Nelson, J. and Menelaus, M. (1987). Effect of combined implants of estradiol and testosterone on libido in post menopausal women. *Br. Med. J.*, **294**, 936–7
7. Lipsett, M. B. (1978). Steroid hormones. In Yen, S. S. C. and Jaffe, R. B. (eds.) *Reproductive Endocrinology*, pp. 140–53. (Philadelphia: W. B. Saunders)
8. Bardin, C. W. and Lipsett, M. B. (1967). Testosterone and androstenedione rates in normal women and in women with idiopathic hirsutism or polycystic ovaries. *J. Clin. Invest.*, **46**, 891–5
9. Baird, D. T., Burger, P. E., Heavon-Jones, G. D. and Scaramuzzi, R. J. (1974). The site of androstenedione production in non-pregnant women. *J. Endocrinol.*, **63**, 201–12
10. Reiter, E. O., Fuldauer, V. G. and Root. A. W. (1977). Secretion of the adrenal androgen, dehydroepiandrosterone sulfate during normal infancy, childhood and adolescence in sick infants and in children with endocrinologic abnormalities. *J. Paediatr.*, **90**, 766–70
11. Hopper, B. R. and Yen, S. S. C. (1975). Circulating concentrations of dehydroepiandrosterone and dehydroepiandrosterone sulfate during puberty. *J. Clin. Endocrinol. Metab.*, **40**, 458–61
12. Anderson, D. C. (1974). Sex hormone binding globulin. *Clin. Endocrinol.*, **3**, 39–52
13. Baird, D. T. and Fraser, I. S. (1974). Blood production and secretion rates of estradiol 17β in women throughout the menstrual cycle. *J. Clin. Endocrinol. Metab.*, **38**, 1009–14
14. Judd, L. H. and Yen, S. S. C. (1973). Serum androstenedione and testosterone levels during the menstrual cycle. *J. Clin. Endocrinol. Metab.*, **36**, 475–81
15. Abraham, G. E. (1974). Ovarian and adrenal contribution to peripheral androgens during the

menstrual cycle. *J. Clin. Endocrinol. Metab.*, **39**, 340–6

16. Adams, D. B., Gold, A. R. and Burt, A.D. (1978). Rise in female-initiated sexual activity at ovulation and its suppression by oral contraceptives. *N. Engl. J. Med.*, **299**, 1145–50

17. Buckler, H. M., Evans, C. A., Mantora, H., Burger, H. G. and Anderson, D. C. (1991). Gonado-tropin, steroid and inhibin levels in women with incipient ovarian failure during anovulatory rebound cycles. *J. Clin. Endocrinol. Metab.*, **72**, 116–24

18. Zumoff, B., Stain, G. W., Miller, L. K. and Rosner, W. (1995). Twenty-four hour mean plasma testosterone concentration declines with age in normal premenopausal women. *J. Clin. Endocrinol. Metab.*, **80**, 1429–30

19. Mushayandebvu, T., Castracane, V. D., Gimpel, T., Tovaghgol, A. and Santoro, N. (1996). Evidence for diminished midcycle ovarian androgen production in older reproductive aged women. *Fertil. Steril.*, **65**, 721–3

20. Longcope, C., Franz, C., Morello, C., Baker, K. and Johnston, C. C. Jr. (1986). Steroid and gonadotrophin levels in women during the peri-menopausal years. *Maturitas*, **8**, 189–96

21. Rannevik, G., Jeppsson, S. and Johnell, O. (1995). A longitudinal study of the perimenopausal transition: altered profiles of steroid and pituitary hormones, SHBG and bone mineral density. *Maturitas*, **21**, 103–13

22. Adashi, E. Y. (1994). The climateric ovary as a functional gonadotropin driven androgen producing gland. *Fertil. Steril.*, **62**, 20–7

23. Zumoff, B., Rosenfield, R. S., Strain, G. W., Levin, J. and Fukushima, D. K. (1980). Sex differences in the twenty-four hour mean plasma concentrations of dehydroisoandrosterone (DHA) and dehydroisoandrosterone sulfate (DHAS) and DHA to DHAS ratio in normal adults. *J. Clin. Endocrinol. Metab.*, **51**, 330–3

24. Judd, H. L., Lucas, W. E. and Yen, S. S. C. (1974). Effect of oophorectomy on circulating testosterone and androstenedione levels in patients with endometrial cancer. *Am. J. Obstet. Gynecol.*, **118**, 793–8

25. Baulieu, E. E. (1996). Dehydroepiandrosterone (DHEA) – a fountain of youth. *J. Clin. Endocrinol. Metab.*, **81**, 3146–51

26. Handelsman, D. J., Conway, A. J. and Boylan, L. M. (1990). Pharmacokinetics and pharmacology of testosterone pellets in men. *J. Clin. Endocrinol. Metab.*, **71**, 216–22

27. Jockenhovel, F., Vodel, E. Kreutzer, M. Rheinhardt, W., Lederbogen, S. and Reinwein, D. (1996). Pharmacokinetics and pharmaco-dynamics of subcutaneous testosterone implants in hypogonadal men. *Clin. Endocrinol.*, **45**, 61–71

28. Nieschlag, E. (1996). Testosterone replacement therapy; something old, something new. *Clin. Endocrinol.*, **45**, 261–2

29. Morales, A. J., Nolan, J. J. Nelson, J. C. and Yen, S. S. C. (1994). Effects of replacement dose of dehydroepiandrosterone in men and women of advancing age. *J. Clin. Endocrinol. Metab.*, **78**, 1360–7

30. Davis, S. R., McCloud, P., Strauss, B. J. G. and Burger, H. G. (1995). Testosterone enhances oestradiol effects on post-menopausal bone density and sexuality. *Maturitas*, **21**, 227–36

31. Cantrill, J. A., Dewis, P., Large, D. M., Newman, M. and Anderson, D. C. (1984). Which testosterone replacement therapy? *Clin. Endocrinol.*, **21**, 97–107

32. Thom M. H., Collins, W. P. and Studd, J. W. W. (1981). Hormonal profiles in post menopausal women after therapy with subcutaneous implants. *Br. J. Obstet. Gynaecol.*, **88**, 426–33

33. Burger, H.G., Hales, J., Menelaus, M., Nelson, J., Hudson, B. and Balazs, N. (1984). The management of persistent menopausal symptoms with oestradiol–testosterone implants – clinical, lipid and hormonal results. *Maturitas*, **6**, 351–8

34. Buckler, H. M., Kalsi, P. K., Cantrill, J. A. and Anderson, D. C. (1985). An audit of oestradiol levels and implant frequency in women undergoing subcutaneous implant therapy. *Clin. Endocrinol.*, **42**, 445–50

35. Behre, H. M., Oberpenning, F. and Nieschlag, E. (1990). Comparative pharmacokinetics of androgen preparations: application of computer analysis and stimulation. In Nieschlag, E. and Behre, H. M. (eds.) *Testosterone Action. Deficiency Substitution*, pp. 115–35. (Berlin: Springer-Verlag)

Androgens and bone function 38

S. R. Davis

Introduction

In women androgens are produced by the ovaries and the adrenal glands which secrete androstenedione (A), testosterone (T) and dehydroepiandrosterone (DHEA), with the latter also producing DHEA-sulfate (DHEA-S). The peripheral conversion of preandrogens to testosterone accounts for at least 50% of circulating T, with A being the main peripheral precursor[1]. In regularly ovulating women the mean plasma levels of both A and T increase during the middle third of the menstrual cycle[2]. However, increasing age is associated with a decline in total circulating androgens partly resulting from lessened ovarian androgen secretion after menopause, and partly due to the age-related decline in adrenal androgen and preandrogen production[3-5].

Androgens and bone mass

The anabolic effects of androgens in premenopausal women have been demonstrated in various studies. Mauras and colleagues observed that prepubertal hypogonadal girls with Turner's syndrome did not have any change in whole-body protein turnover or increased whole-body synthesis when treated with ethinylestradiol even though insulin-like growth factor I (IGF-I) concentrations increased[6]. These findings were in contrast to the effects of T therapy in prepubertal boys. In the latter study, T replacement had anabolic effects measured by parameters of protein metabolism[7]. Thus, estrogen replacement alone may not be sufficient for young adolescent females to attain their growth potential in terms of body protein and muscle mass. Furthermore, young hyperandrogenic women have been found to have higher bone mineral density (BMD) at the hip and lumbar spine than normoandrogenic, non-hirsute controls[8]. BMD in the lumbar spine and proximal femur was correlated with total T and free T but not with either A or DHEA-S[8]. In premenopausal women, BMD is positively correlated with percentage of free T[9]. After controlling for body weight Nilas and Christiansen found a significant negative correlation between sex hormone binding globulin (SHBG) and BMD but no relationship between BMD and free estradiol (E2)[9]. In premenopausal women BMD is also strongly correlated with body weight[9]. Obesity is associated with suppressed SHBG levels and increases in the percentage of free T[10]; hence the relationship between obesity and BMD may be partly due to the increased free T levels which directly enhance bone mass. However, Simberg and co-workers[8] observed a higher BMD in hyperandrogenic women after correction for body mass index.

Androgen receptors (ARs) have been demonstrated in human osteoblastic cells[11], and androgens appear to directly stimulate human bone-cell proliferation via fibroblast growth factor (FGF) and IGF-I and differentiation via transforming growth factor beta (TGF-β)[12]. Androgens increase the uptake of calcium and the formation of inositol triphosphate and diacylglycerol by osteoblasts, and thus potentially strengthen bone[13]. AR concentrations in osteoblasts appear to be up-regulated by androgens via an increase in gene expression, mediated by sequences in the 5'-flanking region of the AR gene[14].

Several clinical studies support the direct anabolic effects of androgens on bone. Savvas and associates studied the effects of combined estradiol (E) and testosterone (T) implants in postmenopausal women and found that combined E and T implants prevented bone loss more effectively than oral estrogen replacement[15]. Need and colleagues observed significant increases in vertebral BMD in postmenopausal osteoporotic women treated with nandrolone decanoate[16]. We have studied the long-term effects of estradiol and testosterone implants on BMD in a prospective 2-year trial[16]. The women were randomized to single-blind treatment with either estradiol implants 50 mg alone or estradiol 50 mg plus testosterone 50 mg administered 3-monthly for 2 years. BMD was measured by dual energy X-ray absorptiometry (DEXA) at 6-monthly intervals. BMD (DEXA) of total body, lumbar vertebrae (L1–L4) and hip area increased significantly in both treatment groups. BMD increased more rapidly in the E plus T-treated group at all sites. A substantially greater increase in BMD occurred in the E plus T group for the total body ($p < 0.008$), vertebral L1–L4 ($p < 0.001$) and trochanteric ($p < 0.005$) measurements[17]. These favorable effects on bone were achieved with preservation of the cholesterol-lowering effects of parenteral estrogen replacement. Raisz and co-workers[18] observed a similar reduction in total cholesterol with oral E plus T therapy, but this was associated with reductions in high-density lipoprotein (HDL) 2 and HDL3 and triglycerides, and no change in low-density lipoprotein (LDL)-cholesterol.

Watts and associates[19] studied surgically menopausal women who were treated with either oral esterified estrogen (1.25 mg) or esterified estrogen (1.25 mg) and methyl-testosterone (2.5 mg) daily for 2 years. Bone loss at the spine and hip was prevented by both treatment regimens; however, combined estrogen/androgen therapy was associated with an increase in spinal BMD compared with baseline[19]. The effects of estrogen alone, and estrogen plus androgen, on biochemical markers of bone formation and resorption in postmenopausal women have also been investigated[18]. Postmenopausal women were treated for 9 weeks with either a combination of 1.25 mg esterified estrogen and 2.5 mg methyltestosterone orally, or 1.25 mg conjugated equine estrogen (CEE) given alone. A similar decrease in the urinary excretion of the bone absorption markers deoxy-pyridinoline, pyridinoline and hydroxyproline occurred in both groups. However, women treated with CEE had a reduction in the serum markers of bone formation, bone-specific alkaline phosphatase, osteocalcin and C-terminal procollagen peptide, whereas the women treated with estrogen plus androgen had increases in all of these markers of bone formation.

It can be concluded from the above clinical studies that E therapy alone appears to have an antiresorptative effect on bone in postmenopausal women whereas the addition of an androgen either orally or parenterally results in an increase in BMD.

Most recently, the extent to which androgen action in bone is due to a direct AR mediated action, or by aromatization to estrogen and an estrogen receptor (ER)-mediated action, has been questioned. The enzyme aromatase is a product of the CYP 19 gene and is a microsomal member of the cytochrome P450 super family of genes. It converts T to E and A to estrone (E1). Aromatase activity and P450 aromatase mRNA have been demonstrated in human osteoblast[20]. It is believed that serum adrenal preandrogens and circulating T may be converted by aromatase in bone to estrogens which then have direct paracrine effects on bone tissue[20].

That estrogens are the main sex steroids for the maintenance of bone density has been suggested by the findings of osteopenia in a male with normal T and a defective ER[21], and an aromatase deficiency in a male with elevated circulating T[22]. In these studies the men were tall (both 204 cm) with a juvenile bone age and normal or elevated T and free T levels (Table 1). The man with the E receptor mutation had a significantly reduced BMD at the lumbar spine when compared with young adults, but had

Table 1 Summary of body composition, hormonal and bone metabolic parameters of two men with biological estrogen lack due to P450 aromatase enzyme (AROM) deficiency and mutation of estrogen receptor (ER)

	Estrogen-resistant men	
	P450 AROM deficiency	ER mutation
Age (years)	24	28
Height (cm)	204	204
Arm span (cm)	210.6	213
Upper : lower body ratio (~0.96)	0.84	0.88
Bone age (years)	14	15
Bone mineral density (g/cm²)		
lumbar spine	0.931 (–1.68SD)	0.745 (–3.1SD, adult)
(right) neck of femur	0.920 (–0.36SD)	(–2.0SD, 15 years)
distal radius	0.570 (–4.65SD)	—
Serum testosterone	↑	N
Free testosterone	N	N
5αDHT	↑	N
SHBG	N	↑
Serum estrone	↓	↑
Serum estradiol	↓	↑
ALP (adult 35–95, puberty 50–375 u/l)	241	205
Bone-specific ALP (4.3–19 ng/ml)	—	34.2
Osteocalcin (3–13 ng/ml)	19.8	18.7
Pyridinium X-links (20–61 nmol/mmolCr)	101.7	110.0

DHT, dihydrotestosterone; SHBG, sex hormone binding globulin; ALP, alkaline phosphatase; N, normal

borderline osteopenia when his bone density was compared with that of boys of the same biological age. The young man with aromatase deficiency[22] had osteoporosis of the distal radius when compared with young adults, but in fact had BMDs of the lumbar spine and hip region well within the normal range. Interestingly, both young men studied demonstrated increases in the serum markers of bone formation, namely alkaline phosphatase, bone-specific alkaline phosphatase and osteocalcin, indicative of enhanced bone-forming activity.

Thus it appears that the apparent osteopenia in these men may well be the result of their extensive lineal growth due to failure of epiphyseal closure, combined with ongoing bone resorption due to estrogen deficiency in excess of their bone forming capacity, and failure to correct for their young biological bone age.

It may be that androgens can only exert a measurable direct anabolic effect on bone in men and women when there is sufficient circulating estrogen to facilitate skeletal maturation and epiphyseal closure, and prevent bone resorption.

Androgens and the mechanical properties of bone

Many studies have examined the effects of sex steroid deprivation on skeletal BMD. However there is a paucity of data regarding the effects of hormones on the mechanical properties of bone. Feral adult female cynomologus monkeys treated for 2 years with T were found to have significant increases in energy absorption capacity and maximum sheer stress of the tibiae measured by torsion tests, and cortical bone density[23]. T treatment significantly increased torsional rigidity and bending stiffness of the tibiae. The maximum compressive stress of the treated trabecular bone samples was significantly higher than those of bone samples from the normal adult female monkeys. Trabecular bone density also increased after T treatment. In this study however the circulating T levels in the treated female monkeys were consistently in the normal to high range for male age-matched monkeys throughout the study period. Furthermore, both E and progesterone levels were suppressed to 25% of the normal values of the female controls, resulting in a hormonally induced menopause. Consistent with this the animals were reportedly annovulatory. Therefore this study reflects the effects of supraphysiological T levels in the female primate model, and extrapolation to pre- or postmenopausal women is not possible.

Adrenal androgens and bone density

Circulating DHEA and DHEA-S have been positively correlated with BMD in aging women[20,24,25], and the progressive decline in DHEA with increasing age is believed to contribute to senile osteoporosis[15]. It is not clear whether these adrenal preandrogens directly influence bone function or if the effects are mediated indirectly after conversion to E2, A or T. Older women treated with oral DHEA have restoration of circulating A, T and dihydro-testosterone (DHT) to premenopausal levels as well as increases in DHEA and DHEA-S, with no changes in circulating levels of E1 or E2 from baseline[26]. Nawata and colleagues[20] observed a positive correlation between BMD and serum DHEA-S in postmenopausal women but no correlation between BMD and serum E2. Administration of DHEA to oophorectomized (OVX) rats restored the femoral BMD level to that of sham-operated animals[20]. Interestingly in this study, the OVX rats treated with T for 12 weeks achieved a mean femoral BMD greater than that of either the sham-operated or DHEA-treated animals. The authors concluded that circulating adrenal DHEA may act via conversion to estrogen in bone. However the greater increase in BMD in OVX rats with T therapy suggests an anabolic action of T on

bone cells which is independent of local aromatization to E2.

DHEA therapy may be an alternative method of administering estrogen and androgen replacement to postmenopausal women. Women treated with oral DHEA reportedly experience enhanced well-being and increased energy[26]. Clearly further study of the effects of DHEA therapy in older women on bone metabolism, general well-being and sexuality is warranted, as well as evaluation of the potential risks of this treatment in the long term.

Conclusion

Women are more likely to develop osteoporosis than men[24,25], and it is well established that sex steroids play an important role in the development of osteoporosis with increasing age. Androgens are important hormones and have diverse actions in women as well as in men. Androgen levels start to decline in women in the decade preceding the average age of natural menopause, and this may impact significantly on long-term health. Many studies have addressed the effects of estrogen deprivation on bone mass and bone turnover, but the direct effects of androgens on bone-cell metabolism, particularly in women, has to date been little researched.

Osteoblastic cells have been demonstrated to possess both estrogen and androgen receptors as well as aromatase activity. It is therefore reasonable to conclude that both estrogens and androgens have direct effects on bone function, and that the effects of the preandrogens DHEA and A, and also some of the effects of T, are the result of the conversion locally of these hormones by aromatase to estrogens and are then mediated via the ER.

Although estrogen appears to be essential for skeletal maturation and epiphyseal closure in both sexes and has a lifelong role in preventing bone resorption, adequate androgen levels are most likely necessary for attainment of peak bone density and maximization of mechanical bone strength.

The clinical sequelae of androgen deficiency in women and the benefits of testosterone replacement are being increasingly acknowledged. Androgen replacement in postmenopausal women is potentially an effective alternative therapeutic approach to osteopenia and osteoporosis, however prospective data confirming a reduction in fracture rate with such therapy in women are lacking. Further basic scientific and clinical research into the role of androgens in bone function is required, in order to define the appropriate clinical application of androgen replacement in postmenopausal women.

References

1. Kirschner, M. A. and Bardin, C. W. (1972). Androgen production and metabolism in normal and virilized women. *Metabolism*, **21**, 667–88

2. Judd, H. L. and Yen, S. S. C. (1973). Serum androstenedione and testosterone levels during the menstrual cycle. *J. Clin. Endocrinol. Metab.*, **36**, 475–81

3. Zumoff, B., Strain, G. W., Miller, L. K. and Rosner, W. (1995). Twenty-four hour mean plasma testosterone concentration declines with age in normal premenopausal women. *J. Clin. Endocrinol. Metab.*, **80**, 1429–30

4. Zumoff, B., Rosenfeld, R. S., Strain, G. W., *et al.* (1980). Sex differences in the 24-hour mean plasma concentrations of dehydroepiandrosterone (DHA) and dehydroepiandrosterone sulfate (DHAS) and the DHA to DHAS ratio in normal adults. *J. Clin. Endocrinol. Metab.*, **51**, 330–4

5. Meldrum, D. R., Davidson, B. J., Tataryn, I. V. and Judd, H. L. (1981). Changes in circulating steroids with aging in post-menopausal women. *Obstet. Gynecol.*, **57**, 624–8

6. Mauras, N. (1995). Estrogens do not affect whole-body protein metabolism in the prepubertal female. *J. Clin. Endocrinol. Metab.*, **80**, 2842–5

7. Mauras, N., Haymond, M. W., Darmaun, D., Vieira, N. E., Abrams, S. A. and Yergey, A. L. (1994). Calcium and protein kinetics in prepubertal boys: positive effects of testosterone. *J. Clin. Invest.*, **93**, 1014–19

8. Simberg, N., Tiitenen, A. and Silfrast, A. (1995). High bone density in hyperandrogenic women: effect of gonadotropin- releasing hormone agonist alone or in conjunction with estrogen–progestin replacement. *J. Clin. Endocrinol. Metab.*, **80**, 646–51

9. Nilas, L. and Christiansen, C. (1987). Bone mass and its relationship to age and the menopause. *J. Clin. Endocrinol. Metab.*, **65**, 697–9

10. Heiss, C. J., Sanborn, C. F. and Nichols, D. L. (1995). Associations of body fat distribution circulating sex hormones and bone density in postmenopausal women. *J. Clin. Endocrinol. Metab.*, **80**, 1591–6

11. Colvard, D. S., Eriksen, E. F., Keeting, P. E., *et al.* (1989). Identification of androgen receptors in normal human osteoblast-like cells. *Proc. Natl. Acad. Sci. USA*, **86**, 854–7

12. Kasperk, C. H., Wergedal, J. E., Farley, J. R., Llinkhart, T. A., Turner, R. T. and Baylind, D. G. (1989). Androgens directly stimulate proliferation of bone cells *in vitro*. *Endocrinology*, **124**, 1576–8

13. Liebherr, M. and Grosse, B. (1994). Androgens increase intracellular calcium concentration and inositol 1,4,5-triphosphate and diacylglycerol formation via a pertussis toxin-sensitive G-protein *J. Biol. Chem.*, **269**, 7217–23

14. Wiren, K. M., Keenan, E. J. and Orwoll, E. S. (1996). Regulation of androgen receptor promotor by androgens in osteoblastic cells. *Proc. Int. Congr. Endocrinol.*, (abstr. P1–214)

15. Savvas, M., Studd, J. W. W., Fogelman, I., Dooley, M., Montgomery, J. and Murby, B. (1988). Skeletal effects of oral oestrogen compared with subcutaneous oestrogen and testosterone in postmenopausal women. *Br. Med. J.*, **297**, 331–3

16. Need, G. A., Horowitz, M. and Bridges, A. (1989). Effects of nandrolone decanoate and antiresorptive therapy on vertebral density in osteoporotic women. *Arch. Intern. Med.*, **149**, 57–60

17. Davis, S. R., McCloud, P., Strauss, B. J. G. and Burger, H. G. (1995). Testosterone enhances estradiol's effects on postmenopausal bone density and sexuality. *Maturitas*, **21**, 227–36

18. Raisz, L. G., Wiita, B., Artis, A., *et al.* (1995). Comparison of the effects of estrogen alone and estrogen plus androgen on biochemical markers of bone formation and resorption in postmenopausal women *J. Clin. Endocrinol. Metab.*, **81**, 37–43

19. Watts, N. B., Notelovitz, M. and Timmons, M. C. (1995). Comparison of oral estrogens and estrogens plus androgen on bone mineral

density, menopausal symptoms and lipid–lipoprotein profiles in surgical menopause. *Obstet. Gynecol.*, **85**, 529–37

20. Nawata, H., Tariaka, S. and Tariaka, S. (1995). Aromatase in bone cell: association with osteoporosis in post menopausal women *J. Steroid. Biochem. Mol. Biol.*, **53**, 165–74

21. Smith, E. P., Boyd, J., Frank, G. R., *et al.* (1994). Estrogen resistance caused by a mutation in the estrogen-receptor gene in a man. *N. Eng. J. Med.*, **331**, 1056–61

22. Morishima, A., Grumbach, M. M. and Simpson, E. R. (1995). Aromatase deficiency in male and female siblings caused by a novel mutation and the physiological role of estrogens. *J. Clin. Endocrinol. Metab.*, **80**, 3689–98

23. Kasra, M. and Grynpas, M. D. (1995). The effects of androgens on the mechanical properties of primate bone. *Bone*, **17**, 265–70

24. Taelman, P., Kayman, J. M., Janssens, X. and Vermeulen, A. (1989). Persistence of increased bone resorption and possible role of dehydroepiandrosterone as a bone metabolism determinant in osteoporotic women in late menopause. *Maturitas*, **11**, 65–73

25. Nordin, B. E. C., Robertson, A., Seamark, R. F., *et al.* (1985). The relation between calcium absorption, serum DHEA and vertebral mineral density in postmenopausal women. *J. Clin. Endocrinol. Metab.*, **60**, 651–7

26. Morales, A. J., Nolan, J. J., Nelson, J. C. and Yen, S. S. C. (1994). Effects of replacement dose of dehydroepiandrosterone in men and women of advancing age. *J. Clin. Endocrinol. Metab.*, **78**, 1360–7

The use of androgens in the postmenopause: evidence from clinical studies

39

B. B. Sherwin

Introduction

The efficacy of estrogen replacement therapy in reversing estrogen-dependent symptoms and in preventing osteoporosis and coronary heart disease in the postmenopause is now well established. Less well understood are the possible benefits of adding androgen to the postmenopausal estrogen replacement regimen. Although there is substantially less information available with regard to the effects of combined estrogen–androgen preparations on a variety of end-points compared to estrogen alone, research findings on combined therapy have been accumulating over the past 15 years. This small but growing body of literature allows the opportunity to estimate purported benefits and possible side-effects of combined estrogen–androgen preparations in postmenopausal women. Moreover, this literature also addresses the actual functional role of androgens in women which provides the rationale for combined therapy under specific conditions.

Female androgen production

In women, both the adrenal gland and the ovary contain the biosynthetic pathways necessary for androgen synthesis and secretion. It has been estimated that in premenopausal women, 49% of testosterone, the most potent androgen, is of adrenal origin, 17% arises from peripheral conversion of other steroid precursors and 33% is produced by the ovary[1]. The ovary also produces approximately 60% of androstenedione and 20% of dehydroepiandrosterone (DHEA). After the menopause, the ovarian production of androstenedione decreases profoundly, and secretion of testosterone declines as well, due to atrophy of ovarian stromal tissue[2]. The fall in the secretion of androstenedione, a major source of testosterone, results in a further decline in circulating testosterone in most postmenopausal women.

Neurobiological effects of androgens

Autoradiographic studies have demonstrated that neurons containing specific receptors for testosterone are predominantly found in the preoptic area of the hypothalamus, with smaller concentrations in the limbic system (amygdala and hippocampus) and in the cerebral cortex[3].

In male rats, there is evidence that serotonin-receptor subtypes mediate androgen effects on sexual behavior. The type of androgen treatment which induces male sexual behavior increases 5HT1A receptor binding in the preoptic area and decreases 5HT3 receptors in the amygdala[4]. No such studies have been undertaken in female rats whose sexual behavior is largely under the control of estrogen and progesterone acting on the ventromedial nucleus. On the other hand, effects of testosterone on various components of mating behavior have been studied intensively in female non-human primates. On the whole, these studies show that the administration of testosterone to ovariectomized rhesus monkeys increased proceptive behavior (i.e. increased attempts to solicit mounts from the male). Implantation of minute amounts of testosterone into the anterior hypothalamus of estrogen-treated ovariectomized and adrenalectomized unreceptive female rhesus monkeys also resulted in restoration of their proceptivity without affecting other aspects of sexual behavior such as attractivity[5].

These studies on testosterone and sexual behavior in female non-human primates serve to underline two points. One is that there is a specificity of action of testosterone on components of sexual behavior such that it enhances proceptivity (the animal's motivation to engage in sexual behavior) but has no effect on its attractivity or receptivity to males. Second, the efficacy of the very small dose of testosterone implanted into the hypothalamus in restoring sexual desire in rhesus monkeys in the Everitt and Herbert study[5], suggests that testosterone exerts its effect on sexual desire in female rhesus monkeys via a direct effect on the brain, and not by an influence on peripheral tissues.

Androgens and sexuality in postmenopausal women

Survey data on the frequency of sexual dysfunctions in the postmenopause generally show that from one-third to two-thirds of women experience a decrease in sexual interest around the time of menopause, while fewer complain of decreases in frequencies of coitus and/or orgasm around this time (for review, see Sherwin[6]). However, none of these epidemiological studies empirically assessed the relationship between circulating levels of the sex hormones and the reported changes in sexual behavior.

The paradigm that is perhaps most powerful for the study of specificity of the sex steroids on female sexuality, involves administering hormone replacement therapy to women who have just undergone total abdominal hysterectomy (TAH) and bilateral salpingo-oophorectomy (BSO). When both ovaries are removed from premenopausal women, circulating testosterone levels decrease significantly within the first 24–48 h

postoperatively[2]. The fact that these women are deprived of ovarian androgen production following this surgical procedure has provided a rationale for administering both estrogen and androgen as replacement therapy.

In Britain and Australia, subcutaneous implantation of pellets containing estradiol and testosterone has been used as a treatment for menopausal symptoms for several decades. This route of sex steroid administration results in a slow constant release of the sex hormones over a period of at least 6 months. Women complaining of decreased libido despite treatment with estrogen received subcutaneous implants of 40 mg estradiol and 100 mg testosterone[7]. Patients reported a significant increase in libido by the third postimplantation month. These findings gained support from a double-blind study of women complaining of loss of libido despite treatment with oral estrogens[8]. They randomly received a subcutaneous implant containing either estrogen alone or estrogen plus testosterone. After 6 weeks, the loss of libido in the estrogen-alone implant group remained, whereas the combined estrogen–testosterone group showed significant symptomatic relief.

During the past decade, several prospective, controlled studies of general and sexual effects of combined estrogen–androgen parenteral preparations in surgically menopausal women were carried out in our laboratory. These studies have shown that the addition of testosterone to an estrogen-replacement regimen induces a greater sense of energy level and well-being, and is associated with fewer somatic and psychological symptoms compared to the administration of estrogen alone[9–11]. Furthermore, the intramuscular administration of testosterone, either alone or in combination with estradiol, increased motivational aspects of sexual behavior (such as desire and fantasies) compared with the administration of estrogen alone or a placebo[12]. Levels of sexual desire and interest covaried with plasma testosterone level throughout a treatment month as the intramuscular drug was being metabolized[9]. The androgenic enhancement of sexual motivation in women treated with the combined intramuscular drug has been shown to persist with long-term chronic administration of monthly injections that cause an initial surge in testosterone levels and metabolize slowly over a period of several weeks[11].

In a recent prospective study, we tested the effects of a combined oral estrogen–androgen drug compared with estrogen alone. Premenopausal women underwent TAH and BSO and received either esterified estrogens 0.625 mg/day orally, or a combined tablet containing esterified estrogens 0.625 mg and methyltestosterone 1.25 mg/day for 4 months[13]. Women who received the estrogen–androgen combined drug reported a significant increase in the number of times they left the house for work or social reasons (taken to be an index of physical activity) compared to those given estrogen alone. Also, patients in the combined group experienced increased sexual arousal after the sixth postoperative treatment, whereas the estrogen only-treated women's sexual arousal was unchanged.

Taken together, the findings from the subcutaneous implant pellet studies and the prospective studies on oophorectomized women provide compelling evidence that testosterone acts to increase the overall energy level, and also to enhance sexual desire and arousal in women, although frequency of sexual activity and of orgasm are unaffected. These findings allow the conclusion that in women, just as in men[14], testosterone has its major impact on the cognitive motivational, or libidinal aspects of sexual behavior such as desire and fantasies, and not on physiological responses. Moreover, studies of non-human primates suggest the likelihood that testosterone exerts this effect on sexual desire via mechanisms that impact directly on the brain, rather than by any effect on peripheral tissues[5].

Possible adverse effects

Hirsutism

Empirical data from controlled studies on the incidence of hirsutism in postmenopausal women treated with combined estrogen–androgen preparations could not be located. However, our own extensive clinical experience suggests that approximately 20% of women who receive 150 mg testosterone enanthate intramuscularly every 4 weeks along with estrogen, will develop mild hirsutism manifested by an increased growth of hair on the chin and/or upper lip. When the dose is reduced to 75 mg testosterone enanthate per month, less that 5% of women have any increased hair growth. Moreover, hair growth decreases or usually stops entirely when the patient is switched to treatment with estrogen alone. There is little doubt that, in women, hirsutism is a dose-dependent side-effect of exogenous testosterone. Its development would depend also on the amount of estrogen given in combination, since both sex steroids influence the production of sex hormone binding globulin (SHBG) which, in turn, determines the concentration of free, or biologically available testosterone.

Lipoprotein lipids

It has been well established that orally administered estrogens provide protection against coronary heart disease in postmenopausal women. A portion of this cardioprotective effect is due to the estrogenic increase of high-density lipoprotein cholesterol (HDL) and its ability to decrease low-density lipoprotein cholesterol (LDL). On the other hand, male athletes who self-administer large doses of anabolic–androgenic steroids experience a significant decrease in HDL and an increase in LDL[15].

Several studies have reported on the effects of combined estrogen–androgen preparations on lipid fractions in postmenopausal women. Teran and Gambrell[16] treated women with subcutaneous implants of pellets containing 25 mg estradiol and 150 mg testosterone. After 12 months of treatment, there were no changes in total cholesterol, HDL, LDL or in VLDL compared with preimplantation values. In oophorectomized women who had been receiving a combined intramuscular estrogen–androgen preparation chronically for 4 years, total cholesterol, LDL and HDL values were not different from those in oophorectomized women treated with intramuscular estrogen alone, or from those in women who had remained untreated since their bilateral oophorectomy 4 years earlier[17]. These findings are not surprising in view of the fact that parenteral routes of administration of the sex hormones bypass the so-called 'first-pass hepatic effect'. Since sex steroid influences on lipoprotein fractions occur in the liver, they are largely attenuated by parenteral routes of hormone administration.

Recently, effects of an oral combined regimen on lipoprotein lipids were tested in postmenopausal women[18]. Subjects randomly received either esterified estrogen 0.625 mg alone or esterified estrogen 0.625 mg and methyltestosterone 1.25 mg daily. Following 6 months of continuous treatment, there was a significant decrease in total cholesterol, HDL, HDL_2, HDL_3 and apolipoproteins A1 compared to baseline, in the group that received esterified estrogens plus methyltestosterone. Low-density lipoprotein cholesterol decreased in both treatment groups. There were no adverse effects of low-dose androgen on other parameters of hepatic function such as total bilirubin, or γ-glutamyl transferase with combined therapy.

Conclusions

There is still a paucity of well-controlled studies on psychological and biological effects of combined estrogen–androgen replacement in postmenopausal women. However, the consistencies among available studies allow several conclusions. First, testosterone administered along with estrogen to surgically menopausal women increases energy level and general well-being, over and above estrogen alone. Second, testosterone has its major impact on libido or sexual desire and interest in women, just as it does in men. Finally, adverse effects of exogenous testosterone on hair growth and on lipoprotein lipids are not only dose dependent in women but are related also to route of administration. There is evidence to show that

such adverse effects are attenuated, or possibly even precluded, by parenteral routes of administration.

Female life expectancy has been increasing profoundly and rapidly over the past century, and there is every reason to believe it will continue to climb. Therefore medical professionals, society, and of course women themselves, have grown increasingly concerned about protecting quality of life into old age. In addition to its purported beneficial effects on aspects of bone metabolism (see Chapter 2 in this volume by S. Davis), testosterone plays a functional role in the maintenance of sexual desire, energy level and well-being in women. All of these androgenic effects are related to current and future quality of life. It is also important to remember, however, that so far, research findings point to a specificity of testosterone effects. That is, exogenous testosterone enhances sexual desire and energy level in postmenopausal women over and above estrogen alone, but there is no evidence that it ameliorates other symptoms commonly associated with the menopause such as hot flushes, atropic vaginitis or irritability, to name a few.

Finally, it should also be acknowledged that human sexuality is multidetermined and that personal, psychological, relationship, and other hormonal and non-hormonal biological factors may all influence sexual functioning. For example, hypoestrogenism may lead to atropic vaginitis and dyspareunia which, in turn, can contribute to loss of sexual desire. Adverse life circumstances and stresses also undoubtedly influence sexual behavior. Therefore, prior to the treatment of postmenopausal women experiencing loss of sexual desire, it is important to assess the possible contribution of these other factors in the etiology of the symptom so that the various causes can be considered and treated appropriately.

Acknowledgement

The preparation of this manuscript was supported by a grant from The Medical Research Council of Canada (No. MA-11623) awarded to B. B. Sherwin.

References

1. Longcope, C. (1986). Adrenal and gonadal androgen secretion in normal females. *Clin. Endocrinol. Metab.*, **15**, 213–28
2. Longcope, C., Franz, C., Morello, C., Baker, R. and Johnson, C. Jr (1986). Steroid and gonadotropin levels in women during their perimenopausal years. *Maturitas*, **8**, 189–96
3. McEwen, B.S. (1980). The brain as a target organ of endocrine hormones. In Kreiger, D. T. and Hughes, J. S. (eds.) *Neuroendocrinology*, pp. 33–42. (Sunderland, MA: Sinauer Association)
4. Mendelson, S. and McEwen, B. S. (1990). Testosterone increases the concentration of (H^3 8-hydroxy-2-propylamine) tethelin binding at 5-HT$_3$A receptors in the medial preoptic nucleus of the castrated male rat. *Eur. J. Pharmacol.*, **181**, 329–31
5. Everitt, B. J. and Herbert, J. (1975). The effects of implanting testosterone propionate in the central nervous system on the sexual behavior of the female rhesus monkey. *Brain Res.*, **86**, 109–20
6. Sherwin, B. B. (1991). The psychoendocrinology of aging and female sexuality. *Ann. Rev. Sex. Res.*, **2**, 181–98
7. Burger, H. G., Hailes, J., Menelaus, M., Nelson, J., Hudson, B. and Balazs, N. (1984). The management of persistent menopausal symptoms with oestradiol testosterone implants: clinical, lipid and hormonal results. *Maturitas*, **6**, 351–8
8. Burger, H. G., Hailes, J., Nelson, J. and Menelaus, M. (1987). Effects of combined implants of estradiol and testosterone on libido in postmenopausal women. *Lancet*, **294**, 936–7
9. Sherwin, B. B. and Gelfand, M. M. (1984). Effects of parenteral administration of estrogen and androgen on plasma hormone levels and hot flushes in surgical menopause. *Am. J. Obstet. Gynecol.*, **148**, 552–7
10. Sherwin, B. B. and Gelfand, M. M. (1985). Differential symptom response to parenteral estrogen and/or androgen administration in the surgical menopause. *Am. J. Obstet. Gynecol.*, **151**, 153–60
11. Sherwin, B. B. and Gelfand, M. M. (1987). The role of androgen in the maintenance of sexual functioning in oophorectomized women. *Psychosom. Med.*, **49**, 397–409
12. Sherwin, B. B., Gelfand, M. M. and Brender, W. (1985). Androgen enhances sexual motivation in females: a prospective cross-over study of sex steroid administration in the surgical menopause. *Psychosom. Med.*, **7**, 339–51
13. Sherwin, B. B., Youngs, D., Daly, R. and Jergens, R. (1993). Effects of a combined estrogen–androgen preparation on sexual behavior and lipid metabolism in surgically menopausal women. Proceedings of the *4th Annual Meeting of the North American Menopausal Society*, Washington, DC, September abstr. 5–10
14. Bancroft, J. and Wu, F. C. W. (1983). Changes in erectile responsiveness during androgen replacement therapy. *Arch. Sex. Behav.*, **12**, 59–66
15. Webb, O. L., Laskarzewski, P. M. and Glueck, C. J. (1984). Severe depression of high-density lipoprotein cholesterol levels in weight lifters and body builders by self-administered exogenous testosterone and anabolic–androgenic steroids. *Metabolism*, **33**, 971
16. Teran, A. Z. and Gambrell, R. D. Jr (1988). Androgens in clinical practice. In Speroff, L. (ed.) *Androgens in the Menopause*, pp. 14–22. (New York: McGraw-Hill)
17. Sherwin, B. B. and Gelfand, M. M. (1987). Postmenopausal estrogen and androgen replacement and lipoprotein lipid concentrations. *Am. J. Obstet. Gynecol.*, **156**, 414–19
18. Hickok, L. R., Toomey, R. N. and Speroff, L. (1993). A comparison of esterified estrogens with and without methyltestosterone: effects on endometrial histology and serum lipoproteins in post-menopausal women. *Obstet. Gynecol.*, **82**, 919–24

8

Phytoestrogens and their influence on menopause

40

The effect of soy on menopausal symptoms

G. Wilcox

Introduction

Estrogenic activity in plants has been documented in the scientific literature for over 70 years[1,2], including more than half of the species of plants used as food by human populations over the millennia[3]. In some situations, certain plants have traditional uses probably as a result of their estrogenic properties. For example *Pueraria Mirifica*, a woody vine native to Thailand, has been used as a rejuvenant and an aphrodisiac over the centuries; its active principle, miroestrol, has a potency three times that of diethylstilbestrol[4]. Ginseng is used by Chinese herbalists to treat hot flushes[5] and has been associated with mastalgia[6] and changes in vaginal cytology in postmenopausal women; a crude methanolic extract has been shown to compete with estradiol for binding to human myometrial cytosol receptors[7].

Now that the majority of our population is reaching old age, health and well-being after menopause have assumed greater importance. The significance of these dietary estrogen-like compounds in menopausal and postmenopausal women therefore warrants investigation.

This paper will discuss the effect of soy on menopausal symptoms and, where data exist, the effects of other phytoestrogen-containing foods on menopausal symptoms. There are three main lines of evidence linking dietary phytoestrogens with menopausal symptoms: epidemiological data, animal studies and studies of humans including the limited number of published clinical trials in postmenopausal women.

Epidemiology of menopausal symptoms in relation to diet

While the menopause is a universal phenomenon, the characteristic symptoms associated with it are reported to vary considerably between different populations[8]. Figure 1 combines data from three major studies: one looking at seven South-East Asian countries[9], one looking at the incidence of menopausal hot flushes in Japan[10] and another looking at the incidence of hot flushes in the Netherlands[11]. While hot flushes affect between 70 and 85% of menopausal women in Western countries, in Japan fewer than 5–10% of women are affected. In fact in Japanese there is no word for 'hot flush'[10]. The incidence in other South-East Asian countries is also lower than in Western women.

These differences in hot-flush symptoms are not explained by the levels of endogenous estrogens in Oriental women. Goldin and colleagues, looking at recent immigrants to Hawaii, reported that the Oriental women had lower levels of estrone and estradiol both premenopausally (0.24 nmol/l, 0.14 nmol/l vs. 0.32 nmol/l ($p < 0.02$), 0.25 nmol/l ($p < 0.001$)) and postmenopausally (0.13 nmol/l, 0.03 nmol/l vs. 0.14 nmol/l (NS), 0.10 nmol/l ($p < 0.001$)) than age-matched Caucasian women, respectively[12]. Key and co-workers looked at plasma estradiol levels in women premenopausally, perimeno-pausally and postmenopausally in rural China and in Britain. The Chinese women had lower levels of estradiol at all age groups compared with the British women, but the relative drop in estradiol levels was similar in both populations[13].

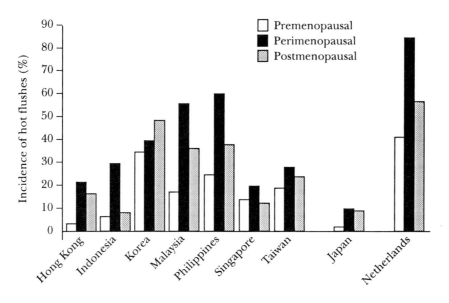

Figure 1   Reported prevalence of vasomotor symptoms across menopausal transition in different populations. Adapted from references 9, 10 and 11

Dietary factors are thought to account for many of these differences, via short-term effects of macronutrients such as dietary fat[14,15], protein[16] and dietary fiber[17] on sex-steroid hormone metabolism and intestinal flora[18], their long-term effects on body composition[19] and possibly, the modulating effects of non-nutrient phytochemicals on sex-steroid metabolism[17].

Legumes are a particularly important and rich source of the isoflavonoid phytoestrogens. If one looks at legume consumption world-wide, there appears to be an inverse association between the incidence of hot flushes and the intake of legumes. The intake reported in Western countries is very low (5–15 g/person per day) and as a consequence, there are very low levels of isoflavonoids in the diet. The Japanese have the highest legume consumption in the group of countries considered here (50–90 g /person per day), largely due to soy, which is a dietary staple. The intake of legumes in other countries such as those of the Mediterranean, is also considerably higher (30–60 g/person per day) than in Western populations[20].

The urinary phytoestrogen levels in Japanese women were compared with those of Finnish and North American women by Adlercreutz and Hamalainen in Helsinki, and Gorbach and Goldin in Boston, who demonstrated that the levels in the urine of equol, daidzein and genistein (all mainly derived from soy) were vastly higher than in the Western women. The excretion in the urine was of the order of 1000-fold that in the Western women, and it is interesting to note that this level was also about 1000-fold that of the endogenous estrogens[21].

Effects of phytoestrogens in various animal species

In Australia and elsewhere until recently, isoflavonoid phytoestrogens were best known for their adverse effects on animal reproduction. Fifty years ago in Western Australia there were massive outbreaks of infertility in sheep grazing on clover which comprised 90% of their fodder. The clinical and pathological features of this disorder were consistent with excessive exposure to estrogen-like compounds[22]. Equol, an isoflavone metabolite formed in the sheep rumen, was ultimately found to be responsible[23].

Concerning the effects of soy, this substance was first reported as being estrogenically active by Walz in 1931[24]. Many early studies looked at the maturation of immature or ovariectomized female rats and mice, using the end-points of increased uterine weight and cornification of the vaginal epithelium[1,2,25,26]. In 1987 Setchell and colleagues reported that the high incidence of liver disease and infertility seriously affecting captive cheetahs in North American zoos may have been due to the high soy diet these naturally carnivorous animals were being given[27].

Experimental evidence in humans

The discovery of equol in human urine in the early 1980s aroused much interest[28]. Subsequently, a study published by Setchell and associates in 1984 demonstrated a dramatic rise in urinary equol excretion in human subjects, following supplementation of the diet with 40 g of textured vegetable (soy) protein daily. Although equol has no more than one-thousandth the potency of estradiol, the levels seen following soy supplementation were of the order of 1000 times those of the endogenous estrogens, and at this point, a biological effect in humans was thought plausible[29].

When extrapolating from animal data to humans there are many limitations as species differ in their diets, their digestive systems and their reproductive systems, and phytoestrogens interact with all three. Furthermore there are differences in relative binding affinity to estrogen receptors with different compounds, in different tissues and in different species. For example, the isoflavonoid coumestrol has a relative binding affinity of 9.8 (where estradiol = 100) in human MCF7 breast-cancer cell lines. Conversely, in the rabbit uterine cytosol model it has a relative binding of 1.4[30]. There are additional limitations in extrapolating from *in vitro* to *in vivo* data. For these and other reasons, it is essential to study humans.

The first published clinical trial in humans of foods reported to be estrogenic in other animal species, was published by Vague and colleagues in 1957[31]. Vague was very much ahead of his time, and in fact is best known for his early work on abdominal obesity and vascular risk. After screening several oils for estrogenic activity in experimental animals, corn oil and olive oil were selected. Corn oil was administered to only three women, limiting statistical analysis. However, 11 postmenopausal women were given 100 g of olive oil daily for 10 days. The percentage of superficial cells prior to the oil administration was of the order of 5%. During the olive-oil supplementation period this percentage increased to between 35 and 40% on average, with considerable variation within the group. Following the completion of the olive-oil supplementation the levels returned to baseline. Vague and co-workers noted that such a large dose of oil so early in the morning 'est un peu désagréable' – is somewhat unpleasant – and they thought they would lose the co-operation of their patients if they continued this for much longer! However, it was suggested that had they been able to persist with a higher dose for a longer period of time a total suppression of menopausal symptoms may have been possible. They further commented that in their experience, women in the South of France where large quantities of unrefined olive oil were consumed appeared to suffer less during the menopause[31]. It is interesting to note that this quantity of olive oil is very similar to that reported to be consumed by traditionally living communities in the Mediterranean such as the Greek Islands[32], and it could be suggested, if this estrogenic activity is confirmed, that it may at least partially account for olive oil's favorable effect on vascuiar disease and, possibly, menopausal symptoms in these populations.

Regarding soy and menopausal symptoms, to date three studies have been published in peer-reviewed journals, at least five more have been presented in abstract form in the past 12 months and many more studies are currently in progress. Studies have varied in the number of subjects, the selection of subjects, the duration of soy administration (which ranged from 2 to 12 weeks) and also the study design. Different soy products have been used: in some situations full-fat soy flour[33–35] has been used, in others, textured vegetable protein[35,36], soy-protein isolate[37,38] or soy grits[39], whereas still other studies have used the more traditional soy products[40]. Approaches to the background diets have also differed. In the first two published studies the background diet was replicated following a 2-week lead-in period where subjects had to record their daily intake. This became their menu for the remainder of the study to which were added additional foods[33,34]. A different method was used by Baird and co-workers, where one-third of the diet was substituted with soy products[35]. Reported isoflavone doses in these studies have varied between 40 and 165 mg daily (Table 1).

Nine years ago we undertook a study to see whether foods known to be rich in phyto-estrogens could have estrogenic effects in postmenopausal women[33]. Twenty-five post-menopausal women were fed 25 g of soy, 25 g

of linseed and 10 g of seeds which were then sprouted (10 g dry seed sprouted (per person per day) → 45–75 g of fresh sprouts), each for 2 weeks at a time over a total period of 6 weeks. Vaginal cytology was assessed by three experienced cytologists blinded to treatment groups. During the food supplementation period, there was a progressive increase in the maturation index of the group of women, and this was significant at the conclusion of the food-supplementation period ($p < 0.01$). This effect persisted for 2 weeks after cessation of the last food ($p < 0.02$); however, in this study the women acted as their own controls, and their maturation indices were not significantly different from baseline values 8 weeks after the last food supplement (Figure 2). Analysis of the effects of individual foods was limited because of the study design[33] with the potential for carry-over effects.

In collaboration with Morton and Griffiths from Tenovus Cancer Research Centre in Cardiff, plasma levels of phytoestrogens in the same aforementioned women during food supplementation were measured. With soy and

Table 1 Summary of methods used in studies reporting effects of soy on menopausal symptoms

Study	n	Duration (weeks)	Design	Test food(s) ± placebo	Diet	Isoflavone dose (mg/day)
Wilcox et al. (1990)[33]	25	3 × 2	modified Latin square	full-fat soy flour, 45 g	usual diet supplemented	80–138
Murkies et al. (1995)[34]	58	12	randomized double blind	full-fat soy vs. white flour, 45 g	usual diet supplemented	80–138
Baird et al. (1995)[35]	97	4	randomized control diet	soy splits, TVP, full-fat soy flour	usual diet ¹/₃ substituted	165
Cassidy (1996)[36]	6	4	open	TVP, 60 g	usual diet supplemented	160
Burke (1996)[37]	51	6	double blind crossover	soy protein vs. CHO drink	usual diet supplemented	—
Brzezinski et al. (1996)[40]	165	12	randomized control diet	tofu, soymilk, miso + linseed	—	40–60 + lignans
Dalais et al. (1996)[39]	21	12	double blind crossover	45 g soy grits vs. wholewheat	usual diet supplemented	80–138
Harding et al. (1996)[38]	20	8	double blind crossover	soy protein vs. casein drink	usual diet supplemented	80

TVP, textured vegetable protein; CHO, carbohydrate

271

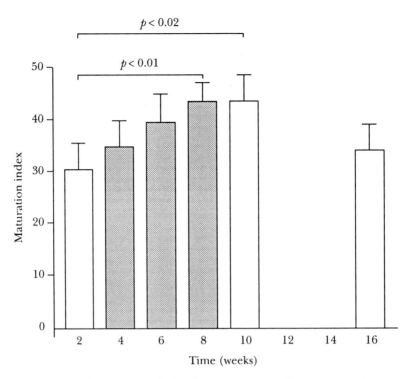

Figure 2 Changes in vaginal maturation index in postmenopausal women supplemented sequentially with soy flour, linseed and red clover sprouts over total period of 6 weeks (shaded bars). Adapted from reference 33

red clover, there was an increase in the levels of isoflavones, daidzein and equol in the plasma, and during linseed supplementation, an increase in the levels of the lignans, entero-lactone and enterodiol. The levels of these compounds in the plasma were of the order of 5000–10 000 times those of endogenous estradiol in this population[41], and about 1000 times the reference range for estrone.

Intrigued by these preliminary findings Murkies and colleagues carried out a further study to investigate whether or not soy-flour supplementation could reduce hot flushes in symptomatic postmenopausal women[34]. Fifty-eight postmenopausal women were randomized to receive either 45 g of full-fat soy flour or 45 g of unbleached refined wheat flour daily. Refined unbleached wheat flour was chosen as a placebo because of its fairly similar appearance and texture compared with soy, and anticipated low levels of phytoestrogen precursors due to the milling process. When we looked at the women treated with soy there was a 27% reduction in hot flushes at 6 weeks ($p < 0.001$) and 42% at 12 weeks ($p < 0.001$). A similar pattern was seen for the menopausal symptom score ($p < 0.05$). However, the vaginal maturation index did not change. A dramatic rise in urinary daidzein excretion ($p < 0.001$) confirmed compliance with the soy-flour supplement; in fact levels of daidzein, equol and enterolactone were all increased significantly. When we looked at the effect of wheat on menopausal symptoms, the wheat-flour group also showed improvements; however, they had not changed significantly at the 6-week time-point. By 12 weeks there had been about a 25% reduction in hot flushes ($p < 0.001$), and again a similar pattern with menopausal symptoms by 12 weeks ($p < 0.05$). Again there was no change in vaginal cytology. Interestingly there was about a 10% fall in follicle stimulating hormone (FSH) which was statistically significant ($p < 0.05$), but the levels of daidzein, equol and enterolactone did not change, confirming that the wheat flour was not a source of these compounds[34]. Explanations for this could merely reflect a placebo effect, or the spontaneous improvement in hot flushes that is known to occur with time. However, the possibility that there may have been un-measured estrogenically active compounds in the wheat flour has not been ruled out.

In a recent study published by Baird and co-workers, soy was fed for 4 weeks in a higher dosage. Despite a trend towards an increase in the percentage of superficial cells in the soy-treated group, this failed to reach significance ($p = 0.06$)[35].

Differences in subject selection (e.g. inclusion vs. exclusion of cigarette smokers, symptomatic vs. asymptomatic postmenopausal women), duration of soy administration or chance variability in responsiveness of vaginal epithelium to estrogens or phytoestrogens within the groups of women may have con-tributed to these differing results. A wide spectrum of variation in vaginal cytological response to various phytoestrogen-containing food supplements was seen in the initial study (Wilcox and colleagues, unpublished obser-vations).

There are currently very limited data on the effects of other phytoestrogen-containing foods on menopausal symptoms. Bourbon extract (de-ethanolized), a source of the estrogenic plant sterol β-sitosterol and the isoflavone biochanin A, was administered to four postmenopausal women in a dosage equivalent of 1–2 'shots' daily for 28 days. Luteinizing hormone (LH) and FSH levels fell by about 25% compared with controls ($p < 0.05$), prolactin rose by 30% ($p < 0.05$), but menopausal symptoms such as hot flushes and vaginal dryness were not assessed in this small group of women[42]. Dalais and associates have looked at linseed and whole wheat and found decreases in hot flushes with both ($p = 0.02$, $p = 0.003$ respectively)[43]. Brzezinski and co-workers reported significant improvements in vaginal dryness ($p < 0.005$), hot flushes ($p < 0.001$) and menopausal symptom score ($p < 0.0001$) and rise in sex hormone-binding globulin (SHBG) ($p < 0.005$) in 165 symptomatic postmenopausal women given a high phytoestrogen diet which included linseed as well as soy products (soy milk and miso). Notably, the control group also showed significant improvements in hot flushes ($p < 0.005$) and menopausal symptom score ($p < 0.005$), but not vaginal dryness or SHBG[40].

Conclusions

To summarize the effect of soy on menopausal symptoms it can be seen that additional work in this area is giving further evidence of weak estrogenic effects in postmenopausal women.

Three out of five studies report a significant improvement in vaginal cytology. Four out of five studies report reductions in hot flushes and three out of five report small changes in serum gonadotropin levels. Only one study reports a rise in sex hormone-binding globulin, and notably this study included linseed in the protocol. Lipid levels showed either no change or improvement, and data on bone metabolism and osteoporosis are very scant, though the findings by Dalais and colleagues[39] of an increase in bone mineral content in the soy-treated group are worthy of further research (Table 2).

Clearly the role of these compounds in the treatment of menopausal symptoms is still being established, with the need for longer-term studies, a wider range of doses, a greater variety of end-points, investigation of other food sources and of course an assessment of safety. It may be that these foods and/or their active compounds are of some use to women with mild to moderate symptoms, for those in whom hormone replacement therapy is contra-indicated or unacceptable, and of course the potential therapeutic combination of these compounds with steroidal estrogens is under active investigation.

As far as the long-term complications of the menopause are concerned, there is epi-demiological evidence and experimental data from the elegant studies reported by Hughes and co-workers that are clearly in favor of soy

Table 2 Summary of findings in studies reporting effects of soy on menopausal symptoms. FSH, follicle-stimulating hormone; LH, luteinizing hormone; SHBG, sex hormone-binding globulin

Study	Vaginal cytology	Hot flushes	FSH and LH	SHBG	Lipids	Bone
Wilcox et al. (1990)[33]	+ $p < 0.05$		FSH 5% ↓ $p < 0.05$	NS	NS	
Murkies et al. (1995)[34]	−	40% ↓ $p < 0.001$	NS	NS	NS	Ur OHProline NS
Baird et al. (1995)[35]	+ NS, $p = 0.06$		NS	NS		
Cassidy (1996)[36]			LH ↓ $p < 0.01$		NS	
Burke (1996)[37]		↓			improved	
Brzezinski et al. (1996)[40]	+ $p < 0.005$	↓ $p < 0.004$		↑ $p < 0.005$		
Dalais et al. (1996)[39]	+ $p = 0.03$	NS				BMC 5% ↑ $p = 0.03$
Harding et al. (1996)[38]		↓ $p < 0.03$	LH 20% ↓ $p < 0.006$		TChol 8% ↓ $p < 0.02$	

NS, not significant; TChol, total cholesterol; Ur OHProline, urinary hydroxyproline; BMC, bone mineral content

phytoestrogens having a beneficial role in protection from cardiovascular disease[44]. Effects on osteoporosis need much more investigation.

Studies to date have been limited by design problems inherent in this area, such as the spontaneous improvement in untreated controls and the confounding effects in all nutritional studies of adding or substituting dietary components. The current availability of purified compounds and isoflavone-free soy products is rapidly facilitating work in this area.

Acknowledgements

The author would like to thank Ms Judy Preston for invaluable assistance with the typing, and Dr Boyd J. G. Strauss for the proofreading of this manuscript.

References

1. Dohrn, M., Faure, W., Poll, H. and Blotevogel, W. (1926). Tokokinine, Stoffe mit Sexual-hormonartiger Wirkung aus Pflanzenellen. *Med. Klin.*, **22**, 1417–19
2. Loewe, S., Lange, F. and Spohr, E. (1927). Uber weibliche Sexualhormone (Thelytropine). *Biochem. Zeitschr.*, **180**, 1–26
3. Farnsworth, N. R., Bingel, A. S., Cordell, G. A., Crane, F. A. and Fong, H. H. S. (1975). Potential value of plants as sources of new antifertility agents II. *J. Pharm. Sci.*, **64**(5), 717–54
4. Bickoff, E. M. (1963). Estrogen-like substances in plants. In Hisaw, F. L. (ed.) *Physiology of Reproduction*. (Corvallis: Oregon State University Press)

5. Ginsburg, E. S. (1994). Hot flushes – physiology, hormonal therapy and alternative therapies. *Obstet. Gynecol. Clin. N. Am.*, **21**(2), 381–90

6. Palmer, B. V., Montgomery, A. C V. and Monteiro, J. C. M. P. (1978). Ginseng and mastalgia (letter). *Br. Med. J.*, **1**, 1284

7. Punnonen, R. and Lukola, A. (1981). Oestrogen-like effect of ginseng. *Br. Med. J.*, **281**, 1110

8. Lock, M. (1991). Contested meanings of the menopause. *Lancet*, **337**, 1270–2

9. Boulet, M. J., Oddens, B. J., Lehert, P., Vemer, H. M. and Visser, A. (1994). Climacteric and menopause in seven south east Asian countries. *Maturitas*, **19**, 157–76

10. Lock, M., Kaufert, P. and Gilbert, P. (1988). Cultural construction of the menopausal syndrome: the Japanese case. *Maturitas*, **10**, 317–32

11. Oldenhave, A. and Netelenbos, C. (1994). Pathogenesis of climacteric complaints: ready for the change? *Lancet*, **343**, 649–53

12. Goldin, B. R., Adlercreutz, H., Gorbach, S., Woods, M. N., Dwyer, J. T., Conlon, T., Bohn, E. and Gershoff, S. N. (1986). The relationships between estrogen levels and diets of Caucasian American and Oriental immigrant women. *Am. J. Clin. Nutr.*, **44**, 945–53

13. Key, T. J. A., Chen, J., Wang, D. Y., Pike, M. C. and Boreham, J. (1990). Sex hormones in rural China and in Britain. *Br. J. Cancer*, **62**, 631–6

14. Longcope, C., Gorbach, S., Goldin, B., Woods, M., Dwyer, J., Morrill, A. and Warram, J. (1987). The effect of a low fat diet on estrogen metabolism. *J. Clin. Endocrinol. Metab.*, **64**, 1246–50

15. Reed, M. J., Cheng, R. W., Simmonds, M., Richmond, W. and James, V. H. T. (1987). Dietary lipids: an additional regulator of plasma levels of sex hormone binding globulin. *J. Clin. Endocrinol. Metab.*, **64**, 1083–5

16. Anderson, K. E., Kappas, A., Conney, A. H., Bradlow, H. L. and Fishman, J. (1984). The influence of dietary protein and carbohydrate on the principal oxidative biotransformations of estradiol in normal subjects. *J. Clin. Endocrinol. Metab.*, **59**, 103–7

17. Adlercreutz, H. (1990). Western diet and Western diseases: some hormonal and biochemical mechanisms and associations. *Scand. J. Clin. Lab. Invest.*, **50** (Suppl. 201), 3–23

18. Reddy, B. S., Weisburger, J. H. and Wynder, E. L. (1974). Fecal b-glucuronidase: control by diet. *Science*, **183**, 416–17

19. Bruning, P. F. (1987). Endogenous estrogens and breast cancer – a possible relationship between body fat distribution and estrogen bioavailability. *J. Steroid Biochem.*, **27**, 487–92

20. Kelly, G. (1993). Patent Application Number PCT/AU93/000230

21. Adlercreutz, H., Hamalainen, E., Gorbach, S., and Goldin, B. (1992). Dietary phyto-oestrogens and the menopause in Japan (letter). *Lancet*, **339**, 1233

22. Bennets, H. W., Underwood, E. J. and Shier, F. L. (1946). A specific breeding problem of sheep on subterranean clover pastures in Western Australia. *Aust. Vet. J.*, **22**, 2–11

23. Shutt, D. A. and Braden, A. W. H. (1968). The significance of equol in relation to the oestrogenic responses in sheep ingesting clover with a high formononetin content. *Aust. J. Agr. Res.*, **19**, 545–53

24. Walz, E. (1931). Isoflavon und sapogenin glucoside in sojahispida. *Justus Liebigs Ann. Chem.*, **489**, 118–55

25. Allen, E. and Doisy, E. A. (1923). An ovarian hormone. Preliminary report on its localization, extraction and partial purification, and action in test animals. *J. Am. Med. Assoc.*, **81**, 819–21

26. Bradbury, R. B. and White, D. E. (1954). Estrogens and related substances in plants. *Vitam. Horm.*, **12**, 207–33

27. Setchell, K. D. R., Gosselin, S. J., Welsh, M. B., Johnston, J. O., Balisten, W. F., Kramer, L. W., Dresser, B. L. and Tarr, M. J. (1987). Dietary estrogens – a probable cause of infertility and liver disease in captive cheetahs. *Gastroenterology*, **93**, 225–33

28. Axelson, M., Kirk, D. N., Farrant, R. D., Cooley, G., Lawson, A. M. and Setchell, K. D. R. (1982). The identification of the weak oestrogen equol [7-hydroxy-3-(4'hydroxyphenyl)chroman] in human urine. *Biochem. J.*, **201**, 353–7

29. Setchell, K. D. R., Borriello, S. P., Kirk, D. N. and Axelson, M. (1984). Non-steroidal estrogens of dietary origin: possible roles in hormone dependent disease. *Am. J. Clin. Nutr.*, **40**, 569–78

30. Verdeal, K. and Ryan, D. S. (1979). Naturally occurring oestrogens in plant foodstuffs – review. *J. Food Prot.*, **42**, 577–83

31. Vague, J., Garrigues, J. C., Berthet, J. and Favier, G. (1957). Note sur l'action de divers corps gras. *Ann d'Endocr.*, **78**, 309–12

32. Keys, A. (1970). Coronary heart disease in seven countries. *Circulation*, **41** (Suppl. 1) 1–211

33. Wilcox, G., Wahlqvist, M. L., Burger, H. G., and Medley, G. (1990). Oestrogenic effects of plant foods in postmenopausal women. *Br. Med. J.*, **301**, 905–6

34. Murkies, A., Lombard, C., Strauss, B. J. G., Wilcox, G., Burger, H. G. and Morton, M. S. (1995). Dietary flour supplementation decreases post-menopausal hot flushes: effect of soy and wheat. *Maturitas*, **21**, 189–95

35. Baird, D. D., Umbrach, D M., Lansdell, L., Hughes, C. L., Setchell, K. D. R., Weinberg, L. R., Haney, A. F., Wilcox, A. J. and McLachlan, J. A. (1995). Dietary intervention study to assess estrogenicity of dietary soy among post-menopausal women. *J. Clin. Endocrinol. Metab.*, **80**(5), 1685–90

36. Cassidy, A. (1996). Hormonal effects of isoflavones in humans. Presented at the *Second International Symposium on the Role of Soy in Preventing and Treating Chronic Disease*, Brussels, September

37. Burke, G. L. (1996). The potential use of a dietary soy supplement as a post-menopausal hormone replacement therapy. Presented at the *Second International Symposium on the Role of Soy in Preventing and Treating Chronic Disease*, Brussels, September

38. Harding, C., Morton, M. S., Gould, V., McMichael-Phillips, D., Howell, A. and Bundred, N. J. (1996). Dietary soy supplementation is oestrogenic in menopausal women (poster). Presented at the *Second International Symposium on the Role of Soy in Preventing and Treating Chronic Disease*, Brussels, September

39. Dalais, F. S., Rice, G. E., Bell, R. J., Murkies, A. L., Medley, G., Strauss, B. J. G. and Wahlqvist, M. L. (1996). Dietary soy supplementation increases vaginal cytology maturation index and bone mineral content in postmenopausal women (poster). Presented at the *Second International Symposium on the Role of Soy in Preventing and Treating Chronic Disease*, Brussels, September

40. Brzezinski, A., Adlercreutz, H., Sheoul, R., Shmuel, A., Roosler, A. and Schenker, J. G. (1996). Phytoestrogen-rich diet for post-menopausal women. Presented at the *5th World Congress on Gynecological Endocrinology*, Barcelona

41. Morton, M. S., Wilcox, G., Wahlqvist, M. L. and Griffiths, K. (1994). Determination of lignans and isoflavonoids in human female plasma following dietary supplementation. *J. Endocrinol.*, **142**, 251–9

42. Gavaler, J. S. (1993). Alcohol and nutrition in postmenopausal women. *J. Am. Coll. Nutr.*, **12**(4), 349–56

43. Dalais, F. S., Rice, G., Murkies, A. L., Bell, R. J., Strauss, B. J. G. and Wahlqvist, M. L. (1996). Effects of dietary phytoestrogens in post-menopausal women (poster). In *Proceedings of the 8th International Congress on the Menopause*. (Carnforth, UK: Parthenon Publishing)

44. Hughes, C. L. (1996). Phytoestrogens. Presented at the *8th International Congress on the Menopause*, Sydney, Australia, November

9

Hormones and brain function

Effects of sex steroids on brain cells   41

L. M. Garcia-Segura, M. C. Fernandez-Galaz, J. A. Chowen and F. Naftolin

Introduction

The central nervous system of vertebrates, including mammals and humans, plays a pivotal role in the success of reproduction by assuring complex forms of social and mating behaviors and an integrated neuroendocrine regulation. Evolutionary mechanisms have assured an appropriate intercommunication between brain and neuroendocrine organs, including the gonads. Sex steroids, one of the major players in the communication between the gonads and brain, are involved in the regulation of central nervous system development and adult neural function.

The mechanism of action of hormonal steroids in the nervous system, as in other tissues, involves the activation of specific intranuclear receptors that act as transcription factors for specific genes[1,2]. In addition, steroid hormones may modulate neuronal excitability by having rapid non-genomic actions[3]. Neural activity is also modulated by sex-steroid metabolites produced by nerve cells, and by local steroids that are synthesized *de novo* in the brain from cholesterol[4]. Hormonal and endogenous steroids modulate behavior, brain physiology and neuroendocrine function by exerting a variety of different effects on specific neuronal populations. In this chapter we review evidence generated in studies on rodents indicating that sex steroids may act as trophic factors for neural cells and as promoters of neural plasticity. This trophic and plastic effect of sex steroids may be mediated in part by interaction with other trophic molecules of peptidergic nature. In particular, complex interactions of one such factor, insulin-like growth factor-I (IGF-I), and estradiol have been documented recently in hypothalamic neurons.

The implication of such findings for estrogen effects on the human brain are still far from being completely understood. However, evidence accumulated in the rodent brain suggests that estradiol and other sex steroids may be important physiological factors necessary to sustain neural function.

Sex hormones influence neurons and glia

Owing to the complex pattern of cell interactions in the development of the central nervous system, it is difficult to determine whether the effect of sex steroids on a given neural cell type is directly exerted on that cell or mediated by other neurons or glial cells. Since many neurons express receptors for gonadal steroids and since a gonadal hormone and its metabolites may have a variety of direct rapid effects on neuronal membranes, it is presumable that steroids will directly affect many different neurons throughout the brain. However, indirect effects are probably very important as well. Indeed, acting on a given cell the hormone may in turn influence other cells. For instance, acting on its target neurons, a gonadal hormone may induce the release of neurotransmitters and trophic factors that may affect the development and function of other neurons. Furthermore, by promoting neuronal survival and differentiation of its target cells, a gonadal hormone may also affect the survival and differentiation of the neurons that contact these cells.

Glial cells are also affected by sex hormones and their metabolites[5]. Several laboratories have shown that glial cells in culture express receptors for sex steroids[6,7]. Furthermore, it has been reported that hypothalamic glia *in situ* express estrogen receptors, based on immuno-histochemical evidence[8]. Sex hormones and neurosteroids affect myelination by acting on oligodendrocytes and Schwann cells[9,10], and modulate the response of nerve tissue to injury by acting on microglia and astroglia[5,11]. In addition to being a target for sex steroids, glial cells are also involved in their metabolism[12] and in the synthesis of neurosteroids[10,13–15], and participate in the organizational and activational effects of sex steroids on synapse formation[16,17] and synaptic plasticity[18,19].

Sex hormones act as neurotrophic factors

It is classically recognized that sex steroids exert organizational effects during the critical period for brain sexual differentiation, and activational effects in the adult brain[20]. During the development of the central nervous system, gonadal steroids determine the number of neurons in several structures, resulting in a sexually dimorphic development. One of the best studied examples is the sexually dimorphic nucleus of the preoptic area in rodents, which is larger in volume in males than in females[21,22]. This difference in nuclear size is at least partially due to the action of gonadal steroids during the critical period, promoting the survival of a specific population of neurons[23]. Another example of a sexually dimorphic structure in the central nervous system of rodents is the spinal nucleus of the bulbocavernosus[24]. Androgens prevent normal cell death of motoneurons of this nucleus[25]. These studies suggest that sex steroids may act as neurotrophic factors, promoting the survival of specific neurons or regulating apoptosis.

Neurotrophic effects of sex steroids have been characterized *in vitro*. Estradiol promotes the survival of cultured neurons from the amygdala, the hypothalamus and the spinal cord[26–29]. The effect of estradiol on the survival of cultured hypothalamic neurons is mimicked by testosterone, but not by the non-aromatizable

androgen dihydrotestosterone[28]. The effect appears to be mediated in part through the estrogen receptor since it is saturable and can be blocked by estrogen receptor antagonists, such as tamoxifen and ICI 182,780, and by the inhibition of estrogen receptor synthesis in the cultures by using an antisense oligonucleotide against estrogen receptor mRNA[28,29].

In addition to the effects on cell number, sex steroids also affect neuronal differentiation in several brain areas, modulating the growth of axons, the number and branching of dendrites and the number of dendritic spines. For instance, estradiol modulates the growth of neurites in hypothalamic neurons in explant cultures[30,31] and in monolayer cultures[29,32,33], while in the spinal nucleus of the bulbocavernosus, androgens regulate dendritic outgrowth during the neonatal period and dendritic retraction during the pubertal period[34,35]. Gonadal steroid-dependent sex differences in neuronal processes have been detected in other brain structures, including the preoptic area[36] and hippocampus[37]. These effects of gonadal hormones on the differentiation of neuronal processes are mediated, at least in part, by the modulation of cytoskeletal proteins[29,32,38].

Sex hormones regulate the formation of neuronal connections and promote neural plasticity

Hormonal modifications in the growth of neuronal processes may result in changes in the pattern of neuronal connectivity. It is well established that during the critical period gonadal steroids influence the formation of synaptic contacts among neurons, resulting in specific sex differences in neuronal connectivity. Furthermore, the effect of sex hormones on synapses is not restricted to the developmental period. Synapses are plastic structures that may be modified in the adult brain in response to changing physiological conditions, including modifications in hormone levels[18,39]. Gonadal hormones influence synapse formation in areas of the central nervous system involved in the control of reproductive behavior, such as the ventromedial hypothalamic nucleus, lateral septum and the amygdala, and in areas involved in the control of the release of pituitary hormones, such as the hypothalamic arcuate nucleus and the preoptic area. In addition, gonadal hormones may affect neuronal connectivity in cognitive areas, such as the hippocampal formation and the cerebral cortex[18,37,39].

Cellular mechanisms mediating steroid actions on synapses in the adult brain have been extensively studied in the rat arcuate nucleus, a hypothalamic center involved in the feedback regulation of gonadotropins. Estradiol induces a transient disconnection of inhibitory gamma-aminobutyric acid-(GABA)ergic inputs to the somas of arcuate neurons during the preovulatory and ovulatory phases of the estrous cycle[18,40,41]. This synaptic remodeling is blocked by progesterone and begins with the onset of female puberty[18].

Effects of sex hormones on brain cells may be mediated in part by polypeptide neurotrophic factors

The complexity of gonadal steroid action on the brain is not only a consequence of the complexity of cellular interactions in the neural tissue. Interactions between the signaling cascades of membrane receptors for peptidic factors and the steroid hormone receptors should also be taken into consideration.

One of the best characterized neurotrophic factors, and the first one to be discovered, is nerve growth factor (NGF). In some brain areas and during specific developmental stages estradiol and NGF may affect on the same target neurons. Genes encoding NGF and the low-affinity receptor for NGF (p75) are expressed in subpopulations of neurons of hypothalamic neuroendocrine areas[42]. Furthermore, it has been shown that estrogen receptors co-localize with low-affinity NGF receptors in cholinergic neurons of the basal forebrain of developing rodents[43]. Estradiol may therefore exert part of its trophic effects modulating the action of NGF. This is further supported by the fact that estradiol

is able to modulate the levels of NGF receptors in PC12 cells, in cerebral cortical cultures and in dorsal root ganglion neurons of adult female rats[44-46]. Moreover, putative estrogen-responsive elements have been identified in the NGF gene and in the genes for NGF receptors of high (trkA) and low affinity[46]. By regulating trkA or p75 levels, estradiol may affect programmed neuronal death[47].

A putative estrogen-receptor element has been identified also in the gene encoding brain-derived neurotrophic factor (BDNF)[48]. The receptor (trkB) for this neurotrophin is expressed in neurons from hypothalamic neuroendocrine areas, as well as trkC, which is the receptor for neurotrophin-3[42].

In addition to neurotrophins, other trophic factors may also be relevant with regard to the action of sex steroids in the brain. These include basic fibroblast growth factor (bFGF) and transforming growth factors α (TGF-α) and β (TGF-β), which appear to be involved in the maturation of the neuroendocrine hypothalamus and/or in the regulation of luteinizing hormone-releasing hormone (LHRH) neurons[49-52]. Sex steroids may interact with some of these factors to exert their effects on neurons and glial cells. For instance, estrogen modulates the expression of TGF-α in the hypothalamus[50]. This factor is produced by hypothalamic glial cells and appears to regulate LHRH neurons[49,50,53]. Gene expression of TGF-α increases in glial cells at the time of puberty in regions of the hypothalamus involved in LHRH control[50].

Another factor that may be involved in the effects of gonadal hormones on the brain is IGF-I. IGF-I is locally synthesized by glia and neurons of the hypothalamus and other brain areas[54,55] and has prominent trophic actions, stimulating the survival and differentiation of specific neural cell populations, including hypothalamic neurons in culture[28,56]. IGF-I may also act as a hormonal signal and may be involved in the feedback regulation of growth hormone by affecting the synthesis or release of growth hormone-releasing hormone or somatostatin by hypothalamic neurons[57,58]. IGF-I may also affect the reproductive axis by modulating the secretion of gonadotropin-releasing hormone[59,60].

Estradiol and insulin-like growth factor-I signaling pathways interact in neurons

In several tissues and cell types estrogen up-regulates IGF-I gene expression[61-67] and modulates IGF-I action by affecting the levels of IGF-I receptors[62,68] and IGF binding proteins (IGFBPs)[69-72]. Likewise, IGF-I may regulate steroid hormone action by stimulating the synthesis of steroid hormones[73-75] and steroid hormone receptors[76-78]. Furthermore, IGF-I, as other peptidic factors, may activate the estrogen receptor in different cell lines, including neuroblastoma cells[79-84]. This activation of the estrogen receptor occurs in the absence of the hormone, is mediated by IGF-I receptor membrane-associated signaling pathways[81,84], and involves the activation function 2 domain of the estrogen receptor in neuroblastoma cells[84] and the activation function 1 domain in other cell lines[80,81].

The first evidence of an interaction between IGF-I and estrogen on neural cells was obtained in explant cultures of fetal rodent hypothalamus where estrogen and insulin have synergistic effects on neurite growth, an effect that is probably mediated through IGF-I receptors[85]. Furthermore, estrogen modulates IGF-I receptors and binding proteins in monolayer hypothalamic cultures[86] and IGF-I immuno-reactive levels in tanycytes, a specialized form of glial cells, in the arcuate nucleus and median eminence[87]. IGF-I immunoreactive levels in tanycytes increase in male and female rats at the time of puberty[87]. In females there is an abrupt increase in IGF-I immunoreactivity between the morning and the afternoon of the first proestrus. Henceforth, IGF-I immuno-reactivity fluctuates in tanycytes according to the different stages of the estrus cycle. IGF-I immunoreactive levels are high in the afternoon of proestrus, after the peak of estrogen in plasma, remain increased on the morning of the following day and then decrease to basal conditions by the morning of metestrus[87]. In addition, IGF-I levels decrease in tanycytes by ovariectomy and increase in a dose-dependent manner when ovariectomized rats are injected with 17β-estradiol[87]. These changes, linked to fluctuations of gonadotropins, suggest that the levels of IGF-I in tanycytes may be related to LHRH regulation.

We have recently studied whether the effects of estrogen on hypothalamic neuronal survival and neurite growth are mediated by IGF-I[29]. Hypothalamic cultures exposed to estradiol or IGF-I show a significant increase in neuronal survival and in the growth of neuronal processes. Inhibition of IGF-I synthesis in the cultures with an antisense oligonucleotide to IGF-I mRNA results in a significant decrease in the stimulatory effects of 17β-estradiol on the number of neurons and the extension of neuronal processes[29]. This indicates that IGF-I is necessary for the manifestation of the hormonal effect, suggesting that estradiol may induce neuronal survival and differentiation by activation of IGF-I signaling cascades. We have also studied whether the effect of IGF-I on the survival and differentiation of hypothalamic neurons is dependent on the estrogen receptor[29]. Both the pure estrogen receptor antagonist ICI 182,780 or an antisense oligodeoxynucleotide to the estrogen receptor mRNA blocked the effects of estradiol. This indicates that estrogen receptors are necessary for the action of IGF-I on hypothalamic survival and neuritic growth, suggesting that IGF-I may activate, either directly or indirectly, estrogen receptors. The interaction of estradiol and insulin-like growth factor-I (IGF-I) signaling cascades in hypothalamic neuronal survival and differentiation provides a good example of the complexity of the mechanism of action of sex steroids in the brain. Further studies are necessary to establish the possible physiological and physiopathological significance of this interaction.

Acknowledgements

This work was supported by Fundación Ramón Areces, DGICYT, NIH (HD13587), and Fundación Endocrinología y Nutrición.

References

1. Beato, M. (1989). Gene regulation by steroid hormones. *Cell*, **56**, 335–44
2. Evans, R. M. (1988). The steroid and thyroid hormone receptor superfamily. *Science*, **240**, 889–95
3. McEwen, B. S. (1991). Non-genomic and genomic effects of steroids on neural activity. *Trends Pharmacol. Sci.*, **12**, 141–7
4. Baulieu, E. E. and Robel, P. (1990). Neurosteroids: a new brain function? *J. Steroid Biochem. Mol. Biol.*, **37**, 395–403
5. Garcia-Segura, L. M., Chowen, J. A. and Naftolin, F. (1996). Endocrine glia: roles of glial cells in the brain actions of steroid and thyroid hormones and in the regulation of hormone secretion. *Front. Neuroendocrinol.*, **17**, 180–211
6. Jung-Testas, I., Renoir, J. M., Gasc, J. M. and Baulieu, E. E. (1991). Estrogen-inducible progesterone receptor in primary cultures of rat glial cells. *Exp. Cell Res.*, **193**, 12—19
7. Santagati, S., Melcangi, R. C., Celotti, F., Martini, L. and Maggi, A. (1994). Estrogen receptor is expressed in different types of glial cells in culture. *J. Neurochem.*, **63**, 2058–64
8. Langub, M. C. and Watson, R. E. (1992). Estrogen receptor-immunoreactive glia, endothelia, and ependyma in guinea pig preoptic area and median eminence: electron microscopy. *Endocrinology*, **130**, 364–72
9. Jung-Testas, I., Schumacher, M., Robel, P. and Baulieu, E. E. (1994). Actions of steroid hormones and growth factors on glial cells of the central and peripheral nervous system. *J. Steroid Biochem. Mol. Biol.*, **48**, 145–54
10. Koenig, H. L., Schumacher, M., Ferzaz, B., Do Thi, A. N., Ressouches, A., Guennoun, R., Jung-Testas, I., Robel, P., Akwa, Y. and Baulieu, E. E. (1995). Progesterone synthesis and myelin formation by Schwann cells. *Science*, **268**, 1500–3
11. Garcia-Estrada, J., Del Rio, J. A., Luquin, S., Soriano, E. and Garcia-Segura, L. M. (1993). Gonadal hormones down-regulate reactive gliosis and astrocyte proliferation after a penetrating brain injury. *Brain Res.*, **628**, 271–8
12. Melcangi, R.C., Celotti, F., Castano, P. and Martini, L. (1993). Differential localization of the 5α-reductase and the 3α-hydroxysteroid dehydrogenase in neuronal and glial cultures. *Endocrinology*, **132**, 1252–9
13. Akwa, Y., Sananes, N., Gouezou, M., Robel, P. I., Baulieu, E. E. and Le Goascogne, C. (1993). Astrocytes and neurosteroids: metabolism of pregnenolone and dehydroepiandrosterone. Regulation by cell density. *J. Cell Biol.*, **121**, 135–43
14. Hu, Z. Y., Bourreau, E., Jung-Testas, I., Robel, P. and Baulieu, E. E. (1987). Neurosteroids: oligodendrocyte mitochondria convert cholesterol to pregnenolone. *Proc. Natl. Acad. Sci. USA*, **84**, 8215–19
15. Kabbadj, K., El-Etr, M., Baulieu, E. E. and Robel, P. (1993). Pregnenolone metabolism in rodent embryonic neurons and astrocytes. *Glia*, **7**, 170–5
16. Chowen, J. A., Busiguina, S. and Garcia-Segura, L. M. (1995). Sexual dimorphism and sex steroid modulation of glial fibrillary acidic protein messenger RNA and immunoreactive levels in the rat hypothalamus. *Neuroscience*, **69**, 519–32
17. Garcia-Segura, L. M., Dueñas, M., Busiguina, S., Naftolin, F. and Chowen, J. A. (1995). Gonadal hormone regulation of neuronal–glial interactions in the developing neuroendocrine hypothalamus. *J. Steroid Biochem. Mol. Biol.*, **53**, 293–8
18. Garcia-Segura, L. M., Chowen, J. A., Parducz, A. and Naftolin, F. (1994). Gonadal hormones as promoters of structural synaptic plasticity: cellular mechanisms. *Prog. Neurobiol.*, **44**, 279–307
19. Garcia-Segura, L. M., Luquin, S., Parducz, A. and Naftolin, F. (1994). Gonadal hormone regulation of glial fibrillary acidic protein immunoreactivity and glial ultrastructure in the rat neuroendocrine hypothalamus. *Glia*, **10**, 59–69
20. Arnold, A. P. and Breedlove, S. M. (1985). Organizational and activational effects of sex steroids on brain and behavior: a reanalysis. *Horm. Behav.*, **19**, 469–98
21. Gorski, R. A., Gordon, J. H., Shryne, J. E. and Southam, A. M. (1978). Evidence for a morphological sex difference within the medial preoptic area of the rat brain. *Brain Res.*, **148**, 333–46
22. Gorski, R. A., Harlan, R. E., Jacobson, C. D., Shryne, J. E. and Southam, A.M. (1980). Evidence for the existence of a sexually dimorphic nucleus in the preoptic area of the rat. *J. Comp. Neurol.*, **198**, 529–39
23. Dodson, R. E., Shryne, J. E. and Gorski, R. A. (1988). Hormonal modification of the number of total and late-arising neurons in culture: sex differences and estrogen effects. *J. Neurosci. Res.*, **33**, 266–81
24. Breedlove, S. M. and Arnold, A. P. (1983). Hormonal control of developing neuromuscular

system. I. Sensitive periods for the androgen-induced masculinization of the rat spinal nucleus of the bulbocavernosus. *J. Neurosci.*, **3**, 424–32

25. Nordeen, E. J., Nordeen, K. W., Sengelaub, D. R. and Arnold, A. P. (1985). Androgens prevent normally occurring cell death in a sexually dimorphic spinal nucleus. *Science*, **229**, 671–3

26. Arimatsu, Y. and Hatanaka, H. (1986). Estrogen treatment enhances survival of cultured fetal rat amygdala neurons in a defined medium. *Dev. Brain Res.*, **26**, 151–9

27. Hauser, K. F. and Toran-Allerand, C. D. (1989). Androgen increases the number of cells in fetal mouse spinal cord cultures: implications for motoneuron survival. *Brain Res.*, **485**, 157–64

28. Chowen, J. A., Torres-Aleman, I. and Garcia-Segura, L. M. (1992). Trophic effects of estradiol on fetal rat hypothalamic neurons. *Neuroendocrinology*, **56**, 895–901

29. Dueñas, M., Torres-Aleman, I., Naftolin, F. and Garcia-Segura, L. M. (1996). Interaction of insulin-like growth factor-I and estradiol signalling pathways on hypothalamic neuronal differentiation. *Neuroscience*, **74**, 531–9

30. Toran-Allerand, C. D. (1976). Sex steroids and the development of the newborn mouse hypothalamus and preoptic area *in vitro*: implications for sexual differentiation. *Brain Res.*, **106**, 407–12

31. Toran-Allerand, C. D., Hashimoto, K., Greenough, W. T. and Saltarelli, N. (1983). Sex steroids and the development of the newborn mouse hypothalamus *in vitro*: III. Effects of estrogen on dendritic differentiation. *Dev. Brain Res.*, **7**, 97–101

32. Ferreira, A. and Cáceres, A. (1991). Estrogen-enhanced neurite growth: evidence for a selective induction of tau and stable microtubules. *J. Neurosci.*, **11**, 392–400

33. Díaz, H., Lorenzo, A., Carrer, H. F. and Cáceres, A. (1992). Time lapse study of neurite growth in hypothalamic dissociated neurons in culture: sex differences and estrogen effects. *J. Neurosci. Res.*, **33**, 266–81

34. Kurz, E. M., Sengelaub, D. R. and Arnold, A. P. (1986). Androgens regulate the dendritic length of mammalian motoneurons in adulthood. *Science*, **232**, 395–8

35. Goldstein, L. A., Kurz, E. M. and Sengelaub, D. R. (1990). Androgen regulation of dendritic growth and retraction in the development of a sexually dimorphic spinal nucleus. *J. Neurosci.*, **10**, 935–46

36. Raisman, G. and Field, P. M. (1973). Sexual dimorphism in the neuropil of the preoptic area of the rat and its dependence on neonatal androgen. *Brain Res.*, **54**, 1–29

37. Gould, E., Woolley, C. S., Frankfurt, M. and McEwen, B. S. (1990). Gonadal steroids regulate dendritic spine density in hippocampal pyramidal cells in adulthood. *J. Neurosci.*, **10**, 1286–91

38. Lorenzo, A., Díaz, H., Carrer, H. and Cáceres, A. (1992). Amygdala neurons *in vitro*: neurite growth and effects of estradiol. *J. Neurosci. Res.*, **33**, 418–35

39. Matsumoto, A. (1991). Synaptogenic action of sex steroids in developing and adult neuroendocrine brain. *Psychoneuroendocrinology*, **16**, 25–40

40. Olmos, G., Naftolin, F., Pérez, J., Tranque, P. A. and Garcia-Segura, L. M. (1989). Synaptic remodelling in the rat arcuate nucleus during the estrous cycle. *Neuroscience*, **32**, 663–7

41. Párducz, A., Pérez, J. and Garcia-Segura, L. M. (1993). Estradiol induces plasticity of GABAergic synapses in the hypothalamus. *Neuroscience*, **53**, 395–401

42. Berg von der Emde, K., Dees, W. L., Hiney, J. K., Hill, D. F., Dissen, G. A., Costa, M. E., Moholt-Siebert, M. and Ojeda, S. R. (1995). Neurotrophins and the neuroendocrine brain: different neurotrophins sustain anatomically and functionally segregated subsets of hypothalamic dopaminergic neurons. *J. Neurosci.*, **15**, 4223–37

43. Toran-Allerand, C. D., Miranda, R. C., Bentham, W., Sohrabji, F., Brown, E. J., Hochberg, R. B. and MacLusky, N. J. (1992). Estrogen receptors co-localize with low-affinity NGF receptors in cholinergic neurons of the basal forebrain. *Proc. Natl. Acad. Sci. USA*, **89**, 4668–72

44. Sohrabji, F., Greene, L. A., Miranda, R. C. and Toran-Allerand, C. D. (1994). Reciprocal regulation of estrogen and NGF receptors by their ligands in PC12 cells. *J. Neurobiol.*, **25**, 974–88

45. Sohrabji, F., Miranda, C. and Toran-Allerand, C. D. (1994). Estrogen differentially regulates estrogen and nerve growth factor receptor mRNA in adult sensory neurons. *J. Neurosci.*, **14**, 459–71

46. Toran-Allerand, C. D. (1996). Mechanisms of estrogen action during neural development: mediation by interactions with the neurotrophins and their receptors? *J. Steroid Biochem. Mol. Biol.*, **56**, 169–78

47. Frade, J.M., Rodriguez-Tébar, A. and Barde, Y.-A. (1996). Induction of cell death by endogenous nerve growth factor through its p75 receptor. *Nature (London)*, **383**, 166–8

48. Sohrabji, F., Miranda, R. C. and Toran-Allerand, C. D. (1995). Identification of a putative estrogen receptor element in the gene encoding brain-derived neurotrophic factor. *Proc. Natl. Acad. Sci. USA*, **92**, 11110–14

49. Ojeda, S. R., Dissen, G. A. and Junier, M. P. (1992). Neurotrophic factors and female sexual development. *Front. Neuroendocrinol.*, **13**, 120–62

50. Ma, Y. J., Junier, M. P., Costa, M. E. and Ojeda, S. R. (1992). Transforming growth factor-α gene expression in the hypothalamus is developmentally regulated and linked to sexual maturation. *Neuron*, **9**, 657–70

51. Melcangi, R. C., Galbiati, M., Messi, E., Piva, F., Martini, L. and Motta, M. (1995). Type 1 astrocytes influence luteinizing hormone-releasing hormone release from the hypothalamic cell line GT1-1: is transforming growth factor β the principle involved? *Endocrinology*, **136**, 679–86

52. Wetsel, W. C., Hill, D. F. and Ojeda, S. R. (1996). Basic fibroblast growth factor regulates the conversion of pro-luteinizing hormone-releasing hormone (pro-LHRH) to LHRH in immortalized hypothalamic neurons. *Endocrinology*, **137**, 2606–16

53. Voigt, P., Ma, Y. J., Gonzalez, D., Fahrenbach, W. H., Wetsel, W. C., Berg von der Emde, K., Hill, D. F., Taylor, K. G., Costa, M. E., Seidah, N. G. and Ojeda, S. R. (1996). Neural and glial-mediated effects of growth factors acting via tyrosine kinase receptors on luteinizing hormone-releasing hormone neurons. *Endocrinology*, **137**, 2593–605

54. Bondy, C., Werner, H., Roberts, C. T. and LeRoith, D. (1992). Cellular pattern of type-I insulin-like growth factor receptor gene expression during maturation of the rat brain: comparison with insulin-like growth factors I and II. *Neuroscience*, **46**, 909–23

55. Garcia-Segura, L. M., Perez, J., Pons, S., Rejas, M. T. and Torres-Aleman, I. (1991). Localization of insulin-like growth factor I (IGF-I)-like immunoreactivity in the developing and adult rat brain. *Brain Res.*, **560**, 167–74

56. Torres-Aleman, I., Naftolin, F. and Robbins, R. J. (1990). Trophic effect of insulin-like growth factor-I on fetal rat hypothalamic cells in culture. *Neuroscience*, **35**, 601–8

57. Berelowitz, M., Szabo, M., Frohman, L. A., Firestone, S., Chu, L. and Hintz, R. L. (1981). Somatomedin C mediates growth hormone negative feedback by effects on both the hypothalamus and the pituitary. *Science*, **212**, 1279–81

58. Tannenbaum, G. S., Guyda, H. J. and Posner, B. I. (1983). Insulin-like growth factors: a role in growth hormone negative feedback and body weight regulation via brain. *Science*, **220**, 77–9

59. Bourguignon, J. P., Gerard, A., Alvarez Gonzalez, M. L. and Franchimont, P. (1993). Acute suppression of gonadotropin-releasing hormone secretion by insulin-like growth factor I and subproducts: an age-dependent endocrine effect. *Neuroendocrinology*, **58**, 525–30

60. Hiney, J. K., Ojeda, S. R. and Les Dees, W. (1991). Insulin-like growth factor I: a possible metabolic signal involved in the regulation of female puberty. *Neuroendocrinology*, **54**, 420–3

61. Gahary, A., Chakrabarti, S. and Murphy, L. J. (1990). Localization of the sites of synthesis and action of insulin-like growth factor-I in the rat uterus. *Mol. Endocrinol.*, **4**, 191–5

62. Hernandez, E. R. (1995). Regulation of the genes for insulin-like growth factor (IGF) I and II and their receptors by steroids and gonadotropins in the ovary. *J. Steroid Biochem. Mol. Biol.*, **53**, 219–21

63. Kapur, S., Tamada, H., Dey, S. K. and Andrews, G. K. (1992). Expression of insulin-like growth factor-I (IGF-I) and its receptor in the peri-implantation mouse uterus, and cell-specific regulation of IGF-I gene expression by estradiol and progesterone. *Biol. Reprod.*, **46**, 208–19

64. Michels, K. M., Lee, W. H., Seltzer, A., Saavedra, J. M. and Bondy, C. A. (1993). Up-regulation of pituitary [125I] insulin-like growth factor-I (IGF-I) binding and IGF-I gene expression by estrogen. *Endocrinology*, **132**, 23–9

65. Murphy, L. J., Murphy, L. C. and Friesen, H. G. (1987). Estrogen induces insulin-like growth factor-I expression in the rat uterus. *Mol. Endocrinol.*, **1**, 445–50

66. Simmen, R. C. M., Simmen, F. A., Hofig, A., Farmer, S. J. and Bazer, F. W. (1990). Hormonal regulation of insulin-like growth factor gene expression in pig uterus. *Endocrinology*, **127**, 2166–74

67. Umayahara, Y., Kawamori, R., Watada, H., Imano, E., Iwama, N., Morishima, T., Yamasaki, Y., Kajimoto, Y. and Kamada, T. (1994). Estrogen regulation of the insulin-like growth factor I gene transcription involves an AP-1 enhancer. *J. Biol. Chem.*, **269**, 16433–42

68. Wimalasena, J., Meehan, D., Dostal, R., Foster, J. S., Cameron, M. and Smith, M. (1993). Growth factors interact with estradiol and gonadotrophins in the regulation of ovarian cancer cell growth and growth factor receptors. *Oncol. Res.*, **5**, 325–37

69. Krywicki, R. F., Figueroa, J. A., Jackson, J. G., Kozelsky, T. W., Shimasaki, S., Von Hoff, D. D. and Yee, D. (1993). Regulation of insulin-like growth factor binding proteins in ovarian cancer cells by oestrogen. *Eur. J. Cancer*, **29A**, 2015–19

70. Molnar, P. and Murphy, L. J. (1994). Effects of oestrogen on rat uterine expression of insulin-like growth factor-binding proteins. *J. Mol. Endocrinol.*, **13**, 59–67

71. Owens, P. C., Gill, P. G., De Young, N. J., Weger, M. A., Knowels, S. E. and Moyse, K. J. (1993). Estrogen and progesterone regulate secretion of insulin-like growth factor binding proteins by human breast cancer cells. *Biochem. Biophys. Res. Commun.*, **193**, 467–73

72. Yallampalli, C., Rajaraman, S. and Nagamani, M. (1993). Insulin-like growth factor binding proteins in the rat uterus and their regulation by oestradiol and growth hormone. *J. Reprod. Fertil.*, **97**, 501–5

73. Constantino, C. X., Keyes, P. L. and Kostyo, J. L. (1991). Insulin-like growth factor-I stimulates steroidogenesis in rabbit luteal cells. *Endocrinology*, **128**, 1702–8

74. Erickson, G. F., Garzo, V. G. and Magoffin, D. A. (1989). Insulin-like growth factor-I (IGF-I) regulates aromatase activity in human granulosa luteal cells. *J. Clin. Endocrinol. Metab.*, **69**, 716–24

75. Hernandez, E. R., Resnick, C. E., Svoboda, M. E., Van Wyk, J., Payne, D. W. and Adashi, E. Y. (1988). Somatomedin-C/insulin-like growth factor I as an enhancer of androgen biosynthesis by cultured rat ovarian cells. *Endocrinology*, **122**, 1603–12

76. Aronica, S. M. and Katzenellenbogen, B. S. (1991). Progesterone receptor regulation in uterine cells: stimulation by estrogen, cyclic adenosine 3',5'-monophosphate, and insulin-like growth factor I and suppression by antiestrogens and protein kinase inhibitors. *Endocrinology*, **128**, 2045–52

77. Cho, H., Aronica, S. M., Katzenellenbogen, B. S. (1994). Regulation of progesterone receptor gene expression in MCF-7 breast cancer cells: a comparison of the effects of cyclic adenosine 3',5'-monophosphate, estradiol, insulin-like growth factor I, and serum factors. *Endocrinology*, **134**, 658–64

78. Katzenellenbogen, B. S. and Norman, M. J. (1990). Multihormonal regulation of the progesterone receptor in MCF-7 human breast cancer cells: interrelationships among insulin/insulin-like growth factor-I, serum, and estrogen. *Endocrinology*, **126**, 891–8

79. Aronica, S. M. and Katzenellenbogen, B. S. (1993). Stimulation of estrogen receptor-mediated transcription and alteration in the phosphorylation state of the rat uterine estrogen receptor by estrogen, cyclic adenosine monophosphate, and insulin-like growth factor-I. *Mol. Endocrinol.*, **7**, 743–52

80. Ignar-Trowbridge, D. M., Pimentel, M., Parker, M. G., McLachlan, J. A. and Korach, K. S. (1996). Peptide growth factor cross-talk with the estrogen receptor requires the A/B domain and occurs independently of protein kinase C or estradiol. *Endocrinology*, **137**, 1735–44

81. Kato, S., Endoh, H., Masuhiro, Y., Kitamoto, T., Uchiyama, S., Sasaki, H., Masushige, S., Gotoh, Y., Nishida, E., Kawashima, H., Metzger, D. and Chambon, P. (1995). Activation of the estrogen receptor through phosphorylation by mitogen-activated protein kinase. *Science*, **270**, 1491–4

82. Ma, Z. Q., Santagati, S., Patrone, C., Pollio, G., Vegeto, E. and Maggi, A. (1994). Insulin-like growth factor activates estrogen receptor to control the growth and differentiation of the human neuroblastoma cell line SK-ER3. *Mol. Endocrinol.*, **8**, 910–18

83. Newton, C. J., Buric, R., Trapp, T., Brockmeier, S., Pagotto, U. and Stalla, G. K. (1994). The unligand estrogen receptor (ER) transduces growth factor signals. *J. Steroid Biochem. Mol. Biol.*, **48**, 481–6

84. Patrone, C., Ma, Z. Q., Pollio, G., Agrati, P., Parker, M. G. and Maggi, A. (1996). Cross-coupling between insulin and estrogen receptor in human neuroblastoma cells. *Mol. Endocrinol.*, **10**, 499–507

85. Toran-Allerand, C. D., Ellis, L. and Pfenninger, K. H. (1988). Estrogen and insulin synergism in neurite growth enhancement *in vitro*: mediation of steroid effects by interactions with growth factors? *Dev. Brain Res.*, **41**, 87–100

86. Pons, S. and Torres-Aleman, I. (1993). Estradiol modulates insulin-like growth factor I receptors and binding proteins in neurons from the hypothalamus. *J. Neuroendocrinol.*, **5**, 267–71

87. Dueñas, M., Luquin, S., Chowen, J. A., Torres-Aleman, I., Naftolin, F. and Garcia-Segura, L. M. (1994). Gonadal hormone regulation of insulin-like growth factor-I-like immunoreactivity in hypothalamic astroglia of developing and adult rats. *Neuroendocrinology*, **59**, 528–38

Neurosteroids: metabolism and activities 42

E. E. Baulieu

Neurosteroids: the beginning

The work to describe the synthesis and metabolic pathways of neurosteroids, and establish their physiological and pathological function and mechanism(s) of action has encountered some major difficulties:

(1) Many analytical problems, qualitative and quantitative, were encountered because of the low concentration and the lipoidal nature of neurosteroids, which have to be separated from the highly lipidic constituents of neural tissues. Strictly controlled conditions had to be established, since neurosteroid concentrations vary according to the time of day, the lighting schedule, the food, the presence of other animals, the habituation to handling, and so on.

(2) The overall dynamics of the synthesis of neurosteroids is unknown, since their turnover cannot be determined and no appropriate techniques are available for describing their compartmentation.

(3) Quantitative aspects are particularly difficult to master since many neurosteroids are also secreted by peripheral glands, may cross the blood–brain barrier and also easily attain peripheral nerves, eventually mixing with neurosteroids. In fact, the respective distribution and contribution of steroids imported into the nervous system and of those synthetized *in situ* remain difficult to assess and consequently, we do not necessarily know what the respective targets are.

(4) Binding studies and thus the search for receptors are especially hard in a lipid-rich milieu, as often encountered in work with nervous tissue and its membranes, again because of the liposolubility of steroids.

We essentially followed two strategic lines. The first consisted of establishing the synthesis and metabolic pathways of steroids in the nervous system (Figure 1), including the characterization of the corresponding enzymes and receptors. The second series of studies was to determine changes and, if possible, function of neurosteroids under various physiological or pathological conditions.

In initial experiments, we measured steroids remaining in the brain after removal of potential glandular sources of steroids, that is after adrenalectomy and gonadectomy (Table 1). In rats, we essentially noted the persistency of dehydroepiandrosterone (DHEA) and its conjugates after several weeks, and the decrease of pregnenolone (PREG) and its conjugates, though this was only partial, as if the ablation of endocrine glands had led to the suppression of only the imported steroid (PREG is a circulating steroid in the rat, and is also synthesized in the brain). In male rats, after operation, we observed the persistency of a low but easily measured level of progesterone (PROG), while in contrast, testosterone and testosterone sulfate disappeared rapidly from the brain tissue[1-3].

Consistent with the hypothesis that the persistency of steroids after adrenalectomy–gonadectomy is not due to retention of compounds originally circulating in the blood, we observed the rapid release of uptaken radioactive DHEA and PREG following their peripheral administration[2]. A circadian cycle of brain PREG and DHEA, unrelated to blood steroid levels, was also observed[4,5], and brain PREG was found to be high for several days after

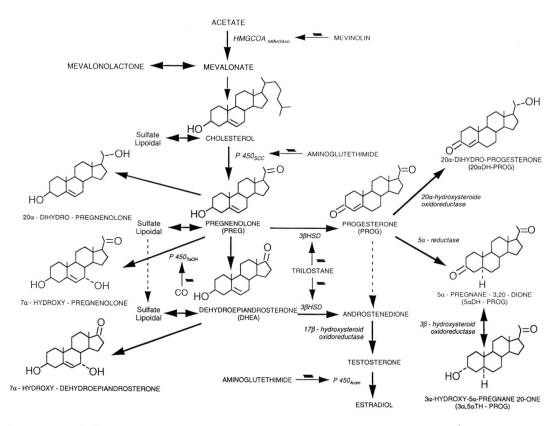

Figure 1 Metabolism of steroids. Most biosynthetic and metabolic reactions cited in text are indicated with corresponding enzymes and some of their pharmacological blockers (marked ▬)

Table 1 Neurosteroid levels in the male rat brain and blood plasma before and after orchidectomy (orx) and adrenalectomy (adx). Values are given as mean ± SD

	PREG	PREGS	PREGL	DHEA	DHEAS	DHEAL	PROG
Brain							
Intact (ng/g)	8.9 ± 2.4	14.2 ± 2.5	9.4 ± 2.9	0.24 ± 0.33	1.70 ± 0.32	0.45 ± 0.13	2.2 ± 1.1
Orx/adx (ng/g)	2.6 ± 0.8	16.9 ± 4.6	4.9 ± 1.3	0.14 ± 0.13	1.64 ± 0.43	0.29 ± 0.12	3.2 ± 1.6
Plasma							
Intact (ng/ml)	1.2 ± 0.6	2.1 ± 0.9	2.4 ± 0.9	0.06 ± 0.06	0.20 ± 0.08	0.18 ± 0.05	1.9 ± 0.7
Orx/adx (ng/ml)	0.3 ± 0.1	ND	1.3 ± 0.3	nm	nm	nm	0.1 ± 0.1

PREG, pregnenolone; PREGS, PREG sulfate; PREGL, lipoidal PREG; DHEA, dehydroepiandrosterone; DHEAS, DHEA sulfate; DHEAL, lipoidal DHEA; PROG, progesterone; ND, not determined; nm, not measured

birth in rats even when the adrenal steroid output is low[6]. Interestingly, in adrenalectomized–orchidectomized male rats (and in sham-operated animals), 2 days after surgery a temporary increase of dehydroepiandrosterone sulfate (DHEAS) was found in the brain, possibly due to a local neural response to stress[1].

Essentially the same results have been obtained with other laboratory animals including monkeys, of which a limited study suggested that there is DHEA or DHEAS of both adrenal and cerebral origins in the brain[7]. Brain steroid concentrations measured in a few human cadavers were in the same $10^{-8\pm1}$ mol/l range; the values, however, varied due to the heterogeneity of samples available[8,9]. Globally, it may be observed that in primates, which have sizable concentrations of DHEA and DHEAS in the blood, brain DHEA(S) is more abundant and PREG (or its sulfate, S) less abundant than in rodents. Also note that DHEA, PREG and their conjugates are found everywhere in the brain, even if there are some differences between certain regions (i.e. relatively more PREG in the olfactory bulb, more DHEA(S) in the hypothalamus in rats). As a whole, the concentrations of several steroids such as DHEA, PREG, their conjugates, and PROG and its 5α-metabolites, expressed in moles/volume equivalent of brain tissue weight, are relatively high in many instances, and possibly even higher than they appear because of compartmentation, the brain tissues being targets for paracrine/autocrine products.

Biosynthesis and metabolism of neurosteroids

3β-hydroxy-$\Delta5$-steroids PREG and DHEA are, in steroidogenic glands, intermediary compounds between cholesterol and active 3-oxo-$\Delta4$-steroids such as PROG and testosterone.

Cholesterol itself can be synthesized in many cells of the nervous system from low molecular weight precursors (for example mevalonate $\rightarrow$ cholesterol, PREG and metabolites in cultured glial cells)[10-12]. There is also evidence for lipoprotein receptors favoring cholesterol uptake, and thus availability for potential steroidogenesis (for example in glial cells)[13]. At the mitochondrial outer membrane level there is a protein, also a benzodiazepine binding entity[14,15], which favors the access of cholesterol to the inner membrane-linked side-chain cleavage enzymatic complex[16] transforming cholesterol (27 carbon atoms) into PREG (21 carbon atoms)[17]. The possibility of a link between pharmacological drug activity and neurosteroid synthesis is of striking interest. After a number of unsuccessful experiments to demonstrate enzymatic conversion of cholesterol to PREG in brain tissues and extracts, immunocytochemical evidence for the presence of the cytochrome P450scc, the specific hydroxylase involved in cholesterol side-chain cleavage, was obtained at the level of the white matter throughout the brain[18-20] (Figure 2), in rat and human. The two associated enzymes, adrenodoxin and adrenodoxin reductase, were correlatively observed. The presence and activity of P450scc in myelinating cells was verified in isolated oligodendrocytes (Figure 3) and Schwann cells, and biochemically confirmed in oligodendrocyte mitochondria[21]. Conversely, we have not yet found PREG synthesizing neurons, but some astrocytes are labelled in P450scc immuno-cytochemical detection experiments. These results have recently been confirmed by the detection of P450scc mRNA in oligodendrocytes[22,23]. Interestingly the P450scc gene

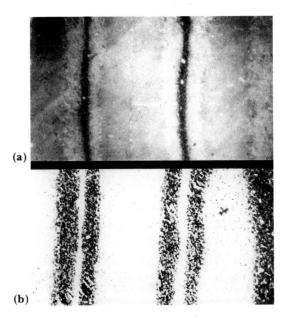

(a)

(b)

Figure 2 Rat cerebellum white matter stained with anti-P450scc antibody: (a) immuno-peroxidase staining, (b) histological staining. The same white matter staining is obtained throughout brain. Data from reference 18

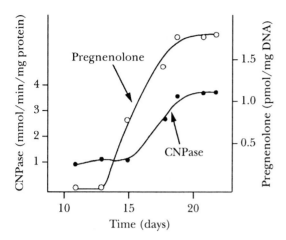

Figure 3 Newborn rat mixed glial cell cultures. Oligodendrocytes differentiated *in vitro*, as indicated by 2',3'-cyclic nucleotide phosphodiesterase (CNPase) activity, can synthesize (radioactive) pregnenolone (PREG) from (radioactive) mevalonate. Data from reference 10

expression may not involve the steroidogenic factor-1[24]. However, the available data are not quantitatively satisfactory, considering the relatively high level of PREG in the central nervous system (CNS)[25], and the regulatory mechanisms governing P450scc function are unknown (even though some cyclic adenosine monophosphate (cAMP)-induced increase in activity has been observed[7], particularly in retina[26]). Although the protein hormones stimulating steroid synthesis in peripheral glands are probably not involved, it remains to investigate the activities of a number of peptidic factors, such as insulin-like growth factor-1 (IGF-1), nerve growth factor (NGF), etc. in this respect.

Paradoxically, the formation of DHEA and of DHEAS in the CNS has not yet been clearly documented, even though the isolation of these steroids in the brain was at the origin of the neurosteroid concept[27], and the recognized precursor in glandular cells, PREG, was rapidly identified at a higher concentration, as indeed a biosynthetic precursor should be[2]. Currently, the possibility that DHEA (or conjugates) derives from cholesterol via unconventional pathways remains open[28].

Both PREG and DHEA are found in conjugated forms, sulfate esters and fatty acid esters ('lipoidal'), whose concentrations are frequently equal or superior to those of the corresponding free steroids (Table 1). Preliminary evidence has been obtained for a low sulfotransferase activity (Rajkowski and co-workers, in press); however, it can not be excluded that there is formation of steroid sulfate-containing lipidic complexes ('sulfolipids')[28]. The enzymes corresponding to the widely distributed steroid sulfatase activities of the brain have not been cloned. Major conjugation forms of PREG and DHEA in the brain are their fatty acid esters[29], designated 'lipoidal' derivatives[30]. The acyltransferase responsible for their formation is enriched in the microsomal fraction of the brain[31] and its activity is highest at the time of myelin formation.

While PREG (and PROG) can be largely reduced to give 20α-hydroxy-metabolites in glial cells and many neurons, no evidence for 17β-reduction of DHEA to give the weak estrogen Δ5-androsten-3β-17β-diol has been documented. The 7α-hydroxylation of 3β-hydroxy-Δ5-steroids can be performed by an enzyme distinct from the classical cholesterol hydroxylase found in the liver[32]. The 7α-hydroxy derivatives are of unknown biological significance.

As in steroidogenic gland cells and many peripheral tissues[33,34], DHEA and PREG can be oxidized to 3-oxo-Δ4-steroids (to Δ4-androstenedione and PROG, respectively) in the nervous system by the 3β-hydroxysteroid dehydrogenase-isomerase enzyme (3β-HSD)[35], which can be inhibited by specific steroidal compounds such as trilostane[36]. The 3β-HSD isoforms are present in most parts of the brain and in the peripheral nervous system (PNS), and are found in glial cells and neurons[37,38]. The metabolism of PREG and DHEA in astroglial cells is regulated by cell density: 3β-HSD activity is strongly inhibited at high cell density[39].

The formation and metabolism of PROG in the brain has been the subject of a number of studies since 5α-reduced PROG metabolites attracted the attention of pharmacologists in the context of their effects on γ-aminobutyric acid receptor (GABA$_A$R) function. Type-1 isozyme predominates in the brain. The 5α-reduced (dihydrogenated) metabolite of PROG, 5α-DHPROG, is in turn converted to 3α- and 3β-hydroxy-5α-pregnane-20-ones (3α/β, 5α-THPROG).

To date, there has been no demonstration of the synthesis of corticosteroids in the nervous system. For the synthesis of estrogens, the discovery of aromatase (P450$_{arom}$)[40,41] in the brain may be viewed as the first evidence for a steroid metabolism of physiological significance in the nervous system, and therefore the formation of estradiol from testicular testosterone in hypothalamic structures may be considered as that of a neurosteroid in males of several species. However, there has been no systematic study of Δ4-androstenedione which could be formed from neurosteroidal DHEA or PROG and is also an aromatase substrate. Other enzymatic reactions have been suggested, such as those involving 11β-, 18- and 19-hydroxylases[42–46]. Whether or not there may be formation of odorous Δ16-androstene derivatives is unknown[47].

In summary, even if many results are available, the global picture of neurosteroid metabolism is still incomplete and patchwork-like. The formation of PREG and PROG in myelinating glial cells is well established qualitatively, but its quantitative and regulatory aspects remain to be documented. The biosynthetic pathway of the neurosteroid DHEA is poorly understood. Sulfates of 3β-hydroxy-Δ5-steroids have been duly identified, but the related enzymology is obscure, whereas the metabolism and the significance of fatty acid esters are completely unknown. The 3β-HSD and 5α-reductase enzymes are definitively active in the nervous system, probably in many cell types, and are crucial to the formation of neurosteroids in appropriate amounts to be neuroactive[3], such as PROG and 3α,5α-THPROG. A number of questions remain, including the possible transfers of steroids from one cell type to another with successive further metabolism during these passages since the relevant enzymes are differentially located in neurons and glial cells[7,48,49], and also the important possibility that steroids entering the nervous system from the blood may not follow the same metabolic pathways as the same steroids synthesized in the nervous system. In that case, different effects on nervous function may be discovered.

Receptors of neurosteroids

To the diversity of neurosteroids themselves should be added that of the receptor systems.

Intracellular receptors

The distribution of intracellular receptors (Rs) in the brain has been described mainly on the basis of binding measurements, autoradiography of tritiated steroids and immunocytochemistry of receptor proteins[50]. Naturally these techniques do not distinguish between receptors for peripheral steroids and neurosteroids, and in any case very little has been done in terms of cloning and sequencing to determine whether receptors in the nervous system are or are not the same as in peripheral target tissues. We have biochemically and immunologically documented the presence of a PROGR in myelinating glial cells (oligodendrocytes of rats of both sexes and mouse and rat Schwann cells) and cloned it (Fiddes and colleagues, in preparation). In addition to the very remarkable presence of active PROGR in glial cells, two notions are of particular interest. The first is the capability of these cells to synthetize PROG from PREG (which itself may derive from cholesterol); therefore the cellular systems include a potential autocrine mechanism which could operate under controlling factors yet unknown. We shall see the functional significance of such a mechanism in Schwann cells in the appropriate section of this paper. The second notion is that the cloning of the ligand-binding domain of the glial PROGR from oligodendrocytes or Schwann cells indicates several aminoacid differences compared with both the uterine and the neuronal PROGR from the same animal.

Whether the pharmacology of PROG analogs may differ when interacting with the sexual (uterine, hypothalamic) or the glial (in CNS and peripheral nervous system (PNS)) PROG receptors is yet conjectural (unpublished data).

Membrane receptors

Some steroid metabolites can produce a rapid depression of the CNS activity, and it was reported in 1984[51] that alphaxalone (5α-pregnane-3α-ol-11,20-one) specifically and potently enhances GABA$_A$R-mediated hyperpolarization, when the 3β-hydroxy isomer is inactive.

A large number of biochemical and electrophysiological experiments have followed, demonstrating that natural (including neurosteroids) and synthetic steroids of very

specific structure are in fact potent allosteric modulators of GABA$_A$R function[52] (Figure 4). Now, besides the anesthetic and anticonvulsant activities of neurosteroids, hypnotic, anxyolytic and analgesic effects of these compounds have been reported[53–58]. Neurosteroids may also play an unexpected endocrine regulatory role via the GABA$_A$R[59–61].

The steroid 3α,5α-THPROG and its 5β-isomer, but not the corresponding 3β-hydroxy-steroid, enhance GABA-evoked currents at concentrations as low as 1 nmol/l. There is no absolute GABA$_A$R subunit specificity yet demonstrated for neurosteroids as there is for benzodiazepine binding. The polymorphism of GABA$_A$R in terms of subunit composition across the different cells of the nervous system, in neurons and glial cells, deserves more study in

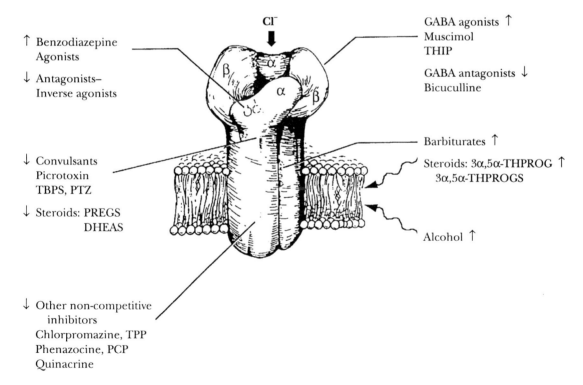

↑ Benzodiazepine
  Agonists

↓ Antagonists–
  Inverse agonists

↓ Convulsants
  Picrotoxin
  TBPS, PTZ

↓ Steroids: PREGS
  DHEAS

↓ Other non-competitive
  inhibitors
  Chlorpromazine, TPP
  Phenazocine, PCP
  Quinacrine

Cl⁻

GABA agonists ↑
Muscimol
THIP

GABA antagonists ↓
Bicuculline

Barbiturates ↑

Steroids: 3α,5α-THPROG ↑
         3α,5α-THPROGS

Alcohol ↑

Figure 4 Schematic cartoon of ligands stimulating (↑) or inhibiting (↓) γ-aminobutyric acid agonist receptor (GABA$_A$R) function (for review see reference 85). PREGS, pregnenolone sulfate; DHEAS, dehydroepiandrosterone sulfate; THPROG, trihydrogenated progesterone metabolite; TBPS, t-butylbicyclophorothionate; PTZ, pentylene tetrazole; TPP, tetraphenyl-phosphorium; PCP, phenylclidine; THIP, 4,5,6,7-tetrahydroisoxazolo(5,4c)pyridine-3-ol

order to discover steroid derivatives with specific functions. Another type of complexity comes from data obtained when considering the interaction of PREGS with GABA$_A$R. At very low concentrations, in the nanomolar range, the steroid is a weak enhancer of GABA-evoked currents, but at a micromolar concentration it produces a non-competitive voltage-independent inhibition[62] (due to reduced frequency of channel opening[63]). These effects may be observed *in vivo*[64] (Figure 5). DHEAS also is an allosteric inhibitor of the GABA$_A$R[65].

A global understanding of the potential effects of neurosteroids on neurotransmission should also take into account other modulatory activities displayed by the steroids. PREGS appears to allosterically potentiate the *N*-methyl-*D*-aspartate (NMDA) receptor[66] (Figure 6), and this effect may functionally reinforce the antagonistic effect of the same steroid on GABA$_A$R and on the glycine receptor. PREGS also inhibits non-NMDA glutamate receptors. Other modulatory activities of neurosteroids have been described on glycine-activated chloride channels[67], on neural nicotinic acetylcholine receptors reconstituted in *Xenopus laevis* oocytes[68], and on voltage-activated calcium channels[69]. Sigma receptors, as pharmacologically defined by their effect on NMDA receptor (NMDAR) activity, have been studied in rat hippocampal preparations: here DHEAS acts as a sigma receptor agonist, differently from PREGS which appears as a sigma inverse agonist (Figure 7), and PROG which behaves as a sigma antagonist[70].

Are there other specific membrane receptors the ligands of which are primarily neurosteroids, in contrast with the preceding examples indicating an allosteric effect upon neurotransmitter receptors and ion channels? Rapid effects of steroids may be explained by such novel receptors[71,72]. A G-protein coupled corticosteroid receptor has been identified in synaptic membranes from an amphibian brain[73]. Studies have indicated specific binding of PROG conjugated with a macromolecule (albumin in general) to different cellular or membrane preparations, but its biological relevance has not been determined[74]. We also

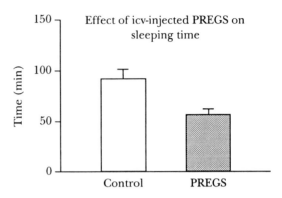

Figure 5 Pregnenolone sulfate (PREGS) inhibits γ-aminobutyric acid receptor (GABA$_A$R) function *in vivo*. Data from reference 64

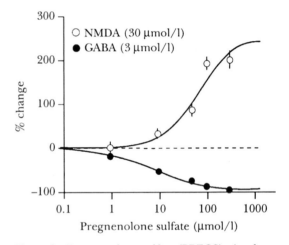

Figure 6 Pregnenolone sulfate (PREGS) stimulates NMDA receptor (NMDAR) function. GABA, γ-aminobutyric acid. Data from reference 66

found selective binding of steroid sulfates to purified neural membranes of yet unknown biological significance[75].

Physiological and pathological aspects

Behavior

We observed an increase of brain DHEAS related to surgical (adrenalectomy and gonadectomy) stress conditions in the rat[1].

We also observed that the exposure of male rats to females (Figure 8) leads to a decrease of PREG in the rat olfactory bulb, an effect

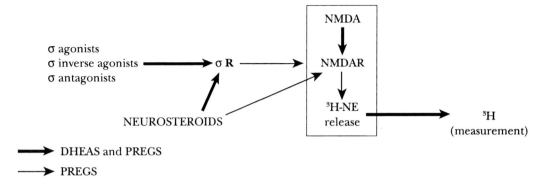

Figure 7 Neurosteroids modulate NMDAR function via sigma receptor (σR). NMDA evokes ^{3}H-norepinephrine (NE) release from preloaded rat hippocampal slices. DHEAS, dehydroepiandrosterone sulfate; PREGS, pregnenolone sulfate

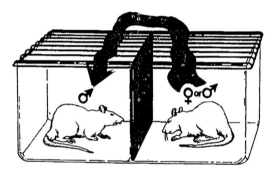

Figure 8 Pregnenolone (PREG) is selectively decreased in olfactory bulb of male rat exposed to 'odor' (pheromone?) of female rat. Data from reference 76

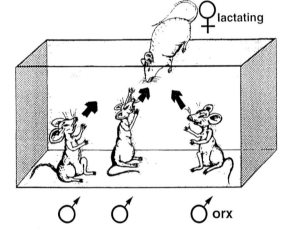

Figure 9 Pregnenolone sulfate (PREGS) is selectively decreased in brain when aggression of castrated (orx) male mice towards female intruder is inhibited by dehydroepiadrosterone (DHEA) administration. Data from reference 36

apparently due to a pheromonal stimulus, ovarian-dependent in the females, and testosterone-dependent in males (orchidectomy suppresses the response and testosterone re-establishes it)[76].

A particular model of aggression in castrated male mice (Figure 9), inhibited by testosterone or estrogen administration, has also been studied[77,78]. The stimulus is the introduction of a lactating female into a cage containing three resident orchidectomized males. The administration of DHEA (280 nmol for 15 days) decreases the males' aggression. This does not seem to be due to a transformation of DHEA into brain testosterone (which has been measured), and indeed a DHEA derivative (3β-methyl-Δ5-androsten-17-one), which is not converted to androgens or estrogens and is devoid of any hormonal activity, is at least as active as DHEA itself. Interestingly we found a progressive and significant decrease of PREGS in the brain, which may be related to the decrease of aggression (experiments have excluded the possibility that an increase of 3α-5α-THPROG, activating the calming GABA$_A$R, was responsible).

Other behavioral changes have been found correlated to changes of neurosteroid concentrations in the brain. In particular, in the cases of increased production or administration of PROG or deoxycorticosterone, in the brain elevation has occurred of the related 3α-hydroxy-5α-reduced tetrahydro-metabolites (3α-5α-THPROG and 3α,5α-tetrahydrodeoxy-corticosterone), both agonists for the GABA$_A$R, which may therefore be responsible for corresponding behaviors in pregnancy or stress, respectively[53,79].

Cognitive performance

The study of cognitive performance in deficient aging rats has been particularly rewarding (Vallée and colleagues, submitted) (Figure 10). We found that PREGS is significantly lower in the hippocampus of aged (24-month-old rats) than in young (male) animals (Figure 10). Interestingly, the individual concentration (ng/g) of PREGS in the hippocampus of aged animals was widely distributed, between ~2 and ~28 ng/g of tissue. The animals had previously been classified according to their performance in two tasks for spatial memory, the Morris water maze and the two-trial test in a Y maze (Figure 10b)[80]: low levels of PREGS in hippocampus were correlated with poor performance in both tasks (Figure 10c). When aged rats which had been classified as memory-impaired received a single dose (by intraperitoneal injection) of PREGS, their performance was significantly improved, albeit transiently (Figure 10d). Both the physiological approach (measurement of endogenous neurosteroid levels) and the pharmacological approach (effect of administered PREGS) suggest strongly that hippocampal PREGS is involved in the maintenance of cognitive performances. These observations are consistent with the results of systemic or intracerebral administration of PREG or derivatives in rodents, enhancing their natural memory performances or antagonizing pharmacologically induced amnesia[81,82]. In most experiments, however, the procedure involves alteration of the motivational or emotional states of the animals, and the direct relationship between the administered dose and endogenous steroid concentration has yet to be established. We have thus described, for the first time, changes of a neurosteroid with age, individual differences and the correlation of these differences with behavioral performance, plus the improvement of performance in impaired PREGS-deficient aged animals by administration of the steroid.

These results are determinant in attributing a physiological significance to a neurosteroid. However, the molecular aspects of the involvement of PREGS in memory, i.e. the steroid's metabolism as well as receptors and enzymes involved, remain to be worked out.

Trophic action: myelination

In a completely different field, namely myelin repair in a wounded peripheral nerve, there is also a clear-cut demonstration of the physiological function of a neurosteroid. We found PREG in the sciatic nerve of human cadavers at a mean concentration ≥ 100-fold the plasma level of the steroid[83], suggesting a possible biosynthesis that we guessed to be in Schwann cells, by analogy with that which has previously been obtained in oligodendrocytes. The experimental simplicity of working with the PNS led to studying the regeneration of cryolesioned sciatic nerve in mice. We measured PREG and PROG in the sciatic nerve of normal animals and after adrenalectomy and gonadectomy (Figure 11). The levels of the two steroids are much higher in the nerve than in the plasma, while the corticosterone concentration is much lower in nerve than in plasma. After surgical endocrine ablation, PREG and PROG remained high in nerve and corticosterone decreased in blood.

After cryolesion[84] (Figure 12a), axons and their accompanying myelin sheaths degenerate quickly in the frozen zone and the distal segments (Wallerian degeneration). However, the intact basal lamina tubes provide an appropriate environment for regeneration. Schwann cells start to proliferate and myelinate

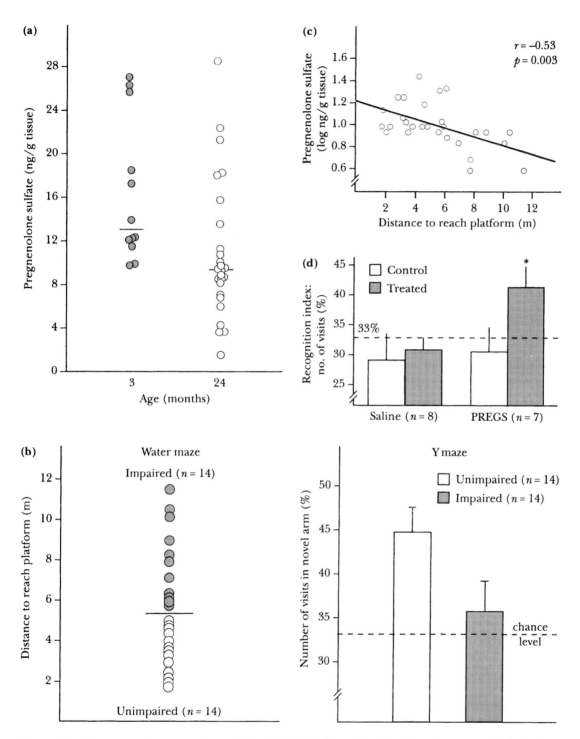

Figure 10 Hippocampal pregnenolone sulfate (PREGS) is lower in old rats than in young rats, but values are scattered (a); memory tasks classify old rats in impaired and unimpaired animals (b); hippocampal PREGS and memory-task impairment (water maze) are inversely correlated (c); administration of PREGS temporarily improves memory performance in two-trial task for impaired rats (d)

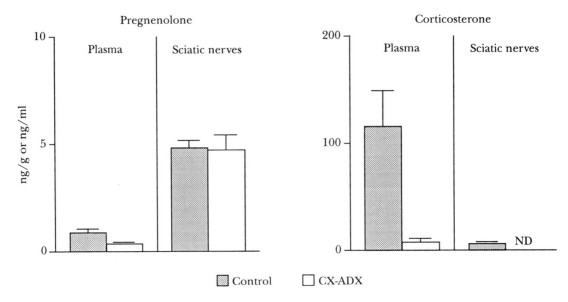

Figure 11 Pregnenolone in male rat sciatic nerve measured by radioimmunoassay: castration (CX) and adrenalectomy (ADX) have no effect. Data from reference 84

the regenerating fibers after 1 week, and, 2 weeks after surgery, myelin sheaths have reached about one-third of their final width. In the damaged portion of the nerve, PREG and PROG levels remain high, and even increase 15 days after lesion (if expressed in pg/cm).

The role of PROG in myelin repair, assessed after 2 weeks, was indicated by the decrease of thickness (number of lamellae) of myelin sheaths when trilostane, an inhibitor of 3β-HSD involved in the PREG to PROG transformation, was applied to the lesioned nerve (Figure 12b), or alternatively, when RU486 was locally delivered in order to competitively antagonize PROG action at the receptor level (Figure 12c) (as indicated before, we had detected a PROG-R immunologically and by binding studies in Schwann cells). The inhibitory action of trilostane (Figure 12b) could not be attributed to toxicity since its effect was reversed by the simultaneous administration of PROG. We could even enhance remyelination with a high dose of either PREG or PROG. In this *in vivo* system, the structure of the myelin sheaths formed in response to neurosteroids, as

determined by electron microscopy, was morphologically normal.

Such an effect was also apparent in cultures of rat dorsal-root ganglia (DRG). After 4 weeks in culture, neurite elongation and Schwann cell proliferation had ceased and, in the appropriate medium, the presence of a physiological concentration of PROG (20 nmol/l) for 2 weeks did not further increase the area occupied by the neurite network, the density of neurites, or the number of Schwann cells, but it did increase the number of myelin segments and the total length of myelinated axons about six-fold (Figure 13).

Mechanistically, several hypotheses may be raised: PROG produced by Schwann cells may act on adjacent neurons and activate the expression of neuronal signalling molecules required for myelination. Alternatively, PROG may function as an autocrine trophic factor and directly enhance the formation of new myelin sheaths. We are currently studying the effect of PROG on the expression of myelin specific proteins. We also analyze the reciprocal influences of neurons and Schwann cells on each other, in terms of Schwann cell

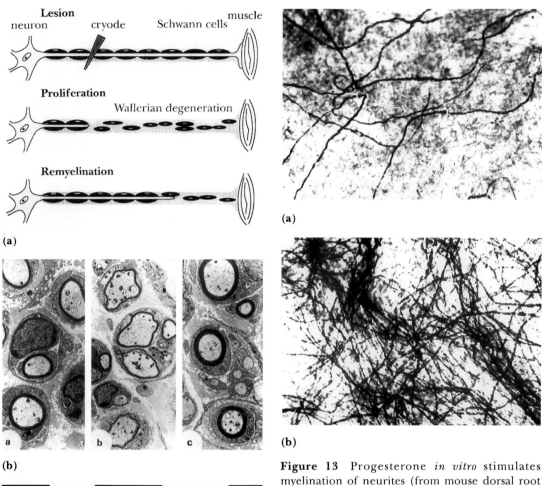

(a)

(b)

(c)

Figure 12 Cryolesion of sciatic nerve occurs in three steps (a); remyelination: effect of the blockade of 3β-hydroxysteroid dehydrogenase (HSD) by trilostane (b); antagonism of progesterone (PROG) at PROG receptor by RU486 (c). Data from reference 84

Figure 13 Progesterone *in vitro* stimulates myelination of neurites (from mouse dorsal root ganglia in culture). (a) No progesterone; (b) progesterone 20 nmol/l. Data from reference 84

proliferation and protein synthesis, and metabolism of PREG and PROG in both cell types (Figure 14). It is worth noting that the rather high concentrations of PROG in intact adult nerves suggest a role for this neurosteroid in the slow but continuous renewal of peripheral myelin. It is quite interesting that PROG, a classical sex steroid, is also an active neurosteroid very probably synthesized and active independently of any sexual context. If similar results are obtained with CNS elements of human origin, we may soon have to work on the possible therapeutic effect of PROG analogs, for treating or preventing certain demyelinating pathological conditions.

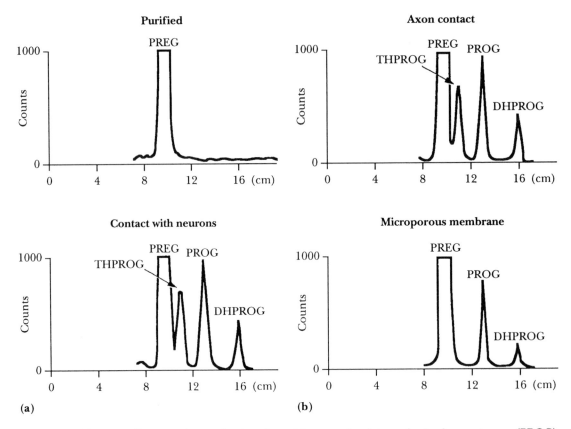

Figure 14 Schwann cell–neuron interaction in culture. Neurons stimulate synthesis of progesterone (PROG) from pregnenolone (PREG) by a diffusible substance (a), while formation of 3α,5α-trihydrogenated progesterone metabolite (THPROG) necessitates axonal contact (b). DHPROG, dihydrogenated PROG

Conclusions

Neurosteroids are synthesized in the central and peripheral nervous system, particularly in myelinating glial cells, but also in astrocytes and many neurons, and act in the nervous system. Synthetic pathways may start from cholesterol or from steroidal precursor(s) imported from peripheral sources. Measured concentrations of neurosteroids are consistent with the affinities of receptor systems with which they interact in the nervous system. Both intracellular and membrane receptors responding to neurosteroids can be distinguished (Figure 15). For the former, receptors are identical or similar to those of steroid hormones found in peripheral target organs; a PROG-R in particular has been found in oligodendrocytes

and Schwann cells, evoking the possibility of an autocrine system for PROG action. For the latter, neurosteroids in the brain are in fact allosteric modulators of neurotransmitter receptors, and their levels are compatible with their playing a physiological neuromodulatory role; this is the case with the GABA$_A$R, and also the NMDAR, sigma 1-R and others. Besides numerous experiments of a pharmacological nature consistent with well-defined properties of several neurosteroids, there are now results which demonstrate a contribution of steroids formed endogenously and accumulated in the nervous system independently, at least in part, of any contribution from the steroidogenic glands. PROG synthesized in Schwann cells has 'trophic' activity; it contributes to the synthesis of myelin in regenerating sciatic nerve in rats

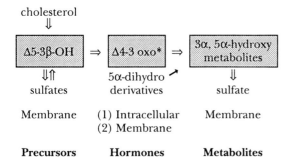

cholesterol
⇓

Δ5-3β-OH ⇒ Δ4-3 oxo* ⇒ 3α, 5α-hydroxy metabolites

⇓⇑   5α-dihydro ↗   ⇓
sulfates   derivatives   sulfate

Membrane   (1) Intracellular   Membrane
           (2) Membrane

Precursors   **Hormones**   **Metabolites**

Figure 15 In the nervous system, steroidal precursors, metabolites of hormones and hormones themselves exert activity through either membrane or intracellular receptors, or both

and mice, and the effect can be demonstrated *in vivo* and *in vitro*. PREGS has a behavioral effect in aged (2-year-old) rats: the concentration of PREGS in the hippocampus (and not in other parts of the brain) is inversely correlated with the quantified impairment of an individual's accomplishment of each of two memory tasks in a Y maze and a water maze, and we obtained temporary improvement after PREGS administration. Therefore it is important to study the neuromodulatory role of neurosteroids in situations such as the estrous cycle, pregnancy, menopause and stress and their influence on sexual behavior, memory and the developmental and aging processes. Available data suggest that the neurosteroid concept may also be applicable to humans, and the robust and specific activities of neurosteroids may become useful for enlarging therapeutic approaches to functional and trophic alterations of the nervous system.

Acknowledgements

I would like to thank researchers and students of my laboratory, and colleagues from many others institutions who helped to collect the data reported in this presentation. I would especially like to thank first of all P. Robel and his wise and persistent contributions, and for many years C. Corpéchot, I. Jung-Testas, B. Eychenne, M. El-Etr and C. Le Goascogne and more recently Y. Akwa, K. Rajkowski and M. Schumacher.

Laboratory work has been mainly supported by INSERM. I gratefully acknowledge the help of the Centre National pour la Recherche Scientifique (CNRS), the College de France, Roussel-Uclaf, l'Association pour la Recherche de la Sclérose en Plaque (ARSEP), l'Association Française contre les Myopathies (AFM), the Mathers Foundation, the Myelin Project and Mme P. Schlumberger. I also thank F. Boussac, C. Legris and J.C. Lambert for preparing the manuscript.

References

1. Corpéchot, C., Robel, P., Axelson, M., Sjövall, J. and Baulieu E. E. (1981). *Proc. Natl. Acad. Sci.*, **78**, 4704–7
2. Corpéchot, C., Synguelakis, M., Talha, S., Axelson, M., Sjövall, J., Vihko, R., Baulieu, E. E. and Robel, P. (1983). *Brain Res.*, **270**, 119–25
3. Corpéchot, C., Young, J., Calvel, M., Wehrey, C., Veltz, J. N., Touyer, G., Mouren, M., Prasad, V. V. K., Banner, C., Sjövall, J., Baulieu, E.E. and Robel, P. (1993). *Endocrinology*, **13**, 1003–9
4. Synguelakis, M., Halberg, F., Baulieu, E. E. and Robel, P. (1985). *C.R. Acad. Sci. Paris*, **301**, 823–6
5. Robel, P., Synguelakis, M., Halberg, F. and Baulieu, E. E. (1986). *C.R. Acad. Sci. Paris*, **303**, 235–8
6. Robel, P. and Baulieu, E. E. (1985). *Neurochem. Int.*, **7**, 953–8
7. Robel, P., Bourreau, E., Corpéchot, C., Dang, D. C., Halberg, F., Clarke, C., Haug, M., Schlegel, M. L., Synguelakis, M., Vourc'h, C. and Baulieu, E. E. (1987). *J. Steroid Biochem.*, **27**, 649–55
8. Lanthier, A. and Patwardhan, V. V. (1986). *J. Steroid Biochem.*, **25**, 445–9
9. Lacroix, C., Fiet, J., Benais, J.P., Gueux, B., Bonete, R., Villette, J. M., Gourmet, B. and Dreux, C. (1987). *J. Steroid Biochem.*, **28**, 317–25
10. Jung-Testas, I., Hu, Z. Y., Baulieu, E. E. and Robel, P. (1989). *Endocrinology*, **125**, 2083–91
11. Hu, Z. Y., Jung-Testas, I., Robel, P. and Baulieu, E. E. (1989). *Biochem. Biophys. Res. Commun.*, **161**, 917–22

12. Jurevics, H. and Morell, P. (1995). *J. Neurochem.*, **64**, 895–901

13. Jung-Testas, I., Weintraub, H., Dupuis, D., Eychenne, B., Baulieu, E. E. and Robel, P. (1992). *J. Steroid Biochem. Mol. Biol.*, **42**, 597–605

14. Yanagibachi, K., Ohno, Y., Kawamura, M. and Hall, P. F. (1988). *Endocrinology*, **123**, 2075–82

15. Costa, E., Romeo, R., Auta, J., Papadopoulos, V., Kozilowski, A. and Guidotti, A. (1991). In Costa, E. and Paul, S. M. (eds.) *Neurosteroid and Brain Function*, pp. 171–6. Fidia Research Foundation Symposium Series. (New York: Thieme Medical Publishers)

16. Oftebro, H., Stormer, F. C. and Pederson, J. I. (1979). *J. Biol. Chem.*, **264**, 4331–4

17. Papadopoulos, V. (1993). *Endocr. Rev.*, **14**, 222–40

18. Le Goascogne, C., Robel, P., Gouezou, M., Sananes, N., Baulieu, E. E. and Waterman, M. (1987). *Science*, **237**, 1212–15

19. Le Goascogne, C., Gouezou, M., Robel, P., Defaye, G., Chambaz, E., Waterman, M.R. and Baulieu, E. E. (1989). *J. Neuroendocrinol.*, **1**, 153–6

20. Iwahashi, K., Ozaki, H. S., Tsubaki, M., Ohniski, J., Taheuchi, Y. and Ichikawa, Y. (1990). *Biochim. Biophys. Acta*, **1035**, 182–9

21. Hu, Z. Y., Jung-Testas, I., Robel, P. and Baulieu, E. E. (1987). *Proc. Natl. Acad. Sci. USA*, **84**, 8215–19

22. Mellon, S. H. and Deschepper, C. F. (1993). *Brain Res.*, **629**, 283–92

23. Compagnone, N. A., Bulfone, A., Rubenstein, J. R. and Mellon S. H. (1995). *Endocrinology*, **136**, 2689–96

24. Zhang, P., Rodriguez, H. and Mellon, S. L. (1995). *Mol. Endocrinol.*, **9**, 1571–82

25. Warner, M. and Gustafsson, J. A. (1995). *Front. Neuroendocrinol.*, **16**, 224–36

26. Guarneri, P., Guarneri, R., Cascia, C., Paravant, P., Piccoli, F. and Papadopoulos, V. (1994). *J. Neurochem.*, **63**, 86–96

27. Baulieu, E. E. (1981). In Fuxe, K., Gustafsson, J. A. and Wetterberg, L. (eds.) *Steroid Hormone Regulation of the Brain*, pp. 3–14. (Oxford: Pergamon)

28. Prasad, W. W. K., Raju Vegesnas, S., Welsch, M. and Lieberman, S. (1994). *Proc. Natl. Acad. Sci. USA*, **91**, 3220–3

29. Jo, D. H., Abdallah, M. A., Jung, I., Baulieu, E. E. and Robel, P. (1989). *Steroids*, **54**, 287–97

30. Hochberg, R. B., Bandy, L., Ponticorvo, L. and Lieberman, S. (1976). *Proc. Natl. Acad. Sci. USA*, **74**, 941–5

31. Vourc'h, C., Eychenne, B., Jo, D. H., Raulin, J., Lapous, D., Baulieu, E. E. and Robel, P. (1992). *Steroids*, **57**, 210–15

32. Akwa, Y., Morfin, R. F., Robel, P. and Baulieu, E. E. (1992). *Biochem. J.*, **228**, 959–64

33. Vande Wiele, R. L., McDonald, P. C., Gurpide, E. and Lieberman, S. (1965). *Rec. Prog. Horm. Res.*, **19**, 275–305

34. Labrie, F. (1991). *Mol. Cell. Endocrinol.*, **78**, C113–18

35. Labrie, F., Simard, J., Luu The, V., Belanger, A., Lachana, Y., Zhao, F., Labrie, C., Breton, N., De Launoit, Y., Dupont, I. M., Rhéaume, M., Martel, C., Couët, J. and Trudel, C. (1992). *J. Steroid Biochem. Mol. Biol.*, **41**, 421–35

36. Young, J., Corpéchot, C., Perche, F., Haug, M., Baulieu, E. E. and Robel, P. (1994). *Endocrinology*, **2**, 505–9

37. Guennoun, R., Fiddes, R. J., Gouezou, M., Lombes, M. and Baulieu, E. E. (1995). *Mol. Brain Res.*, **30**, 287–300

38. Sanne, J. L. and Krueger, K. E. (1995). *Neurochemistry*, **65**, 528–36

39. Akwa, Y., Sananes, N., Gouezou, M., Robel, P., Baulieu, E. E. and Le Goascogne, C. (1993). *J. Cell. Biol.*, **121**, 135–43

40. Naftolin, F., Ryan, K. J., Davies, I. J., Reddy, V. V., Flores, F., Petra, Z., Kuhn, M., White, R. J., Takaoka, Y. and Wolin, J. (1975). *Rec. Prog. Horm. Res.*, **31**, 295–319

41. MacLusky, N. J., Walters, M. J., Clark, A. S. and Toran-Allerand, C. D. (1994). *Mol. Cell. Neurosci.*, **5**, 691–8

42. Osaki, H. S., Iwahashi, K., Tsukaki, M., Fukui, Y., Ichikawa, Y. and Takeuchi, J. (1991). *J. Neurosci. Res.*, **28**, 518–24

43. Iwahashi, K., Kawai, Y., Suwaki, H., Hosokawa, K. and Ichikawa, Y. (1993). *J. Steroid Biochem. Mol. Biol.*, **44**, 163–9

44. Compagnone, N. A., Bulfone, A., Rubenstein, J. R. and Mellon, S. H. (1995). *Endocrinology*, **136**, 5212–23

45. Gomez-Sanchez, C.E., Morita, H., Zhou, M., Cozza, E.N. and Gomez-Sanchez, E.P. (1996). *Endocr. Soc. Meet. Poster*, P2–788

46. Miyairi, S., Sugita, O., Sassa, S. and Fishman, J. (1988). *Biochem. Biophys. Res. Commun.*, **150**, 311–5

47. Gower, D. B. and Ruparalia, B. A. (1993). *J. Endocrinol.*, **137**, 167–87

48. Melcangi, R. C., Celotti, F. and Martini, L. (1994). *Brain Res.*, **639**, 202–6

49. Pelletier, G., Luu The, V. and Labrie, F. (1994). *Mol. Cell. Neurosci.*, **5**, 394–9

50. McEwen, B. S. (1991). *Trends Pharmacol. Sci.*, **12**, 141–6

51. Harrison, N. L. and Simmonds, M. A. (1984). *Brain Res.*, **323**, 287–92

52. Majewska, M. D., Harrison, N. L., Schwartz, R. D., Barker, J. L. and Paul, S. M. (1986). *Science*, **232**, 1004–7

53. Majewska, M. D. (1992). *Prog. Neurobiol.*, **38**, 379–95

54. Gee, K. W., McCauley, L. D. and Lan, N. C. (1995). *Crit. Rev. Neurobiol.*, **9**, 207–27

55. Bäckström, T. (1995). *Non-Reproductive Actions of Sex Steroids*, CIBA Foundation Symposium No. 191, pp. 171–80. (Chichester: Wiley)

56. Lambert, J., Belelli, D., Hill-Venning, C., Callachan, H. and Peters, J. A. (1996). *Cell. Mol. Neurobiol.*, **16**, 155–74

57. Purdy, R. H., Morrow, A. L., Moore, P. H. Jr and Paul, S. M. (1991). *Proc. Natl. Acad. Sci. USA*, **88**, 4553–7

58. Schumacher, M., Coirini, H., Johnson, A. E., Flanagan, L. M., Frankfurt, M., Pfaff, D. W. and McEwen, B. S. (1993). *Regul. Pept.*, **45**, 115–19

59. Brann, D. W., Hendry, L. B. and Mahesh, V. B. (1995). *J. Steroid Biochem. Mol. Biol.*, **52**, 113–33

60. El-Etr, M., Akwa, Y., Fiddes, R. J., Robel, P. and Baulieu E. E. (1995). *Proc. Natl. Acad. Sci. USA*, **92**, 3769–73

61. Genazzani, A. R., Salvestroni, C., Guo, A. L., Palumbo, M., Cela, V., Casarosa, E., Luisi, M., Genazzani, A. D. and Petraglia, F. (1996). In Genazzani, A. R., Petraglia, F. and Purdy, R. H. (eds.) *The Brain: Sources and Target for Sex Steroid Hormones*, pp. 83–91. (Casterton, UK: Parthenon Publishing)

62. Majewska, M. D., Mienville, J. M. and Vicini, S. (1987). *Neurosci. Lett.*, **90**, 279–84

63. Mienville, J. L. and Vicini, S. (1989). *Brain Res.*, **489**, 190–4

64. Majewska, M. D., Bluet-Pajot, M. T., Robel, P. and Baulieu, E. E. (1989). *Pharmacol. Biochem. Behav.*, **33**, 701–3

65. Majewska, M. D., Demirgören, S., Spiwak, C. E. and London, E. D. (1990). *Brain Res.*, **526**, 143–6

66. Wu, F. S., Gibbs, T. T. and Farb, D. H. (1991). *Mol. Pharmacol.*, **40**, 333–6

67. Prince, R. J. and Simmonds, M. A. (1992). *Neuropharmacology*, **31**, 201–5

68. Valera, S., Ballivet, M. and Bertrand, D. (1992). *Proc. Natl. Acad. Sci. USA*, **89**, 9949–53

69. ffrench-Mullen, J. M. H., Danks, P. and Spence, K. (1994). *J. Neurosci.*, **14**, 1963–77.

70. Monnet, F. P., Mahé, V., Robel, P. and Baulieu, E. E. (1995). *Proc. Natl. Acad. Sci. USA*, **92**, 3774–8

71. Smith, S. S., Waterhouse, B. D. and Woodward, D. J. (1987). *Brain Res.*, **422**, 40–51

72. Schumacher, M., Coirini, H., Pfaff, D. W. and McEwen, B. S. (1990). *Science*, **250**, 691–4

73. Orchinik, M., Murray, T. and Moore, F. L. (1991). *Science*, **252**, 1848–51

74. Tischkau, S. A. and Ramirez, V. D. (1993). *Proc. Natl. Acad. Sci. USA*, **90**, 1285–9

75. Robel, P. and Baulieu, E. E. (1994). *Trends Endocrinol. Metab.*, **5**, 1–18

76. Corpéchot, C., Leclerc, P., Baulieu, E. E. and Brazeau, P. (1985). *Steroids*, **45**, 229–34

77. Haug, M., Ouss-Schlegel, M. L., Spetz, J. F., Brain, P. F., Simon, V., Baulieu, E. E. and Robel, P. (1989). *Physiol. Behav.*, **46**, 955–9

78. Young, J., Corpéchot, C., Haug, M., Gobaille, S., Baulieu, E. E. and Robel, P. (1991). *Biochem. Biophys. Res. Commun.*, **174**, 892–7

79. Paul, S. M. and Purdy, R. H. (1992). *FASEB J.*, **6**, 2311–22

80. Mayo, W., Dellu, F., Robel, P., Cherkaoui, J., Le Moal, M., Baulieu, E. E. and Simon, H. (1993). *Brain Res.*, **607**, 324–8

81. Flood, J. F., Morley, J. F. and Roberts, E. (1992). *Proc. Natl. Acad. Sci. USA*, **89**, 1567–71

82. Mathis, C., Paul, S. M. and Crawley, J. (1994). *Psychopharmacology*, **116**, 201–6

83. Morfin, R., Young, J., Corpéchot, C., Egestad, B., Sjövall, J. and Baulieu, E. E. (1992). *Proc. Natl. Acad. Sci. USA*, **89**, 6790–3

84. Koenig, H., Schumacher, M., Ferzaz, B., Do-Thi, A. N., Ressouches, A., Guennoun, R., Jung-Testas, I., Robel, P., Akwa, Y. and Baulieu, E. E. (1995). *Science*, **268**, 1500–3

85. MacDonald, R. L. and Olsen, R. W. (1994). *Ann. Rev. Neurosci.*, **17**, 569–602

Estrogen treatment for senile dementia-Alzheimer's type

H. Honjo, M. Urabe, K. Iwasa, T. Okubo, H. Tsuchiya, N. Kikuchi, T. Yamamoto, S. Fushiki, T. Mizuno, K. Nakajima, M. Hayashi and K. Hayashi

Introduction

With the aging of the population, senile dementia-Alzheimer's type (AD) has become one of the most serious diseases in the world. However, there are no effective drugs which improve cognitive functions in AD, i.e. immediate, recent and remote memories. Estrogen may be an effective method to treat and prevent AD. This paper explains the background, clinical effects, mechanisms and possible prevention using estrogen.

Endogenous level of estrogen in AD

Senile dementia-Alzheimer's type is more common among women than men. In women, the incidence of AD increases after the menopause. Fillit and colleagues[1] reported the first open trial of estradiol-17β (E_2) therapy for AD. They administered micronized E_2, 2 mg/day, over a 6-week period to seven women with AD. Three of the seven women responded. Clinical symptoms, including attention, orientation, mood and social interaction were improved.

The main form of estrogen in women before menopause is E_2, but after menopause the main form of estrogen is estrone sulfate (E_1-S) which comes from dehydro-epiandrosterone (DHEA) and/or its sulfate after aromatization mainly in peripheral fat tissues. The level of serum estrone sulfate in postmenopausal women without any hormonal treatment was measured by direct radioimmunoassay[2,3]. The serum level of E_1-S in 18 women with AD was significantly lower than that in age-matched women without AD.

Estrogen treatment for AD

Thus, we treated seven women (80.1 ± 2.9 years, Mean ± SD), suffering from probable AD, with conjugated estrogen (CE, main content: E_1-S) at a dose of 1.25 mg/day over a 6-week period, and improvements in memory, orientation and calculation were observed from the 3rd week[4]. A simple screening test for dementia, the Hasegawa scale (HDS), showed increased scores, indicating improvement of symptoms in five women. Another new screening test for dementia developed by the Japanese National Institute of Mental Health (NSD)[5] also showed increased scores, indicating improvement of symptoms in six women. Untreated women with AD did not show any improvement.

Another eight women with probable AD were treated with a low dose of CE, cyclically (0.625 mg/day for 3 weeks plus no estrogen for 1 week) over a period of six cycles. Both HDS and the mini mental status examination (MMS)[6] indicated improvements.

Double-blind study

To confirm the effect, a placebo-controlled double-blind study[7,8] was performed in 14 women (83.7 ± 4.5 years, Mean ± SD) with probable AD. Conjugated estrogen (1.25 mg/day) or placebo was given for 3 weeks. Three psychometric tests, the revised version of Hasegawa's dementia scale (HDS-R)[9], NSD and MMS were administered just before the trial, and during the 3rd week of the study. Only the group treated with estrogen (seven women) showed significant improvements in the scores. In the HDS-R and MMS, significant ($p < 0.05$)

improvement was seen in immediate memory. None of the HDS-R, NSD and MMS scores in the placebo group were significantly changed.

Side-effects

Estrogen treatments cause uterine bleeding even in 71% of older women[4]. To reduce uterine bleeding and to inhibit estrogen-induced tumors, we administered estrogen in combination with progestogen: CE (1.25 mg/day) was given for 7 weeks to 13 women with AD, and 2.5 mg/day of medroxyprogesterone acetate was added during the 4th to the 7th week. The scores in HDS-R and NSD were increased (improved, $p < 0.05$) in the 3rd week, but slightly decreased in the 6th week compared with the 3rd week. Breakthrough bleeding occurred in eight patients (62%, 83.4 ± 6.5 years, Mean $\pm$ SD) and withdrawal bleeding occurred in three patients (86.0 ± 3.6 years). No bleeding was noted in two patients (80 and 90 years). There was no significant difference between patients due to age. Uterine bleeding occurred in 11 of 13 patients (85%) which was not significantly different from the 71% shown previously.

In the next study, CE (0.625 mg/day) was given for 7 weeks to another nine women with AD, and 1 mg/day of norethisterone and 50 µg/day of mestranol were added during the 4th to the 7th week. The scores on HDS-R, NSD and MMS were increased (improved, $p < 0.05$, $p < 0.01$ and $p < 0.05$, respectively) in the 3rd week, but again decreased in the 6th week compared with scores in the 3rd week. Breakthrough bleeding was reduced to 22% (two of nine patients), but withdrawal bleeding was not reduced (56%, five of nine). Uterine bleeding still occurred in 78% (seven of nine). Other kinds of progestogen and various ways of administering them should be further examined, but at present, estrogen only without progestogen might be used to improve the quality of life for women with AD.

Mechanisms of improvement with estrogen

The mechanisms by which estrogen has ameliorative effects in AD are still unknown. At present, the following mechanisms are considered. Some mechanisms may be combined, contributing to beneficial effects on clinical symptoms.

Improvement of depressive status

Klaiber and co-workers[10] reported that large doses of CE therapy (5–25 mg/day) gave pharmacological benefits to premenopausal and postmenopausal women suffering from depression. Gerdes and associates[11] showed significant improvements in depression and anxiety in climacteric women with a regimen including the usual dose of CE (1.25 mg/day). We frequently encountered improvements of mood and depressive status in climacteric women with the usual doses of CE (0.625–1.25 mg/day). A depressive state frequently occurs in patients with AD, especially in the early stage when the patient becomes aware of her disabilities. An improvement in the depressive status by administering estrogen may make the patient more active and improve scores on psychometric tests for AD.

Improvement of cerebral blood flow

By single-photon emission computerized tomography, Ohkura and colleagues[12,13] observed an improvement of regional cerebral blood flow in the right lower frontal region and primary motor area resulting from long-term treatment with CE. Recently, Rosano and co-workers[14] administered 1 mg E_2 sublingually, and reported direct, immediate and beneficial effects of estrogen on exercise-induced myocardial ischemia in women with coronary artery disease. Sarrel[15] reported one patient who complained of migraine. A dose of E_2 1 mg was administered sublingually, and systolic and diastolic blood flow were measured using transcranial Doppler ultrasound. Four minutes later, E_2 appeared in the blood circulation. Seven minutes later, systolic and diastolic blood flow began to increase in the middle cerebral artery and the migraine began to disappear.

Acute and chronic improvement of cerebral blood flow by estrogen administration may have beneficial effects on cognitive impairment.

Direct effect on neural cells

Several investigators have shown that estrogen affects neural cells[16-18]. An acceleration of acetylcholine transferase by estrogen was reported in the substantia innominata[19]. In our study[20], estrogen treatment promoted the development of acetylcholinesterase-positive basal forebrain neurons transplanted in the anterior eye chamber of the rat. The stimulation may be transmitted via cholinergic fibers[21] to some regions of the frontal lobe that are related to AD.

Differentiation of astrocytes

Diencephalons were dissected from newborn ICR mice. After trypsin/EDTA treatment, the dispersed cells were incubated for 10 days at 37°C in DMEM including 10% horse serum, under 5% CO_2 + 95% air. The cells adhering to the bottom of the culture flask were separated with trypsin treatment and collected. The collected cells were incubated for another 7 days under the same conditions. The re-adhered cells were collected and used for an experiment to determine estrogen effects. The collected cells were incubated for another 4 days under the same conditions with E_1-S in various concentrations (0, 10^{-9}–10^{-6} mol/l). More than 95% of cells were flat and glial fibrillary acidic protein (GFAP)(+) in immunohistochemistry and were thought to be astrocytes. The astrocytes were divided morphologically into three types, i.e. epithelioid type, radial type and stellate type. The stellate type of astrocyte, which is thought to be a more developed type, increased significantly ($p < 0.01$) with E_1-S. *In vivo*, estrogen may increase the number of developed astrocytes and support greater neural function.

Suppression of apolipoprotein E: a possibility of preventing AD

The senile plaques in AD consist of amyloid. The main component of amyloid is β-protein. Apolipoprotein E (Apo E) accelerates precipitation of β-protein[22-24] (Figure 1). The

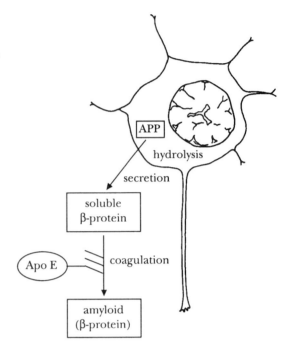

Figure 1 Schematic diagram showing precipitation of β-protein, which is the main component in the senile plaques in the senile plaques in senile dementia-Alzheimer's type. Estrogen suppresses apoliprotein E (apo-E), which is one of the factors to precipitate β-protein in the senile plaque. APP, β-amyloid protein precursor

ε4 allele of Apo E is a risk factor for late-onset AD[25]. Apolipoproteins were analyzed in 68 women (37–67 years)[26]. Apo E was higher in the patients with a serum E_2 level of < 20 pg/ml. Apo E was remarkably suppressed by hormone replacement therapy (HRT) in postmenopausal women (3.41 ± 0.75 mg/dl, Mean ± SD < 4.87 ± 1.63, $p < 0.01$). In our other study, CE therapy significantly suppressed Apo E from the 4th week (unpublished). With ethinylestradiol administration[27], Apo E was significantly decreased.

A mass screening for AD was performed in a northern town in Kyoto prefecture. The phenotype of Apo E was analyzed. E3/4 was found in 35% of 20 women suffering from AD. E4/4 (1%), E2/4 (1%) and E3/4 (16%) were found in 68 normal women. The serum level of estrone (E_1) was significantly ($p < 0.01$) lower in women with AD than in normal women. Obese women produce more E_1 by aromatization of androgen in peripheral fatty tissue. The produced E_1 may be useful in preventing AD.

Genotype of Apo E was analyzed with polymerase chain reaction–restriction fragment length polymorphism (PCR–RFLP) with restriction enzyme (Cfo I). Of another 20 women with AD, ε4 carrier was found in 35% (ε4/4 5%, ε3/4 30%). In 158 normal female outpatients in our department, ε4 carrier was significantly ($p < 0.01$) lower (12.6%; ε4/4 0.6%, ε2/4 1.2%, ε3/4 10.8%). Low-dose CE (0.625 mg/day, 3 weeks) was given to nine women with AD. They showed ameliorative effects in clinical symptoms and significant improvement of NSD ($p < 0.01$) and MMS ($p < 0.05$). Apo E was suppressed remarkably ($p < 0.01$) with estrogen.

Recently, Paganini-Hill and colleagues[27] reported that two separate epidemiologic studies supported the hypotheses that estrogen replacement therapy (ERT) decreased the risk of AD in women, and improved their cognitive performance. Tang and co-workers[28] also reported that estrogen use in postmenopausal women might delay the onset and decrease the risk of AD. Kampen and Sherwin[29] examined memory and estrogen status of postmenopausal women. They found that the ERT group performed significantly better than the control group on the 30-minute delayed paragraph recall subtest of the Wechsler memory scale. The ERT group also performed significantly better on the letter fluency test. Higher levels of estrogen were associated with higher memory scores in postmenopausal women. Sherwin[30] showed that exogenous E_2 specifically enhanced short-term memory in surgically menopausal women, and suggested that E_2 may be important in the maintenance of short-term memory in women. Limouzin-Lamothe and colleagues[31] performed a randomized, open, 6-month comparison of HRT (E_2 transdermal system plus chlormadinone) and symptomatic treatment (verapipride). In their Women's Health Questionnaire, cognition and depression improved significantly ($p < 0.01$ and $p < 0.001$) after HRT.

The ε4 allele of Apo E seems to be a risk factor for late-onset AD. Estrogen treatment for postmenopausal women, especially those with the ε4 allele detected by screening, may prevent AD.

Acknowledgements

This study was supported in part by a Grant-in-Aid for General Scientific Research (No. 03454401 and No. 07557366), Research Institute for Neurological Diseases and Geriatrics and Works of Scientific Research and Technical Development, Public Health Department of Kyoto Prefectural Government.

References

1. Fillit, H., Weinref, H., Cholst, I., Luine, V., McEwen, B., Amador, R. and Zabriskie, J. (1986). Observations in a preliminary open trial of estradiol therapy for senile dementia-Alzheimer's type. *Psychoneuroendocrinology*, **11**, 337–45

2. Honjo, H., Kitawaki, J., Itoh, M., Yasuda, J., Yamamoto, T., Yamamoto, T., Okada, H., Ohkubo, T. and Nambara, T. (1986). Serum and urinary oestrone sulphate in pregnancy and delivery measured by a direct radioimmunoassay. *Acta Endocrinol. (Copenhagen)*, **112**, 423–30

3. Honjo, H., Kitawaki, J., Itoh, M., Yasuda, J., Iwasaku, K., Urabe, M., Naitoh, K., Yamamoto, T., Okada, H., Ohkubo, T. and Nambara, T. (1987). Serum and urinary estrone sulfate during the menstrual cycle, measured by a direct radioimmunoassay, and fate of exogenously injected estrone sulfate. *Horm. Res.*, **27**, 61–8

4. Honjo, H., Ogino, Y., Naitoh, K., Urabe, M., Kitawaki, J., Yasuda, J., Yamamoto, T., Ishihara, S., Okada, H., Yonezawa, T., Hayashi, K. and Nambara, T. (1989). *In vivo* effects by estrone sulfate on the central nervous system-senile dementia (Alzheimer's type). *J. Steroid Biochem.*, **34**, 521–5

5. Otsuka, T., Shimonaka, J., Kitamura, T., Nakazato, K., Maruyama, S., Yaguchi, K., Sato, S. and Ikeda, H. (1987). A new screening test for dementia. *Clin. Psychiatry*, **29**, 395–402

6. Folstein, M. F., Folstein, S. E. and McHugh, P. R. (1975). 'Mini-Mental State': a practical method for grading the cognitive state of patients for the clinician. *J. Psychiatr. Res.*, **12**, 189–98

7. Honjo, H., Ogino, Y., Tanaka, K., Urabe, M., Kashiwagi, T., Ishihara, S., Okada, H., Araki, K., Fushiki, S., Nakajima, K., Hayashi, K., Hayashi, M. and Sasaki, T. (1993). An effect of conjugated estrogen to cognitive impairment in women with senile dementia-Alzheimer's type: A placebo-controlled double blind study. *J. Jpn. Menopause Soc.*, **1**, 167–71

8. Honjo, H., Tanaka, K., Kashiwagi, T., Urabe, M., Okada, H., Hayashi, M. and Hayashi, K. (1995). Senile dementia-Alzheimer's type and estrogen. *Horm. Metab. Res.*, **27**, 204–7

9. Katoh, S., Simogaki, H., Onodera, A., Ueda, H., Oikawa, K., Ikeda, K., Kosaka, A., Imai, Y. and Hasegawa, K. (1991). Development of the revised version of Hasegawa's Dementia Scale (HDS-R). *Jpn. J. Geriatr. Psychiatry*, **2**, 1339–47

10. Klaiber, E. L., Broverman, D. M., Vogel, W. and Kobayashi, Y. (1979). Estrogen therapy for severe persistent depressions in women. *Arch. Gen. Psychiatry*, **36**, 550–4

11. Gerdes, L. C., Sonnendecker, E. W. and Polakow, E. S. (1982). Psychological changes effected by estrogen–progestogen and clonidine treatment in climacteric women. *Am. J. Obstet. Gynecol.*, **142**, 98–103

12. Ohkura, T., Isse, K., Akazawa, K., Hamamoto, M., Yaoi, Y. and Hagino, N. (1994). Evaluation of estrogen treatment in female patients with dementia of the Alzheimer type. *Endocr. J.*, **41**, 361–71

13. Ohkura, T., Teshima, Y., Isse, K., Matsuda, H., Inoue, T., Sakai, Y., Iwasaki, N. and Yaoi, Y. (1995). Estrogen increases cerebral and cerebellar blood flows in postmenopausal women. *Menopause*, **2**, 13–18

14. Rosano, G. M. C., Sarrel, P. M., Poole-Wilson, P. A. and Collins, P. (1993). Beneficial effect of oestrogen on exercise-induced myocardial ischaemia in women with coronary artery disease. *Lancet*, **342**, 133–6

15. Sarrel, P. M. (1990). Ovarian hormones and the circulation. *Maturitas*, **590**, 287–98

16. McEwen, B. S., Biegon, A., Fischetee, C. T., Luine, V. N., Parsons, B. and Rainbow, T. C. (1984). Towards a neurochemical basis of steroid hormone action. In Martini, L. and Ganong, W. (eds.) *Frontiers in Neuroendocrinology*, pp. 1153–76. (New York: Raven Press)

17. Toran-Allerand, C. D. (1980). Sex steroids and the development of the newborn mouse hypothalamus and preoptic area *in vitro*. II Morphological correlates and hormonal specificity. *Brain Res.*, **189**, 413–27

18. Arimatsu, Y. and Hatanaka, H. (1986). Estrogen treatment enhances survival of cultured amygdala neurons in a defined medium. *Dev. Brain Res.*, **26**, 151–9

19. Pearson, R. C. A., Sofroniew, M. V., Cuello, A. C., Powell, T. P. S., Eckemstein, F., Esiri, M. M. and Willcock, G. K. (1983). Persistence of cholinergic neurons in the basal nucleus in a brain with senile dementia of the Alzheimer's type demonstrated by immunohistochemical staining for choline acetyl transferase. *Brain Res.*, **289**, 375–9

20. Honjo, H., Tamura, T., Matsumoto, Y., Kawata, M., Ogino, Y., Tanaka, K., Yamamoto, T., Ueda, S. and Okada, H. (1992). Estrogen as a growth factor to central nervous cells. Estrogen treatment promotes development of acetylcholinesterase-positive basal forebrain neurons transplanted in the anterior eye chamber. *J. Steroid Biochem. Mol. Biol.*, **41**, 633–5

21. Coyle, J. T., Price, D. L. and Delong, M. R. (1983). Alzheimer's disease: a disorder of cortical cholinergic innervation. *Science*, **219**, 1184—90

22. Yamaguchi, H. and Hasegawa, K. (1994). Senile dementia-Alzheimer's type. *J. Jpn. Med. Assoc.*, **111**, 152–9

23. Peacock, M. L. and Fink, J. K. (1994). Apo E ε4 allelic association with Alzheimer's disease: independent confirmation using denaturing gradient gel electrophoresis. *Neurology*, **44**, 339–41

24. Hardy, J. (1994). Apo E, amyloid and Alzheimer's disease. *Science*, **263**, 454–5

25. Anwar, N., Lovestone, S., Cheetham, M. E., Levy, R. and Powell, F. (1993). Apolipoprotein E-ε4 allele and Alzheimer's disease. *Lancet*, **342**, 1308–9

26. Urabe, M., Yamamoto, T., Kashiwagi, T., Okubo, T., Tsuchiya, H., Iwasa, K., Hosokawa, K., Kikuchi, N. and Honjo, H. (1996). Effect of estrogen replacement therapy on HTGL, LPL and lipids including apolipoprotein E in climacteric and elderly women. *Endocr. J.*, in press

27. Paganini-Hill, A., Buckwalter, J. G., Logan, C. G. and Henderson, V. W. (1993). Estrogen replacement and Alzheimer's disease in women. *Soc. Neurosci.*, **19**, 1046, abstr.

28. Tang, M., Jacobs, D., Stern, Y., Marder, K., Schofield, P., Gurland, B., Andrews, H. and Mayeux, R. (1996). Effect of oestrogen during menopause on risk and age at onset of Alzheimer's disease. *Lancet*, **348**, 429–32

29. Kampen, D. and Sherwin, B. (1992). Differences in memory functioning in postmenopausal women taking and not taking estrogen. *3rd Annual Meeting. The North American Menopause Society,* Cleveland, September, p. 97, abstr.

30. Sherwin, B. B. (1992). Estrogen and memory in postmenopausal women. *3rd Annual Meeting. The North American Menopause Society,* Cleveland, September, p. 50, abstr.

31. Limouzin-Lamothe, M.-A., Mairon, N., Joyce, C. R. B. and Le Gal, M. (1994). Quality of life after the menopause: influence of hormonal replacement therapy. *Am. J. Obstet. Gynecol.,* **170,** 618–24

10

Management of women with chronic medical diseases

Epilepsy and sex hormones

44

E. R. Somerville

Introduction

The relationships between neurological conditions and sex hormones are numerous and varied (Table 1). These are exemplified by epilepsy (Table 2).

Puberty

Some epileptic syndromes, including juvenile myoclonic epilepsy and juvenile absence epilepsy, appear around puberty while others,

Table 1 Chronic neurological conditions influenced by sex hormones

---

Epilepsy
Migraine
Multiple sclerosis
Chorea
Parkinson's disease
Cerebrovascular disease
Carpal tunnel syndrome

Table 2 Aspects of relationships between epilepsy and sex hormones

---

Puberty
Menstruation
  catamenial epilepsy
  hormonal therapy
  menstrual disorders
Fertility
Pregnancy
Menopause
Oral contraceptives
  effect on epilepsy
  effect on antiepileptic drugs
  contraceptive failure
Prolactin

---

most notably benign Rolandic epilepsy, disappear. However, the lack of major gender differences suggests that the timing is due more to age than hormonal changes.

Menstruation and epilepsy

In most patients with epilepsy, seizures occur unpredictably and apparently haphazardly. This factor alone contributes significantly to the disability and inconvenience of seizures. However, it is not infrequent for seizures to occur in clusters or apparent cycles. In women, such cycles are often associated with menstruation: catamenial epilepsy. Locock, who introduced the first effective drug treatment for epilepsy, noted in 1857 that seizures were often associated with menstruation[1]. Gowers in 1885 found that in more than half of his female patients with epilepsy, seizures were worse premenstrually[2]. More recent studies have confirmed and extended these observations[3–5]. The timing of seizures corresponds to phases of the menstrual cycle when estrogen levels are relatively high or progesterone levels low[6,7]. Seizures therefore occur predominantly during or a few days before menstruation. A mid-cycle peak in seizures may also occur, while anovulatory cycles may be associated with an increased frequency of seizures throughout the cycle[4] or with the exception of the follicular phase[8].

Hormonal therapy of catamenial epilepsy with progestogens by injection or suppository[9–12] has been successful, while oral administration has not[13]. Gonadotropin-releasing hormone analogs[14] may also reduce seizures. However, all clinical trials published to date have been uncontrolled and included only a small number of subjects.

Another approach has been the use of the benzodiazepine antiepileptic drug clobazam perimenstrually[15].

Menstrual disorders are more common in women with epilepsy[6,16,17]. This may relate to abnormal cyclic hormone release due to intermittent abnormal stimulation of the hypothalamus by epileptic neuronal discharges, and may also relate to antiepileptic drug therapy[18].

Fertility

Fertility is slightly decreased in women with epilepsy[19,20]. This may relate to an increase in anovulatory cycles[21], polycystic ovaries[18] and reproductive endocrine disorders[16].

Epilepsy and pregnancy

Approximately one-half of patients with epilepsy experience no change in their seizure frequency during pregnancy, one-quarter improve and one-quarter deteriorate[22]. Deterioration may be due to a number of factors, including hormonal changes, decreased antiepileptic drug levels[23,24], sleep deprivation and non-compliance through fear of teratogenesis.

Epilepsy and menopause

There have been few studies in this area. Rosciszewska[25] studied 59 women and found an average age at last menstruation of 45.7 years, which was 2 years earlier than controls. In 12 patients, epilepsy first appeared at menopause. However, in the whole group, epilepsy more often improved than deteriorated. Another small study suggested equal numbers of menopausal women with epilepsy experienced improvement and deterioration[26]. It has also been suggested that epilepsy beginning at menopause is most commonly idiopathic rather then due to a specific cause other than hormone changes[27].

Catamenial epilepsy would be expected to improve after menopause but there are no adequate data. The effect of hormone replacement therapy on epilepsy has not been studied in large numbers of women but a small study suggested that approximately 30% of women taking hormone replacement therapy deteriorate[26].

Postmenopausal osteoporosis increases the risk of serious skeletal trauma during seizures, including fractures of the humerus and spine.

The increased prevalence of epilepsy in the elderly[28] and the aging of the population will substantially increase the number of post-menopausal women with epilepsy.

Effect of sex hormones on antiepileptic drugs

Serum levels of phenytoin slightly decline premenstrually[29], although the magnitude of the fall is unlikely to be sufficient to be the sole causative factor in catamenial epilepsy. In pregnancy, both phenytoin and carbamazepine levels fall[30].

Effect of antiepileptic drugs on sex hormones

Enzyme-inducing antiepileptic drugs raise sex hormone-binding globulin (SHBG) levels, resulting in reduced levels of free hormone[31]. This may be responsible for the increased prevalence of menstrual disorders in women with epilepsy[32]. Valproate therapy has been associated with polycystic ovaries[18].

In males, the lower free androgen levels due to raised SHBG levels may be associated with impotence and hyposexuality. In these men, therapy with testosterone and an aromatase inhibitor to block conversion to estrogen may be effective[33].

Antiepileptic drugs and contraceptives

As with endogenous sex hormones, the metabolism of estrogens and progestogens administered as contraceptive agents is accelerated in women taking enzyme-inducing antiepileptic drugs[34]. Elevated SHBG levels also reduce free hormone levels[35]. These changes may lead to breakthrough bleeding or contraceptive failure[36,37]. Increasing the dose of hormone arbitrarily or titrating the dose of hormone to suppress breakthrough bleeding have been suggested. However, pregnancy may still occur and women should be informed accordingly. Progesterone-only, as well as combined estrogen–progesterone oral contraceptives have been associated with contraceptive failure[38]. Depot medroxy-progesterone may be an effective alternative[37]. Non-enzyme-inducing antiepileptic drugs, including valproate and the newer agents, vigabatrin, gabapentin, lamotrigine and tiagabine do not significantly affect hormone levels and should not produce breakthrough bleeding or contraceptive failure.

Hormones and seizures

A number of animal and human studies indicate that estrogen has convulsant properties while progesterone is anticonvulsant. Estrogen administered to animals reduces seizure threshold and progesterone elevates it[39,40]. Estrogen applied topically to the brain is effective in creating an epileptic focus[41]. In humans, epileptiform discharges in the electroencephalograph (EEG) have been actived by intravenously administered estrogen[42] and suppressed by intravenous progesterone[43]. These immediate effects imply a mechanism other than that of traditional steroid hormones. Progesterone appears to exert its antiepileptic effects by interacting with gamma-aminobutyric acid (GABA) receptors; GABA is the principal inhibitory neurotransmitter and many antiepileptic drugs act by enhancing GABA activity. Progesterone metabolites, including allopregnanolone possess potent agonist properties at the GABA-A receptor[44,45]. Estrogen may act via excitatory amino-acid receptors, enhancing the action of the neurotransmitter glutamate[46].

Prolactin

Neuronal stimulation of the hypothalamus during epileptic seizures frequently results in transient but marked elevations in serum prolactin levels[47]. Prolactin rises after generalized tonic–clonic seizures and in about 60% of partial seizures[48]. Postictal prolactin measurement may be useful in distinguishing generalized tonic–clonic epileptic seizures from psychogenic pseudoseizures, which do not affect prolactin levels. However, a normal postictal prolactin level in a patient with partial seizures is of no diagnostic significance.

References

1. Locock, C. (1857). Discussion of paper by E. Sieveking. Analysis of fifty-two cases of epilepsy observed by the author. *Lancet*, 1, 527
2. Gowers, W. R. (1901). *Epilepsy and Other Chronic Convulsive Diseases: their Causes, Symptoms and Treatment*, pp. 204–8. (New York: William Wood)
3. Newmark, M. E. and Penry, J. K. (1980). Catamenial epilepsy: a review. *Epilepsia*, 21, 281–300
4. Mattson, R. A., Kamer, J. M., Cramer, J. A. and Caldwell, B. V. (1981). Seizure frequency and the menstrual cycle: a clinical study. *Epilepsia*, 22, 242
5. Tauboll, E., Lundervold, A. and Gjerstad, L. (1991). Temporal distribution of seizures in epilepsy. *Epilepsy Res.*, 8, 153–65
6. Backstrom, T. (1976). Epileptic seizures in women related to plasma estrogen and progesterone during the menstrual cycle. *Acta Neurol. Scand.*, 54, 321–47
7. Herkes, G. K., Eadie, M. J., Sharbrough, F. and Moyer, T. (1993). Patterns of seizure occurrence in catamenial epilepsy. *Epilepsy Res.*, 15, 47–52
8. Herzog, A. G. and Klein, P. (1996). Three patterns of catamenial epilepsy. *Epilepsia*, 37 (Suppl. 5), 83
9. Zimmerman, A. W., Holden, K. R., Reiter, E. O. and Dekaban, A. S. (1973). Medroxyprogesterone acetate in the treatment of seizures associated with menstruation. *J. Pediatr.*, 83, 959–63
10. Mattson, R. A., Cramer, J. A., Caldwell, B. V. and

Siconolfi, B. C. (1984). Treatment of seizures with medroxyprogesterone acetate: preliminary report. *Neurology*, **34**, 1255–8

11. Herzog, A. G. (1986). Intermittent progesterone therapy and frequency of complex partial seizures in women with menstrual disorders. *Neurology*, **36**, 1607–10

12. Herzog, A. G. (1995). Progesterone therapy in women with complex partial and secondary generalized seizures. *Neurology*, **45**, 1660–2

13. Dana-Haeri, J. and Richens, A. (1983). Effect of norethisterone on seizures associated with menstruation. *Epilepsia*, **24**, 377–81

14. Bauer, J., Hocke, A. and Elger, C. E. (1995). Catamenial seizures – an analysis. *Nervenarzt*, **66**, 760–9

15. Feely, M., Calvert, R. and Gibson, J. (1982). Clobazam in catamenial epilepsy. A model for evaluating anticonvulsants. *Lancet*, **2**, 71–3

16. Herzog, A. G., Seibel, M. M., Schomer, D. L., Vaitukaitis, J. L. and Geschwind, N. (1986). Reproductive endocrine disorders in women with partial seizures of temporal lobe origin. *Arch. Neurol.*, **43**, 341–6

17. Bilo, L., Meo, R. and Nappi, C. (1988). Reproductive endocrine disorders in women with primary generalized epilepsy. *Epilepsia*, **29**, 612–19

18. Isojarvi, J. I. T., Laatikainen, T. J., Pakarinen, A. J., Juntunen, K. T. and Myllyla, V. V. (1993). Polycystic ovaries and hyperandrogenism in women taking valproate for epilepsy. *N. Engl. J. Med.*, **329**, 1383–8

19. Dansky, L. V., Andermann, E. and Andermann, F. (1980). Marriage and fertility in epileptic patients. *Epilepsia*, **21**, 261–71

20. Webber, M. P., Hauser, W. A., Ottman,, R. and Annegers, J. F. (1986). Fertility in persons with epilepsy: 1935–1974. *Epilepsia*, **27**, 746–52

21. Cummings, L. N., Giudice, L. and Morrell, M. J. (1995). Ovulatory function in epilepsy. *Epilepsia*, **36**, 355–9

22. Schmidt, D. (1982). The effects of pregnancy on the natural history of epilepsy : review of the literature. In Janz, D., Bossi, L., Dam, M., Helge, H., Richens, A. and Schmidt, D. (eds.) *Epilepsy, Pregnancy and the Child*, pp. 3–14. (New York: Raven Press)

23. Mygind, K. I., Dam, M. and Christiansen, J. (1976). Phenytoin and phenobarbitone plasma clearance during pregnancy. *Acta Neurol. Scand.*, **54**, 160–6

24. Lander, C. M., Edwards, V. E., Eadie, M. J. and Tyrer, J. H. (1977). Plasma anticonvulsant concentrations during pregnancy. *Neurology*, **27**, 128–31

25. Rosciszewska, D. (1987). Epilepsy and menstruation. In Hopkins, A. (ed.) *Epilepsy*, pp. 373–81. (London: Chapman and Hall)

26. Purves, S. J., Wolff, D., La Valleur, J., Leppik, I., DeBlieck, S. and Frazer, C. (1996). Effect of menopause and hormone replacement therapy on seizures. *Epilepsia*, **37** (Suppl. 5), 96

27. Abbasi, F., Krumholz, A., Kittner, S. J. and Langenberg, P. (1996). New onset epilepsy in older women is influenced by menopause. *Epilepsia*, **37** (Suppl. 5), 97

28. Hauser, W. A. (1992). Seizure disorders: the changes with age. *Epilepsia*, **33** (Suppl. 4), S6–14

29. Herkes, G. K. and Eadie, M. J. (1990). Possible roles for frequent salivary antiepileptic drug monitoring in the management of epilepsy. *Epilepsy Res.*, **6**, 146–54

30. Lander, C. M. and Eadie, M. J. (1991). Plasma antiepileptic drug concentrations during pregnancy. *Epilepsia*, **32**, 257–66

31. Barragry, J. M., Makin, H. L., Trafford, D. J. and Scott, D. F. (1978). Effect of anticonvulsants on plasma testosterone and sex hormone binding globulin levels. *J. Neurol. Neurosurg. Psychiatry*, **41**, 913–14

32. Isojarvi, J. I., Laatikainen, T. J., Pakarinen, A. J., Juntunen, K. T. and Myllyla, V. V. (1995). Menstrual disorders in women with epilepsy receiving carbamazepine. *Epilepsia*, **36**, 676–81

33. Klein, P., Jacobs, A. R. and Herzog, A. G. (1996). A comparison of testosterone versus testosterone and testolactone in the treatment of reproductive/sexual dysfunction in men with epilepsy and hypogonadism. *Neurology*, **46**, 177

34. Crawford, P., Chadwick, D. J., Martin, C., Tjia, J., Back, D. J. and Orme, M. (1990). The interaction of phenytoin and carbamazepine with combined oral contraceptive steroids. *Br. J. Clin. Pharmacol.*, **30**, 892–6

35. Back, D. J., Breckenridge, A. M. and Crawford, F. E. *et al.* (1980). The effect of oral contraceptive steroids and enzyme inducing drugs on sex hormone binding globulin capacity in women. *Br. J. Clin. Pharmacol.*, **9**, 115

36. Mattson, R. H., Cramer, J. A., Darney, P. D. and Naftolin, F. (1986). Use of oral contraceptives by women with epilepsy. *J. Am. Med. Assoc.*, **256**, 238–40

37. Krauss, G. L., Brandt, J., Campbell, M., Plate, C. and Summerfield, M. (1996). Antiepileptic medication and oral contraceptive interactions: a national survey of neurologists and obstetricians. *Neurology*, **46**, 1534–9

38. Haukkamaa, M. (1986). Contraception by Norplant subdermal capsules is not reliable in epileptic patients on anticonvulsant treatment. *Contraception*, **33**, 559–65

39. Holmes, G. L. and Donaldson, J. O. (1987).

Effect of sexual hormones on the electro-encephalogram and seizures. *J. Clin. Neurophysiol.*, **4**, 1–22

40. Herzog, A. G. (1989). A hypothesis to integrate partial seizures of temporal lobe origin and reproductive endocrine disorders. *Epilepsy Res.*, **3**, 151–9

41. Marcus, E. M., Watson, C. W. and Goldman, P. L. (1966). Effects of steroids on cerebral electrical activity. Epileptogenic effects of conjugated estrogens and related compounds in the cat and rabbit. *Arch. Neurol.*, **15**, 521–32

42. Logothetis, J., Harner, R., Morrell, F. and Torres, F. (1959). The role of estrogens in catamenial exacerbation of epilepsy. *Neurology*, **9**, 352–60

43. Backstrom, T., Zetterlund, B., Blom, S. and Romano, M. (1984). Effects of intravenous progesterone infusions on the epileptic discharge frequency in women with partial epilepsy. *Acta Neurol. Scand.*, **69**, 240–8

44. Deutsch, S. I., Mastropaolo, J. and Hitri, A. (1992). GABA-active steroids: endogenous modulators of GABA-gated chloride ion conductance. *Clin. Neuropharmacol.*, **15**, 352–64

45. Gee, K. W., McCauley, L. D. and Lan, N. C. (1995). A putative receptor for neurosteroids on the GABAA receptor complex: the pharmacological properties and therapeutic potential of epalons. *Crit. Rev. Neurobiol.*, **9**, 207–27

46. Smith, S. S. (1989). Estrogen administration increases neuronal responses to excitatory amino acids as a long-term effect. *Brain Res.*, **503**, 354–7

47. Dana-Haeri, J., Trimble, M. R. and Oxley, J. (1983). Prolactin and gonadotropin changes following generalised and partial seizures. *J. Neurol. Neurosurg. Psychiatry*, **46**, 331–5

48. Bauer, J. (1996). Epilepsy and prolactin in adults: a clinical review. *Epilepsy Res.*, **24**, 1–7

Hormone replacement therapy in diabetes

45

J. C. Stevenson and I. F. Godsland

Introduction

Hormone replacement therapy (HRT) is increasingly being used for various indications in healthy women. However, there are concerns about its use in women with certain existing clinical conditions. This stems largely and inappropriately from the adverse side-effects seen with the synthetic high-estrogen dose oral contraceptives used in the 1960s. Among these side-effects was impairment of glucose tolerance, resulting in cautions being issued against their use in diabetics. Oral contraceptive therapy and postmenopausal HRT resemble each other in that both involve administration of estrogens, usually in combination with a progestogen. However, they are entirely different in that the former requires supraphysiological estrogenic activity for suppression of ovulation, whereas the latter only requires that a state of hormone deficiency be alleviated. As well as suppressing ovulation, excessive estrogen action induces metabolic disturbances which lead to impairment of carbohydrate metabolism. Principal among these is an increase in corticosteroid activity[1], which causes resistance to the glucoregulatory actions of insulin. These changes are not seen with physiological estrogen replacement. In fact, to the contrary, physiological estrogen replacement appears to be associated with an improvement in carbohydrate metabolism.

In contrast to vascular disease, there appears to be no epidemiological information with respect to the effects of estrogens on the incidence of diabetes. Diabetes in older women may remain undiscovered for many years, and reliable epidemiological information requires repeated blood glucose testing in any cohort under investigation. As yet, there are still few studies of the effects of HRT, either with estrogen alone or with estrogen and progestogen combination therapy, in diabetic women. However, there is accumulating information on the effects of different HRT regimens on glucose and insulin metabolism in healthy postmenopausal women, and there is appreciable information on factors which might affect the development of diabetic complications. It may be possible, therefore, to predict the effect different HRT regimens may have in postmenopausal women with diabetes. Such inferences can provide a preliminary basis for prescribing while studies are undertaken in diabetics.

Effects of menopause on glucose and insulin metabolism

No effect of menopause on fasting plasma glucose levels was found in women who became postmenopausal during the course of the Framingham Study[2]. Similarly, there was no effect of menopause on fasting or 2-h oral glucose tolerance test (OGTT) glucose or insulin levels in the prospective study of Matthews and colleagues[3]. The problem with such studies is that women just before and just after the menopause are likely to have similar hormonal status, and comparisons of these groups may be meaningless. It is also difficult to distinguish effects of menopause from effects of aging. Our own studies, therefore, have involved comparisons of large groups of pre- and postmenopausal women, with statistical standardization of data in each group to a common age. In this way, differences in the relationship between the variable in question and age in each group can be distinguished, and any distinct effect of menopause can be quantified[4]. In comparing 66 premenopausal women with 92 postmenopausal women, we found that menopause was associated with no effect on the plasma insulin response during an intravenous glucose tolerance test (IVGTT), but there was a significant reduction in pancreatic insulin secretion[5]. This was accompanied by an increase in the plasma insulin half-life, which corrected for the deficiency in insulin secretion (Figure 1). There was no apparent effect of menopause on insulin resistance, although this finding may result from the tests in the premenopausal women having been carried out during the luteal phase of the menstrual cycle when there may be some increase in insulin resistance. Further analysis revealed a progressive increase in insulin resistance in the postmenopausal women (Figure 2), accompanied by increasing insulin secretion that related to time since menopause rather than chronological age[6]. This finding has been confirmed in a subsequent study[7].

Menopause, therefore, appears to be associated with the emergence of two major risk factors for diabetes, namely impaired insulin secretion and insulin resistance. National surveys in the USA have shown that the incidence of diabetes dramatically increases in women over 50 years of age. This increase is considerably greater than that seen in men of comparable age, the total prevalence of diabetes in white women aged 55–64 years being 62% higher than in men[8]. Whether menopause contributes to this increased incidence in women remains unknown.

Effects of estrogen on glucose and insulin metabolism

Studies of the effects of estrogens on glucose and insulin metabolism in postmenopausal women may complement findings from studies of the menopause. Estrogen replacement would be expected to have the opposite effect to the

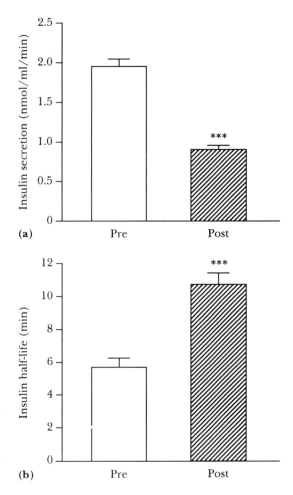

Figure 1 Pancreatic insulin secretion (a) and insulin elimination (b) in pre- (open bars) and post- (hatched bars) menopausal women. ***$p < 0.001$. Reproduced from reference 5, with permission

changes seen in postmenopausal women due to estrogen deficiency. Cagnacci and associates studied the effects of transdermally administered 17β-estradiol (50 μg/day) on OGTT glucose, insulin and C-peptide responses in 15 postmenopausal women followed for 3 months[9]. There was no change in glucose response, insulin response fell significantly and C-peptide response increased significantly. The increase in C-peptide response with no change in glucose response suggests an improved sensitivity of pancreatic insulin secretion to glucose; the increase in C-peptide response with

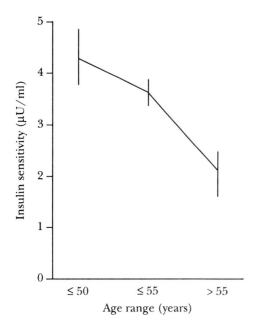

Figure 2 Age and insulin sensitivity in postmenopausal women. Reproduced from reference 5, with permission

a reduction in insulin response suggests an improvement in insulin elimination; and the reduction in insulin response with no change in glucose response suggests a reduction in insulin resistance. Thus, these effects of estradiol were indeed the opposite of the effect seen with the menopause.

Evidence for improvements in pancreatic insulin secretion in response to estrogens dates back many years. For example, in extensive work on the effects of estrogens in animal models of diabetes, estrogens were found to reduce the incidence of diabetes in the partially pancreatectomized rat by up to 60%, and this was associated with a hypertrophic and hyperplastic response of the pancreatic islet[10]. Similar improvements were seen when cultures of isolated pancreatic islets from oophorectomized animals were treated with estrogens. They showed a significantly higher insulin response to glucose than those from untreated animals[11-13].

Estrogens have also been shown to improve the sensitivity of various insulin-dependent

metabolic processes to insulin in tissues isolated from animals treated with estrogens. Reduced insulin resistance has thus been demonstrated in skeletal muscle, diaphragm muscle and adipose tissue in response to estrogens[14-16]. Similarly, the majority of studies of the effects of estradiol alone in postmenopausal women show an improvement in glucose or insulin levels consistent with a reduction in insulin resistance[9,17-20].

Effects of hormone replacement therapy on glucose and insulin metabolism

Hormone replacement therapy regimens prescribed for postmenopausal women with an intact uterus comprise continuous estrogen with progestogen addition, while estrogen alone is given to hysterectomized postmenopausal women. The effects of estradiol alone have been described above. There are only a few studies of the effects of conjugated equine estrogens at the usual dose of 0.625 mg/day, and these are equally divided between those showing an improvement in carbohydrate metabolism and those showing no effect[9,21-23]. The higher dose of 1.25 mg/day causes significant deterioration in glucose tolerance and insulin resistance.

Four of the progestogens commonly used in European combined HRT regimens are norethisterone acetate, levonorgestrel, medroxyprogesterone acetate and dydrogesterone. They have been studied with respect to their effects on glucose and insulin metabolism. Norethisterone acetate appears to be entirely neutral, whereas levonorgestrel and medroxyprogesterone acetate induce insulin resistance[21,24]. When they are combined with estrogens, these progestogens are associated with effects that might be expected from the effects they have when given alone, although some novel features emerge. Norethisterone acetate combinations appear to be neutral with regard to carbohydrate metabolism[24,25]. In contrast, levonorgestrel and medroxyprogesterone acetate combinations are associated with a deterioration in glucose tolerance[22–24]. In a detailed evaluation of the effects of two HRT combinations on glucose metabolism and insulin action, we found that the reduction in glucose tolerance seen in users of an orally administered combination of conjugated equine estrogens (0.625 mg/day) and cyclical ± norgestrel (0.15 mg/day) was associated with an increase in the insulin response to glucose during an IVGTT (Figure 3(a)), which in turn resulted from a reduction in the initial insulin response (Figure 3(b))[24]. There is evidence for a similar reduction in the early insulin response when conjugated equine estrogens are given with medroxyprogesterone acetate[22]. In combination therapy with dydrogesterone, some of the beneficial effects of 17β-estradiol on insulin levels can still be seen[26].

Effects of hormone replacement therapy on factors involved in diabetic complications

Various explanations have been proposed for the development of vascular disease, retinopathy, nephropathy and neuropathy in diabetics. Glycosylation of proteins continuously increases with increasing glucose levels. The degree of hyperglycemia, independent of any other metabolic disturbance in diabetics, has been linked to the development of diabetic complications[27]. The formation of advanced glycosylation end products provides a single mechanism whereby the manifold complications of diabetes might be explained, and provides a mechanistic basis for the current practice of tight glycemic control in diabetic patients[28].

Much attention is currently focused on the possible role of dyslipidemia, particularly increased triglyceride levels and decreased high-density lipoprotein (HDL) levels, in the increased risk of coronary heart disease (CHD) seen in diabetics[29]. This is the leading cause of death in diabetics, and women appear to be particularly susceptible. The advantage that females enjoy over males with regard to CHD is entirely lost when they become diabetic[30]. It has

been noted that women with diabetes have significantly higher triglyceride levels and lower HDL levels than men with diabetes[31], and these disturbances are particularly strong predictors of CHD in women[32]. Hormone replacement with transdermal 17β-estradiol probably reduces triglyceride levels[33] and may effect small increases in HDL levels in the important HDL_2 subfraction[34]. Conjugated equine estrogens increase triglyceride levels but also increase HDL concentrations[33,34]. Norethisterone acetate and levonorgestrel oppose any estrogen-induced increase in triglycerides and their use may result in an absolute decrease in triglyceride levels. Levels of HDL tend to be reduced with these progestogens but this reduction appears primarily to be in the less important HDL_3 subfraction[33]. Medroxyprogesterone acetate has less of a triglyceride-lowering effect but can diminish any estrogen-induced increase in HDL levels[23]. Dydrogesterone also has little effect on triglycerides but permits the estrogen-induced increase in HDL[26].

Increased susceptibility to oxidative damage and endothelial dysfunction are two further disturbances which have been suggested as potential causative agents in the development of diabetic complications, particularly with regard to the vasculature[35,36]. Lipid peroxidation is reduced in postmenopausal women taking estradiol[37], and the improvements in endothelium-dependent vascular function that accompany estrogen administration are now well documented[38]. Other factors which may affect vascular function and are influenced by estrogens and progestogens include calcium-dependent mechanisms[39] and angiotensin-1 converting enzyme (ACE) activity[40].

Hormone replacement therapy in diabetics

The great majority of postmenopausal women with diabetes who might wish to use HRT will have non-insulin-dependent (maturity-onset) diabetes, and the effects of female sex steroids on insulin resistance and insulin secretion described above relate to these women.

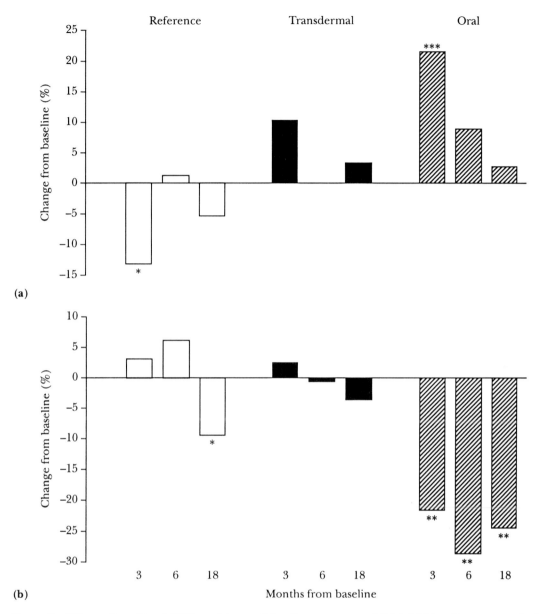

Figure 3 Effects of combined HRT on (a) overall insulin response and (b) initial insulin response during intravenous glucose tolerance test in postmenopausal women: 29 women received no therapy (open bars), 30 women received transdermally administered 17β-estradiol (50 μg/day) and cyclical transdermal norethisterone acetate (0.25 mg/day, solid bars), and 30 women received orally administered conjugated equine estrogens (0.625 mg/day) and cyclical oral ± norgestrel (0.15 mg/day, hatched bars). $*p < 0.05$, $**p < 0.01$, $***p < 0.001$. Reproduced from reference 24, with permission

However, postmenopausal women with insulin-dependent diabetes also experience similar metabolic and vascular disturbances. Thus, all diabetic women could receive the same benefits of HRT as non-diabetic women. Few studies of HRT in postmenopausal diabetics have been published, but there is some epidemiological evidence that HRT brings a reduction in CHD in diabetes similar to that seen in healthy postmenopausal women[41].

With regard to which HRT to use, in the first instance, prescription of HRT combinations that do not have an adverse effect on some of the factors involved in the development or progression of diabetes would appear logical. If these combinations prove unsuitable, there may be recourse to other combinations, albeit with some additional attention being given to control of blood glucose levels. In general, there would seem to be little need for additional surveillance of diabetic women commencing HRT, beyond the routine monitoring of diabetic control. Until there is more knowledge of the effects of different HRT regimens in diabetics, it might be prudent to pay some attention to triglyceride levels, particularly in women who are overweight.

Conclusions

Estrogen deficiency has adverse effects on glucose and insulin metabolism and may contribute to the increased incidence of diabetes seen in older women. Estrogens have beneficial effects on glucose and insulin metabolism, and these can be seen during physiological estrogen replacement in postmenopausal women. Estrogen/progestogen combination HRT regimens affect glucose and insulin metabolism in different ways, depending on the type of estrogen and progestogen used. In general, combinations containing norethisterone acetate or dydrogesterone do not adversely affect glucose and insulin metabolism, whereas combinations containing medroxyprogesterone acetate or levonorgestrel can cause deterioration in glucose tolerance. Estrogen replacement and HRT combinations can also have beneficial effects on some of the factors that may contribute to diabetic complications, particularly with regard to vascular disease. Thus, rather than HRT being contraindicated in diabetic postmenopausal women, it may be positively beneficial to their diabetes. Detailed investigations of the effects of HRT in postmenopausal women with diabetes are clearly needed, including studies of continuous combined HRT and estrogen-like molecules.

References

1. Burke, C. W. (1969). Biologically active cortisol in plasma of oestrogen-treated and normal subjects. *Br. Med. J.*, **2**, 798–800
2. Hjortland, M. C., McNamara, P. M. and Kannel, W. B. (1976). Some atherogenic concomitants of the menopause: the Framingham Study. *Am. J. Epidemiol.*, **103**, 304–11
3. Matthews, K. A., Meilahn, E., Kuller, L. H., Kelsey, S. F., Caggiula, A. W. and Wing, R. R. (1989). Menopause and risk factors for coronary heart disease. *N. Engl. J. Med.*, **321**, 641–6
4. Godsland, I. F., Walton, C. and Stevenson, J. C. (1993). Impact of menopause on metabolism. In Diamond, M. P. and Naftolin, F. (eds.) *Metabolism in the Female Life Cycle*, pp. 171–89. (Rome: Ares Serono Symposia)
5. Walton, C., Godsland, I. F., Proudler, A. J., Wynn, V. and Stevenson, J. C. (1993). The effects of the menopause on insulin sensitivity, secretion and elimination in nonobese, healthy women. *Eur. J. Clin. Invest.*, **23**, 466–73
6. Proudler, A. J., Felton, C. and Stevenson, J. C. (1992). Ageing and the response of plasma insulin, glucose and C-peptide concentrations to intravenous glucose in postmenopausal women. *Clin. Sci.*, **83**, 489–94
7. Godsland, I. F., Crook, D., Stevenson, J. C., Collins, P., Rosano, G. M. C., Lees, B., Sidhu, M. and Poole-Wilson, P. A. (1995). The insulin resistance syndrome in postmenopausal women with cardiological syndrome X. *Br. Heart J.*, **74**, 47–52
8. Harris, M. I., Hadden, W. C., Knowler, W. C. and Bennett, P. H. (1987). Prevalence of diabetes and impaired glucose tolerance and plasma glucose levels in US population aged 20–74 years. *Diabetes*, **36**, 523–34
9. Cagnacci, A., Soldani, R., Carriero, P. L., Paoletti, A. M., Fioretti, P. and Melis, G. B. (1992). Effects of low doses of transdermal 17β-estradiol on carbohydrate metabolism in postmenopausal women. *J. Clin. Endocrinol. Metab.*, **74**, 1396–400

10. Rodriguez, R. R. (1965). Influence of oestrogens and androgens on the production and prevention of diabetes. In Leibel, B. and Wrenshall, G. (eds.) *On the Nature and Treatment of Diabetes*, pp. 288–307. (New York: Excerpta Medica)

11. Bailey, C. J. and Ahmed-Sorour, H. (1980). Role of ovarian hormones in the long-term control of glucose homeostasis. *Diabetologia*, **19**, 475–81

12. El Seifi, S., Green, I. C. and Perrin, D. (1981). Insulin release and steroid-hormone binding in isolated islets of Langerhans in the rat: effects of ovariectomy. *J. Endocrinol.*, **90**, 59–67

13. Faure, A., Haourari, M. and Sutter, B.-C.-J. (1985). Insulin secretion and biosynthesis after oestradiol treatment. *Horm. Metab. Res.*, **17**, 378

14. McKerns, K. W., Coulomb, B., Kaleita, E. and DeRenzo, E. C. (1958). Some effects of *in vivo* administered oestrogens on glucose metabolism and adrenal cortical secretion *in vitro*. *Endocrinology*, **63**, 709–22

15. Gilmour, K. E. and McKerns, K. W. (1966). Insulin and estrogen regulation of lipid synthesis in adipose tissue. *Biochim. Biophys. Acta*, **116**, 220–8

16. Rushakoff, R. J. and Kalkhoff, R. K. (1981). Effects of pregnancy and sex steroid administration on skeletal muscle metabolism in the rat. *Diabetes*, **30**, 545–50

17. Talaat, M., Habib, Y. A., Higazy, A. M., Abdel Naby, S., Malek, A. Y. and Ibrahim, Z. A. (1965). Effect of sex hormones on the carbohydrate metabolism in normal and diabetic women. *Arch. Int. Pharmacodyn.*, **154**, 402–11

18. Notelovitz, M., Johnston, M., Smith, S. and Kitchens, C. (1987). Metabolic and hormonal effects of 25 mg and 50 mg 17β-estradiol implants in surgically menopausal women. *Obstet. Gynecol.*, **70**, 749–54

19. Silfverstolpe, G., Gustafson, A., Samsioe, G. and Svanborg, A. (1980). Lipid metabolic studies in oophorectomised women: effects induced by two different estrogens on serum lipids and lipoproteins. *Gynecol. Obstet. Invest.*, **11**, 161–9

20. Lindheim, S. R., Duffy, D. M., Kojima, T., Vijod, M. A., Stancyk, F. Z. and Lobo, R. A. (1994). The route of administration influences the effect of estrogen on insulin sensitivity in postmenopausal women. *Fertil. Steril.*, **62**, 1176–80

21. Lindheim, S. R., Presser, S. C., Ditkoff, E. C., Vijod, M. A., Stanczyk, F. Z. and Lobo, R. A. (1993). A possible bimodal effect of estrogen on insulin sensitivity in postmenopausal women and the attenuating effect of added progestin. *Fertil. Steril.*, **60**, 664–7

22. Lobo, R. A., Pickar, J. H., Wild, R. A., Walsh, B. and Hirvonen, E. (1994). Metabolic impact of adding medroxyprogesterone acetate to conjugated estrogen therapy in postmenopausal women. *Obstet. Gynecol.*, **84**, 987–95

23. The Writing Group for the PEPI Trial (1995). Effects of estrogen or estrogen/progestin regimens on heart disease risk factors in postmenopausal women: the Postmenopausal Estrogen/Progestin Interventions (PEPI) Trial. *J. Am. Med. Assoc.*, **273**, 199–208

24. Godsland, I. F., Gangar, K. F., Walton, C., Cust, M. P., Whitehead M. I., Wynn, V. and Stevenson, J. C. (1993). Insulin resistance, secretion and elimination in postmenopausal women receiving oral or transdermal hormone replacement therapy. *Metabolism*, **42**, 846–53

25. Luotola, H., Pyörälä, T. and Loikkanen, M. (1986). Effects of natural oestrogen/progestogen substitution therapy on carbohydrate and lipid metabolism in post-menopausal women. *Maturitas*, **8**, 245–53

26. Crook, D., Godsland, I. F., Hull, J. and Stevenson, J. C. (1997). Hormone replacement therapy with dydrogesterone and estradiol-17β: effects on serum lipoproteins and glucose tolerance. *Br. J. Obstet. Gynaecol.*, **104**, 298–304

27. Singer, D. E., Nathan, D. M., Anderson, K. M., Wilson, P. W. F. and Evans, J. C. (1992). Association of HbA1c with prevalent cardiovascular disease in the original cohort of the Framingham Heart Study. *Diabetes*, **41**, 202–8

28. Nathan, D. M. (1996). The pathophysiology of diabetic complications: how much does the glucose hypothesis explain? *Ann. Intern. Med.*, **124**, 86–9

29. Betteridge, D. J. (1994). Diabetic dyslipidemia. *Am. J. Med.*, **96** (Suppl. 6A), 25S–31S

30. Barrett-Connor, E. L., Cohn, B. A., Wingard, D. L. and Edelstein, S. L. (1991). Why is diabetes mellitus a stronger risk factor for fatal ischemic heart disease in women than in men? The Rancho Bernardo Study. *J. Am. Med. Assoc.*, **265**, 627–31

31. Walden, C. E., Knopp, R. H. and Wahl P. W. (1984). Sex differences in the effect of diabetes mellitus on lipoprotein triglyceride and cholesterol concentrations. *N. Engl. J. Med.*, **311**, 953–9

32. Miller Bass, K., Newschaffer, C. J., Klag, M. J. and Bush, T. L. (1993). Plasma lipoprotein levels as predictors of cardiovascular death in women. *Arch. Intern. Med.*, **153**, 2209–16

33. Crook, D., Cust, M. P., Gangar, K. F., Worthington, M., Hillard, T. C., Stevenson, J. C., Whitehead, M. I. and Wynn, V. (1992). Comparison of transdermal and oral estrogen–progestin replacement therapy: effects on serum lipids and lipoproteins. *Am. J. Obstet. Gynecol.*, **166**, 950–5

34. Walsh, B. W., Schiff, I., Rosner, B., Greenberg, L., Ravnikar, V. and Sacks, F. M. (1991). Effects of postmenopausal estrogen replacement on the concentrations and metabolism of plasma lipoproteins. *N. Engl. J. Med.*, **325**, 1196–204

35. Wolff, S. P. (1993). Diabetes mellitus and free radicals. *Br. Med. Bull.*, **49**, 642–52

36. Cohen, R. A. (1993). Dysfunction of vascular endothelium in diabetes mellitus. *Circulation*, **87** (Suppl V), V67–76

37. Sack, M. N., Rader, D. J. and Cannon, R. O. III (1994). Oestrogen and inhibition of oxidation of low-density lipoproteins in postmenopausal women. *Lancet*, **343**, 269–70

38. Collins, P., Shay, J., Jiang, C. and Moss, J. (1994). Nitric oxide accounts for dose-dependent estrogen-mediated coronary relaxation after acute estrogen withdrawal. *Circulation*, **90**, 1964–8

39. Jiang, C., Poole-Wilson, P. A., Sarrel, P. M., Mochizuki, S. and Collins, P. (1992). Effects of 17β-oestradiol on contraction, Ca^{2+} current and intracellular free Ca^{2+} in guinea-pig isolated cardiac myocytes. *Br. J. Pharmacol.*, **106**, 739–45

40. Proudler, A. J., Ahmed, A. I. H., Crook, D., Fogelman, I., Rymer, J. M. and Stevenson, J. C. (1995). Hormone replacement therapy and serum angiotensin-converting-enzyme activity in postmenopausal women. *Lancet*, **346**, 89–90

41. Psaty, B. M., Heckbert, S. R., Atkins, D., Lemaitre, R., Koepsell, T. D., Wahl, P. W., Siscovick, D. S. and Wagner, E. H. (1994). The risk of myocardial infarction associated with the combined use of estrogens and progestins in postmenopausal women. *Arch. Intern. Med.*, **154**, 1333–9

Arthritis, menopause and estrogens   46

G. H. M. George and T. D. Spector

Introduction

It is well established that autoimmune, connective tissue and other rheumatic disorders, such as rheumatoid arthritis and systemic lupus erythematosus, are more common in women. As a consequence, attention by researchers has been focused on the interactive effects of sex hormones on inflammatory and immune pathways, in order to perceive disease mechanisms and explore the potential of hormonal manipulation as a therapeutic tool. The following summarizes the evidence to date of the influence of the menopause on common rheumatic disorders, and the effect of hormone replacement on these.

Rheumatoid arthritis

There is a three-fold difference in the prevalence of rheumatoid arthritis (RA) in women, with slightly increased levels of severity and disability. In the early 19th century, Haygarth noted the 'nodosities of the joints' that occur at the menopause, and in 1928 Weil pointed to the inevitability of arthritis following female castration. The age of disease onset in women seems to adopt a Gaussian-type distribution, with a peak between the ages of 45 and 55 years and a relative decline in later years[1], suggesting that the menopausal transition may play an important role in the etiopathogenesis of this disease. Up to one-third of women first report rheumatoid symptoms within 2 years of the menopause. Pregnancy and exogenous estrogens also seem to influence RA. Over 75% of all pregnant women with RA experience disease remission during preg-nancy[2]; however more than 80% will have relapsed by 3 months postdelivery. Most studies have found that nulliparous women are two to three times more likely to develop RA[3], and a recent study of the effect of oral contraception, parity and breast-feeding in women with at least one child on the severity of RA, suggests that parity and to a lesser extent breast-feeding before RA onset worsened RA prognosis[4]. The effect of the oral contraceptive (OC) pill is more contentious, but it seems that there may be a modest beneficial effect on disease severity and a reduction in incidence in OC users[3]. These studies, although supportive of a hormonal influence in RA, do not provide an indication of the relative importance of individual hormones, interaction between hormones or other factors such as genetic composition. Studies of the biological effects of sex hormones have helped to provide a more detailed insight into the possible mechanisms behind these clinical observations[5-9].

Human trials of hormone replacement therapy

Attempts to correct estrogen insufficiency in women with menopausally related RA were made by Hall[10] and Cohen and associates[11] using intramuscular estradiol. Although end-points were not reported, they described improvements in up to 50% of their patients. The first controlled study of combined hormone replacement therapy (HRT) in RA was that of Gilbert and colleagues[12] who treated 13 females and four males with Enovid®, a combination of norethynodrel and small amounts of the estrogen, mestranol. Four patients responded favorably, and five were able to halve their dose of corticosteroid. A larger study of the same preparation in 44 patients found significant improvements in 18 subjects, another 11 having withdrawn because of side-effects[13].

In 1987, a cross-over study of ethinylestradiol in ten pre- and postmenopausal women found significant improvements in hemoglobin, thrombocytosis and 30-meter walking time[14], but another study of a high-dose combined contraceptive pill in ten premenopausal women found no positive effects[15].

Hall and co-workers carried out a 6-month controlled trial of transdermal estradiol in 200 postmenopausal women with RA[16]. There was no statistically significant overall improvement in patients receiving HRT, but we found that many patients allocated to the HRT arm did not have appropriate serum estradiol levels. In patients with estradiol levels above 100 pmol/l, as expected with the HRT preparation used, there were significant improvements in the articular index and the visual analog pain-scale compared with controls. Daily self-reported assessments of pain and morning stiffness suggested that RA symptoms were worse during the progestogen phase of treatment compared with the estrogen phase. The same HRT preparation was used by MacDonald and colleagues in a double-blind controlled trial in 62 patients[17]. After 48 weeks there were significant improvements in articular index and the Nottingham Health Care Profile (assessing well-being). However, van den Brink and associates reported on 40 postmenopausal women with active RA treated with oral estradiol in a double-blind controlled trial, and found no improvements in any parameter of disease activity[18].

The two studies using transdermal estrogen replacement provide weak evidence of a positive effect of estrogen in RA, at least in some individuals, but the oral estradiol trial did not, however, support these findings.

Trials using progesterone have been limited. The studies using Enovid in the 1960s were of a combined HRT that was predominantly progestogenic and produced mixed results, as previously discussed. Earlier, a report of high-dose progesterone administration to RA patients, given in an uncontrolled trial, found a substantial improvement in over one-third[19]. An interesting study of intra-articular progesterone in 12 patients with severe rheumatoid knee synovitis found that a lasting anti-inflammatory effect could be induced in the majority of patients[20].

Clinical studies of HRT in RA have been few and often uncontrolled. As yet they have not supported promising animal and *in vitro* studies.

Systemic lupus erythematosus

The incidence of systemic lupus erythematosus (SLE) in females is approximately ninefold that in males, and the onset of the disease is most common during the fertile years with exacerbations frequently occurring pre-menstrually. The effect of pregnancy in SLE is variable, producing both exacerbations and remissions. Why SLE appears to be more estrogen-driven than RA is unclear. The immunological pathways in SLE are very much different; the disease is characterized by a greater B-cell lymphocyte response than seen in RA, itself mainly driven by T-cells[21]. The illness tends to abate at the menopause, although elderly-onset SLE is well recognized. A prospective cohort study by Sanchez-Guerrero and colleagues noted an increase in the risk for SLE related to the duration of use of post-menopausal hormones[22]. Despite this and the improvement at the menopause, it should be noted that HRT is not a contraindication in stable SLE patients as there is no evidence that it leads to a disease flare, or, in the small numbers studied, is associated with thrombo-embolism[23].

Osteoarthritis

The frequent onset of generalized osteoarthritis (OA) around the time of the menopause, along with the inverse relationship with postmeno-pausal osteoporosis[24] and the faster rise in prevalence of OA with age in women than in men, suggest a role for reproductive hormones in OA. The effect of HRT on OA has been studied, and a weak non-significant effect in knee OA was observed in the elderly[25]. More recently, a study of 985 women showed that current use of HRT is associated with a threefold reduction in risk of knee OA, and a modest reduction in distal interphalangeal but not carpo–metacarpal joint OA[26]. A cross-sectional study by Nevitt and co-workers examined the association of radiographic evidence of OA of the hip with postmenopausal estrogen replacement in 4366 women[27]: 17.2% had evidence of hip OA. Those currently using estrogen replacement had a significantly reduced risk of any hip OA, and this effect was greatest in those women who had taken estrogen replacement for 10 years or longer.

Further studies are undoubtedly required to uncover the possible mechanisms of action and to clarify the potential benefits of HRT in OA.

Carpal tunnel syndrome

Carpal tunnel syndrome (CTS) is five times more common in women than in men, with a preponderance for postmenopausal and oophorectomized women[28]. Changes in forearm fat content known to occur at the menopause may account for this increased incidence[29]. A study by Hall and Steadman[30] looking at the frequency and response of rheumatic conditions to HRT in menopausal women, found 17% of 42 women had CTS and a further 5% had symptoms without signs. There was an impressive response to estrogen replacement therapy. Confino-Cohen and associates describe two postmenopausal women with CTS who responded to estrogen replacement therapy[31], suggesting a reversal of the increased forearm fat associated with the menopause.

Fibromyalgia

Women predominate at all ages among patients diagnosed as having fibromyalgia. A study of 100 women with fibromyalgia by Waxman and Zatzkis[32] found the average age of onset to be 46 years. Of 65 patients in whom menopause occurred before diagnosis of fibromyalgia, the average age of menopause was 42 years, and most of these had menopause related to surgery and insufficient estrogen therapy. They conclude not surprisingly that estrogen therapy should be added to the treatment armamentarium for fibromyalgia. The study by Hall and Steadman[30] set in a menopause clinic found 14% had fibromyalgia, and those with persistent symptoms had low estrogen concentrations. After 6 months' HRT there was a modest improvement in symptoms, pain and examination scores. However, as yet no randomized prospective studies of the use of HRT in fibromyalgia have been performed.

Gout

Although more common in men than in women, gout occurs most frequently in women after the menopause. Retrospective reviews by Puig and colleagues[33] and Lally and co-workers[34] found 86% and 91%, respectively, of cases of gout in women diagnosed after the menopause. In addition, gout is rare in pregnancy[35]. There have not been studies, however on the response of gout to estrogen replacement therapy, but this may yield interesting results.

Conclusion

The menopause is a time of hormonal change that results in the manifestation of many different rheumatic diseases. From the evidence presented it can be extrapolated that the use of estrogen replacement may have preventive and therapeutic benefits, although further controlled studies are needed to consolidate the theoretical benefits in rheumatic diseases.

References

1. Goemaere, S., Ackerman, C., Goethals, K., De Keyser, F., van der Straeten, C., Verbruggen, G., Mielants, H. and Veys, E. M. (1990). Onset of symptoms of rheumatoid arthritis in relation to age, sex and menopausal transition. *J. Rheumatol.*, **17**, 1620-2

2. Klipple, G. L. and Cecere, F. A. (1989). Rheumatoid arthritis and pregnancy. *Rheum. Dis. Clin. N. Am.*, **15**, 213–39

3. Spector, T. D., Roman, E. and Silman, A. J. (1990). The pill, parity and rheumatoid arthritis. *Arthritis Rheum.*, **33**, 782–9

4. Jorgensen, C., Picot, M. C., Bologna, C. and Sany, J. (1996). Oral contraception, parity, breast feeding, and severity of rheumatoid arthritis. *Ann. Rheum. Dis.*, **55**, 94–8

5. Holmdahl, R., Jansson, L., Meyerson, B. and Klareskog, L. (1987). Oestrogen induced suppression of collagen arthritis: 1. Long-term oestradiol treatment of DBA/1 mice reduces severity and incidence of arthritis and decreases the anti type II collagen immune response. *Clin. Exp. Immunol.*, **70**, 372–8

6. Da Silva, J. A. P., Colville-Nash, P., Spector, T. D., Scott, D. L. and Willoughby, D. A. (1993). Inflammation induced cartilage degradation in female rodents. Protective role of sex hormones. *Arthritis Rheum.*, **36**, 1007–13

7. Cutolo, M., Accardo, S., Villagio, B., Clerico, P., Bagnasco, M., Coviello, D. A., Carruba, G., Io Casto, M. and Castagnetta, L. (1993). Presence of estrogen-binding sites on macrophage like synoviocytes and CD8+, CD29+, CD45RO+ T lymphocytes in normal and rheumatoid synovium. *Arthritis Rheum.*, **36**, 1087–97

8. Paavonen, T. (1987). Hormonal regulation of lymphocyte function. *Med. Biol.*, **65**, 229–40

9. Pacifici, R., Rifas, L., McCracken, R., McMurty, C., Avioli, L. V. and Peck, W. A. (1989). Ovarian steroid treatment blocks a postmenopausal increase in monocyte interleukin-1 release. *Proc. Natl. Acad. Sci. USA*, **86**, 2398–402

10. Hall, F. C. (1938). Menopausal arthralgia. *N. Engl. J. Med.*, **219**, 1015–26

11. Cohen, A., Dubbs, A. W. and Myers, A. (1940). The treatment of atrophic arthritis with estrogenic substance. *N. Engl. J. Med.*, **222**, 140–2

12. Gilbert, M., Rotstein, J., Cunningham, C., Estrin, I., Davidson, A. and Pincus, G. (1964). Norethynodrel with mestranol in treatment of rheumatoid arthritis. *J. Am. Med. Assoc.*, **190**, 235

13. Demers, R., Blais, J. A. and Pretty, H. (1966). Arthrite rhumatoide traitée par norethynodrel associée à mestranol. *Can. Med. Assoc.*, **95**, 350–4

14. Bijlsma, J. W. J., Huber-Bruning, O. and Thijssen, A. H. J. (1987). Effect of estrogen treatment on clinical and laboratory manifestations of rheumatoid arthritis. *Ann. Rheum. Dis.*, **46**, 777–9

15. Hazes, J. M. W., Dijkmans, B. A. C., Vandenbroucke, J. P. and Cats, A. (1989). Oral contraceptive treatment for rheumatoid arthritis: an open study in 10 patients. *Br. J. Rheumatol.*, **28** (Suppl.), 28–30

16. Hall, G. M., Daniels, M., Huskisson, E. C. and Spector, T. D. (1994). A randomised controlled trial of the effect of hormone replacement therapy on disease activity in postmenopausal rheumatoid arthritis. *Ann. Rheum. Dis.*, **53**, 112–16

17. MacDonald, A. G., Murphy, E. A., Capell, H. A., Bankowska, U. Z. and Ralston, S. H. (1994). Effects of hormone replacement therapy in rheumatoid arthritis: a double-blind placebo controlled study. *Ann. Rheum. Dis.*, **53**, 54–7

18. van den Brink, H. R., van Everdingen, A. A., van Wijk, M. J., Jacobs, J. W. and Bijlsma, J. M. (1993). Adjuvant oestrogen therapy does not improve disease activity in postmenopausal patients with rheumatoid arthritis. *Ann. Rheum. Dis.*, **52**, 862–5

19. Vignos, P. J. Jr and Dorfman, R. I. (1951). Effect of large doses of progesterone in rheumatoid arthritis. *Am. J. Am. Sci.*, **222**, 29–34

20. Cuchacovich, M., Tchernitchin, A., Gatica, H., Wurgraft, R., Valenzuela, C. and Cornejo, E. (1988). Intra-articular progesterone: effects of a local treatment for rheumatoid arthritis. *J. Rheumatol.*, **15**, 561–5

21. Ansar Ahmed, S., Penhale, W. J. and Talal, N. (1985). Sex hormones, immune responses and autoimmune diseases. Mechanisms of sex hormones actions. *Am. J. Pathol.*, **121**, 531–51

22. Sanchez-Guerrero, J., Liang, M. H., Karlson, E. W., Hunter, D. J. and Colditz, G. A. (1995). Postmenopausal estrogen therapy and the risk for developing systemic lupus erythematosus. *Ann. Intern. Med.*, **122**, 430–3

23. Arden, N. K., Lloyd, M. E., Spector, T. D. and Hughes, G. R. V. (1994). Safety of hormone replacement therapy in systemic lupus erythematosus. *Lupus*, **3**, 11–13

24. Hart, D. J., Mootooswamy, I., Doyle, D. V. and Spector, T. D. (1994). The relationship between osteoarthritis and osteoporosis in the general population: the Chingford Study. *Ann. Rheum. Dis.*, **54**, 158–62

25. Hannan, M. T., Felson, D. T., Anderson, J. J., Naimark, A. and Kannel, W. B. (1990). Estrogen

use and radiographic osteoarthritis of the knee in women. *Arthritis Rheum.*, **33**, 525–32

26. Spector, T. D., Nandra, D., Hart, D.J. and Doyle, D. V. (1996). Is hormone replacement therapy protective for hand and knee osteoarthritis in women?: the Chingford Study. *Ann. Rheum. Dis.*, in press

27. Nevitt, M. C., Cummings, S. R., Lane, N. E., Hochberg, M. C., Scott, J. C., Pressman, A. R., Genant, H. K. and Cauley, J. A. (1996). Association of estrogen replacement therapy with the risk of osteoarthritis of the hip in elderly white women. *Arch. Intern. Med.*, **156**, 2073–80

28. Pascual, E., Girer, V., Arostegni, A., Conill, J., Ruiz, M. T. and Pico, A. (1991). Higher incidence of carpal tunnel syndrome in oophorectomized women. *Br. J. Rheumatol.*, **30**, 60–2

29. Hasseger, C. and Christiansen, C. (1989). Estrogen/gestagen therapy changes soft tissue body composition in postmenopausal women. *Metabolism*, **38**, 662–5

30. Hall, G. M. and Steadman, J. W. W. (1992). Carpal tunnel syndrome and hormone replacement therapy. *Br. Med. J.*, **304**, 382

31. Confino-Cohen, R., Lishner, M., Savin, H., Lang, R. and Ravid, M. (1991). Response of carpal tunnel syndrome to hormone replacement therapy. *Br. Med. J.*, **303**, 1514

32. Waxman, J. and Zatzkis, S. M. (1986). Fibromyalgia and menopause. Examination of the relationship. *Postgrad. Med.*, **80**, 165–7, 170–1

33. Puig, J. G.,Michan, A. D., Jimenez, M. L., Perez de Ayala, C., Mateos, F. A., Capitan, C. F., de Miguel, E. and Gijon, J.B. (1991). Female gout. Clinical spectrum and uric acid metabolism. *Arch. Intern. Med.*, **151**, 726–32

34. Lally, E. V., Ho, G. Jr and Kaplan, S. R. (1986). The clinical spectrum of gouty arthritis in women. *Arch. Intern. Med.*, **146**, 2221–5

35. Kelsall, J. T. and O'Hanlon, D. P. (1994). Gout during pregnancy. *J. Rheumatol.*, **21**, 1365–6

Hormone replacement therapy following myocardial infarction, stroke and venous thromboembolism

47

A. Pines

Recently published large-scale epidemiological studies confirmed that prolonged hormone replacement therapy reduces the risk for future cardiovascular events by 30–50%[1,2]. Other clinical studies demonstrated that hormone users had a better cardiovascular risk profile when compared with that of non-users or of women receiving placebo[3–5]. According to Grady and colleagues the lifetime probability for coronary artery disease in a 50-year-old white woman treated with long-term hormone replacement is 12% lower than that in non-users[6].

Cardioprotection by hormonal therapy is more pronounced in women with high-risk profiles (hypertension, hypercholesterolemia, diabetes mellitus or smoking) than in women without risk factors for coronary artery disease[1]. This finding is interesting since endothelial dysfunction appears early during the course of the above diseases, and the ability of estrogen to restore endothelial function and improve arterial-wall reactivity may be one mechanism by which estrogens induce a reduction in cardiovascular morbidity and mortality[7].

However, little information is available on the effects of long-term hormone therapy in women already experiencing a heart condition, namely, on secondary prevention by hormones. In fact, until recently, many physicians considered arterial or cardiac disease a contraindication for hormone substitution. Even hypertension was listed among the relative contraindications, while in fact the epidemiological data, such as in the Post-menopausal Estrogen/Progestin Interventions (PEPI) trial[5], showed that blood pressure was not influenced by postmenopausal hormonal treatment.

The Coronary Drug Project reported in the early 1970s that post myocardial infarction, males who received 5 mg of conjugated estrogens daily suffered an increased number of cardiovascular events[8]. This did not happen with a daily dose of 2.5 mg, although there were more cancers in this group than in the placebo arm. Following this study, estrogens were labeled as hazardous for coronary patients, especially men. In contrast with the above results, during the past 10 years, studies in women with ischemic heart disease have shown that those women who took estrogens at a traditional dose level (0.625 mg conjugated estrogens) did have a clear-cut benefit with regards to cardiac morbidity and mortality.

The unique studies carried out by Clarkson and colleagues investigating atherosclerosis in monkeys, demonstrated the capability of estrogens to retard or even reverse the development of arterial plaques[9,10]. In keeping with these results, Espeland and co-workers[11] studied postmenopausal women with early carotid artery atherosclerosis over a 4-year follow-up period. Women taking estrogen showed a regression in the intima–media thickness, which was similar to the effect of lipid-lowering medications. During the same time, a placebo group showed a progression of the atherosclerotic lesions. Several studies on women undergoing coronary angiography revealed that the extent of coronary atherosclerosis among hormone users was relatively small, namely that there were less

328

stenosed coronary arteries when compared with non-users of hormones[12,13].

Two long-term observational studies on women with cardiovascular disease at baseline, showed that the survival benefit conveyed by estrogens was greater in that group than in women who were initially free of cardiovascular disease. The first study, the Lipid Research Clinics Program[14], included a cohort of 23 000 women followed for 8.5 years. In women with prevalent cardiovascular disease, the cardio-vascular death rate was 14 per 10 000 in users, versus 66 per 10 000 in non-users. In the second study, the Leisure World Study[15], about 9000 women were followed for 7.5 years. In women with a positive history of angina or myocardial infarction, the all-cause mortality was 27 per 1000, versus 42 per 1000 in non-users. However, more exciting was the study of Sullivan and colleagues[16] who followed more than 2000 women with angiographically documented coronary artery disease during a 10-year period. Survival rate was far better among hormone users compared with non-users, and also among the users, protection was more pronounced in those women with severe coronary disease at baseline. The same group of investigators also found that the prognosis for hormone users among women undergoing coronary-artery bypass grafting was again much better than that for non-users[17].

Relating to stroke, the epidemiological data are inconsistent. Some studies demonstrated a reduction in the incidence of stroke in hormone users[18,19], while the largest study, the Nurses' Health Study[1], concluded that the incidence of stroke was similar among users and non-users of estrogens. There are almost no data on secondary prevention of stroke by estrogens. In a trial on women with prior transient cerebral ischemic attack who were taking aspirin, estrogen users among the participants had a relative risk for stroke of 0.2, compared with non-users[20].

Menopause has been associated with ele-vation in plasma concentrations of fibrinogen, factor VII and plasminogen activator inhibitor-1 (PAI-l), and a reduction in antithrombin

III[3,5,21]. This creates a change in hemostatic balance which is in favor of the coagulatory activity. Estrogens have a complex effect on hemostasis: they reverse some of the above-mentioned menopause-related alterations, but may also increase the activity of other coagulation factors. According to Winkler[22], the net effect of postmenopausal estrogen replacement is in favor of fibrinolysis. Despite a lack of carefully designed studies on the consequences of hormone therapy post thrombophlebitis or pulmonary embolism, most experts in the field of menopause believe that hormones can be given safely in these situations unless there is clear-cut evidence for a major coagulopathy. However, this view might change following three research articles which recently appeared in Lancet. The first study[23], a retrospective screening of hospital records of idiopathic venous thrombosis in women aged 45–64 years, demonstrated an odds ratio of 3.5 in current hormone users compared with current non-users. Risk was highest among short-term users, while past use was not associated with increased risk. The second study[24] used the database of a large health-providing organization. Current use of hormones was associated with a threefold increase in risk for idiopathic venous throm-bosis, as compared to non-users, in women aged 50–74 years. Estimates of risk positively correlated with the daily estrogen dosage. The third article, on pulmonary embolism, comes from the Nurses' Health Study[25]. Although primary pulmonary embolism was uncommon in their cohort, the authors found a twofold risk in current users of hormone replacement therapy compared with non-users. Although the above relative risk figures probably amount to only one additional case per year among 5000 hormone users, these data should at least increase caution in high-risk situations for venous thrombosis, and should be incorporated into the benefit versus risk calculations performed before starting hormonal replace-ment.

To conclude, the diversity of actions of female sex hormones, primarily estrogens, on lipid profile, on endothelial and vascular function, and on the development of atherosclerosis, all point to the expected benefit of such treatment in women with established coronary artery disease. Several studies on the secondary prevention by estrogens are now in progress, and when these data become available, we will be able to better understand and estimate the importance of hormone substitution in the treatment of women with ischemic heart disease. In the meantime, the American and European guidelines clearly suggest that hormone replacement should be advised for secondary prevention of coronary artery disease[26,27].

References

1. Grodstein, F., Stampfer, M. J., Manson, J. F., *et al.* (1996). Postmenopausal estrogen and progestin use and the risk of cardiovascular disease. *N. Engl. J. Med.*, **335**, 453–61
2. Ettinger, B., Friedman, G. D., Bush, T. and Quesenberry, C. P. Jr (1996). Reduced mortality associated with long-term postmenopausal estrogen therapy. *Obstet. Gynecol.* **87**, 6–12
3. Nabulsi, A. A., Folsom, A. R., White, A., *et al.* (1993). Association of hormone replacement therapy with various cardiovascular risk factors in postmenopausal women. *N. Engl. J. Med.*, **328**, 1069–75
4. Manolio, T. A., Furberg, C. D., Shemanski, L., *et al.* (1993). Association of postmenopausal estrogen use with cardiovascular disease and its risk factors in older women. *Circulation*, **88** (part 1), 2163–71
5. The Writing Group for the PEPI Trial. (1995). Effects of estrogen or estrogen/progestin regimens on heart disease risk factors in postmenopausal women: the Postmenopausal Estrogen/Progestin Interventions (PEPI) Trial. *J. Am.. Med.. Assoc.*, **273**, 199–208
6. Grady, D., Rubin, S. M., Petiti, D. B., *et al.* (1992). Hormone therapy to prevent disease and prolong life in postmenopausal women. *Ann. Intern. Med.*, **117**, 1016–37
7. White, M. M., Zamudio, S., Stevens, T., *et al.* (1995). Estrogen, progesterone, and vascular reactivity: potential cellular mechanisms. *Endocr. Rev.*, **6**, 739–51
8. The Coronary Drug Project Research Group. (1970). The Coronary Drug Project. Initial findings leading to modifications of its research protocol. *J. Am. Med. Assoc.*, **214**, 1303–13
9. Adams, M. R., Kaplan, J. R., Manuck, S. B., *et al.* (1990). Inhibition of coronary artery atherosclerosis by 17-beta estradiol in ovariectomized monkeys: lack of effect of added progesterone. *Arteriosclerosis*, **10**, 1051–7
10. Williams, J. K., Anthony, M. S., Honore, E. K. (1995). Regression of atherosclerosis in female monkeys. *Arterioscler. Thromb. Vasc. Biol.*, **15**, 827–36
11. Espeland, M. A., Applegate, W., Furberg, C. D., Lefkowitz, D., Rice, L. and Huninnghake, D. (1995). Estrogen replacement therapy and progression of intimal–medial thickness in the carotid arteries of postmenopausal women. *Am. J. Epidemiol.* **142**, 1011–19
12. Gruchow, H. W., Anderson, A. J., Barboriak, J. J. and Sobocinsky, K. A. (1988). Postmenopausal use of estrogen and occlusion of coronary arteries. *Am. Heart J.*, **115**, 954–63
13. Hong, M. K., Romm, P. A., Reagen, K., Green, C. E. and Rackley, C. E. (1992). Effects of estrogen replacement therapy on serum lipid values and angiographically defined coronary artery disease in postmenopausal women. *Am. J. Cardiol.* **69**, 176–8
14. Bush, T. L., Barrett-Connor, E., Cowan, L. D. *et al.* (1987). Cardiovascular mortality and non-contraceptive use of estrogen in women. Results from the Lipid Research Clinics Program Follow Up Study. *Circulation*, **75**, 1102–9
15. Henderson, B. E., Paganini-Hill, A. and Ross, R. K. (1991). Reduced mortality in users of estrogen replacement therapy. *Arch. Intern. Med.*, **151**, 75–8
16. Sullivan, J. M., Vander Zwaag, R., Hughes, J. P., *et al.* (1990). Estrogen replacement and coronary artery disease: effect in survival in postmenopausal women. *Arch. Intern. Med.* **150**, 2557–62
17. Sullivan, J. M., El-Zeky, E., Vander Zwaag, R. and Ramanathan, K. B. (1994). Estrogen replacement therapy after coronary artery bypass surgery: effect on survival. *J. Am. Coll. Cardiol.*, **23**, 49A
18. Falkeborn, M., Persson, I., Tereni, A., Adami, H. O., Lithell, B. and Bergstrom, R. (1993). Hormone replacement therapy and the risk of stroke. Follow-up of a populatlon-based cohort in Sweden. *Arch. Intern. Med.*, **153**, 1201–9
19. Finucane, F. F., Madans, J. H., Bush, T. L., Wolf,

P. H. and Kleinman, J. C. (1993). Decreased risk of stroke among postmenopausal hormone users. Results from a national cohort. *Arch. Intern. Med.*, **153**, 73–9

20. American–Canadian Cooperative Study Group. (1986). Persantine aspirin trial in cerebral ischemia. Part 3: risk factors for stroke. *Stroke*, **17**, 12–18

21. Mijatovic, V., Pines, A., Stehouwer, C. D. A., van der Mooren, M. J., and Kenemans, P., (1996). The effects of oestrogen on vessel wall and cardiac function, haemostasis and homocysteine metabolism. *Eur. Menopause J.*, **3**, 209–18

22. Winkler, U. H. (1992). Menopause, hormone replacement therapy and cardiovascular disease: review of haemostaseological findings. *Fibrinolysis*, **6**, (Suppl. 3), 5–10

23. Daly, E, Vessey, M. P., Hawkins, M. M., Carson, J. L. Gough, P. and Marsh, S. (1996). Risk of venous thromboembolism in users of hormone replacement therapy. *Lancet*, **348**, 977-80

24. Jick, H., Derby, L. E., Myers, M. W., Vasilakis, C. and Newton, K. M. (1996). Risk of hospital admission for idiopathic venous thrombo-embolism among users of postmenopausal oestrogens. *Lancet*, **348**, 981–3

25. Grodstein, F., Stampfer, M. J., Goldhaber, S. Z., *et al.* (1996). Prospective study of exogenous hormones and risk of pulmonary embolism in women. *Lancet*, **348**, 983–7

26. American College of Physicians. (1992). Guidelines for counseling postmenopausal women about preventive hormone therapy. *Ann. Intern. Med.*, **117**, 1038–41

27. Vessey, M., Stampfer, M., Breart, G., Godsland, I., Pines, A., Samsioe, G., Sullivan, J. and the European consensus development conference on menopause. (1996). Cardiovascular disease and menopause. *Hum. Reprod.*, **11**, 975–9

11

The aging male

Factors determining androgen levels in aging males

A. Vermeulen

Introduction

In middle-aged women the menopause, characterized by ovarian depletion of oocytes, signals the end of ovulatory cycles and hence the irreversible end of both reproductive life as well as of cyclic hormonal activity of the ovaries. In men, however, spermatogenesis and fertility are maintained until very old age and a sudden fall in sex hormone levels does not occur. Hence the male equivalent of the menopause, the andropause, does not exist. This does not imply, however, that testicular function remains uninfluenced by the aging process, as both exocrine (i.e. spermatogenesis and fertility) as well as endocrine function decrease slowly but progressively with age.

Carefully collected data concerning the influence of age on plasma androgen levels, obtained in both cross-sectional (for review see reference 1) and longitudinal[2,3] studies involving large groups of subjects, have shown that in healthy males testosterone (T) levels decrease by about 30% between age 25 and 75 years, whereas free testosterone (FT) levels decrease by ±50% over the same period. The more important decrease of FT levels than of total T levels is the consequence of the age-associated increase in sex hormone-binding globulin (SHBG) binding capacity[4].

At any age there exists, however, a very wide dispersion of the T and FT levels, such that even at very old age, some men have values which fall entirely within the range for young adults, whereas others have levels well in the hypogonadal range. In a study involving 300 healthy men aged 20–100 years, one out of 105 men aged 20–40, 7% of males aged 40–60

($n = 68$), 21% aged 60–80 years ($n = 87$) and 35% over 80 years ($n = 40$) had T values below the lower normal limit (11 nmol/l[5].) The latter is, however, rather arbitrary and it is probable that the sensitivity threshold for androgens is variable from tissue to tissue. What then are the factors responsible for this variability of T levels, accounting for the wide range of normal values in healthy males?

Factors influencing testosterone levels

Whereas many systemic diseases such as renal failure, cirrhosis of the liver, diabetes mellitus, rheumatoid arthritis and AIDS[6] may accelerate and accentuate the age-associated decrease of T levels, several factors appear to influence T levels in healthy males.

Genetic factors

Among these, genetic factors appear to have considerable influence on plasma testosterone concentration. Meikle and colleagues[7], comparing the variability of T levels in mono- and dizygotic twins, concluded that 80% of variability of T levels was attributable to genetic factors, whereas a heritability of over 40%[8] was found for the variability of the production rates of T, normalized for body surface area. One assumption in these studies is that the environmental correlation between monozygotic twin pairs is equal to the environmental correlation between dizygotic twins. Also the variability between SHBG levels, which codetermine total T levels, was largely determined by genetic factors.

Seasonal variations

Whereas the well-known circadian variation in T levels with maximum in the early morning and minimum in the late afternoon should not play a role in the wide range of normal T values, plasma samples being taken in the early morning, it is well known that plasma levels show circannual variations with highest levels generally in autumn, around October; the amplitude of the circannual variation is about 25% of the annual mesor[9,10].

Pulsatile secretion of testosterone

It has been reported[11,12] that testosterone is secreted in a pulsatile manner, with a pulse interval of 112 ± 14 min, an amplitude of 910 ± 92 ng/dl and a lag time, with respect to the luteinizing hormone (LH) pulse, of ± 60 (50–70) min. It should be mentioned, however, that the relationship between LH pulses and T levels is not always evident and that several authors have not observed any relation between these phenomena.

Smoking

Another factor influencing T levels is smoking: smokers and ex-smokers have higher T levels than non-smokers[13–15]; the difference persists when corrected for body mass index (BMI) and age, and corresponds to about 10 % of the levels in non smokers.

Obesity

The body mass index (relative obesity) is another important determinant of plasma T levels[16]. There exists a highly significant inverse correlation between body mass index (BMI) and plasma T, and this over the whole range of BMI. The decrease of T levels as a function of the BMI is related to the decrease in SHBG levels with increasing BMI, most probably as a consequence of increased insulin levels[15,17–21]. Whereas as long as BMI remains below 35–40 (moderate obesity) the FT levels remain comparable to levels in non-obese men of similar age, at higher BMI, i.e. morbid obesity, FT levels are decreased, indicating impairment of the feedback set point of the gonadostat[18], as evidenced by the decreased amplitude of the LH pulses in these subjects

Growth hormone levels

There exists also a strong negative correlation between the 24 hr growth hormone (GH) and insulin-like growth factor-I (IGF-I) levels on the one hand and the SHBG levels. Acromegalics have lower SHBG levels than controls[22] and GH administration to adult men with isolated GH deficiency results in a decrease of SHBG and total T levels[5,23,24].

Growth hormone therapy as well as hypersomatotropism induces, however, insulin resistance, and part of the effect of GH on SHBG levels might be mediated by hyperinsulism. In adult patients with isolated GH deficiency treated with physiologic doses of GH, we observed a significant decrease in SHBG levels without any increase in insulin level[5] and Riedl and co-workers[25] reported that total insulin secretion during an oral glucose tolerance test remained unchanged after 6 months of GH treatment. As GH and IGF-I decrease with aging, it is probable that the age-associated increase in SHBG levels and decrease of FT levels is in part the consequence of the decrease in GH levels[5].

Thyroid hormone levels

Also thyroid hormone levels are important determinants of SHBG and total T levels, FT levels remaining generally unaffected. In clinical hyperthyroidism, SHBG levels and consequently also total T levels are increased by a factor of 3–5 resulting in increased T levels[26,27]. Even in subclinical hyperthyroidism, characterized by isolated suppression of thyroid stimulating hormone (TSH) levels, without clinical symptoms of hyperthyroidism, SHBG and T levels are significantly increased.

Diet

As to the influence of diet on T levels most authors report an increase of SHBG levels when a vegetarian diet is taken. Key and associates[28] observed that vegetarians have a 23% higher SHBG concentration than omnivores, whereas their total T was only 7% higher and their FT 3% lower; they concluded that a vegan diet has little effect on total T and FT but increases SHBG.

Based on studies carried out for about 15 years in his department, Adlercreutz[29] claims that a Western-type diet elevates plasma levels of sex hormones and decreases SHBG concentration, increasing the bioavailability of these steroids. Belanger and colleagues[30] reported higher SHBG levels in vegetarians than in omnivores, but in this study no correction for differences of BMI was applied. Reed and co-workers[31] reported a decrease in SHBG when subjects were switched from a very low-fat (< 20 g/day) to a very high-fat diet (< 100 g/day). The latter diet, although isocaloric to the low-fat diet, was certainly low in carbohydrates and fiber; hence the respective role of these factors cannot be evaluated.

Surprisingly, Meikle and associates[32], in an acute experiment, observed that administration of a fat-containing meal resulted in a significant reduction of total and free testosterone, while Schultz and colleagues[33] found that a 6-week consumption of fiber-rich, flax-seed fortified bread high in lignan precursors did not affect free or total testosterone ((F) T) or SHBG levels. Field and colleagues[15] did not find an association between energy, alcohol or fat intake and sex hormone levels, but SHBG showed an inverse correlation with dietary fiber.

Insulin resistance

In how far the changes in diet induce changes in insulin secretion and plasma levels is not clear from these studies. It has been reported that low SHBG levels are a risk factor for the development of non-insulin-dependent diabetes mellitus (NIDMM)[34].

However, NIDDM is characterized by insulin resistance, and several authors reported an inverse correlation between SHBG and T levels on the one hand and insulin levels on the other hand[5,35,36]. *In vitro* studies by Singh and co-workers[37] as well as by Plymate and associates[38] have shown a direct inhibitory effect of insulin/IGF-I on SHBG production by hepatoma cells.

Alcohol

Alcohol abuse, even without cirrhosis of the liver, may also accentuate the age-associated decrease of testosterone levels[39,40], plasma levels of estradiol being increased.

Other factors

Other factors influencing (F)T levels are *stress situations*, whether physical (fever, for example) or psychological (depression), which generally depress T levels. This of course is most evident in acute critical illness[41,42], surgical injury[43] or acute myocardial infarction[43]. Interestingly, Phillips and colleagues[44] in a study involving 55 males without previous myocardial infarction, reported an inverse correlation between (F)T levels and the degree of *coronary artery disease*. Moreover, most authors[45–49] reported that male survivors of myocardial infarction have lower T levels then controls. On the other hand, in a longitudinal study involving 1000 Caucasian men aged 40–59 years, followed for 12 years, Barrett-Connor and Khaw[50] observed no correlation between plasma T and cardiovascular mortality; a similar observation was made by Cauley and co-workers[51] as well as by Haffner and associates[52]. Low T levels, therefore, appear to be accompanied by an increase of risk factors for cardiovascular disease but not with increased cardiovascular mortality.

Also *strenuous physical activity* decreases plasma T, eventually to clearly hypogondal levels. As expected, cortisol levels increase dramatically, the increase in dehydroepiandrosterone(sulfate) (DHEA(S)), although significant, being only modest. LH levels decrease only modestly and the response to gonadotropin-releasing hormone (GnRH) is reported to be increased, the T response to human chorionic gonadotropin (hCG) stimulation being reduced by 25%[53,54].

Albumin concentration may also affect total T levels: about 20–40% of T is albumin bound and a decrease of albumin decreases also total T levels[5].

Conclusion

In summary, while chronic diseases do accelerate and accentuate the age-associated decrease in (F) T levels, the variability of these levels in adult healthy males seems to be largely attributable to a complex interplay of genetic, seasonal, social (smoking, alcohol) and environmental (stress) factors, as well as to subtle variations in general health status (obesity, insulin resistance, atherosclerosis).

References

1. Vermeulen, A. (1991). Androgens in the aging male. Clinical Review 24. *J. Clin. Endocrinol. Metab.*, **73**, 221–4

2. Pearson, U. J. D., Blackman, M. R., Metter, E. J., Wachawiw, Z., Carter, H. B. and Harman, S. M. (1995). Effect of age and cigarette smoking on longitudinal changes in androgens and SHBG in healthy males. *77th Annual Meeting of the Endocrine Society*, Washington DC, abstr. P2–129

3. Morley, J. E., Kaiser, F. E., Perry, H. M., Patrick, P., Stauber, P. M., Vellas, B., Baumgartner, R. N. and Garry, P. J. (1996). Longitudinal changes in testosterone, SHBG, LH, and FSH in healthy older males. *10th International Congress on Endocrinology*, San Francisco, June, abstr. P1–158

4. Vermeulen, A. and Verdonck, L. (1972). Some studies on the biological significance of free testosterone. *J. Steroid Biochem.*, **3**, 421–6

5. Vermeulen, A., Kaufman, J. M. and Giagulli V. A. (1996). Influence of some biological indices on sex hormone binding globulin and androgen levels in aging or obese males. *J. Clin. Endocrinol. Metab.*, **81**, 1821–6

6. Handelsman, D. J. (1994). Testicular dysfunction in systemic disease. *Endocrinol. Metab. Clin. N. Am.*, **23**, 839–52

7. Meikle, A. W., Bishop, D. T., Stringham, J. D. and West, D. W. (1986). Quantitating genetic and non genetic factors to determine plasma sex steroid variation in normal male twins. *Metabolism*, **35**, 1090–5

8. Meikle, A. W., Stringham, J. D., Bishop, T. and West, D. W. (1988). Quantitation of genetic and non genetic factors influencing androgen productions and clearance rates in men. *J. Clin. Endocrinol. Metab.*, **67**, 104–9

9. Reinberg, A., Lagoguey, M., Chauffoumier, J. M. and Cesselin, F. (1975). Circannual and circadian rhythms in plasma testosterone in five healthy, young Parisian males. *Acta Endocrinol.*, **80**, 723–43

10. Smals, A. G. H., Kloppenburg, P. W. C. and Benraad, Th.J. (1976). Circannual cycle in plasma testosterone levels in man. *J. Clin. Endocrinol. Metab.*, **42**, 979–82

11. Naftolin, E., Judd, J. H. and Yen, S. C. C. (1973). Pulsatile pattern of gonadotropin and testosterone in men. Effects of clomiphene with and without testosterone. *J. Clin. Endocrinol. Metab.*, **36**, 285–8

12. Veldhuis, J. D., King, J. C., Urban, R. J., Rogol, A. D., Evans, W. S., Kolp, L. A. and Johnson, M. L. (1987). Operating characteristics of male hypothalamo–pituitary–gonadal axis. Pulsatile release of testosterone and follicle stimulating hormone and their temporal coupling with luteinizing hormone. *J. Clin. Endocrinol. Metab.*, **68**, 929–47

13. Deslypere, J. P. and Vermeulen, A. (1984). Leydig cell function in normal men. Effect of age, life style, residence, diet and activity. *J. Clin. Endocrinol. Metab.*, **59**, 955–61

14. Dai , W. S., Gutai, J. P. and Cauley, J. A. (1988). Cigarette smoking and serum sex hormones in men. *Am. J. Epidemiol.*, **128**, 796–808

15. Field, A. E., Colditz, G. A., Willett, W. C., Longcope, C. and McKinley, J. B. (1994). The relation of smoking, age, relative weight and dietary intake to serum adrenal steroids, sex hormones and sex hormone binding globulin in middle age men. *J. Clin. Endocrinol. Metab.*, **79**, 1310–16

16. Demoor, P. and Goossens, J. V. (1970). An inverse correlation between body weight and the activity of the steroid binding β globulin in human plasma. *Steroidologia*, **1**, 129–36

17. Vermeulen, A., Rubens, R. and Verdonck, L. (1972). Testosterone secretion and metabolism

in male senescence. *J. Clin. Endocrinol. Metab.*, **39**, 730–40

18. Giagulli, V. A., Kaufman, J. M. and Vermeulen, A. (1994). Pathogenesis of decreased androgen levels in obese men. *J. Clin. Endocrinol. Metab.*, **79**, 997–1000

19. Haffner, J. M., Katz, M. S., Stern, M. P. and Dunn, J. F. (1988). The relationship of sex hormones to hyperinsulinemia and hyperglycemia. *Metabolism*, **7**, 686–8

20. Strain, G., Zumoff, S., Rossner W. and Pi Sunyer, X. (1994). The relationship between serum levels of insulin and sex hormone binding globulin in man: the effect of weight loss. *J. Clin. Endocrinol. Metab.*, **79**, 1173–6

21. Simon, D., Preziosi, P., Bennett-Connor, F., Roger, M., Saint Paul, M., Nahoul, K. and Papoz, L. (1991). Interrelations between plasma testosterone and plasma insulin in healthy adult men: The Telecom Study. *Diabetologia*, **35**, 173–7

22. Demoor, P., Heyns, W. and Bouillon, R. (1972). Growth hormone and the steroid binding β-globulin in human plasma. *J. Steroid Biochem.*, **3**, 593–600

23. Erfurth, E. M., Hagmart, L. E., Sääf, M., Halt, K. (1996). Serum levels of insulin like growth factor 1 and insulin like growth factor binding protein 1 correlate with serum free testosterone and sex hormone binding globulin in healthy young and middle aged men. *Clin. Endocrinol.*, **44**, 654–64

24. Pfeilschifter, J., Scheidt-Nave, C., Leidig-Bruckner, G., Woitge, H. W., Blum, W. F., Wuster, C., Haack, and Ziegler, R. (1996). Relationship between circulating insulin-like growth factor components and sex hormones in a population based sample of 50–80 year old men and women. *J. Clin. Endocrinol. Metab.*, **81**, 2534–40

25. Riedl, M., Kotzman, H., Clodi, M., *et al.* (1995). The effect of 3 months of recombinant growth hormone replacement therapy on glucose metabolism in growth hormone deficient adults. *77th Annual Meeting of the Endocrine Society*, Washington DC, abstr. P2-268

26. Dray, F., Mowszowisz, I., Ledru, M. J., Crepy, O., Delzant, G. and Sebaoun, J. (1969). Anomalies de l'affinité de liaison de la testostérone dans le sérum de sujets thyréotoxicosiques. *Ann. d'Endocrinol.*, **30**, 223–32

27. Vermeulen, A., Stoica, T. and Verdonck, L. (1971). The apparent free testosterone concentration, an index of androgenicity. *J. Clin. Endocrinol. Metab.*, **33**, 759–67

28. Key, T., Roe, L., Thorogood, M., Moore, J. W., Clark, G. M. and Wang, D. Y. (1990). Testosterone, sex hormone binding globulin, calculated free T and estradiol in male vegans and omnivores. *Br. Med. J.*, **64**, 111–19

29. Adlercreutz, H. (1990). Western diet and Western diseases: some hormonal and biochemical mechanisms and associations. *Scand. J. Clin. Lab. Invest.*, **201** (Suppl.), 3–23

30. Belanger, A., Locong, A., Noel, C., Cusan, L., Dupont, A., Prevost, J., Caron, S. and Sevigny, J. (1989). Influence of diet on plasma steroid and plasma binding globulin levels in adult males. *J. Steroid Biochem.*, **32**, 829–33

31. Reed, M. J., Cheng, R. W., Simmonds, M., Richmond, W. and James V. H. T. (1987). Dietary lipids: an additional regulator of plasma levels of sex hormone binding globulin. *J. Clin. Endocrinol. Metab.*, **64**, 1083–5

32. Meikle, A. W., Stringham, J. D., Woodward, M. G. and McMurray, M. P. (1990). Effects of fat containing meal on sex hormones in men. *Metabolism*, **39**, 943–6

33. Schultz, T. D., Bonorden, W. R. and Seaman, W. R. (1991). Effect of short time flax-seed consumption on lignan and sex hormone metabolism in men. *Nutr. Res.*, **11**, 1089–100

34. Lindstedt, G., Lundberg, P. A., Lapidus. L., Lundgren, H., Bengtsson, C. and Björntorp, P. (1991). Low sex hormone binding globulin concentration an independent risk factor for the development of NIDDM. *Diabetes*, **40**,123–8

35. Simon, D., Nahoul, K. and Charles, M. A. (1995). Sex hormones, aging, ethnicity and insulin serum levels in men: an overview of the TELECOM study. In Oddens, B. and Vermeulen, A. (eds.) *Androgens and the Aging Male*, pp. 85–101. (Carnforth: Parthenon Publishing

36. Haffner, S. M., Valdez, R. M., Mykkanen, L., Stern, M. P. and Katz, M. S. (1994). Decreased testosterone and dehydroepiandrosterone sulfate concentration are associated with increased insulin and glucose concentration in non diabetic men. *Metabolism*, **43**, 599-603

37. Singh, A., Hamilton, F. D., Koistinen, R., Seppälä, M., James, V. H. T., Franks, S. and Reed, M. J. (1990). Effect of insulin-like growth factor type 1 (IGF-1) and insulin on the secretion of sex hormone binding globulin and IGF-1 binding protein by human hepatoma cells. *J. Endocrinol.*, **124**, R1–3

38. Plymate, S. R.,Matej, L. A., Jones, R. E. and Friedl, K. E. (1988). Inhibition of sex hormone binding globulin production in the human hepatoma cell line. *J. Clin. Endocrinol. Metab.*, **67**, 460–4

39. Irwin, M., Dreyfus, E., Baird, D., Smith, T. L. and Schuckit, M. (1988). Testosterone in chronic alcoholic disease. *Br. J. Addict.*, **83**, 949–53

40. Cicero, T. J. (1982). Alcohol induced defects in the hypothalamo-pituitary luteinizing hormone action in the male. *Alcoholism*, **6**, 207–15

41. Dong, Q., Hawker, F., William, D., *et al.* (1992). Circulating inhibin and testosterone levels in

men with critical illness. *Clin. Endocrinol.*, **36**, 399–404

42. Woolf, F. D., Hamill, R. W., McDonald, J. V., Lee, L.A. and King, M. (1985). Transient hypogonadotropic hypogonadism caused by critical illness. *J. Clin. Endocrinol. Metab.*, **60**, 444–50

43. Wang, C., Chan ,V. and Yeung, R. T. T. (1978). Effect of surgical stress on pituitary testicular function. *Clin. Endocrinol.*, **9**, 255–66

44. Phillips, G. B., Pinkernell, B. J., Jing, T. Y. (1994). The association of hypotestosteronemia with coronary heart disease. *Arterioscl. Thromb.*, **14**, 701–6

45. Poggi, U. I., Arguelles, A. E., Rosner, J., de Laborde, M. P., Cassini, J. H. and Volmer, M. C. (1976). Plasma testosterone and serum lipids in male survivors of myocardial infarction. *J. Steroid Biochem.*, **7**, 229–31

46. Swartz, C. M. and Young, M. A. (1987). Low serum testosterone and myocardial infarction in geriatric male patients. *J. Am. Geriatr. Soc.*, **35**, 39–44

47. Lichtenstein, M. J., Yarnell, J. W. G., Elwood, P. C., Beswick, A. D., Sweetnam, P. M., Marks, V., Teale, D. and Raid Fahmy, D. (1987). Sex hormones, insulin, lipids and prevalent ischemic disease. *Am. J. Epidemiol.*, **12**, 647–57

48. Mendoza, S. G., Zerpa, A., Carrasco, H., Colmenares, O., Rangel, A., Gartside, P. S. and Kashyap, M. L. (1983). Estradiol, testosterone, apolipoproteins, apolipoprotein cholesterol and lipolytic enzymes in men with premature myocardial infarction and angiographically assessed coronary occlusion. *Artery*, **2**, 1–23

49. Sewdarsen, M., Vythilingum, S., Sialal, I., Desai, R. K. and Becker P. (1990). Abnormalities in sex hormones are a risk factor for premature manifestation of coronary artery disease in South African Indian men. *Atherosclerosis*, **83**, 111–17

50. Barrett-Connor, F. and Khaw, K. S. (1988). Endogenous sex hormone levels and cardiovascular disease in men: a prospective population based study. *Circulation*, **78**, 539–43

51. Cauley, S. A., Gutai, J. P., Kuller, L. H. and Dai, S. (1987). Usefulness of sex steroid hormone levels in predicting coronary artery disease in men. *Am. J. Cardiol.*, **60**, 771–7

52. Haffner, S. M., Moss, S. E., Klein, B. E. K. and Klein, R. (1996). Sex hormones and DHEASO$_4$ in relation to ischemic heart disease in diabetic subjects: a WESDR study. *Diabetes Care*, **19**, 1045–50

53. Bernton, E., Hoover, D., Galloway, R. and Popp, K. (1995). Adaptation to chronic stress in military trainees. Adrenal androgens, testosterone, glucocorticoids, IGF-l and immune function. *N.Y. Acad. Sci.*, **774**, 217–31

54. Opstad, P. R. (1992). The hypothalamo-pituitary regulation of androgen secretion in young men, after prolonged physical stress combined with energy and sleep deprivation. *Acta Endocrinol.*, **127**, 231–6

The benefits and risks of androgen therapy in the aging male: prostate disease, lipids and vascular factors

49

L. J. G. Gooren

Introduction

It is now well established that there is a statistically significant decline of levels of biologically available androgens in aging men. This is more manifest in the free testosterone levels than in the values of total testosterone routinely measured in the laboratory[1]. Notwithstanding this statistical decline, testosterone values of aged men will often be found to lie within the range of reference values of eugonadal men. They may have fallen significantly in a person's lifetime but this cannot be assessed in an individual presenting for clinical evaluation. Determination of luteinizing hormone (LH) levels may be of help, since most studies have found that LH levels are elevated in response to the decline of testosterone levels with aging[2], though less so than is observed in younger men with similarly decreased testosterone levels[3].

Thus a substantial number of elderly men continue to have serum testosterone levels within the range found in much younger men, and the question arises whether the observed decline of androgen levels has any clinical significance. The question could be phrased differently: do aging men have complaints or physical characteristics that would imply androgen deficiency? The next question is whether androgen supplementation would be beneficial in the sense that it reverses or ameliorates the presumed expressions of this androgen deficiency in aging men; and would this be a safe medical practice? None of these questions can presently be answered definitively.

Aging of androgen-dependent systems and functions

On closer examination aging men show physical signs reminiscent of androgen deficiency and maybe also growth hormone deficiency. This had already been noted by pioneers in the field of the study of testicular function and aging such as Brown-Séquard and Steinach, which persuaded them to booster androgen action as was the fashion of their day. Over the past decades target organs of androgens have been extensively studied and there is now some information on how aging affects these androgen targets.

Bone mass and aging

Unlike in women, osteoporosis in men has received much less attention, but similar to the situation in women men show a progressive loss of bone, with an exponential increase in the incidence of bone fractures with aging[4,5]. The role of estrogens in the maintenance of adult bone mass in premenopausal women and in bone loss of postmenopausal women is now widely accepted. The role of androgens in the (patho)physiology in the maintenance of skeletal integrity is much less clear. Also the question of whether the still relatively high androgen levels in aging men are (in)sufficient to prevent bone loss has not been resolved[4,5]. Indeed, both androgen levels and bone mass decline with age, but whether the relative decline of androgen levels with aging is a causal factor in senile osteoporosis remains uncertain[4]. In the elderly some rather weak associations between androgen levels and bone mineral density could be established at some, but not at all skeletal sites[6]. In a recent study of aging men it could be shown that the levels of free testosterone predicted loss of cancellous bone[7]. Others failed to find any correlation[8]. A recent paper found evidence that bioavailable testosterone levels are positively associated with insulin-like growth factors; the latter correlated again with bone mineral density of the femur and the calcaneus[9]. It may well be that growth hormone, in a complex way interrelated with levels of bioavailable androgens, is also a significant factor in bone loss in aging.

A complicating factor for our understanding of the role of androgens in bone metabolism is that (part of) their effects may be mediated through estrogens following aromatization of androgens. But specific androgen binding sites in human osteoblast-like cell lines[10] and a stimulatory effect on osteoblast function as well as bone-cell proliferation and differentiation[11] have been demonstrated. Testosterone administration to female-to-male transsexuals resulted in an increase of serum insulin-like growth factor-1 and biochemical indices of bone formation[12]. In line with this observation is the fact that the underlying process of bone loss in aging is a decreased osteoblast function which appeared to correlate with a marker of free androgens[7].

The available studies in hypogonadal men receiving androgen replacement treatment show that their bone mass increases but does not become normal[13]. This might indicate that testosterone is not capable of inducing a normal male bone mass or, alternatively, that the mode of replacement is inadequate[14]. Further, the timing of testosterone replacement might be crucial. Men with a history of delayed puberty suffer from osteopenia, maybe providing an indication that development of bone mass is critically dependent upon androgen exposure at the normal age of puberty[15].

Some studies have found a beneficial effect of androgen supplementation in old age on biochemical indices of bone turnover. During androgen treatment of elderly males an increase of levels of osteocalcin, a biochemical marker of osteoblast activity, was found[16] and another study found a reduction in the excretion of hydroxyproline, an index of bone resorption[17]. A third study, however, found no effect[4].

In conclusion, the role of the relative hypogonadism of old age in senile osteoporosis has not been clearly established. The first evidence of a beneficial effect of androgen supplementation is encouraging but not undisputed. Only longitudinal studies can clarify both issues satisfactorily.

Lean body mass and muscle strength

Androgens have an anabolic effect on muscles, especially the muscles of the upper body. This effect is mediated by testosterone itself; there is little 5α-reductase activity in muscles. With aging there is a decrease in muscle mass, most of the time associated with an increase in adipose tissue, predominantly in the abdominal and also upper body regions[18,19]. Again, it remains to be established whether the synchronism of the decline of muscle mass and of androgen levels with aging is causally interrelated. Declining levels of growth hormone (correlating with abdominal adiposity and physical fitness) might be another relevant factor[19]. While androgen administration to hypogonadal men increases muscle and alters fat distribution, it is uncertain whether such an effect can be expected in the case of aging men with relatively normal testosterone levels. Two studies that investigated the effect of testosterone supplementation to small groups of aging men found an increase of lean body mass and muscle strength[16,17]. Interestingly, a very recent report[20] sheds light on a long disputed question whether administration of androgenic–anabolic steroids to eugonadal men adds to their muscle mass/strength. This study showed such an effect when 600 mg of testosterone enanthate per week were given to men between 19 and 40 years of age. The effect was more pronounced when testosterone administration was combined with strength training. In view of the potential side-effects it is almost certain that such supraphysiologic doses could not be given in the long term to aging men.

In conclusion, again, the causal role of declining androgen levels with aging in loss of muscle mass/strength has not been proven. The potential benefit of androgen supplementation in a safe dosage for the elderly awaits further study.

Androgens and sexual/psychological functions

Reliable studies on the relationships between androgens and psychological functions are of rather recent date. There is now solid evidence that androgens stimulate sexual appetite. With regard to erectile function the situation is somewhat less clear. Nocturnal and spontaneous erections are clearly androgen-dependent; erections in response to visual erotic stimuli are less androgen dependent though achievement of erections and rigidity show a relationship, while detumescense appears to be prolonged with lower testosterone levels. Erections in response to auditory stimuli and fantasy are probably androgen dependent. It has become clear that in males between 20 and 50 years approximately 60–80% of the normal physiological levels suffice to maintain sexual functions, and that increasing testosterone levels above that threshold adds little to sexual functioning. Whether this holds true for aging men remains to be established. Some believe that the sensitivity to androgens decreases with aging[21]. Most aging men complain rather of erectile failure than of loss of libido; therefore it is not certain that their sexual functioning will improve much upon androgen supplementation.

Administration of high doses of androgens may lead to sexual deviancy in those predisposed to it. However, it seems safe to assume that a modest increase of testosterone levels in aging men will not lead to sexually deviant behavior. The relationship between testosterone and aggression is less well researched, but a relationship with anger proneness and tendencies to aggression is demonstrable. The latter is not identical with overt aggression. Recently there has been a large number of reports on psychological effects of anabolic steroids. They may vary from depression to mania to overt violence specifically in response to provocation. It is likely that these effects are related to the doses used and are unlikely to occur with moderate androgen supplementation.

There is some evidence to suggest that peripheral testosterone levels can influence performance of cognitive tasks[22] which is supported by the finding that testosterone administration to older men enhances performance on a measure of spatial cognition[23].

Benefits and risks of androgen supplementation in old age

The phenomena described above might suggest that some signs and symptoms of aging are related to the (statistically reliably demonstrated) decline of androgen levels with old age. But it is likely that aging itself is the most prominent determinant of this process. The question arises whether androgen supplementation for (selected) aging men might benefit their health. Naturally, before an informed and sound decision can be made the potential benefits and the disadvantages have to be weighed carefully. On balance, androgens enjoy a dubious medical reputation[24]. They have been implicated in some typically age-related medical conditions of men, such as cardiovascular and prostate disease. Though there is certainly truth in these assumptions, some views need to be modified.

Androgens and cardiovascular disease

Traditionally it is thought that the relationship between sex steroids and cardiovascular disease is predominantly determined by the relatively beneficial effects of estrogens and by the relatively detrimental effects of androgens on lipid profiles. Recent research shows that this view is too limited and that effects of sex steroids on other biological systems, such as fat distribution, endocrine/paracrine factors produced by the vascular wall, blood platelets and coagulation must be considered too. It is now generally believed that women until menopause, in comparison to men, are protected against cardiovascular disease. Postmenopausal estrogen use provides further protection[25]. It is then paradoxical that in cross-sectional studies of men elevated levels of estrogens and relatively low levels of testosterone[26] appear to be associated with coronary disease and myocardial infarction. Whether testosterone supplementation of aging men can reverse this cardiovascular risk is an interesting question which cannot be answered yet.

Fat distribution, insulin resistance and cardiovascular disease

From puberty onwards, men and women differ in their distribution of body fat over the subcutaneous and intra-abdominal (or visceral) fat depots. From age 20–30 years onwards men have twice as large visceral fat storage as women with a comparable body mass index. If men store fat, they accumulate it preferentially intra-abdominally, while in women this occurs preferentially subcutaneously on hips and thighs. There is convincing evidence that this storage pattern is androgen-related. Women with high androgen levels have more intra-abdominal fat than controls.

Visceral fat accumulation has been found to be a risk factor for cardiovascular disease and non-insulin-dependent diabetes mellitus. Its mechanism is not fully clear but it appears that visceral fat is metabolically very active with a high turnover of triglycerides possibly induced by testosterone. Testosterone inhibits triglyceride uptake and lipoprotein lipase activity[27]. The subsequent load of triglycerides and/or free fatty acids reaching the liver via the portal vein interferes with hepatic handling of insulin, leading to hyperinsulinism[28] and impaired glucose tolerance, and further to a lowering of high-density lipoprotein (HDL)

cholesterol and to a rise of triglycerides, all constituting cardiovascular risk factors[29,30].

Though the role of testosterone seems certain in the above mechanism, there is a paradox, in the sense that men with lower-than-normal testosterone levels are more at risk of cardiovascular disease[26]. Men with visceral fat accumulation often have relatively low testosterone values, the mechanism of which has not been elucidated, though in the Rancho Bernardo survey it was observed that men with lower levels of gonadal and adrenal androgens were more likely to develop a high waist/hip ratio in the following years[30]. Further it has been shown in several studies that men with low levels of testicular and adrenal androgens have higher insulin levels and an impaired glucose tolerance[31]. It is not known whether low androgen levels or hyperinsulinemia is the primary event in this correlation. Some evidence for both positions has been found. The observation that men with low androgen levels have higher basal insulin levels contrasts with the reports that describe the induction of hyper-insulinemia upon androgen administration in younger subjects[32]. Once men have developed non-insulin-dependent diabetes associated with hyperinsulinemia, they turn out to have lower androgen levels[33].

Androgens and sodium retention

All androgens cause some degree of sodium retention and expansion of extracellular fluid volume[24]. This effect is usually small; weight increases by about 3% in healthy individuals. However, in patients with heart and/or renal disease an already fragile balance may be disturbed, and edema may develop.

Androgens and vasoactive substances

Among the most significant vasoactive substances are the endothelins. Endothelins are a family of peptides which are produced in a variety of tissues where they act as modulators of vasomotor tone, cell proliferation and hormone production. Studies with endothelins

343

and specific endothelin-receptor antagonists have suggested that these peptides are important in vascular physiology and disease. Endothelin should be regarded more as a paracrine than as an endocrine hormone. The production of endothelins is regulated by a variety of hormones, other vasoactive substances and conditions of vascular stress. Endothelin-1 probably has a role in the maintenance of basal vasomotor tone and it is a very potent vasoconstrictor, counteracted by nitric oxide, prostacyclin and atrial natriuretic peptide. It is likely that endothelin-1 plays a role in atherosclerosis and cardiac hypertrophy (for review see Levin, reference 34).

Plasma levels of endothelins are higher in men than in women[35]. In a study we found that testosterone administration to female-to-male transsexuals increased plasma endothelin levels, while androgen deprivation with cyproterone acetate with simultaneous administration of ethinylestradiol decreased endothelin levels[35]. Indeed, in a study of female cynomolgus monkeys it was found that induction of male plasma androgen levels was strongly atherogenic, independently of variations in plasma lipoprotein and non-lipoprotein risk variables, though it reversed atherosclerosis-related impairment of endothelium-dependent vasodilator responses in this study[36]. It is too early to determine whether replacement with physiological doses of androgens does indeed contribute to cardiovascular risks through an endothelin-mediated mechanism, but it seems advisable to pay attention to this factor in future studies of androgen replacement in elderly men.

Androgens and hemostasis

Androgens exert an effect on hemostasis and one of the factors to be considered are the prostaglandins. Platelet aggregation is prevented by prostaglandin I2 (PGI2, prostacyclin), a vasodilatatory and anti-aggregatory eicosanoid, and is stimulated by thromboxane B2 (TXB2), a vasoconstricting and proaggregatory eicosanoid. It has been shown that testosterone inhibits PGI2 production in aortic smooth muscle cell cultures, whereas testosterone significantly increased TXB2 in monkeys[36]. Furthermore, the expression of TXA2 receptors is upregulated by testosterone, which may contribute to the thrombogenicity of androgenic steroids[37]. There have indeed been incidental reports of thrombotic complications associated with androgen administration[38,39]. Such effects were more apparent when high-dose anabolic steroids were used [40]. By contrast, administration of anabolic 17α-alkylated androgens may increase fibrinolytic activity and the natural anticoagulant proteins, protein C, protein S[40] and antithrombin III[41], thereby partly counterbalancing the unfavorable effects of androgens. These observations suggest strongly that androgen administration, apart from its effects on coagulation, also influences vascular factors which play a significant role in the increased thrombosis risks of androgen administration. The von Willebrand factor (vWF) stimulates thrombocyte adhesion and aggregation and carries clotting factor VIII. There are no clear sex differences in health and disease. In a study of female-to-male transsexuals receiving testosterone we found a decrease of vWF levels while testosterone had no effect on tissue-type plasminogen activator and urinokinase-type plasminogen activator, factors in fibrinolysis, and their inhibitor plasminogen activator inhibitor-1 (unpublished observation). By contrast, there are studies that suggest that the higher rate of cardiovascular disease in androgen-deficient patients is mediated by a low baseline fibrinolytic activity via an increased synthesis of plasminogen activator inhibitor PAI 1 (for review see reference 42). In summary, while some effects of testosterone on the cardiovascular system must be viewed as negative, others are neutral or even positive.

Androgens and serum lipids

There is as yet no full consensus on the effect of androgens on serum lipids and lipoproteins. This is (partially) due to differences in study designs and whether endogenous or exogenous androgen effects are investigated. The evaluation is complicated since part of both endogenous and exogenous testosterone is metabolized to estrogens.

There is, however, consensus that the incidence of coronary disease is significantly higher in men than in women until menopause, after which the incidence becomes somewhat similar. Therefore there is at first sight reason to believe that this sex difference in incidence of coronary heart disease is (in part) related to differences in endocrine milieu, causing differences in lipid profiles. Serum HDL cholesterol is lower and triglyceride levels are higher in eugonadal men than in premenopausal women, while these differences are not manifest before puberty.

Very convincing evidence that testosterone is involved in this sex difference comes from experiments wherein androgen levels were severely lowered with a luteinizing hormone-releasing hormone agonist, whereupon HDL cholesterol levels increased. When serum androgen levels subsequently were returned to normal, serum levels of HDL cholesterol decreased to normal male levels[43]. Most, but not all studies in adult men find a positive correlation between plasma testosterone and plasma HDL cholesterol concentrations. Administration of aromatizable androgens to hypogonadal men caused an increase in HDL cholesterol, while non-aromatizable androgens did the opposite. The role of estrogens was corroborated in another study[44]. In our own study the oral (aromatizable) androgen testosterone undecanoate was administered to hypogonadal men and to previously non-treated female-to-male transsexuals. While serum estradiol levels in the females remained three to four times higher during testosterone administration than in men, in both sexes levels of HDL cholesterol and HDL2 cholesterol declined and were eventually of the same magnitude. This led us to conclude that testosterone is indeed the major determinant of the sex difference in HDL cholesterol levels[45]. An alternative explanation is that the oral administration of testosterone may have been a significant variable since the effects of

androgens on lipoproteins are, at least in part, mediated by hepatic lipase, which enhances catabolism of HDL particles. Hepatic lipase may be more stimulated by oral than by parenteral administration of androgens. However, in line with our finding is that women with hyperandrogenism, with endogenous androgen overproduction, show 'male-like' plasma lipoprotein profiles.

Some studies in aging men have shown results that seem to contradict the overall notion that androgens, by their action on lipid profiles, would increase the risk for coronary artery disease. In a study of men with non-insulin-dependent diabetes mellitus these patients showed lower levels of endogenous total and free testosterone; their HDL cholesterol levels were lower but triglyceride levels higher than in controls[33]. In support of this finding another study found that in men with coronary artery disease plasma levels of testosterone correlated positively with HDL cholesterol, and negatively with the cardiovascular risk factors fibrinogen, plasminogen activator inhibitor-1 and insulin levels[26]. In a study of geriatric male patients who had suffered a myocardial infarction it was found that these patients had low testosterone levels in a threshold manner[46]. These studies suggest the intriguing possibility that, in spite of the overall negative effects of androgens on lipid profiles, a lower-than-normal androgen level in aging men is associated with an increase of atherosclerotic disease.

The first results of studies wherein testosterone itself was administered to mildly hypogonadal aging men were comforting. In a double-blind, placebo-controlled, crossover study Tenover[17] found that administering testosterone enanthate (100 mg per week) for 3 months to 13 healthy elderly men with low serum total and non-sex hormone binding globulin bound testosterone levels, decreased total and low density lipoprotein (LDL) cholesterol without changing HDL cholesterol. In agreement with these results are the findings of Morley and colleagues[16]. Administration of 200 mg testosterone enanthate every 2 weeks for 3 months decreased total cholesterol without changing HDL cholesterol levels. Of great interest is the study of Ellyin[47] establishing, in a 2-year study of administration of testosterone cypionate (25 mg per week or 50 mg every 2 weeks) to elderly mildly hypogonadal men, a decrease in total and LDL cholesterol and no change in HDL cholesterol and triglycerides.

In summary, not all results of studies on the relationship between testosterone and lipid profiles indicate that androgens induce a more atherogenic lipid profile; actually, the studies of testosterone administration in aging men point in another direction. When studying the effects of androgens on lipid profiles in relation to cardiovascular disease, it has to be kept in mind that androgens also have direct effects on the vascular wall, on clotting and on insulin sensitivity independently of their effects on lipids, and the latter could also be invoked to explain sex differences in coronary artery disease.

Androgens and hematopoiesis and sleep apnea

From puberty onwards men have higher hemoglobin levels, hematocrits and red blood cell counts than women. Both testosterone and 5α-dihydrotestosterone (DHT) stimulate renal production of erythropoietin. There is evidence for a direct effect of androgens on erythropoietic stem cells[48]. Androgen receptors have been found in cultured erythroblasts[49]. Young hypogonadal men have lower red blood cell counts and hematocrits than age-matched controls. These values increase upon administation of androgens to hypogonadal men[50]. Healthy older men tend to have similar or slightly lower hematocrit values than young adult men[46]. Two studies of older men receiving androgen administration have shown increases of hematocrit of up to 7%[16,17].

In a study of Matsumoto and co-workers[50] it was shown that androgen levels may play an important role in the pathogenesis of obstructive sleep apnea and that this may be a complication of testosterone therapy, though the relevance of androgens for obstructive sleep apnea could not be shown in a study wherein the pure antiandrogen flutamide was used[51]. Since these apneic events and the ensuing oxygen desaturation may lead to cardiovascular complications, it is pertinent to ask older men about this symptom, and to measure and follow up hematocrit values before and during androgen administration. Care must be exercised in men who are overweight, heavy smokers, or who have chronic obstructive airway disease.

In humans androgens appear to enhance platelet aggregation, through a mechanism involving substances secreted by the vascular wall, which is dealt with in a previous section.

Prostate disease and androgen supplementation in old age

An immediate concern of androgen supplementation in old age is the development and/or progression of prostate diseases such as benign prostate hyperplasia (BPH) and prostate carcinoma. It is widely accepted that both conditions do not develop without testosterone exposure early in life up to early adulthood. The present position of experts in the field is that androgens do not truly cause BPH or prostate carcinoma but that they have a 'permissive' role, clearly evidenced by the effects of reduction of the biological effects of androgens on both conditions. Nevertheless, this 'permissive' effect of androgens is reason enough to be careful with androgen supplementation in old age.

Several studies have found that the prevalence of microscopical prostate cancer and its precursor lesions increases strongly with aging. A prevalence of 33–50% has been found in men between 60 and 70 years of age[52]. Yet only a small subset of this men (4–5%) will develop clinically detectable carcinomas. There is presently no evidence that this subset has higher androgen levels[53]. While the prevalence of microscopical prostate cancer is similar in different parts of the world, the progression to clinical cancer varies strongly, with the highest prevalence in those parts with a western lifestyle. So it is probable that life-style factors, such as nutrition, might play a role. With regard to BPH there is no evidence that androgen administration to hypogonadal[54,55] or to eugonadal men[56] increases the incidence of BPH over that observed in control eugonadal men. A number of studies of androgen supplementation in elderly men who were not hypogonadal, have shown that, in the short term, there is only a modest increase in size and in levels of prostate specific antigen (PSA)[16,17,57]. Tissue concentrations of testosterone and DHT in the prostate are substantially higher than serum concentrations; it could be that a modest increase in serum androgens as would be the aim with androgen supplementation in old age, has no large effect on prostate levels.

So, even if there are no reasons for immediate concern, in any case testosterone administration to aging men should be done with caution. At the Second International Androgen Workshop (1995) the following recommendations were formulated with regard to safety of androgen administration to aging men by Snyder[58]. 'Investigators conducting trials of testosterone treatment should screen the men for prostate cancer before entering them in a study and monitor those who enter the study for possible development of prostate cancer, because prostate cancer is, to some extent, testosterone dependent. Screening should include a digital examination and a PSA. Finding a prostate nodule should lead to urological examination. Subjects who have an elevated PSA should be excluded. Using a PSA value of 4.0 ng/ml as the upper limit of normal would be conservative; alternatively, an age-adjusted range of normal or PSA density could be used.' The latter was very well documented in a recent publication[59]. This paper argued convincingly to apply age-specific and race-specific PSA values for the early detection of prostate cancer[60]. Subjects who qualify for and enter the study should also be monitored by digital rectal examination and PSA. An annualized rate of change of > 0.75 ng/ml per year (or the so-called PSA velocity) for 2 years should lead to urologic evaluation and prostate biopsy[58]. This guideline allows clinical studies to be carried out or androgens to be administered to individual hypogonadal aging men with due concern for adverse effects on the prostate.

With regard to how far an androgen that can be aromatized to estradiol but cannot be 5α-reduced to dihydrotestosterone[61] signifies progress with regard to safety for the prostate, remains to be determined.

Androgens and the liver

Most clinicians will encounter few side-effects of present androgen treatment on the liver. Several of the more serious side-effects of androgens on the liver (such as peliosis hepatis, subcellular changes of hepatocytes, hepatocellular hyperplasia and hepatocellular adenomas) turned out to be largely, though not exclusively, associated with the use of 17α-alkylated androgens or abuse of anabolic steroids. There is presumably a relation between side-effects of androgens on the liver and previous liver integrity. With a modest androgen supplementation to the aging male, no serious side-effects need to be expected.

Androgens and gynecomastia

Gynecomastia develops in cases of an increased estrogen/androgen ratio, or more precisely an estrogen/androgen ratio that effectively acts at the breast tissue (for review see Glass, reference 62). The aging process itself is associated with a loss of androgen production, a rise of sex hormone binding globulin, and an increase of adipose tissue, the site of aromatase activity enabling the conversion of androgens to estrogens. The combination of these factors leads already to a prevalence of spontaneous gynecomastia in old age. Administration of aromatizable androgens may lead to gynecomastia in both puberty and old age, in all likelihood when the subsequent increases of estrogens and androgens tip the balance in favor of a higher estrogen/androgen ratio. This side-effect is medically innocent and may subside over time. Patients with liver or renal disease may be particularly predisposed to the development of gynecomastia.

Androgens and skin effects

Androgens have a profound effect on the skin. Androgens regulate by means of receptors the sebaceous glands and hair growth function, and remarkably they do so on two different types of target cells in the skin: the epithelial sebocyte of the sebaceous gland and the mesenchymal cells of the hair follicle dermal papilla. Excessive oiliness of the skin and the development of acne are seen in younger men given androgen replacement. Whether these skin changes will occur in elderly men is not known. Middle-aged men starting on androgen replacement almost never show acne. In genetically predisposed individuals androgens induce male pattern alopecia.

Androgens and interaction with other drugs

Few interactions of androgens with other drugs have been reported. In patients using anticoagulants, anabolic steroids may reduce the dose which a patient requires by up to 25%. This is in part owing to the effect on coagulation factors; they may decrease the synthesis or increase the degradation of coagulation factors. Also, an increase of the natural anticoagulant antithrombin III has been found. Although not all patients are affected equally this should be taken into account when anticoagulants are given to patients using androgenic hormones, requiring a dose reduction of anticoagulants in these patients. There is some evidence from *in vitro* and animal experiments that the inhibitory effect of aspirin on platelet aggregation occurs only in the presence of androgens, an effect distinct from the above action of androgens on coagulation factors[63,64].

Conclusion

It is now well established that there is statistically a decline of androgen levels with aging, of which the clinical significance is not yet clear. Nevertheless, common features of aging in men, such as (abdominal) obesity, insulin resistance, hypertension, dyslipidemia and their increased cardiovascular morbidity, traditionally ascribed to the male–female difference in testosterone levels, appear also to have a relation to low-for-age testosterone levels.

The first reports on androgen supplementation to aging men are rather positive. It is at present difficult to predict whether androgen supplementation with modest dosages carries a significant risk. A reliable evaluation of that risk is hampered by our less than ideal androgen treatment modalities. Ideally, they should provide the aging male with only the amount of testosterone that restores his androgen deficiency. Several indications exist that aromatizable androgens have fewer negative side-effects that non-aromatizable forms. A new formula of an androgen, 7α-methyl-19-nortestosterone, which cannot be 5α-reduced to DHT, might be promising with regard to safety of androgen administration in old age.

With regard to cardiovascular risk factors there are literature data to suggest that androgens influence a number of risk factors in a negative direction although some effects may be more positive. There is no consensus on the negative effects of androgens on lipid profiles and on body fat distribution, but, on balance, effects are negative. Androgens seem to induce insulin resistance although hypoandrogenic men have been found to have hyperinsulinemia. Androgens may alter some, but not necessarily all vascular factors to a higher risk profile. It has been hypothesized that there is a threshold effect below which associations between levels of testosterone and unfavorable cardiovascular effects are stronger, explaining why lower-than-normal testosterone levels in aging carry a higher cardiovascular risk. At this moment no clear evaluation is possible how much these androgen-induced negative shifts in cardiovascular risk factors, assessed by laboratory methods, will in fact contribute to actual clinical cardiovascular morbidity and mortality. In view of the positive effects of the above mentioned studies, further investigations are warranted. Analogous to the studies on estrogen replacement in postmenopausal women, well-designed, long-term studies to monitor beneficial and negative effects are needed.

References

1. Gray, A., Feldman, A., McKinlay, J. B. and Longcope, C. (1991). Age, disease, and changing sex hormone levels in middle-aged men: results of the Massachusetts Male Aging Study. *J. Clin. Endocrinol. Metab.*, **73**, 1016–25

2. Deslypere, J. P. and Vermeulen, A. (1981). Aging and tissue androgens. *J. Clin. Endocrinol. Metab.*, **53**, 430–4

3. Korenman, S. G., Morley, J. E., Moorian, A. D., Davis, S. S., Kaiser, F. E., Silver, A. J., Viosca, S. P. and Garza, D. (1990). Secondary hypogonadism in older men: its relation to impotence. *J. Clin. Endocrinol. Metab.*, **71**, 963–9

4. Orwoll, E. S. and Klein, R. F. (1995). Osteoporosis in men. *Endocr. Rev.*, **16**, 87–116

5. Jones, G., Nguyen, T., Sambrook, P., Kelly, P. J. and Eisman, J. A. (1994). Progressive loss of bone in the femoral neck in elderly people: longitudinal findings from the Dubbo osteoporosis epidemiology study. *Br. Med. J.*, **309**, 691–5

6. Rudman, D., Drinka, P. J., Wilson, C. R., Mattson, D. E., Scherman, F., Cuisinier, M. C. and Schultz, S. (1994). Relations of endogenous anabolic hormones and physical activity to bone mineral density and lean body mass in elderly men. *Clin. Endocrinol.*, **40**, 653–61

7. Clarke, B. L., Ebeling, P. R., Jones, J. D., Wahner, H. W., O'Fallon, W. M., Riggs B. L. and Fitzpatrick, L. A. (1996). Changes in quantitative bone histomorphometry in aging healthy men. *J. Clin. Endocrinol. Metab.*, **81**, 2264–70

8. Drinka, P. J., Olson, J., Bauwens, S., Voeks, S. K., Carlson, I. and Wilson, M. (1993). Lack of association between free testosterone and bone density separate from age in elderly males. *Calcif. Tissue Int.*, **52**, 67–9

9. Pfeilschifter, J., Scheidt-Nave, C., Leidig-Bruckner, G., Woitge, H. W., Blum, F., Wüster, C., Haack, D. and Ziegler, R. (1996). Relationship between circulating insulin-like growth factor components and sex hormones in population-based sample of 50- to 80-year-old men and women. *J. Clin. Endocrinol. Metab.*, **81**, 2534–40

10. Orwoll, E. S., Otribirska, L., Romsey, E. E. and Keenan, E. J. (1991). Androgen receptors in osteoblast-like cell lines. *Calcif. Tissue Int.*, **49**, 182–7

11. Kasperk, Ch., Fitzsimmons, R., Strong, D., Mohan, S., Jennings, J., Wegerdal, J. and Baylink, D. (1990). Studies on the mechanisms by which androgens enhance mitogenesis and differentiation in bone cells. *J. Clin. Endocrinol. Metab.*, **71**, 1322–9

12. Van Kesteren, P., Lips, P., Deville, W., Popp-Snijders, C., Asscheman, H., Megens, J. and Gooren, L. (1996). The effect of one-year cross-sex hormonal treatment on bone metabolism and serum insulin-like growth factor-1 in transsexuals. *J. Clin. Endocrinol. Metab.*, **81**, 2227–32

13. Finkelstein, J. S., Klibanski, A., Neer, R. M., Doppelt, S. H., Rosenthal, D. and Crowley, W. F. Jr (1989). Increase in bone density during treatment of men with idiopathic hypogonadotropic hypogonadism. *J. Clin. Endocrinol. Metab.*, **69**, 776–83

14. Wong, F. H. W., Pun, K. K. and Wang, C. (1993). Loss of bone mass despite sufficient testosterone replacement. *Osteoporosis Int.*, **7**, 281–7

15. Finkelstein, J. S., Neer, R. M., Biller, B. M. K., Crawford, J. D. and Klibanski, A. (1992). Osteopenia in men with a history of delayed puberty. *N. Engl. J. Med.*, **326**, 600–4

16. Morley, J. E., Perry, H. M., Kaiser, F. E., Kraenzle, D., Jensen, J., Houston, K., Mattammal, M. and Perry, H. M. Jr (1993). Effect of testosterone replacement therapy in old hypogonadal males: a preliminary study. *J. Am. Geriatr. Soc.*, **41**, 149–52

17. Tenover, J. S. (1992). Effects of testosterone supplementation in the aging male. *J. Clin. Endocrinol. Metab.*, **75**, 1092–8

18. Swerdloff, R. S. and Wang, C. (1993). Androgens and aging in men. *Exp. Gerontol.*, **28**, 435–46

19. Vahl, N., Jørgensen, J. O. L., Jurik, A. G. and Christiansen, J. S. (1996). Abdominal adiposity and physical fitness are major determinants of the age associated decline in stimulated GH secretion in healthy male adults. *J. Clin. Endocrinol. Metab.*, **22**, 2209–15

20. Bhasin, S., Storer, T. W., Berman, N., Callegari, C., Clevenger B., Phillips, J., Bunnel, T. J., Tricker, R., Shirazi, R. and Casaburi, R. (1996). The effect of supraphysiologic doses of testosterone on muscle size and strength in normal men. *N. Engl. J. Med.*, **335**, 1–7

21. Schiavi, R. C. (1990). Sexuality and aging in men. *Ann. Rev. Sex. Res.*, **1**, 227–50
22. Kimura, D. and Hampson, E. (1994). Cognitive pattern in men and women is influenced by fluctuations in sex hormones. *Am. Psychol. Soc.*, **3**, 57–61
23. Janowsky, J. S., Oviatt, S. K. and Orwoll, E. S. (1994). Testosterone influences spatial cognition in older men. *Behav. Neurosci.*, **108**, 325–32
24. Wilson, J. D. (1988). Androgen abuse by athletes. *Endocr. Rev.*, **9**, 181–99
25. Grady, D., Rubin, S. M., Petitti, D. B., Fox, C. S., Black, B., Ettinger, B., Ernster, V. L. and Cummings, S. R. (1992). Hormone therapy to prevent disease and prolong life in postmenopausal women. *Ann. Intern. Med.*, **117**, 1016–37
26. Phillips, G. B., Pinkernell, B. H. and Jing, T.-Y. (1994). The association between hypo-testosteronemia and coronary artery disease in men. *Arterioscler. Thromb.*, **14**, 701–6
27. Marin, P., Odén, B. and Björntorp, P. (1995). Assimilation and mobilization of triglycerides in subcutaneous abdominal and femoral adipose tissue *in vivo* in men: effects of androgens. *J. Clin. Endocrinol. Metab.*, **80**, 239–43
28. Laws, A. and Reaven, G. M. (1993). Insulin resistance and risk factors for coronary heart disease. *Clin. Endocrinol. Metab.*, **7**, 1063–78
29. Plymate, S. R. and Swerdloff, R. S. (1992). Androgens, lipids and cardiovascular risk. *Ann. Intern. Med.*, **117**, 871–2
30. Khaw, K. T. and Barrett-Connor, E. (1992). Lower endogenous androgens predict central adiposity in men. *Ann. Epidemiol.*, **2**, 675–82
31. Haffner, S. M., Valdez, R. A., Mykkänen, L., Stern, M. P. and Katz, M. S. (1994). Decreased testosterone and dehydroepiandrosterone sulfate concentrations are associated with increased insulin and glucose concentrations in nondiabetic men. *Metabolism*, **43**, 599–603
32. Polderman, K. H., Gooren, L. J. G., Asscheman, H., Bakker, A. and Heine, R. J. (1994). Induction of insulin resistance by androgens and estrogens. *J. Clin. Endocrinol. Metab.*, **97**, 265–71
33. Barrett-Connor, E. (1992). Lower endogenous androgen levels and dyslipidemia in men with non-insulin dependent diabetes mellitus. *Ann. Intern. Med.*, **117**, 895–901
34. Levin, E. R. (1995). Endothelins. *N. Engl. J. Med.*, **333**, 356–63
35. Polderman, K. H., Stehouwer, C. D. A., Kamp, G. J., Dekker, G. A., Verheugt, F. W. A. and Gooren, L. J. G. (1993). Influence of sex hormones on plasma endothelin levels. *Ann. Intern. Med.*, **118**, 429–32
36. Adams, M. R., Williams, J. K. and Kaplan, J. R. (1995). Effects of androgens on coronary artery atherosclerosis and atherosclerosis-related impairment of vascular responsiveness. *Arterioscler. Thromb. Vasc. Biol.*, **15**, 562–70
37. Ajayi, A. A. (1995). Testosterone increases human platelet thromboxane A2 receptor density and aggregation responses. *Circulation*, **91**, 2742–7
38. Nagelberg, S. B., Laue, L., Loriaux, D. L., Liu, L. and Sherin, R. J. (1986). Cerebrovascular accident associated with testosterone therapy in a 20-year old hypogonadal man (letter). *N. Engl. J. Med.*, **314**, 649–50
39. Shizowa, Z., Yamada, H., Mabuchi, C., Hotta, T., Saito, M., Sobue, I. and Huang, Y. P. (1982). Superior sagittal sinus thrombosis associated with androgen therapy. *Ann. Neurol.*, **12**, 57–88
40. Mochizuki, R. M. and Richter, K. J. (1988). Cardiomyopathy and cerebrovascular accident associated with anabolic androgenic steroid use. *Phys. Sportsmed.*, **16**, 109–14
41. Ansell, J. E., Tiarks, C. and Fairchild, V. K. (1993). Coagulation abnormalities associated with the use of anabolic steroids. *Am. Heart J.*, **125**, 367–71
42. Winkler, U. H. (1996). Effects of androgens on hemostasis. *Maturitas*, **24**, 147–55
43. Bagatell, C. J., Knopp, R. H., Vale, W. W., Rivier, J. E. and Bremner, W. J. (1992). Physiological levels of testosterone suppress HDL cholesterol levels in normal men. *Ann. Intern. Med.*, **116**, 967–73
44. Bagatell, C. J., Knopp, R. H. and Bremner, W. J. (1994). Physiological levels of estradiol stimulate plasma high density lipoprotein 2 in normal men. *J. Clin. Endocrinol. Metab.*, **78**, 855–61
45. Asscheman, H., Gooren, L. J. G., Megens, J. A. J., Nauta, J., Kloosterboer, H. J. and Eikelboom, F. (1994). Serum testosterone level is the major determinant of the male–female differences in serum levels of high density lipoprotein cholesterol and HDL2 cholesterol. *Metabolism*, **43**, 935–9
46. Swartz, C. A. and Young, M. A. (1987). Low serum testosterone and myocardial infarction in geriatric male inpatients. *J. Am. Geriatr. Soc.*, **35**, 39–44
47. Ellyin, F. M. (1995). The long term beneficial effect of low dose testosterone in the aging male. In *The Endocrine Society 77th Annual Meeting*, Washingtom DC, June, program and abstracts, pp. 322, P2-127
48. Shahidi, N. T. (1973). Androgens and erythropoiesis. *N. Engl. J. Med.*, **289**, 72
49. Claustres, M. and Sultan, C. (1988). Androgen and erythropoiesis: evidence for an androgen receptor in erythroblasts from human bone marrow cultures. *Horm. Res.*, **29**, 17
50. Matsumoto, A. M., Sandblom, R. E., Schoene,

R. E., Lee, K. A., Giblin, E. C., Pierson, D. J. and Bremner, W. J. (1985). Testosterone replacement in hypogonadal men. *Clin. Endocrinol.*, **22**, 713–21

51. Stewart, D. A., Grunstein, R. R., Berthon-Jones, M., Handelsman, D. J. and Sullivan, C. E. (1992). Androgen blockade does not affect sleep-disordered breathing or chemosensitivity in men with obstructive sleep apnea. *Am. Rev. Resp. Dis.*, **146**, 1389–93

52. Sakr, W. A., Grignon, D. J., Crissman, J. D., Heilbrun, L. K., Cassin, B. J., Pontes, J. J. and Haas, G. P. (1994). High grade prostatic intraepithelial neoplasia (HGPIN) and prostate adenocarcinoma between the ages of 20–69: an autopsy study of 249 cases. *In Vivo*, **8**, 439–43

53. Carter, H. B., Pearson, J. D., Metter, E. J., Chan, D. W., Andres, R., Fozard, J. L., Rosner, W. and Walsh P. C. (1995). Longitudinal evaluation of serum androgen levels in men with and without prostate cancer. *The Prostate*, **27**, 25–31

54. Sasagawa, I., Nakada, T., Kazama, T., Satomi, S., Terada, K., and Katasyama, T. (1990). Volume change of the prostate and seminal vesicles in male hypogonadism after androgen replacement therapy. *Int. Urol. Nephrol.*, **22**, 279–84

55. Behre, H. M., Bohmeyer, J. and Nieschlag, E. (1994). Prostate volume in testosterone-treated hypogonadal men in comparison to age-matched normal controls. *Clin. Endocrinol.*, **40**, 341–9

56. Wallace, E. M., Pye, S. D., Wildt, S. R. and Wu, F. C. (1993). Prostate specific antigen and prostate size in men receiving exogenous testosterone for male contraception. *Int. J. Androl.*, **16**, 35–40

57. Holmäng, S., Marin, P., Lindtstedt, G. and Hedelin, H. (1993). Effect of long-term oral testosterone undecenoate treatment on prostate volume and serum prostate specific antigen in eugonadal middle-aged men. *The Prostate*, **23**, 99–106

58. Snyder, P. J. (1996). Development of criteria to monitor the occurrence of prostate cancer in testosterone clinical trials. In Bhasin, S., Gabelnick, H. L., Swerdloff, R. S. and Wang, C. (eds.) *Pharmacology, Biology, and Clinical Applications of Androgens*, pp. 143–50. (New York: Wiley-Liss)

59. Morgan, T. O., Jacobsen, S. J., McCarthy, W. F., Jacobson, D. J., McLeod, D. G. and Moul, J. W. (1996). Age specific reference ranges for serum prostate specific antigen in black men. *N. Engl. J. Med.*, **335**, 304–10

60. Oesterling, J. E. (1996). Age-specific reference ranges for serum PSA (editorial). *N. Engl. J. Med.*, **335**, 345–6

61. Sundaram, K., Kumar, N. and Bardin, C. W. (1993). 7α-methyl-nortestosterone (MENT): the optimal androgen for male contraception. *Ann. Med.*, **25**, 199–205

62. Glass, A. R. (1994). Gynecomastia. *Endocrinol. Metab. Clin. N. Am.*, **23**, 825–37

63. Westerholm, B. (1988). Sex hormones. In Dukes, M. N. G. (ed.) *Meyler's Side Effects of Drugs*, Chapter 42b, pp. 866–7. (Amsterdam: Elsevier)

64. Spranger, M., Aspey, B. S. and Harrison, M. J. (1989). Sex difference in antithrombotic effects of aspirin. *Stroke*, **20**, 34–7

Adrenal androgens in the adult male 50

K. Carlström

Introduction

Corticosteroids and sex steroids are both vital for mankind: corticosteroids for our survival as individuals and sex steroids for our survival as a species. *De novo* synthesis of steroid hormones in non-pregnant individuals only occurs in the adrenal cortex and in the gonads. The adrenal cortex secretes the vital glucocorticoids and mineralocorticoids, and also androgens. The latter in turn are converted into minor amounts of estrogens by peripheral aromatization. The gonads are only capable of secreting sex steroids. However, gonadal sex-steroid production is fully sufficient for an adequate reproductive function in both sexes. Why do the adrenals secrete androgens?

Adrenal androgens are usually discussed in terms of adrenal hyperandrogenism, e.g. congenital adrenal hyperplasia due to 21- or 11β-hydroxylase deficiency, androgen-secreting adrenal tumors or premature adrenarche. The physiological role of a normal adrenal androgen secretion is unknown. However, in the past decade, adrenal androgens have gained a new interest in two fields. First, the adrenal 'rest androgen' has been suggested to influence the outcome of endocrine treatment of prostatic cancer and second, the main adrenal androgen, dehydroepiandrosterone (DHEA) and its sulfate (DHEAS), are again brought up as being the 'fountain of youth'. In the present article the author will discuss the importance of adrenal androgens for androgen status in the adult male and for the etiology and treatment of prostatic disease, and also suggest a physiological role for circulating DHEA/DHEAS.

Origin of androgens in the adult male

The gonads and the adrenal cortex are the only glands capable of direct secretion of androgens in man. The testes secrete testosterone (T) and also lesser amounts of other androgens including T sulfate, 5-androstene-3β,17β-diol (5-ADIOL), DHEA, DHEAS, 4-androstene-3,17-dione (A-4) and others. T is by far the most important circulating androgen in the human male. More than 95% of circulating T in adult men is due to direct testicular secretion[1]. The remaining part arises by peripheral conversion of adrenal androgens into T. Direct adrenal secretion of T is minimal and the main androgens secreted from the adrenal cortex are the so-called 'adrenal androgens' DHEA, DHEAS, 5-ADIOL and A-4[1,2]. The androgen A-4 is an important substrate for peripheral estrogen synthesis in men and in postmenopausal women. The adrenal androgens have very weak androgenic potency of their own. The relative contribution of the testis and the adrenal cortex to circulating androgen concentrations in healthy adult men is summarized in Table 1. Circulating concentrations of the adrenal androgens are high and for compounds having steroid structure, the serum levels of DHEAS are secondary only to cholesterol (Table 1).

Is there any adrenal–testicular interaction?

Do adrenal steroids affect testicular steroid synthesis?

Besides the adrenal androgens, the adrenal cortex also secretes the vital corticosteroids cortisol and aldosterone, and also minor

Table 1 Relative testicular and adrenal contribution (glandular secretion + peripheral formation from precursors) and typical serum concentrations of circulating androgens, 17α-hydroxyprogesterone (17OHP) and cortisol in adult men[1,12]

Steroid	Serum levels	Testes (%)	Adrenals (%)
T (nmol/l)	10–35	> 95	< 5
A-4 (nmol/l)	3–8	25	75
DHEA (nmol/l)	8–25	10	90
DHEAS (nmol/l)	2000–10 000	15	85
17OHP (nmol/l)	2–10	75	25
Cortisol (nmol/l)	240–740	0	100

T, testosterone; A-4, 4-androstene-3,17-dione; DHEA/S, dehydroepiandrosterone/sulfate

amounts of other C_{21}-steroids. If adrenal steroids affect testicular testosterone synthesis, this may be either by regulating or modulating testicular activity or by providing raw material for testicular androgen synthesis. It is well known that high doses of glucocorticoids inhibit testicular T secretion: Cushing's disease, exogenous adrenocorticotropic hormone (ACTH) stimulation, insulin-induced hypoglycemia and exogenous glucocorticoids are all accompanied by low T levels in men. The inhibitory mechanisms seem to vary with the nature of hypercortisolism and include interference of glucocorticoids with the luteinizing hormone (LH) receptors in the Leydig cells, increased metabolic clearance rate of T and also interference with the pituitary–gonadal axis[3–6]. However, corticosteroids inhibit testicular T secretion only at supraphysiological levels and there are no reports of an influence of normal cortisol levels on testicular T synthesis. In fact, recent studies from some groups including our own rather seem to indicate the reverse (see below).

Do the quantitatively important, but weak adrenal androgens have any significance for androgen status in adult men? Only a minor amount of circulating T in men is formed by peripheral conversion of the adrenal androgens. The possibility of adrenal androgens serving as substrates for gonadal T synthesis has been discussed. Peripheral DHEAS may serve as an important substrate for T production in the ovarian follicles during superstimulation for ovulation induction[7]. Concerning the testis, Parker and Lifrak[8] reported a highly significant correlation between serum T and DHEAS in a group of healthy men having a very narrow age range, and suggested circulating DHEAS as a precursor also for testicular T synthesis. However, as far as we know from the literature, this is the only report of such a correlation and we have ourselves repeatedly failed to demonstrate it in large clinical materials. Nieschlag and Kley[9] reported an impaired T response upon human chorionic gonadotropin (hCG) stimulation in patients with Addison's disease and suggested DHEA/DHEAS as precursors for testicular T synthesis. However, a certain impairment of gonadal function *per se* by autoimmune mechanisms cannot be excluded in this disease. Furthermore, these patients had normal basal T levels, and this is also the case for another group of men with very low or even undetectable DHEAS levels, namely glucocorticoid-treated men with 21-hydroxylase deficiency[10]. This minimizes the role of adrenal steroids as precursors for testicular T synthesis and thereby the importance of the adrenal cortex for androgen status in men.

Do testicular steroids affect adrenal steroid synthesis?

A 'compensatory increase' in adrenal steroids following gonadectomy was frequently discussed and even accepted in older literature[11]. More recent studies including our own have shown slightly decreased or unchanged levels of most adrenal steroids following orchidectomy[11,12] and the decreases in basal steroid levels are entirely due to loss of the gonadal component (Table 1). However, while changes in testicular steroids do not seem significantly to affect basal levels of mainly adrenal steroids, there are indications that androgen status can modulate the response of the adrenal cortex to ACTH stimulation. We have previously demonstrated significantly increased adrenocortical responses in cortisol and 17α-hydroxy-progesterone (∂Cortisol and ∂17OHP) to an ACTH stimulation test in patients with prostatic cancer, 6 months after orchidectomy or chemical castration with gonadotropin releasing hormone (GnRH) agonists. On the other hand, 6 months of monotherapy with flutamide, which increases T levels due to increased pituitary LH secretion, resulted in significantly decreased ∂Cortisol and ∂17OHP levels (Figure 1). Basal cortisol levels and ∂DHEA and ∂A-4 values were not affected by

any of the treatment regimens[13,14]. These findings indicate a modulatory action of testicular T on the adrenocortical 4-ene-C_{21} steroid response to ACTH stimulation. This is further supported by recent reports on a higher responsiveness to ACTH of the female adrenal cortex than its male counterpart in terms of glucocorticoid production[15,16]. Recent data from our own departments indicate that this is the case also for other adrenocortical steroids (Table 2). Finally, in pooled clinical materials of healthy controls and metastase-free patients with prostatic cancer, having normal adrenocortical steroid values, we have found significant negative correlations between ACTH-induced increments in 4-ene-C_{21} steroids on the one hand and basal T and non-sex hormone binding globulin (SHBG)-bound T on the other, without any association to age (Figure 2). Thus androgens seem to modulate the adrenal response to ACTH; however, neither the underlying reason nor the mechanism is known. Interestingly, the

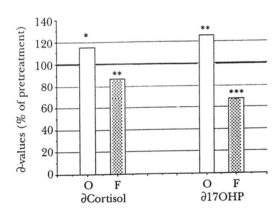

Figure 1 Changes in serum cortisol and 17α-hydroxyprogesterone (17OHP) 120 min after i.v. bolus injection of 250 μg adrenocorticotropic hormone (ACTH) 1–24 to patients with cancer of the prostate (CAP) 6 months after surgical or chemical (GnRH agonists) castration (O; $n = 23$) or after 6 months of monotherapy with flutamide (F; $n = 10$). The values are expressed as per cent of patients' ACTH-induced increase in steroid levels before treatment. *$p < 0.05$; **$p < 0.01$; ***$p < 0.001$, respectively. Data from references 13 and 14

Table 2 Basal serum levels and increments (∂-values) in adrenal steroids after 120 min following bolus i.v. injection of 250 μg adrenocorticotropic hormone (ACTH) 1–24 in healthy men and women. Mean and SEM or median and range. Significances of sex differences: *$p < 0.05$; **$p < 0.01$; ***$p < 0.001$ (unpaired t- or Mann–Whitney U-test)

	Men	Women
n	38	19
Age (years)	62.9 ± 0.4	60.4 ± 2.2
Cortisol (nmol/l)	405 ± 16	384 ± 32
∂Cortisol (nmol/l)	522 ± 25	652 ± 32**
17OHP (nmol/l)	2.8 ± 0.2	1.3 ± 0.1***
∂17OHP (nmol/l)	5.9 ± 0.6	8.9 ± 1.2*
A-4 (nmol/l)	4.2 ± 0.2	4.2 ± 0.3
∂A-4 (nmol/l)	2.3 ± 0.3	4.1 ± 0.5***
DHEA (nmol/l)	6.7 (1.8–15.8)	9.2 (1.8–24.2)*
∂DHEA (nmol/l)	12.6 (1.9–35.0)	17.1 (6.6–53.6)**

17OHP, 17α-hydroxyprogesterone; A-4, 4-androstene-3,17-dione; DHEA, dehydroepiandrosterone

increase in circulating T caused by monotherapy with flutamide decreased the adrenocortical response to ACTH, despite the fact that these patients were under androgen receptor blockade.

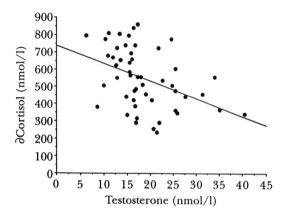

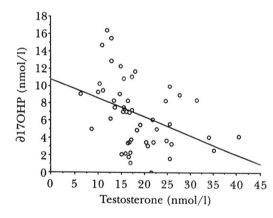

Figure 2 Correlations between adrenocorticotropic hormone (ACTH)-induced increments in serum cortisol (∂Cortisol) and 17α-hydroxyprogesterone (17OHP) (∂17OHP) 120 min after i.v. bolus injection of 250 μg ACTH 1–24 and serum testosterone (T) in a pooled group of 22 healthy men, and 29 untreated patients with newly diagnosed metastase-free prostatic cancer, but otherwise healthy, aged 60–87 years. Spearman's rank correlation coefficients for ∂Cortisol vs. T, −0.458 ($p < 0.01$) and for ∂17OHP vs. T, −0.457 ($p < 0.01$). Corresponding correlation coefficients to non-SHBG-bound T were −0.340 ($p < 0.05$) and −0.479 ($p < 0.001$), respectively. Influence of age was excluded by multiple regression analysis

Adrenal androgens and prostatic disease

Although benign prostatic hyperplasia (BPH) and cancer of the prostate (CAP) are both androgen-dependent diseases, they usually develop at an age when testicular and adrenal androgen levels are decreasing. Most previous case–control studies on hormone levels in patients with prostatic disease have yielded conflicting or inconclusive results owing to the use of improper 'control materials'. However, using carefully selected and matched controls, we found elevated levels of total and non-SHBG-bound T in both BPH and CAP[17,unpublished results] (Figure 3). In BPH also the levels of the adrenal androgens DHEA and DHEAS were distinctly elevated. Although we were not able to measure 5-ADIOL, the elevated DHEA and DHEAS levels are certainly accompanied by increased 5-ADIOL levels due to direct adrenal secretion and to peripheral conversion of DHEA and DHEAS.

The androgen 5-ADIOL has a considerable estrogenic potency itself and binds to the estrogen receptor[18]. The endocrine picture of

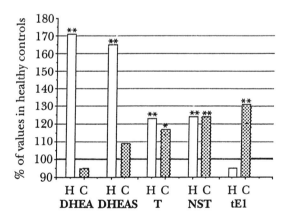

Figure 3 Mean or median serum concentrations of dehydroepiandrosterone/sulfate (DHEA/DHEAS), total testosterone (T) and non-SHBG-bound T (NST) and total estrone (tE1, ≥ 85% estrone sulfate) in patients with benign prostatic hyperplasia (H) and cancer of the prostate (C), expressed as per cent of values for age-matched healthy controls. *, $p < 0.05$; **, $p < 0.01$; and ***, $p < 0.001$, respectively. Data from reference 7 and unpublished results

BPH very much resembles that of endometrial hyperplasia and carcinoma with a combination of elevated 5-ene-C_{19} steroids and total and biologically active T[19,20]. The periurethral glands have the same embryological origin as the uterus and are sensitive to both estrogens and androgens. Elevated levels of the nonclassical 5-ene-C_{19} steroid estrogen 5-ADIOL and its immediate precursors DHEA and DHEAS in combination with hyperandrogenism may therefore stimulate growth of the periurethral glands into a BPH.

Patients with CAP had perfectly normal DHEA/DHEAS levels, but profoundly elevated levels of the 'classical' estrogens estrone and estrone sulfate (Figure 3). High doses of intramuscular depot estrogens are successfully used in the treatment of CAP, but in this case serum levels of T are suppressed to castration values[21,22]. However, there are several reports on synergism between classical estrogens and androgens in their action on the prostate in animals as well as in man[23,24]. Elevated serum estrone levels together with elevated levels of biologically active T are reported in black Americans, who have the highest incidence of CAP[25]. These findings and the results from our study suggest a carcinogenic role for the estrogen–androgen combination also in humans. Since about 60% of circulating estrone in men originates from peripheral aromatization of A-4 from the adrenal cortex[1], the activity of this gland may have some importance also for the etiology of CAP.

The adrenal 'rest androgen' in endocrine treatment of prostatic cancer

Following orchidectomy or chemical castration with intramuscular depot estrogen or GnRH-agonists, less than 5% of the T remains in the circulation in patients with CAP. Androgens of predominantly adrenal origin are of course much less affected. Labrie and co-workers[26] have suggested that this adrenal 'rest androgen' may be important for tumor growth in endocrine-treated patients with CAP, by intratumoral conversion into 5α-dihydrotestosterone, and they

have introduced the concept of 'total androgen blockade', i.e. surgical or chemical castration together with antiandrogens, e.g. flutamide. If this hypothesis is valid, it may be reasonable to find associations between therapy results and adrenal androgen levels during therapy. As far as we know, only one such study has been conducted[27] in which no association whatsoever was found between adrenal rest androgen levels and outcome of treatment (Figure 4). This finding does not support the hypothesis about an important role of the adrenal 'rest androgen' for the outcome of endocrine treatment of CAP. The concept of total androgen blockade in the treatment of CAP is still a debated issue[28].

A physiological role of the 'adrenal androgens'?

Despite its huge concentrations, no vital direct role for circulating DHEA/DHEAS has been demonstrated. A conference entitled 'Dehydro-epiandrosterone (DHEA) and Aging' was held in Washington, DC in 1995 and the proceedings of the conference have recently been published[29]. The volume presents a wealth of nice *in vitro* and

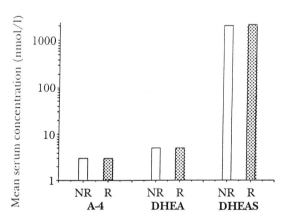

Figure 4 Mean serum concentrations of adrenal androgens in patients with prostatic cancer responding (R) or not responding (NR) upon orchidectomy. Mean observation time 2.25 years. No significant differences between responders and non-responders. A-4, 4-androstene-3,17-dione; DHEA/S, dehydroepiandrosterone/sulfate. Data from reference 27

animal experimental work, and also clinical studies showing beneficial effects of exogenous DHEA in pharmacological doses. However, after reading these proceedings, the present author is still not convinced about a vital direct role for circulating endogenous DHEA/DHEAS. One well-known fact seems to have been forgotten by the enthusiasts: following corticosteroid substitution, individuals with 21-hydroxylase deficiency or Addison's disease can lead a normal life and also have an adequate reproductive function, despite having extremely low or undetectable DHEA/DHEAS levels[30]. In fact, a condition of 'DHEA deficiency' has never been demonstrated.

What is, then, the physiological role of the 'adrenal androgens'? Adrenal androgen and cortisol synthesis are both regulated by ACTH. In contrast with cortisol levels, which are constant throughout life, adrenal androgen levels are very low in childhood, rise during adrenarche to very high levels with maximum values at about 25 years and after that decline continuously to a low plateau value at about 60 years of age (adrenopause). Cortisol and adrenal androgens are synthesized from their common precursor 17α-hydroxy-5-pregnenolone (17OH5P). DHEA and 17OHP represent the first steps after 17OH5P, leading to adrenal androgens and to cortisol respectively (Figure 5). The ∂DHEA values following acute ACTH stimulation show the same age-related change as basal DHEA/DHEAS values, but the ∂17OHP values change in the opposite direction, with minimum values at about 25 years of age (Figure 6). Cortisol levels increase and adrenal androgens decrease in stressful situations such as trauma, chronic disease and malnutrition[10].

The 5-ene-C_{19} steroids DHEA and DHEAS are structurally 'primitive', i.e. structurally similar to cholesterol, and they are physiologically harmless. The increased synthetic capacity for DHEA/DHEAS during the adrenarche may reflect a buildup of a reserve capacity for cortisol synthesis for the adult individual. In unstressed conditions, the intra-adrenal steroid flux from this reserve synthetic capacity is directed towards harmless DHEA/DHEAS. In stressful situations (childbirth, hunting, fighting, trauma,

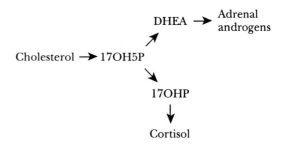

Figure 5 A simplified outline of glucocorticoid and adrenal androgen biosynthesis. 17OH5P, 17α-hydroxy-5-pregnenolone; DHEA, dehydroepiandrosterone; 17OHP, 17α-hydroxyprogesterone

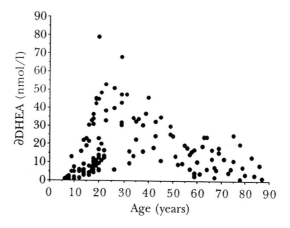

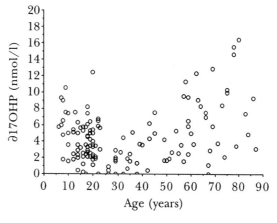

Figure 6 Adrenocorticotropic hormone (ACTH)-induced increments in serum dehydroepiandrosterone (DHEA) (∂DHEA) and 17α-hydroxyprogesterone (17OHP) (∂17OHP) 120 min after i.v. bolus injection of 250 μg ACTH 1–24 in males 6–87 years. Data from references 17 and 33

etc.) the synthesis is shifted over to cortisol production, resulting in increased cortisol and decreased DHEA/DHEAS levels. Similarly, the decreased DHEA/DHEAS levels in older subjects probably reflect the decreased total synthetic capacity of the aging adrenal cortex for the common substrate 17OH5P[31], giving priority to production of vital cortisol. Thus the physiological role of circulating DHEA/DHEAS may simply be to serve as a 'safety valve' for reserve cortisol production in adults during their most active years – and perhaps nothing else.

Conclusions

The role of the adrenal cortex for androgen status in intact adult men is minimal or even non-existent. Rather than affecting testicular androgens, the adrenocortical steroid synthesis may be modulated by testicular testosterone. Adrenal androgens may have a role in the etiology of prostatic disease, but their role for the outcome of endocrine treatment of prostatic cancer may be uncertain. Finally, no vital direct role has been shown for circulating DHEA and DHEAS, but they may reflect a reserve steroidogenic capacity for cortisol mobilization.

Acknowledgements

The author's own work was supported by Riksföreningen mot cancer and Karolinska Institutets fonder.

References

1. Crilly, R. G., Francis, R. M. and Nordin, B. E. C. (1981). Steroid hormones, ageing and bone. *Clin. Endocrinol. Metab.*, **10**, 115–39
2. Vihko, R. and Roukonen, A. (1974). Regulation of steroidogenesis in testis. *J. Steroid. Biochem.*, **5**, 843–8
3. Luton, J.-P., Thiebolt, P., Valcke, J.-C., Mahoudeau, J. A. and Bricaire, H. (1977). Reversible gonadotropin deficiency in male Cushing disease. *J. Clin. Endocrinol. Metab.*, **45**, 488–95
4. Pratt, J. H. and Longcope, C. (1978). Effect of adrenocorticotropin on production rates and metabolic clearance rates of testosterone and estradiol. *J. Clin. Endocrinol. Metab.*, **47**, 307–13
5. Cumming, D. C., Quigley, M. E. and Yen, S. S. C. (1986). Acute suppression of circulating testosterone levels by cortisol in men. *J. Clin. Endocrinol. Metab.*, **57**, 671–3
6. Bambino, T. H. and Hsueh, A. J. W. (1981). Direct inhibitory effect of glucocorticoids upon testicular luteinizing hormone receptor and steroidogenesis *in vivo* and *in vitro. Endocrinology*, **108**, 2142–6
7. Haning, R. V., Hacket, R. J., Flood, C. A., Loughlin, J. S., Zhao, Q. Y. and Longcope, C. (1994). Plasma dehydroepiandrosterone sulfate serves as a prehormone for 48% of follicular fluid testosterone during treatment with menotrophins. *J. Clin. Endocrinol. Metab.*, **76**, 1301–7
8. Parker, L. N. and Lifrak, E. T. (1981). Adrenal and testicular androgen are correlated. *Horm. Metab. Res.*, **13**, 653–4
9. Nieschlag, E. and Kley, H. K. (1975). Possibility of adrenal–testicular interaction as indicated by plasma androgens in response to hCG in men with normal, suppressed and impaired adrenal function. *Horm. Metab. Res.*, **7**, 326–30
10. Parker, L. N. (1989). *Adrenal Androgens in Clinical Medicine.* (San Diego: Academic Press)
11. Parker, L., Lai, M., Wolk, F., Lifrak, E., Kim, S., Epstein, L., Hadley, D. and Miller, J. (1984). Orchidectomy does not selectively increase adrenal androgen concentrations. *J. Clin. Endocrinol. Metab.*, **59**, 547–50
12. Stege, R., Eriksson, A., Henriksson, P. and Carlström, K. (1987). Orchidectomy or oestrogen treatment in prostatic cancer: effects on serum levels of adrenal androgens and related steroids. *Int. J. Androl.*, **10**, 581–7
13. Carlström, K. and Stege, R. (1990). Adrenocortical function in prostatic cancer patients: effects of orchidectomy or different modes of oestrogen treatment on basal steroid levels and on the response to exogenous ACTH. *Urol. Int.*, **45**, 160–3
14. Carlström, K., Pousette, Å. and Stege, R. (1990). Flutamide has no effect on adrenal androgen response to acute ACTH stimulation in patients with prostatic cancer. *The Prostate*, **17**, 219–25

15. Roelfsema, F., van den Berg, G., Frölich, M., Veldhuis, J. D., van Eijk, A., Buurman, M. and Etman, B. H. B. (1993). Sex-dependent alteration in cortisol response to endogenous adrenocorticotropin. *J. Clin. Endocrinol. Metab.*, **77**, 234–40

16. Born, J., Ditschuneit, I., Schreiber, M., Dodt, D. and Fehm, H. (1995). Effect of age and gender on pituitary–adrenocortical responsiveness in humans. *Eur. J. Endocrinol.*, **132**, 705–11

17. Stege, R. and Carlström, K (1992). Testicular and adrenocortical function in healthy men and in men with benign prostatic hyperplasia. *J. Steroid Biochem. Mol. Biol.*, **42**, 357–62

18. Markiewicz, L. and Gurpide, E. (1988). C_{19} adrenal steroids enhance prostaglandin $F_{2\alpha}$ output by human endometrium *in vitro*. *Am. J. Obstet. Gynecol.*, **159**, 500–4

19. Brody, S., Carlström, K., von Uexküll, A.-K., Lagrelius, A., Lunell, N.-O. and Rosenborg, L. (1983). Peripheral hormones and the endometrial condition in postmenopausal women. *Acta. Obstet. Gynecol. Scand.*, **62**, 525–9

20. Möllerström, G., Carlström, K., Lagrelius, A. and Einhorn, N (1993). Is there an altered steroid profile in patients with endometrial carcinoma? *Cancer*, **72**, 173–81

21. Stege, R., Carlström, K., Collste, L., Eriksson, A., Henriksson, P., Pousette, Å. and von Schoultz, B. (1989). Single drug parenteral estrogen treatment in prostatic cancer: a study of different initial and maintenance dose regimens. *The Prostate*, **14**, 183–8

22. Henriksson, P., Blombäck, M., Eriksson, A., Stege, R. and Carlström, K. (1990). Effects of parenteral oestrogen on the coagulation system in patients with prostatic carcinoma. *Br. J. Urol.*, **65**, 282–5

23. Ho, S.-M., Yu, M., Leav, I. and Viccione T. (1992). The conjoint action of androgens and estrogens in the induction of proliferative lesions in the rat prostate. In Li, J. J., Nandi, S. and Li, S. A. (eds.) *Hormonal Carcinogenesis*, pp. 18–25. (New York: Springer-Verlag)

24. Bosland, M. C. (1992). Carcinogenic risk assessment of steroid hormone exposure in relation to prostate cancer risk. In Li, J. J., Nandi, S. and Li, S. A. (eds.) *Hormonal Carcinogenesis*, pp. 225–33. (New York: Springer-Verlag)

25. Ross, S., Bernstein, L., Judd, H., Hanisch, R., Pike, M. and Henderson, B. (1986). Serum testosterone levels in healthy young black and white men. *J. Nat. Cancer Inst.*, **75**, 45–8

26. Labrie, F., Dupont, A. and Belanger, A. (1985). Complete androgen blockade for the treatment of prostate cancer. In Vita, V. T., Hellman, S. R. and Rosenberg, S. A. (eds.) *Important Advances in Oncology*, pp. 193–217. (Philadelphia: J. B. Lippincott)

27. Eriksson, A. and Carlström, K. (1988). Prognostic value of serum hormone concentrations in prostatic cancer. *The Prostate*, **13**, 249–55

28. Crawford, E. D., deAntonio, E. P., Labrie, F., Schroeder, F. and Geller, J. (1995) Endocrine therapy of prostate cancer: optimal form and appropriate timing. *J. Clin. Endocrinol. Metab.*, **80**, 1062–78

29. Bellino, F. L., Daynes, R. A., Hornsby, P. J., Lavrin, D. H. and Nestler, J. E. (eds.) (1995). Dehydroepiandrosterone and aging. *Ann. NY Acad. Sci.*, **774**

30. Helleday, J., Siwers, B., Ritzén, E. M. and Carlström, K.(1993). Subnormal androgen and elevated progesterone levels in women treated for congenital virilizing 21-hydroxylase deficiency. *J. Clin. Endocrinol. Metab.*, **76**, 933–6

31. Vermeulen, A., Deslypere, J.P., Schelfhout, W., Verdonck, L. and Rubens, R. (1982). Adrenocortical function in old age: response to acute adrenocorticotropin stimulation. *J. Clin. Endocrinol. Metab.*, **54**, 187–91

32. Bolme, P., Borgström, B. and Carlström, K. (1995). Adrenocortical function following allogenic bone marrow transplantation in children. *Horm. Res.*, **43**, 279–85

12

Menopausal medicine under difficult conditions

Menopausal medicine under difficult conditions: Pakistan

51

S. Wasti

Introduction

Pakistan as a country came into being in 1947, but the history of its people goes back for several thousand years, beginning with the Indus valley civilization of Mohenjodaro and Harappa (5000 BC). Pakistan today is the land of one predominant religion (Islam) and is primarily a feudal cum tribal society.

The estimated population of Pakistan is 120–130 million, 52% being female. Eighty per cent of the population resides in the rural areas. Female life expectancy is 57.3 years[1], and an increase in life expectancy is going to continue well into the 21st century. If the assumptions underlying the median variant projection of the World Bank[2] are correct, then by the year 2025, 12% of the female population of Pakistan will be postmenopausal.

The portrait of menopause in Pakistan cannot be complete without elucidating the sociocultural perspective of a female's life, as this environment has a marked impact on perceptions and symptomatic manifestations of the menopause.

Sociocultural perspective

Total literacy in Pakistan stands at 36%[3]; female literacy stands at 25% which is 45% that of males. Girls studying at university level constitute only 0.8% of the total female population, while the rural female literacy rate in 1990 stood at an abysmal 11.3%[4].

Despite cultural constraints limiting their acquisition of knowledge and mobility, the majority of women in our country contribute substantially to the rural economy and are active in the urban services and industrial sectors. However, women's employment in remunerated activities is negatively valued. It is widely acknowledged that women's economic contribution is grossly underenumerated. A conservative estimate of women's labour-force participation across the various sectors is actually 35–40%[4]. More relevant is that women lack control over financial and other resources derived from their economic activity.

Thus, lack of economic autonomy reduces their decision-making powers within the family, with implications for population and health programs. At the most mundane level women often need to request and account for expenditures on health. In the final analysis it is not so much whether women work, but the extent to which they exercise control over their income, derive benefits from it and acquire decision-making power, that will enhance their ability to exercise choices in all spheres of their lives including their own health.

Women's health in general is also determined by their level of access, both physical and social, to health services. UNICEF estimates that 55% of the total population and 35% of the rural population lives within 5 km, or an hour's walk, from any fixed health facility[5]. This disturbing estimate may nevertheless be overoptimistic as it overlooks the realities of women's lives.

Physical mobility is a crucial issue for females. Analyzing women's problems of access, one writer clearly illustrated the social restriction on longer-distance travel for women. The males have to go to work and the females do not like to go to the health center or dispensary alone, leaving them to rely on unscientific practices and untrained practitioners immediately placed in their village[6]. Further, the burden of daily household work leaves few Pakistani women adequate time for traveling to a health facility (except in emergencies), let alone the time consumed in waiting at invariably understaffed facilities.

As women cross the threshold of their reproductive age, there is an easing of social restrictions, a possibility of increased mobility and interaction outside the family. At this stage women become more self-assertive, take more decisions and have access to financial resources. They have to do less work, as daughters and daughters-in-law take care of the household. Their opinions are sought, and as age advances they make a place for themselves in society.

However, from the health perspective, menopause remains a neglected life-cycle milestone. With less than 4% of the GNP spent on health, resources are directed towards combating female health issues of the reproductive age group. An estimated maternal mortality rate of 600 maternal deaths per 100 000 live births is an issue which is the focus of attention, compounded by a population growth rate of 2.8% which is one of the highest in the world[1]. In this social, cultural and economic environment, menopausal health is not a priority because health and social planning continue to be for the young and fertile female, rather than the middle-aged woman. Finally, there is the issue of lack of information available on the menopause, because extrapolating data from Western literature will not achieve desirable results in our set-up. Because of this lack of relevant data, we undertook to collect baseline information regarding menopause in urban Karachi.

The mean age of menopause was 47 years in two studies conducted in three distinct socioeconomic groups of urban Karachi. Socioeconomic status has been demonstrated to influence health, nutrition and education[7,8], but it had no bearing on the age of menopause. A retrospective hospital-based study conducted at the Aga Khan University Hospital showed the mean age of hip fracture to be 67.6 years. This result is similar to that reported by our group

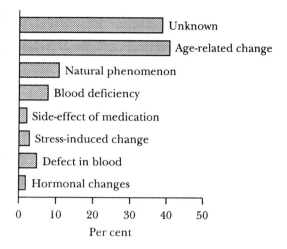

Figure 1 Perceptions of menopause: 'Why do periods stop?'

earlier[7], and is considerable lower than that reported from other parts of the world. This finding is possibly a consequence of early menopause.

We were also interested in a Pakistani female's perception of menopause. A prospective cross-sectional study was conducted in 1996, and 200 females were interviewed. These women were non-patient visitors to the Aga Khan University Hospital. A structured questionnaire was used to interview the ladies and included both open and closed questions, in order to assess their perception of the menopause and its effect on their health. One hundred and fifty (75%) of the women interviewed left school before passing grade 10, and only 50 (25%) had passed grade 10. We asked them, 'Why do periods stop?' The response is shown in Figure 1. When asked 'Does menopause affect female health ?', 59 (29.5%) stated that menopause had no effect on health (Figure 2). Two (0.5%) said they were not aware of any side-effect of loss of menstruation, 20 (10%) thought that the health improves after menopause, 67 (33.5%) thought that weight gain was due to cessation of menstruation, and 52 (25%) said that menopause leads to worsening of female health but they were not aware of how this occurred.

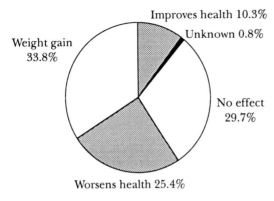

Figure 2 Perceptions of menopause: 'Does menopause affect female health?'

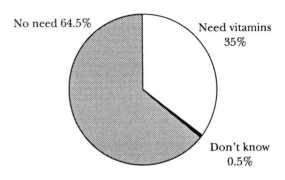

Figure 3 Perceptions of menopause: 'Need for any medication after the menopause?'

We asked if there was a 'Need for any medication after the menopause?' Seventy women (35%) said yes, but they were not aware whether any specific drugs were required and thought that vitamins were needed. One hundred and twenty-nine (64%) said that no medication was required, and one woman (0.5%) replied that she was not aware of any medication (Figure 3).

The first health-care professionals to observe and treat any health problem in a community are general practitioners (GPs). The importance of the role played by general practitioners in taking care of women in middle age is reflected in our early study[7], in which the family doctors were consulted for problems related to the menopause by 25% of the total women interviewed. A cross-sectional knowledge, attitudes and practices survey was conducted in Karachi from March to June 1995. The study population consisted of GPs in Gulshan-e-Iqbal, which is a middle-class residential area of urban Karachi, and doctors undergoing training at three tertiary teaching hospitals. A questionnaire was developed keeping the objectives of the study in mind. Of all the participant GPs, 18 (56%) were males and 14 (44%) were females. Among the trainee doctors, 23 (55%) were males and 19 (45%) were females. Notable findings were that 81% of GPs and 66% of trainee doctors were of the opinion that menopause should not be

interfered with. Less than 50% of GPs thought osteopenia was related to the climacteric, whereas 79% of trainees related it to the climacteric. Only 12.9% of GPs and 23.8% of trainee doctors recommended hormone replacement therapy (HRT) for prevention of osteopenia. Among the GPs only 37.5% prescribed a combination of estrogen and progesterone, and none of them prescribed it for more than 3 years' duration. Few doctors knew the current recommendations for treatment of the climacteric and its related problems. We feel there is a serious need for focused educational programs to increase awareness and knowledge about the climacteric and its problems, and their prevention and treatment, among both general practitioners and doctors training in other specialities (Figures 4–6).

Achievements

There is increased awareness regarding menopausal health, and lectures on menopausal health are delivered to groups of women and to medical personnel all over the country. Menopausal clinics are being conducted in major tertiary units. The model of the menopause that is emerging is the recognition of the interaction of the physiological, sociocultural, religious and economic factors in our set-up.

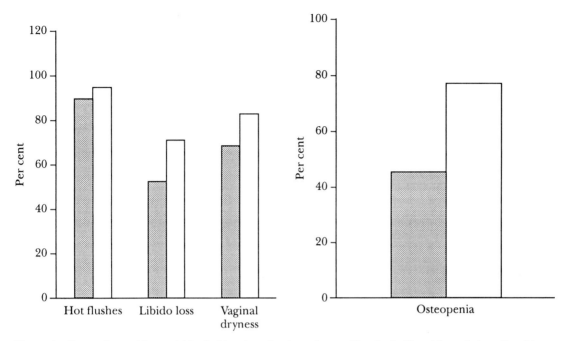

Figure 4 General practitioners' (shaded bars) and trainee doctors' (unshaded bars) knowledge of problems related to menopause

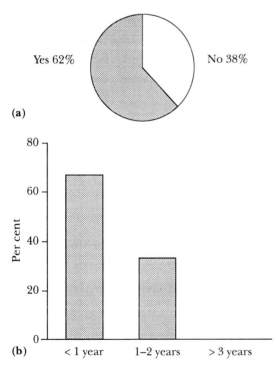

Figure 5 Practices of general practitioners (GPs): (a) GPs prescribing hormone replacement therapy (HRT) and (b) duration of HRT prescription

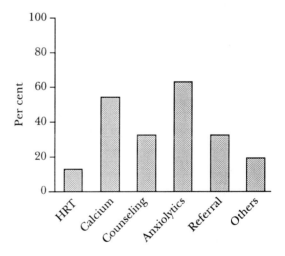

Figure 6 Treatment for osteopenia by general practitioners. HRT, hormone replacement therapy

Conclusions

With less than 4% of the GNP spent on health, the focus of health care is on maternal and child health. Use of scarce resources for non-life threatening conditions such as the menopause do not have a high priority either for individual families or the Government. Yet the possibility that women may respond to the advertising pressure of pharmaceutical firms is of concern. Despite a relatively low life expectancy in many developing countries, the life expectancy at birth in Pakistan is increasing. Early age of menopause could result in related complications affecting more of the aging female population. As resources are limited, through education and simple cost-effective programs, menopausal health can be achieved by targeting middle-aged women as well as health-care providers. Larger sections of the menopausal population need to be studied because extrapolating data from Western studies and hence planning for the future will not give the desired results.

References

1. Government of Pakistan (1991). *Pakistan Demographic Survey*. Federal Bureau of Statistics, Economic Affairs and Statistics Division, Government of Pakistan
2. United Nations (1984). *World Population Prospects: Estimates and Projections as Assessed in 1982. Review and Appraisal of the World Population Plan of Action*, E/Conf. 76/4. (New York: United Nations)
3. United Nations (1994). *Human Development Report, United Nations Development Programme.* (New York: Oxford University Press)
4. Shaheed, F. and Mumtaz, K. (1992). *Women's Economic Participation in Pakistan: a Status Report.* (Pakistan: UNICEF)
5. Government of Pakistan (1992). *Situation Analysis of Children and Women in Pakistan.* (Pakistan: UNICEF)
6. Ansari, R. L. (1980). Problems of access of women, particularly rural women to various services for health. Presented at *National Conference of Health; Problems and Prospects for Women*, Islamabad, Pakistan
7. Wasti, S., Robinson, S. C., Akhtar, Y., Khan, S. and Badruddin, N. (1993). Characteristics of menopause in three socio-economic urban groups in Karachi, Pakistan. *Maturitas*, **16**, 61–9
8. Wasti, S., Kamal, R. and Robinson, S. C. (1993). Characteristics and perceptions of menopause in a Pakistani community. In Berg, G. and Hammar, M. (eds.) *The Modern Management of the Menopause*, pp. 35–45. (Carnforth, UK: Parthenon Publishing)

Menopausal medicine under difficult conditions: the Philippines

52

J. R. Jalbuena

Introduction

In many countries the serious, nationwide interest in modern menopausal medicine might have started many years ago. In the Philippines, however, that kind of interest had been largely limited to a small group, or individual physicians, and it was only 4 years ago that a national society of physicians dedicated to menopausal medicine was formed, the Philippine Society of Climacteric Medicine. The association has a membership of 225 and is an affiliate of the International Menopause Society. It was the author's good fortune to have been given the privilege of being its founding President.

The Philippines is a beautiful country with a tropical climate. It is mainly agricultural but we are fast moving into industrialization. Many parts of the Southern Philippines have marine reserves, remarkable for their pristine waters and home to unique species of flora and fauna indigenous to the region. The Philippines is an archipelago composed of approximately 7100 islands. We always say 'approximately' because the number of our islands varies, depending on whether it is high or low tide.

It is very much the same in the case of what we know about menopausal women in our country: as of now, we can only approximate. Most of the available reading materials and statistics on menopausal women are from Western countries. It is likely that the Philippines is not alone in this situation and that many other developing countries are like ours in still approximating the true, unique and universal characteristics of their menopausal women.

Difficult conditions

The primary difficult condition which physicians in the Philippines have encountered in the treatment of menopause is the absence of data on the climacteric Filipino woman. How can Filipino physicians then approach the problem in terms of treatment and information dissemination?

Two other major barriers to the effective treatment of climacteric women in the Philippines are: the low compliance rate in hormone replacement therapy, and poverty.

Experience of menopause in the Philippines

The Filipino physician has for generations depended on Western data in approaching the problems of the climacteric Filipino woman. Such an approach, of course, is inherently inaccurate because racial, geographic and socioeconomic factors influence the age of menopause and the character of climacteric complaints.

In 1989, the Geneva-based International Health Foundation (IHF) conducted an exploratory study on menopause in seven Southeast Asian countries: Hong Kong, Malaysia, the Philippines, South Korea, Taiwan, Indonesia and Singapore. The question to be answered by the IHF study was[1]: 'Menopause is universal, what about the climacteric?' Four to five hundred women aged 40 to 60 years were surveyed in each country. The task of conducting the study in the Philippines was given to this author, and the results presented at the Sixth Congress on the Menopause in Bangkok in 1990[2].

To broaden the basis for the portrayal of the climacteric Filipino woman, the Philippine sample population was expanded with an additional 515 respondents to form a total of 1015 climacteric subjects[3]. The findings are given in Table 1. The typical respondent experienced menarche in her early teens, and married in her mid-20s. Eighty per cent lived with their husbands and had an average of four children, the youngest of whom was aged 14 years. Twenty-five per cent had grand-children living with them. The average age of menopause was established at 48 years, which is 2–3 years lower when compared with the 50–51 years average age reported in other Southeast Asian countries and most Western countries. Climacteric symptoms were experienced by 87% of the respondents as given in Table 2.

No relationship was found between age of menarche and age of menopause in our studies. At present, we are studying the effects of smoking, prolonged use of contraceptive pills, malnutrition, chronic anemia, tuberculosis and bilateral tubal ligation as possible causes of earlier menopause among Filipino women.

Overall psychological symptoms were more prevalent than vasomotor symptoms. The frequency of climacteric symptoms rose during perimenopause and declined during postmeno-pause. In general however, these symptoms were encountered infrequently and appeared not burdensome enough to motivate the women to seek medical assistance or to continue taking prescribed medication. Only one-quarter consulted a physician for menopause-related ailments, and 88% of them were prescribed medication (Table 3).

The most commonly prescribed medications were tranquilizers (24%), analgesics (20%), vitamins (19%), anti-hypertensives (13%) and hormones (11%).

These 1015 climacteric Filipino women were predominantly living in the urban area of Metro Manila. Recently that survey was expanded by looking into the status of 145 climacteric women in a rural community named Jala-Jala, an agricultural town in the Rizal province, about 75 km south of Manila. Table 4 gives a brief summary of the findings.

Table 1 1015 climacteric Filipino women. Data from reference 3 and expressed as median

Age at survey (range) (years)	48 (35–55)
Menarche age (years)	13.5
Marriage age (years)	24
Pregnancies (–)	5
Live births (–)	4
Menopause age (years)	48

Table 2 1015 climacteric Filipino women: symptoms experienced. Data from reference 3

Climacteric symptoms	87%
psychological	84 %
vasomotor	60 %

Table 3 1015 climacteric Filipino women: rates of consultation, prescription and compliance with medicine. Data from reference 3

Status	Ratio	Percentage
Positive cases	857/983	87
Consulted	212/857	25
Given prescription	186/212	88
Still medicating	56/186	30

Table 4 Climacteric Filipino women in the rural province of Jala-Jala. Data expressed as median unless otherwise indicated

Age (median; range) (years)	59.3 (43–83)
Menopause age (years)	47.4
Children (–)	6
Climacteric symptoms	78%
Consulted	15%

Compared with the respondents in 1989, this group has an average age of 59 years, about 11 years older than the previous predominantly urban group. The average age of menopause among these rural women however, is similar to the urban women in the 1989 study; about 47 years. The median age of menopause is also similar to the findings in 1989: about 48 years.

The women respondents in Jala-Jala have an average of six children almost twice the number of the 1989 respondents.

Climacteric symptoms were experienced by 78% of the respondents in Jala-Jala. Thirty-five per cent had only the combination of vasomotor and psychological symptoms. The intensity and frequency of symptoms were described as tolerable, which perhaps explains why only 22 women or 15% of the 145 subjects consulted a physician for menopause-related symptoms.

The most commonly prescribed medications were tranquilizers, analgesics, vitamins, anti-hypertensives and anti-diabetics. Only one respondent was given HRT, and she discontinued treatment after a month because of withdrawal bleeding (Table 5).

A study of the author's own 216 menopausal patients was also conducted because they represented a specific socioeconomic group, distinct from the group surveyed for the International Health Foundation in 1989. This survey of patients is more particularized, or, as they say, 'up close and personal'. These women's ages ranged from 38 to 87 years, with a median age of approximately 55 years, which is between the ages of the two other groups of respondents. Average age at menopause was 48 years ± 3 years. Seventy per cent or 151 of my patients experienced climacteric symptoms (Table 6).

Of these 151 climacteric women, 110 women or 73% experienced mild symptoms which were tolerable, that lasted for a day or two and did not warrant consultation. In fact, these 110 women did not come to the clinic to complain of menopausal symptoms; these 110 patients were part of a total 130 menopausal women [130/216 = 60%] who came to the clinic for a gynecological check-up and Pap smear.

Forty-one patients, or 27% of those with menopausal symptoms, came with severe climacteric symptoms in the form of dyspareunia, 59%; psychological, 21%; and vasomotor symptoms, 15%. The other 5% had a combination of symptoms.

Fifteen per cent came to the clinic because of abnormal uterine bleeding, 99% underwent fractional curettage (92% of these were not on

Table 5 Prescriptions for climacteric women in the rural province of Jala-Jala

Tranquilizers	20%
Vitamins	19%
Analgesics	18%
Anti-hypertensives	10%
Anti-diabetics	6%
Hormone replacement therapy	0.7%

Table 6 Climacteric Filipino women, author's own clinic

With symptoms	70%
mild	73%
severe	27%
dyspareunia	59%
psychological	21%
vasomotor	15%
combination	5%

Table 7 Incidence of hormone replacement therapy (HRT), author's own clinic

Without HRT	57%
With HRT	43%
continued	79%
discontinued	18%

hormone replacement therapy (HRT)), and 1% underwent panhysterectomy and bilateral salpingo-oophorectomy in the non-HRT group. The histopathological report of the 99% who underwent fractional curettage revealed no malignancy. Six per cent consulted for leukorrhea and pruritus.

While the 1989 survey showed that 11% of the women took HRT, and the Jala-Jala survey showed only one woman (0.7%) had the hormone treatment, among the author's own 216 patients, 92 menopausals or 43% had HRT (Table 7).

Of these 92 cases who were prescribed hormones, 79% continued to take HRT (for 1 year or more), and only 18% have discontinued it. The compliance for the remaining 3% could not be ascertained because they did not return to the clinic often enough. A nationwide survey was also conducted in early 1996 of 1058 menopausal women. The HRT compliance rate of this group is 63%.

These large differences can perhaps be attributed to the variations in the income levels of the four population sets. As mentioned earlier, the author's own patients came from an income bracket that is higher than those of the respondents in 1989, those respondents in the rural area of Jala-Jala, and the 1058 climacteric women surveyed nationwide.

The crushing burden that poverty places on the health of the Philippine population cannot be ignored. Health maintenance entails some expense, and health restoration can be prohibitively expensive when the simple requirements of food and shelter are a day-to-day struggle to attain. In the Philippines, families with a monthly income of more than US$1000 are considered wealthy and rare. Forty per cent of families earn less than US$150 per month, which is the poverty threshold. In stark terms, 28 million Filipinos do not have the means to provide themselves with even the most humble standard of living.

We can certainly offer the complete menopausal medicine package to our wealthy patients, and given the ease with which new medicinal information travels around the world, our practice will be on a par with the best of Western nations. However, that leaves out the vast majority of our population. What can we offer the low-income woman in her later years? Perhaps, not surprisingly, our studies among lower-income women showed a great tolerance for climacteric symptoms. Less than 25% of perimenopausal and menopausal women consulted a physician for menopause-related ailments; 90% of the women surveyed rated their state of health as 'good' to 'excellent'[3]. These observations suggest that the Filipina is better able to cope with menopause than her Western counterpart.

Should we prescribe hormonal therapy to women who have climacteric symptoms but are not concerned about these symptoms? It would be impractical to prescribe HRT among the poor. We are aware, however, that a patient's sense of well-being does not necessarily correspond to the actual physiological state of her health. That sense of well-being does not remove the health risks that she faces.

A telling statistic from the Philippine National Orthopedic Hospital (1979–88) showed that 62% of women over the age of 50 years admitted to the hospital had osteoporotic fractures, mostly hip fracture. This may indicate a high incidence of osteoporosis among our postmenopausal population. Likewise, the increasing incidence of cardiovascular disease as the leading cause of death among older women aged 60 years and above[4], provides a compelling reason to advocate hormonal therapy even among women who do not complain of climacteric symptoms. Moreover, we are aware that hormonal therapy capriciously applied may do more harm than good, because some women who could afford medication may not be able to afford the periodic check-ups, mammograms, uterine ultrasonography, endometrial biopsy and bone densitometry that are part of a prudent course of hormonal therapy.

Confronted with these dilemmas, the Philippine Association of Climacteric Medicine was formed in 1993. We initially instituted a nationwide campaign to increase the awareness of Philippine physicians regarding the health needs of menopausal women, through scientific and postgraduate seminars, the organization of menopause clinics, guest appearances on radio and television and the publication of research work as well as press releases in various newspapers and magazines. Two years after the campaign began, one of the board members, Dr Florante Gonzaga[5] conducted a survey of physicians, both gynecologists and non-gynecologists which included family physicians, surgeons, cardiologists, psychiatrists and general practitioners, to determine their level of awareness (Table 8).

The results were fairly encouraging, with a great majority of the physicians aware of, sympathetic to, and willing to treat the problems of menopause. Gonzaga showed that up to 79%

Table 8 Physicians' perspective on menopause and hormone replacement therapy. CVD, cardiovascular disease; Gyn, gynecological; Non-gyn, non-gynecological. Data from reference 6

	Gyn	Non-gyn
Awareness: risks of		
CVD	94%	82%
osteoporosis	100%	95%
Always asks of symptoms	NA	72%
Regard for symptoms		
not important	0%	1%
no cause – disregard	5%	21%
important	92%	78%
View of menopause		
no treatment needed	9%	31%
treatment needed	88%	69%

Table 9 Reasons for discontinued hormone replacement therapy in the Philippines

Fear of cancer	25 %
Withdrawal bleeding	16 %
Economic reasons	13 %
Other reasons	46 %

of them are aware of the benefits of HRT, and 69% of non-gynecologists and 88% of gynecologists are apt to prescribe HRT.

In general it can be seen that Filipino physicians are nevertheless quite aware of the associated risks of menopause, and the great majority of them take an active approach in treating these risks. Hopefully, the Association's campaign to disseminate information on this subject has contributed to this situation. However, the Association has also interpreted the results to mean that we should increase our co-ordination with non-gynecologists, and this is being done.

The information dissemination campaign was not directed solely to the physicians but to the layman as well, specifically to the menopausal themselves. In this regard, some level of success has also been achieved. In 1989

as noted above, when a survey of more than 1000 climacteric Filipino women was conducted only 11% were prescribed or were undergoing HRT. The recent survey of 1058 Filipino women nationwide showed that 435 of them or 41% were formerly, or are currently on HRT, and 276 of that group or 63% continue to take hormones.

A survey of 162 physicians which was also conducted in 1996 showed that our gynecologists estimated that nearly 26% of their menopausal patients discontinue HRT. That figure would not even include those HRT patients who were lost to follow up, so the actual rate of HRT discontinuation may be higher. In a parallel survey of 1058 patients nationwide, we observed that 36%, about one in every three of them admitted that they discontinued HRT.

Consequently, we looked into these women's reasons for not taking HRT or for discontinuing the treatment. The findings are summarized in Table 9. The single most common reason for those who stopped HRT was fear of cancer. This reason accounted for one of every four (25%) menopausal women who ceased taking hormones. Withdrawal or abnormal bleeding ranked as the second most common reason for discontinuing HRT, accounting for 16% or one of about six women who stopped taking hormones.

Financial reasons, which accounted for 13% or one of eight ranked third. A large proportion of the Philippine population cannot afford HRT, and that is probably the main reason why only a small percentage of our menopausals are taking hormones.

We are only just beginning to expand our research beyond the small samples that mark our initial efforts at defining the problem. At the University of the Philippines College of Medicine and other academic institutions, menopausal clinics are being established not only to treat but also to study the population. We currently use the studies from Western nations to formulate protocols, because of the lack of local data. It is fully realized that cultural genetic and environmental factors in those studies do not apply to our population. Our own research is crucial to validating or amending our therapy, but again we are faced with the problem of lack of funds. High-cost projects such as bone densitometry studies for osteoporosis, and controlled studies of different HRT protocols for efficacy and complications, cannot be funded by local government. The cash resources of our government, quite understandably, are assigned to infrastructures and other projects that directly affect economic growth. Pharmaceutical companies fund studies related to their products. They may be reluctant to underwrite projects that do not directly influence their sale. It is persistently hoped that international health organizations such as the World Health Organization, the International Health Foundation, the Robert Wood Johnson Foundation and others, would consent to join projects with our universities. Both the skills and the manpower are available: we lack only the material resources to study a condition that affects millions of our population.

Our efforts at research and education, while still in their early stages, offer the best hope of improving care for our low-income climacteric population. Even without hormonal therapy, these women will benefit from the increased awareness and knowledge that we can provide. Of course, the treatment of menopause is not all HRT. The woman should be treated as a whole with individualized attention. In the presence of contraindications alternative treatment is prescribed. We stress the preventive strategies for good health during the menopause, such as: proper hygiene; a well-balanced diet rich in calcium, high fibers and low cholesterol; regular physical exercise; having an active non-stressful life, avoidance of smoking, excesses of alcohol and caffeine; and visiting the doctor for routine check-ups and discussion of any difficulties.

In general, Filipino women have accepted menopause-related disorders as an unavoidable and normal stage of a woman's life cycle: a condition they just have to live with like their mothers and grandmothers before them. This attitude is typically Filipino and a cultural trait. Many welcome the relief from the risk of childbirth, fears of unwanted pregnancy and the inconvenience of menstruation. The majority feel that the climacteric symptoms they experience are bearable and not life threatening, and therefore merit very low priority. The exception to these is when a patient shows abnormal uterine bleeding. The patient should be seen by a gynecologist. While the majority of cases of uterine bleeding are due to hormonal imbalance, the possibility of cancer should not be overlooked.

Menopausal medicine is new in the Philippines. Despite the difficulties associated with poverty and lack of funding, we have made unprecedented progress in establishing the specialty by educating the health profession as well as the general public, and in plotting a course for the future. These provide a good foundation from which to tackle the problems of menopause.

Issues and concerns

Basic attitude of Filipino women towards medicine is curative rather than preventive

This attitude is the result of generations of cultural conditioning which makes the Filipina self-sacrificing, in general, thinking of her family first and herself last. Hence, she is likely to seek medical help only when the symptoms become intolerable. It is only the younger and more liberated set who see their doctors as part of the program of looking after their own well-being. These are usually career women who, because they have a career, know the importance of being in top shape.

Surgically induced menopause

There is a tendency towards indiscriminate removal of normal-looking ovaries at the time of hysterectomy for benign conditions in women of 40 years and above. In fairness to the attending physicians, most of these procedures are chosen by the patients themselves, for fear of developing cancer of the ovaries later. Here, new information to help them make an intelligent decision will be invaluable. Earlier onset of menopause of 2–3 years has been observed among more than 1000 women seen in the menopause clinic (Philippine General Hospital, PGH) who underwent bilateral tubal ligation or hysterectomy. In performing these surgical procedures, the blood supply of the ovaries should not be disturbed.

Breast cancer

This is the leading cause of death among women aged 49–59 years[4]. Breast cancer (5.17 per 100 000) is the leading cause of death among cancer patients.

Cardiovascular disease

This is the leading cause of death among women 60 years and above[4]. It would seem then, that the middle-aged and elderly Filipina is faced with the choice of either dying of cancer of the breast or of cardiovascular disease. We should be able to offer them better options than these. Here again, advances in research and management of both diseases will be very helpful.

Poverty

The government's health programs remain focused on primary health care, life threatening ailments, and at alleviating anemia, malnutrition, tuberculosis, parasitism, high infant mortality rate (21.9 per 1000 live births), high maternal mortality rate (0.8 per 1000 live births) and population explosion. The official census places the number of Filipinos at 70 million and growing at an average rate of 2.3% per year. The government distributes contraceptive pills to the poor freely.

If pharmaceutical companies can be convinced to reduce the cost of HRT to the price level of contraceptives, then the poor and marginalized Filipino woman can be provided with free or low-cost HRT to improve her well-being.

It is fortunate that despite the widespread poverty in the Philippines, there is an abundance of natural resources. Thus, even the poor woman in the rural area has access to fresh milk from water buffalos, cows and goats, fresh fish from the sea and sunshine for most of the year. Her depressed economic situation forces upon her weight-bearing chores such as carrying grandchildren and lifting heavy baskets of fish, fruits, vegetables and flowers to the market as sources of income.

Ironically, the poor have a healthier life-style than the upper class. They cannot afford to buy cigarettes, alcohol and coffee in excessive amounts and consider such things as luxuries. Because they live a simple life, they are not subjected to the stresses of the rat race. Again, because of their depressed economic situation, 82%[6] live under the same roof as their children and grandchildren who provide them with tender loving care, especially when they are ill which gives them fewer moments of depression or loneliness.

Conclusion

From the point of view of someone from a Third World country, the biggest challenge is to come up with a program of action that will benefit all women in the world, through a free exchange of relevant data, and the extension of much needed expertise as well as resources to the disadvantaged women of the Philippines and elsewhere. This global effort to advance the well-being of women who are rich in experience, but are hampered needlessly by the complications of menopause is a more positive kind of feminism.

References

1. Boulet, M. J., Oddens, P.L., Lehert, P., Vermer, H. M. and Visser, A. (1994). Climacteric and menopause in seven south-east Asian countries. *Maturitas*, **19**, 157–76

2. Jalbuena, J. R. (1994). Climacteric Filipino women: a preliminary survey in the Philippines. *Maturitas*, **19**, 183–90

3. Jalbuena, J. R. (1991). Climacteric Filipino women: a preliminary survey of 1015 cases. *Philippine J. Obstetr. Gynecol.*, **2**, 75–88

4. Tan, Lim M. (1992). Leading causes of death among women: In *Health Action Information Network. Philippine Health Statistics 1992*, pp. 114–88. (Republic of the Philippines: Department of Health)

5. Serrano, G. P. and Gonzaga, F. P. (1996). Perspectives of Filipino physicians regarding the menopause and hormone replacement therapy: a survey. *J. Philippine Soc. Climacteric Med.*, **4**, 16–21

6. Domingo, L. J., Feranil, I. Z. *et al.* (1990). *Socioeconomic Consequences of the Aging Population: Insights from the Philippine Experience*, p. 80. (Republic of the Philippines: Demographic Research and Development Foundation)

Menopausal medicine under difficult conditions: Yugoslavia

T. Moskovic

53

Introduction

The menopause is associated with symptoms of estrogen deficiency[1] which may be extremely debilitating and seriously reduce the quality of life. Quality of life has many components and one of its aspects, well-being, should not simply be considered as the absence of illness but the presence of 'happiness'. Indeed, the ways in which happiness may be influenced by physiological changes at mid-life should be deliberated. Additionally, the increased risk of cardiovascular disease[2] and osteoporosis[3], which occur with loss of ovarian function, has important implications for a modern society which is looking to prevent these avoidable conditions in an aging population. Hormone replacement therapy (HRT) has a strong positive effect on vasomotor[4], urinary[5] and genital symptoms[6], has an effect on psychological disturbances[7] and sexual functioning[8], and has been shown effectively to reduce the incidence of osteoporosis[9] and cardiovascular disease[10].

Background

Yugoslavia was until recently a developing country, with a current population of 12.5 million. The country has declined economically and lost its 'developing' status as a result of the war situation during the past 6 years. Unemployment, poverty and uncertainty caused people to wonder how they would survive. Some subgroups, especially old people, were often hungry and in the lowest depths of existence. Medical care at all levels depended sometimes only on charity. It was difficult to find and to pay for medicine, diagnostic and therapeutic procedures. Additionally, it was a time when doctors found themselves unable to help their patients, because of the lack of drugs. Medical equipment was very often out of order, laboratory assays were too expensive, and the overall standard of medical care was very low. Many people died for reasons which will be incomprehensible to western developed and even developing countries. In this situation it was very difficult and unrealistic to think and talk about quality of life. The new idea of menopausal medicine which had started to be widespread among gynecologists stagnated during these years but has not disappeared. Menopausal medicine not only improves quality of life, but decreases mortality from cardiovascular disease, and severe invalidity due to osteoporosis.

In all situations doctors must try to improve the quality of life although it may seem impossible and hopeless. The situation in Yugoslavia is now improving slowly, step by step. During all these years of conflict the author has continued to improve his knowledge, to improve menopausal clinic organization, to educate women and colleagues, and practise menopausal medicine despite difficult circumstances. It was a long battle against women's prejudice as well as the opposition of many doctors. Sometimes not only knowledge and energy, but much patience and imagination were required to solve practical problems. It was necessary to think about the economic status of a patient when prescribing a medicine and when advising some diagnostic procedures. Prescribing medicine was rather social choice than the best medical option. Although the best world medical products for use in hormone replacement therapy were on the market, sometimes there was a lack of the drugs, or the available drugs were too expensive.

To date, there have been no long-term studies undertaken in Yugoslavia concerning the menopause and its management. The longevity of the female population has increased dramatically but the average age of the menopause has not altered[11]. Although it is well known that the menopause may occur in women who are in their early twenties and may also be delayed until the late fifties, the average age of a Yugoslav woman at menopause is 48 years. Female life expectancy is now 72 years. By the year 2000, it is estimated that 70% of women in developing countries will reach the age of 65; one in three of this group can be expected to celebrate her 80th birthday. Thus, one in every two or three women can expect about 30 years of postmenopausal life by the year 2000. Yugoslavia is not now a welfare state but we expect development in all aspects of life including health care.

Clinic study

With the aim of giving more data about menopausal problems, an initial study was undertaken in 1995–96 in our outpatient menopause clinic, interviewing 500 women who attended the clinic. The results from 500 respondents showed that:

(1) The average age of menopause was 48.4 years;

(2) 76% of respondents were aged between 45 and 54 years at menopause;

(3) 19.1% menopaused before 45 years; and

(4) 4.9% menopaused after 54 years of age.

Out of all the women who attended the clinic 46.6% were premenopausal and 53.4% postmenopausal. Only 5% of perimenopausal women came seeking help because of vasomotor symptoms, or psychiatric disorders. The main complaint of perimenopausal respondents was irregular periods (63.5%). In a detailed face-to-face questionnaire it was found that 80% of women attending the clinic for any reason experienced some menopausal symptoms: 58% complained of vasomotor symptoms and 61% of psychiatric disturbance; 49% felt their libido had decreased and 1.5% had increased libido. Among the post-menopausal women 86% complained of menopausal symptoms: vasomotor symptoms (71%) and psychiatric disturbance (67%); 51% had decreased libido but only 0.07% had increased libido.

Osteoporosis

There are no statistics available for Yugoslavia as a whole that indicate the prevalence of osteoporosis. Much attention is paid to the prevention and therapy of osteoporosis in our clinic, but it is difficult to estimate how many osteoporotic fractures treated in orthopedic hospitals are as a result of failings in gynecological practice. In our clinic 11.8% of premenopausal women are osteoporotic according to dual energy X-ray absorptiometry (DEXA) measurement of bone mineral density of the lumbar spine. In postmenopausal women 20.6% are osteoporotic according to DEXA. Unfortunately this does not represent the real situation, because many women in the at-risk group who attend our clinic have not undergone densitometry screening. Until very recently there was only one DEXA facility available in Yugoslavia, 350 km away from the capital. It is not surprising that most patients refuse screening mainly because of lack of time. Nowadays there is a DEXA facility in the capital but one machine is not enough for screening all responders. The problem is whether to screen women at risk of osteoporosis or give them preventive therapy anyway. If we decide to screen, who has priority? Is it reasonable to screen established osteoporosis diagnosed already by X-ray? Is it reasonable to measure bone mineral density in an aim to evaluate the effect of therapy? Maybe, when selection is constrained we need to screen peri- or postmenopausal women who are in cryptomenopause but refuse HRT, and in cases where osteoporosis is not easy to diagnose. The only way to reduce the incidence of osteoporotic fracture is widespread screening for osteoporosis using more available densitometers.

Hormone replacement therapy

The quality of life of menopausal women may be dramatically improved by relieving menopausal syndrome. Estrogen replacement therapy also reduces the risk of cardiovascular disease; women at risk of cardiovascular disease are generally prescribed hormone replacement therapy (HRT). If it is possible a lipid profile analysis is advised, but this is extremely expensive and only carried out if necessary for a large number of patients.

Despite growing public and medical interest in the management of the menopause, under 1% of women in Yugoslavia currently receive HRT. There has recently been a major change in opinion among gynecologists favoring the use of HRT. Nevertheless, this change has not yet resulted in any more widespread or consistent use of HRT in practice, possibly because any change has been on the part of only a few gynecologists, while the majority have maintained their more conservative approach. In our clinic 60% of attending women receive HRT, excluding those on local estrogen therapy.

General practitioners are the first line of care for menopausal women, who can then be referred to gynecologists, endocrinologists and other physicians. Unfortunately, many doctors are insensitive to a suffering woman. Most of them do not want to change the course of 'nature', and many of them have 'estrogenophobia', but will easily prescribe antidepressive drugs and tranquilizers to suffering women.

From another point of view, traditional culture in our country led women to believe that the menopause is a natural inevitable change in their life, and they must be strong enough to carry it without any help. Most women reject HRT for 'medical reasons' such as fear of cancer, pollution of the body and interference with nature. But with an increasing number of women remaining in employment well into their fifties and beyond, there is understandably less tolerance of the symptoms which their mothers often suffered without complaint. With an increasing tendency to discuss a subject which was once taboo, and with higher expectations for quality of life, a more informed population is increasingly inclined to opt for treatment rather than to suffer in silence.

Some women who experienced irregular bleeding in perimenopause see the end of menstrual bleeds as a release from an inconvenience and will welcome the menopause, and they refuse to bleed again as a result of HRT. On the other hand, women who have regular bleeding again due to HRT in pre- or perimenopausal years when suffering metrorrhagia are the best candidates for HRT in the postmenopausal years.

HRT in the future

In the future, widespread education about HRT should be given to consultant physicians, obstetricians and gynecologists, and primary health care doctors, both in the private and public sectors. A multi-disciplinary approach must be established with good intercommunication between general practitioners, gynecologists, endocrinologists, physicians, bone specialists, psychologists and psychiatrists.

Public education of men, women and teenagers must use simple explanations to combat myths and to achieve an understanding that HRT is just a replacement of hormones that are normally present in the body, but which fall to a low level in mid-life women. The advantages of HRT must be strongly emphasized.

It is hoped that menopausal women will receive greater education concerning the menopause and HRT and, hence, will be involved increasingly in selecting their own treatment. Moreover, the importance of quality of life should continue to be emphasized. The menopause is only one of the problems that a woman facing mid-life must encounter. With hormone replacement therapy we shall not be able to restore youth, but help to keep women healthy during their autumn years.

References

1. Shurz, B., Wimmer-Greinecker, G., Metka, M., Heytamanek, G., Egarter, C. H. and Knogler, W. (1988). Beta endorphin levels during the climacteric period. *Maturitas*, **10**, 45–50

2. Lobo, R. A. (1990). Cardiovascular implications of estrogen replacement therapy. *Obstet. Gynecol.*, **75**, 18S–25S

3. Browner, W. S., Seeley, D. G., Vogt, T. M. and Cummings, S. R. (1991). Non-trauma mortality in elderly women with low bone mineral density. Study of Osteoporotic Fractures Research Group. *Lancet*, **338**, 355–8

4. Padwick, M. L., Endacott, J. and Whitehead, M. I. (1985). Efficacy, acceptability and metabolic effects of transdermal estradiol in the management of postmenopausal women. *Am. J. Obstet. Gynecol.*, **152**, 1085–91

5. Walter, S., Wolf, H. and Barlebo, H. (1978). Urinary incontinence in postmenopausal women treated with oestrogens: a double-blind clinical trial. *Urol. Int.*, **33**, 135–43

6. Martin, P. L., Greany, M. O. and Burner, A. M. (1984). Estradiol, estrone and gonadotrophin levels after use of vaginal estradiol. *Obstet. Gynecol.*, **63**, 441–4

7. Campbell, S. and Whitehead, M. (1977). Estrogen therapy and the menopausal syndrome. *Clin. Obstet. Gynecol.*, **4**, 31

8. Dennerstein, L. and Burrows, G. D. (1982). Hormone replacement therapy and sexuality in women. *Clin. Endocrinol. Metab.*, **11**, 661–79

9. Felson, D. T., Zhang, Y., Hannan, M. T., Kiel, D. P., Wilson, P. W. F. and Anderson, J. J. (1993). The effect of postmenopausal estrogen therapy on bone density in elderly women. *N. Engl. J. Med.*, **329**, 1141–6

10. Hong, M. J., Romm, P. A. and Reagan, K. (1992). Effects of estrogen replacement therapy on serum lipid values in angiographically defined coronary artery disease in post-menopausal women. *Am. J. Cardiol.*, **69**, 176–8

11. Admudsen, D. W. and Diers, C. I. (1973). The age of menopause in medial Europe. *Hum. Biol.*, **45**, 605–8

13

Hormones and mood change

Neuroendocrinology of the climacteric period and hormonal replacement therapy

54

A. R. Genazzani, M. Stomati, A. Spinetti, M. M. Greco, A. D. Genazzani and F. Petraglia

Introduction

Sex-steroid hormones exert relevant functions in the central nervous system (CNS), controlling the reproductive function and modulating a woman's general psychophysical well-being. These actions occur through specific receptors for estrogens, progestogen and androgens. Receptors for sex hormones have been demonstrated in the cortex, limbic system, hippocampus, cerebellum, locus ceruleus, hypothalamus, preoptic area and amygdala[1,2]. In fact, in the CNS genomic effects of ovarian steroids through specific binding with intracellular receptors have been described. However, recently non-genomic effects have been demonstrated in experimental studies on female rats. Estrogens are able to modulate neuron activity, stimulating dendritic growth, synaptic junction formation, neuronal plasticity and neurotransmission[1-3].

The main actions of gonadal steroids on the CNS are mediated by neuroactive transmitters. Estrogens, progesterone and androgens exert a modulatory effect on the synthesis, release and metabolism of some neuropeptides and neurotransmitters. Moreover, sex steroids modulate the concentrations and the expression of the neurotransmitter receptors. Noradrenaline, dopamine, gamma-aminobutyric acid (GABA), acetylcholine, serotonin and melatonin are the neurotransmitters mainly modulated by sex-steroid hormones. Neuropeptides influenced by sex steroids are opioid peptides, neuropeptide Y, corticotropin-releasing factor (CRF) and galanin[4].

During a woman's reproductive life, the equilibrium and interaction of neuro-transmitters, neuropeptides and gonadal steroids modulate the ovulatory function, electively acting at hypothalamic level on the synthesis and release of gonadotropin-releasing hormone (GnRH). GnRH pulse-generation directly regulates the production and release of pituitary gonadotropins and the consequent secretion of ovarian hormones. Cyclic ovarian-steroid production, controlled by the action of gonadotropins, modulates GnRH and gonadotropin production through feedback mechanisms. This modulation is mediated by the neuroactive transmitters.

Moreover, neuroactive transmitters and sex-steroid hormones are involved in the regulation of other vegetative centers[2,4]. They are involved in the neuroendocrine control at hypothalamic level of the activity of the thermoregulatory, satiety, appetite and blood-pressure centers, and at limbic-system level of the regulation of mood, behavior and psychophysical well-being (Table 1)[4,5].

The failure of ovarian sex-steroid production at the climacteric periods generates neuro-endocrine modifications of the adaptive response at the CNS level associated with neuroendocrine modifications. For this reason, specific symptoms involving CNS derangement occur in postmenopausal women.

Neuroendocrine implications of clinical disturbances

It is possible to separate climacteric and postmenopausal disturbances in relation to the anatomical site of the CNS in which the

Table 1 Physiological function and principal areas modulated by sex steroids

Limbic system
   mood and behavior
   cognitive function

Hypothalamus
   thermoregulation
   satiety
   hunger
   blood pressure

Table 2 Neuroendocrine dysfunction and disorders of hypothalamus and limbic system

Limbic system
   changes of mood and behavior
   anxiety
   depression
   insomnia
   headache/migraine
   modification of cognitive function

Hypothalamus
   hot flushes and sweating
   hypertension
   obesity

withdrawal of sex steroids induces modification of the neuroactive transmitters. At the hypothalamic level, vasomotor symptoms such as hot flushes and sweats, obesity and hypertension are consequences of the postmenopausal neuroendocrine impairment. However, mood changes, anxiety, depression, insomnia, headaches/migraine and alterations of cognitive functions are related to postmenopusal changes in the limbic system (Table 2). In addition, aging women are more affected by chronic and degenerative diseases, such as impairment of motor activity with increased incidence of Parkinson's disease, or reduction of short-term memory and increased incidence of Alzheimer's disease, than age-matched men. The long period of a woman's life associated with estrogen deprivation plays a fundamental role in the physiopathological mechanisms of these CNS-degenerative diseases.

The reduction of gonadal-hormone production exerts relevant modifications of the neuroendocrine control at CNS level. These modifications are expressed by changes in the synthesis, release and activity of the neuroactive transmitters and modifications to their receptors. Moreover, the longer absence of ovarian steroids, typical of the late postmenopausal period, is related to alterations in neuronal plasticity, synaptic junctions, and a reduction of synapsis numbers[6,7].

Vasomotor instability

The hot flush is the hallmark of the climacteric period: it is the most common and typical symptom, occurring in 50–70% of women after the menopause. The hot flush is considered to be like a temporary derangement of the hypothalamic set-point for thermoregulation. The theory that hot flushes originate in the CNS is supported by many experimental studies that evidence important modification of neuro-transmitters and neuropeptides in the development of vasomotor instability[8]. The activation or inhibition of some hypothalamic and suprahypothalamic neurotransmitters and neuropeptides could explain hot flushes and the stimulation of GnRH–luteinizing hormone (LH) pulses.

The lack of estrogens in postmenopausal women provokes an increased activity of the noradrenergic system and the reduction of dopaminergic activity (Figure 1). The noradrenergic and dopaminergic systems modulate both GnRH and LH pulsatile release and the vasomotor/thermoregulator system[9]. These data are supported by the efficacy of clonidine, an α_2 agonist at presynaptic receptors, and veralipride, a dopamine antagonist, in the reduction of postmenopausal vasomotor symptoms[10].

Changes in the noradrenergic and dopaminergic systems could only partially explain the induction of hot flushes in postmenopausal women. Several studies demonstrate a relevant role of opioid peptides in the regulation of GnRH synthesis and pulsatile release, a mechanism mediated by

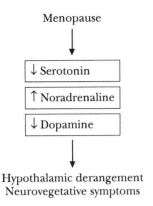

Figure 1 Hypothalamic neurotransmitter impairment at menopause

aminergic release and affecting thermo-regulatory function[11]. The evidence for an opioid inhibitory role on GnRH–LH secretion is the increment in frequency and amplitude of GnRH–LH release with the administration of naloxone, an opioid-receptor antagonist, in normal menstruating women[7]. In post-menopausal women there is a failure of opioid-receptor blockade by naloxone to modify gonadotropin secretion. This phenomenon could in part explain the high frequency and amplitude of gonadotropin pulses in post-menopausal women[7].

The modulatory-positive effect of endogenous opioids on adrenergic neurons explains the similar action of clonidine and naloxone in the reduction of hot flushes, confirming the role of the opioidergic and noradrenergic systems in the modulation of vasomotor instability. During the climacteric period, the lack of sex-steroid activity induces a reduction in β-endorphin plasma level which is restored following hormone replacement therapy[12,13].

Psychological symptoms, cognitive and memory declines

It is known that during the climacteric period psychological symptoms increase, and that at this stage of life the incidence of psychological disorders is greater in women than in age-matched men[14]. An involvement of neuropeptides and neurotransmitters, as a consequence of sex-hormone withdrawal, explains the psychological dysfunction expressed by cognitive, memory, sexuality and sleep disturbances, and instability of mood tonus with irritability, anxiety, depression and insomnia[5,15].

With the reduction of plasma sex-steroid levels there is a parallel decrease of serotoninergic tonus in the CNS. It is known that estrogen increases the rate of degradation of monoamine oxidase, the enzyme that catabolizes the neurotransmitter serotonin[16]. The reduction of serotoninergic tonus seems to be related to depression and the modulation of mood changes in postmenopausal women.

Moreover, estrogen increases the action of choline acetyltransferase, the most important enzyme in acetylcholine synthesis[17]. A reduction in acetylcholine concentrations is the most important expression of Alzheimer's disease. The reduction of cholinergic tone could explain changes in short-term memory in post-menopausal women[18].

Even norepinephrine and dopamine appear to play a significant role in modulating mood, behavior, cognitive ability and motor activity[7]. In fact, it has been found that dopaminergic tone decreases and noradrenergic tone increases in women following gonadectomy. With estrogen withdrawal there is an increase in the norepinephrine/dopamine ratio level.

Hormone replacement therapy and menopausal disturbances

Hormone replacement therapy (HRT) exerts a positive effect on vasomotor instability, reducing the number and intensity of hot flushes and sweats. In fact, estrogens are able to re-equilibrate the change in the neuroendocrine systems. However, the positive effect of HRT on the vasomotor symptoms is not present in about 25% of postmenopausal treated women (Figure 2). In these patients, the use of neuroendocrine therapies has been

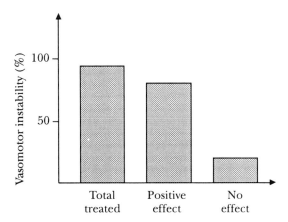

Figure 2 Therapeutical effect of hormone replacement therapy (HRT) on vasomotor symptoms

evaluated; clonidine, an α_2 agonist at presynaptic receptors, and veralipride, a dopamine antagonist, have been found to reduce vasomotor instability (Figure 3).

Regarding psychological disturbances, HRT and in particular estrogen replacement therapy, positively influences depressive symptomatology, pain perception and affective and sexual behavior. Regarding the effect of progestogens, different doses, routes of administration and types of compound influence their different actions.

At the neuroendocrine level, experimental animal studies with HRT have shown a restoration of noradrenergic tone, suggesting a feedback mechanism of sex-steroid action on

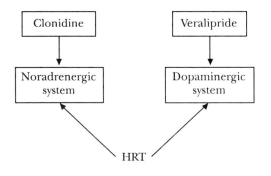

Figure 3 Drugs which modulate neurovegetative postmenopausal instability. HRT, hormone replacement therapy

catecholaminergic neurons[19]. Other studies on castrated female rats demonstrated that estradiol exerts a reduction of noradrenaline release at the hypothalamic level[20]. With regard to the dopaminergic system, estradiol directly modulated dopaminergic neuronal activity, increasing the dopaminergic release at the mediobasal hypothalamus level[21].

Hormone replacement therapy is able to restore plasma choline acetyltransferase levels in postmenopausal women. It is associated with an increase of short-term memory and cognitive functions[18]. Epidemiological studies evidence a reduced incidence of Alzheimer's disease in postmenopausal women using HRT. Estrogen directly increases cerebral flow and neuronal genomic activation through the binding with cholinergic receptors.

Among neuropeptides, the opioidergic system is modulated by gonadal hormones. Estrogen increases the synthesis and release of endogenous opioids (β-endorphin, met-enkephalin and dinorphin) through a direct action on opioidergic-receptor activity[12,13]. Moreover, the beneficial effects of estrogen on opioidergic neurons seem not to be modified by the different regimens and progestogen compounds used during HRT.

Role of neurosteroids

In recent studies it has been demonstrated that steroid hormones can be synthesized *de novo* in the brain[22]. The term neurosteroids was coined for steroids synthesized in the brain, but a more general definition of neurosteroids would include all steroids synthesized in the brain that have an action in the CNS. Neurosteroids could also act non-genomically, modulating classic neurotransmitters in the brain[23]. Some studies have evidenced how some psychological symptoms such as depression, anxiety and irritability, can be related to the fluctuation in synthesis and release of the neurosteroids, and in particular of dehydroepiandrosterone (DHEA)[23]. Physiological doses of DHEA may have a beneficial psychological effect, characterized by an improved sense of well-being[24]. This suggests a possible future clinical application of the steroid in prevention of the

psychological disturbances associated with the climacteric period.

References

1. Smith, S. S. (1993). Hormones, mood and neurobiology – a summary. In Berg, G. and Hammar, M. (eds.) *The Modern Management of the Menopause*, pp. 257–68. (Carnforth, UK: Parthenon Publishing)
2. Maggi, A. and Perez, J. (1985). Role of female gonadal hormones in the CNS: clinical experimental aspects. *Life Sci.*, **37**, 893–906
3. Sherwin, B. B. (1996). Hormones, mood and cognitive functioning in postmenopausal women. *Obstet. Gynecol.*, **87**, 20–6
4. Speroff, L., Glass, R. H. and Kase, N. H. (1995). *Clinical Gynecological Endocrinology and Infertility*, 5th ed. (Baltimore, MD: Williams and Wilkins)
5. Lobo, R. A. (1993). *Treatment of Postmenopausal Women: Basic and Clinical Aspects.* (New York: Raven Press)
6. Panay, N., Sands, R. H. and Studd, J. W. W. (1996). Estrogen and behavior. In Genazzani, A. R., Petraglia, F. and Purdy, R. H. (eds.) *The Brain: Source and Target for Sex Steroid Hormones*, pp. 257–76. (Carnforth, UK: Parthenon Publishing)
7. Yen, S. S. C. and Jaffe, R. B. (1991). *Reproductive Endocrinology.* (Philadelphia: W. B. Saunders)
8. Meldrum, D. L., De Fazio, J., Erlik, Y., Wolfsen, A. *et al.* (1984). Pituitary hormones during the menopausal hot flush. *Obstet. Gynecol.*, **64**, 752–6
9. Toivola, P. T. and Gale, C. C. (1979). Effect of temperature on biogenic amine infusion into hypothalamus of baboon. *Neuroendocrinology*, **6**, 210–19
10. Ginsburg, J. and Hardiman, P. (1987). Adrenergic agonist for menopausal complaints. In Genazzani, A. R., Montemagno, U., Nappi, C. and Petraglia, F. (eds.) *The Brain and Female Reproductive Function*, pp. 623–5. (Carnforth, UK: Parthenon Publishing)
11. Melis, G., Cagnacci, A., Gambacciani, M. *et al.* (1988). Restoration of luteinizing hormone response to naloxone in postmenopausal women by chronic administration of the anti-dopaminergic drug veralipride. *J. Clin. Endocrinol. Metab.*, **66**, 964–9
12. Aleem, F. A. and McIntosh, T. K. (1985). Menopausal syndrome: plasma levels of beta endorphin in postmenopausal women measured by a specific radioimmunoassay. *Maturitas*, **7**, 329–34
13. Genazzani, A. R., Petraglia, F., Facchinetti, F., Grasso, A., Alessandrini, G. and Volpe, A. (1988). Steroid replacement treatment increases β-endorphin and β-lipotropin plasma levels in postmenopausal women. *Gynecol. Obstet. Invest.*, **26**, 153–9
14. Hallstrom, T. (1977). Sexuality in climacteric. In Greenblatt, R. B. and Studd, J. W. W. (eds.) *Clinics in Obstetrics and Gynecology*, pp. 277–89. (Philadelphia: W. B. Saunders)
15. Campbell, S. and Whitehead, M. (1977). Estrogen therapy and menopausal syndrome. *Clin. Obstet. Gynecol.*, **4**, 31
16. Luine, V. N. and McEwen, B. S. (1977). Effect of estradiol on turnover of type A monoamine oxidase in the brain. *J. Neurochem.*, **28**, 1221–7
17. Bartus, R. T., Dean, R. L., Beer, B. and Lippa, A. S. (1982). The cholinergic hypothesis of memory dysfunction. *Science*, **217**, 408–17
18. Phillips, S. and Sherwin, B. B. (1992). Effects of estrogen on memory function in surgically menopausal women. *Psychoneuroendocrinology*, **17**, 485–95
19. Advis, J., McConn, S. and Negro-Vilar, A. (1980). Evidence that catecholaminergic and peptidergic (luteinizing hormone-releasing hormone) neurons in suprachiasmatic-medial preoptic, medial basal hypothalamus and median eminence are involved in estrogen negative feed back. *Endocrinology*, **107**, 892–902
20. Wise, P., Rance, N. and Berraclough, C. (1980). Effect of estradiol and progesterone on catecholamine turnover rates in discrete hypothalamic regions in ovariectomized rats. *Endocrinology*, **108**, 2186–93
21. Sar, M. (1989). Estradiol is concentrated in tyrosine hydroxylase-containing neurons of the hypothalamus. *Science*, **223**, 938–40
22. Bohus, B., Koolhaas, J. M. and Korte, S. M. (1991). Psychological stress, anxiety and depression: physiological and neuroendocrine correlates in animal model. In Genazzani, A. R., Nappi, G., Petraglia, F. and Martignoni, E. (eds.) *Stress and Related Disorders from Adaptation to Dysfunction*, pp. 129–38. (Carnforth, UK: Parthenon Publishing)
23. Mellan, S. H. (1994). Neurosteroids: action and clinical relevance. *J. Clin. Endocrinol. Metab.*, **78**, 1003–8

Estrogens in the treatment of climacteric depression, premenstrual depression, postnatal depression and chronic fatigue syndrome

55

J. J. W. Studd and N. Panay

Background

The effect of hormones on behavior and depression is a major area of controversy because of the disparate views of gynecologists and psychologists. There is now good evidence that estrogens are rapidly effective in the treatment of depression in many women, but this information has not found its way through to those health-care personnel, psychiatrists and psychologists who are principally involved in the treatment of depression.

Depression is more common in women than men regardless of whether one looks at community studies, hospital admission data, suicide attempts or prescriptions for antidepressants. The dilemma is to determine how much this excess in depression is due to the hormonal characteristics of the adult woman rather than the other environmental, domestic or sociological factors which may be more stressful in women than men. The latter would be the view of most psychologists and the view of politically correct feminism, but ignores the fact that increased depression occurs at times of hormonal fluctuation.

Historically there has always been a belief that psychological problems are more common in women, and the philosophy reached its nadir in Victorian times with the belief that menstruation and female physiology seriously limited the capability of women. The fashionable Victorian disorders were neuresthenia, chloris, menstrual insanity, ovarian mania, nymphomania and even masturbation, which 'clearly' caused insanity. This view was supported by the most senior academics in gynecology and psychiatry in Northern Europe and North America. Appalling operations were performed on young women in removing the clitoris and ovaries, to treat these disorders which were mostly in the imaginations of their husbands or more commonly, their devoted fathers. This period of 30 years is a black stain on the story of the treatment of women, and perhaps instinctively there is now a deeply ingrained objection to the view that hormones are at all involved in any sort of mental disease.

Effects of endogenous estrogens on the central nervous system

During fetal life estrogen exerts genomic, organizational effects on brain development that control neural architecture. Estrogen receptors mediating the genomic effects in the central nervous system (CNS) are primarily found in the preoptic area, hypothalamus and amygdala, and to a lesser degree in the hippocampus, cerebellum, septal area and inferior colliculus[1]. Limbic system functions, which subserve emotion and behavior, can therefore be influenced by circulating estrogenic steroids.

Non-genomic, activational effects on brain function are produced via the transitory regulation of brain plasticity[2]. Also, the action of estrogen on CNS neuroreceptors can alter the concentration and availability of neurotransmitter amines, including serotonin and norepinephrine[3]. Estrogen increases the rate of degradation of monoamine oxidase, the enzyme that catabolizes serotonin[4], and has been shown to displace tryptophan from its binding sites to plasma albumin[5] allowing more free tryptophan to be available to the brain where it can be metabolized to serotonin. Finally, estrogen enhances the transport of serotonin. The effect of estradiol on neurotransmitter receptors for excitatory amino acids explains how estrogen may affect mood, particularly as depression is largely due to a serotonin deficit.

Clinical features

The excess of depression in women begins at puberty, but there are three other times of increased depression related to hormonal changes. These are:

(1) Premenstrual depression;

(2) Postnatal depression; and

(3) Climacteric depression;

which have been shown in randomized trials to respond to percutaneous estrogens either in the form of transdermal patches or percutaneous implants. These are the 'triad of responses of mood disorders' which now should be treated in our opinion primarily by estrogens rather than psychoactive drugs. They often occur in the same vulnerable woman. For example, it is common to see a 45-year-old woman with severe perimenopausal depression. She will say that she last felt well when she was pregnant 10 years ago. She then developed postnatal depression which lasted 6–9 months. When the periods returned, the depression became cyclical. The premenstrual syndrome (PMS) became worse with age, and her 7 days of symptoms became 14 days of symptoms. Soon the cyclical depression became continuous, and she was given antidepressants because she was still having periods and the perception was that she could not be estrogen-deficient. The patient

with such a story responds well to moderately large doses of percutaneous estrogens.

The depression is not related to absolute hormone levels, as many studies have shown no difference in hormone profiles of premenopausal women who are not depressed. Similarly there is no difference within groups of postnatal climacteric patients or patients after bilateral oophorectomy which relate to the presence or absence of depression. Thus the determination of hormone-level profiles is not valuable in making this diagnosis. The depression is due to a change of hormone levels, either estradiol or progesterone, in susceptible women. The diagnostic clues come from the women's history. Climacteric women with an estrogen-responsive depression will usually have a history of (1) being well during pregnancy, but pregnancy was followed by (2) postnatal depression. They will often have a history of cyclical symptoms such as (3) premenstrual depression and (4) menstrual headaches. Not all patients will have all four clues in their history, but the presence of (1), (2) and (3) are a fairly sure sign that estrogens will be very helpful.

Menopausal depression

Effect of menopause on mood

The menopause is associated with a reduction of central content and activity of certain neurotransmitters and neuropeptides which is improved by estrogen administration. Climacteric depression is at its worst 2–3 years before the periods stop, and it is the women who are still having regular periods whose depression may respond to estrogens rather than the postmenopausal women[6]. Certainly correction of vasomotor instability, insomnia and painful intercourse will help mood in what is called the 'domino effect', but there is also a mental tonic effect of estrogens that occurs irrespective of other climacteric symptoms. Estrogen replacement appears to enhance mood in a dose-dependent manner, and also enhances or maintains aspects of cognitive functioning.

Therapeutic effects of estrogen therapy

Many studies have evaluated whether mood is worsened during the climacteric by studying overall quality of life. For example, Daly and colleagues[7] found that 63 women with complaints of menopausal symptoms had improved well-being after estrogen therapy. Limouzin-Lamothe and co-workers[8] also showed that general well-being, in 499 women with a mean age of 51 years, was improved by estrogen therapy. Others have used more specific depression-rating scales. Ditkoff and associates[9] produced significantly improved Beck depression scores with conjugated estrogens in 36 asymptomatic women aged 45–60 years, and Best and colleagues[10] observed improved Hamilton depression scores in 16 hysterecto-mized postmenopausal women using estradiol implants.

The effect of estrogen therapy on mood has been studied by many workers, but few have concentrated on patients with major depressive disorder. One of the earliest and most convincing studies as to the benefits of estrogen in depression is that of Klaiber and associates[11], who studied the use of oral equine estrogens in severely depressed inpatients who had been unresponsive to conventional treatments such as electroconvulsive therapy, antidepressants and psychotherapy. According to Diagnostic and Statistical Manual of Mental Disorders (DSM) criteria, these patients all had primary, recurrent unipolar major depressive disorders. Conjugated equine estrogens were commenced in huge doses, starting with a dose of 5 mg and increasing weekly in 5 mg increments to a maximum of 25 mg daily, a dose achieved in 50% of those receiving active treatment. The results were impressive in that there were highly significant reductions in depression scores in the estrogen-treated group, as well as clinically significant improvements in mood as observed by trained personnel (Figure 1). This important study was overlooked because of fears of high-dose estrogens and is only recently being corroborated.

There are few studies that have looked at oral estrogen in adequate doses, but climacteric

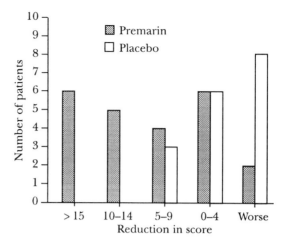

Figure 1 Effect of high dose conjugated equine estrogens on major depression. Improvement in Hamilton depression scores: premarin vs. placebo. Adapted from reference 11

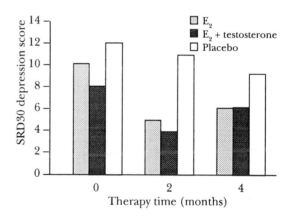

Figure 2 Effect of estradiol/testosterone implants in perimenopausal women. At 2 months, SRD30 depression score for estradiol (E_2) alone and E_2 + testosterone was significantly different from placebo: $p < 0.01$. From reference 6 with permission

depression has been shown to improve with percutaneous estrogens, using either patch or implant. Montgomery and colleagues[6] demonstrated significant elevation of mood in climacteric depression in women treated with estrogen and testosterone implants (Figure 2).

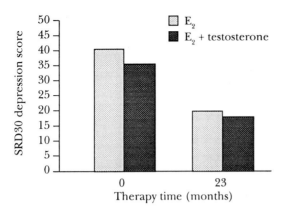

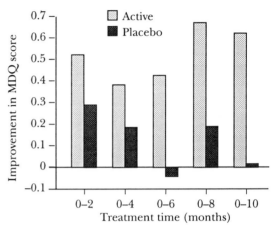

Figure 3 Perimenopausal depression and hormone implants: 23-month results. SRD30 depression score for estradiol (E_2) alone and E_2 + testosterone was significantly different from baseline: $p < 0.05$. From Montgomery, J. and Studd, J. W. W., unpublished data, with permission

Figure 4 Subcutaneous estradiol and premenstrual syndrome (PMS) improvement in total Moos menstrual distress questionnaire (MDQ) score with time: estradiol vs. placebo. At 0–4, 0–8 and 0–10 months, active vs. placebo was significantly different: $p < 0.05$; at 0–6 months: $p < 0.01$. From reference 17, with permission

The benefits were not transient but were maintained until the end of a 23-month follow-up (Figure 3).

The most acceptable treatment for climacteric depression in our opinion is the estradiol patch, 200 µg twice weekly, which will produce estradiol levels of about 600 pmol/l. There are anxieties about overtreatment with estrogens, but these levels are still within the normal range of the ovarian cycle.

Premenstrual depression

Premenstrual syndrome (PMS) has been defined as distressing physical, behavioral and psychological symptoms not due to organic disease, which regularly recur during the same phase of each menstrual (ovarian) cycle and which disappear or significantly regress during the remainder of the cycle[12]. Typical psychological and behavioral problems include depression, anxiety, irritability and loss of concentration and confidence. Many premenstrual women will experience minor emotional changes. Severe PMS with symptoms of depression, irritability, anxiety, bloating,

headaches, mastalgia and even violence can be debilitating factors in domestic life, although surprisingly these women can usually cope within the working environment. These severe symptoms occur in 3–5% of women[13].

Although the underlying cause of PMS remains unknown, cyclical ovarian activity appears to be an important factor[14]. A logical treatment for severe PMS, therefore, is to suppress ovulation and thus suppress the cyclical endocrine/biochemical changes which cause the cyclical symptoms[12]. A number of possible drugs are capable of performing this function such as the combined pill, danazol[15] and gonadotropin analogs[16], but they are not without their own side-effects, which may influence efficacy of treatment or the duration for which they may be given. A treatment of proven efficacy in a placebo-controlled trial which appears suitable for long-term usage, is continuous 17β-estradiol combined with cyclical progestogen. This was first administered as a 100 mg implant, and proved to be highly effective in every Moos cluster of symptoms compared with placebo (Figure 4)[17]. The drawback with this method is that the implants

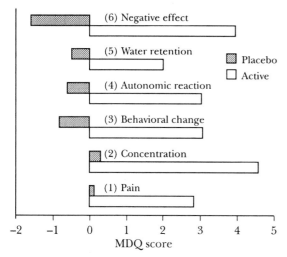

Figure 5 Percutaneous estradiol and premenstrual syndrome (PMS) improvement in adverse Moos symptom clusters. Active vs. placebo significantly different for (1), (2) and (5): $p < 0.001$; and for (3), (4) and (6): $p < 0.01$. From reference 19, with permission

last for a long period of time; this has twofold implications if treatment is to be stopped. First, fertility is suppressed and it may take 12–24 months before fertility is restored as the implant wears out, so implants may not be appropriate for the younger age group. Second, progestogens must continue to be taken for at least 18 months until the stimulatory estrogenic effects on the endometrium have ceased.

Transdermal estradiol patches were subsequently used so that treatment could be discontinued at short notice. In the first study, Estraderm TTS® 200 µg patches were shown to suppress ovulation[18]. This dose was subsequently tested against placebo in a cross-over trial and found to be highly effective in the treatment of PMS[19]. Both the physical and psychological symptoms of PMS were reduced by an average of 60% (Figure 5). A randomized study recently completed by Smith and co-workers[20] showed that estradiol 100 µg twice weekly was as effective as 200 µg twice weekly in reducing symptom levels in severe premenstrual syndrome, and that this dosage was better tolerated. This study also served to further enhance knowledge about the etiology of PMS and ovulation, as it

appeared from day-21 progesterone levels that even the 100 µg estradiol patch suppressed ovulation. An attractive theory is that by suppressing ovarian function, estradiol is preventing production by the ovary of an as yet unidentified PMS-promoting agent[14], probably progesterone or one of its psychoactive metabolites.

Another theory about the action of estradiol in PMS is that it may act directly by elevating mood[21]. It has been shown to do this both in perimenopausal and postmenopausal women[6,8], and its antidepressant effect in high doses has been demonstrated by Klaiber and associates[11]. The observation by Smith and colleagues[20] that estradiol 100 µg was equally as effective as estradiol 200 µg in treating PMS, strongly suggests that the principal mechanism of action is ovarian suppression, although the logical study of luteal-phase support by transdermal or oral estrogen has yet to be performed.

Postnatal depression

Postnatal depression, a dangerous and unpredictable condition, will affect approximately 10–15% of women following childbirth, and will persist for longer than 1 year in approximately 40% of those affected[22]. It is usually unreported and therefore left untreated. The possibility of a biological etiology for postnatal depression has been proposed because of various pieces of evidence. These include: the increasing incidence of mood disorders at times of rapidly fluctuating, mainly falling hormone levels which occur postnatally, premenstrually and perimenopausally; the relatively constant time interval between delivery and the onset of each postpartum disorder; the lack of overall influence of psychosocial and background factors in determining postpartum disorders; the possible association between PMS and postpartum depression; and finally the estrogen responsiveness of both PMS and postnatal depression[23].

Wagner and Davis[24] have postulated that the high circulating estrogen levels of pregnancy protect against depression, and the rapid decline of levels at birth removes this effect. Although a clear link has not as yet been established between the reproductive steroids and postnatal depression in some studies[25,26], this may be because of methodological problems of such research. Alder and Cox[27], who assessed breast-feeding patterns and postpartum contraceptive use, stressed the importance of taking these factors into account when conducting biological studies into postpartum depressive illness.

A number of studies using estrogens[6–11] have produced significant improvements in levels of depression in menopausal women using hormone replacement therapy. There has formerly been no suggestion that hormone therapy can effectively treat postnatal depression, but by extending the hypothesis of the triad of estrogen mood disorders, our department has demonstrated that this also is estrogen-responsive. There are data to support the hypothesis that therapy with 200 μg transdermal estradiol both significantly reduces depression scores and accelerates recovery in women with postnatal depression[28]. Gregoire and co-workers[29] recently showed that 200 μg of Estraderm was more effective than placebo even in patients who had not reacted to psychoactive drugs (Figure 6).

Progestogen

Although estrogens elevate the mood there is still a problem, as women with a uterus would need cyclical progestogen to prevent excess endometrial proliferation. We have previously demonstrated that progestogen may produce depression and irritability, i.e. symptoms of PMS, and depressed women are often progestogen-intolerant[30]. It is often necessary to change the progestogen, or reduce the dose or the duration each month in order to cut down the progestogenic side-effects[31]. Early work suggests that the levonorgestrel-releasing intrauterine system (LNG IUS) may be valuable in this situation. The LNG IUS can prevent endometrial proliferation in perimenopausal women using oral or transdermal estradiol[32,33].

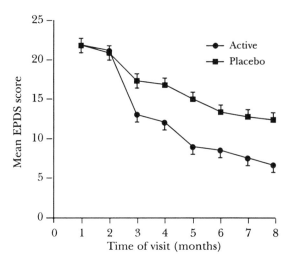

Figure 6 Transdermal estradiol for severe postnatal depression. Subjects' Edinburgh postnatal depression (EPDS) scores are shown before (< 2 months) and after (> 2 months) starting placebo-controlled trial of transdermal therapy with 17β-estradiol, 200 μg per day. Pretreatment scores of two groups are very similar. At third visit, i.e. after 1 month of treatment, there is already significant difference between active and placebo groups, which is then maintained. Mean scores ± SE are shown for each group. Adapted from reference 29

Plasma concentrations of levonorgestrol achieved by the LNG IUS are lower than those seen with oral progestogens; also, unlike with use of oral progestogens, levels with use of the LNG IUS do not display peaks and troughs. It is therefore postulated that using the LNG IUS rather than an oral progestogen to prevent endometrial hyperplasia, would be an ideal way of avoiding progestogenic side-effects in women being treated with estrogens. Work recently completed in our unit showed that adverse progestogenic effects and severity of bleeding were reduced to a minimum when progestogen-intolerant menopausal patients using mainly estradiol implants, even with relatively high serum estradiol levels, were switched from oral progestogens to the LNG IUS. Endometrial suppression was uniform with no cases of endometrial proliferation or hyperplasia at 1 year and a greater than 60% rate of amenorrhea at this time[34].

Table 1 Effect of estrogens on depression: key points

Affect neurotransmitters and their receptors in similar manner to antidepressants

Physiological doses effectively treat premenstrual syndrome

Physiological doses effectively treat postnatal depression

Physiological doses modulate mood in non-depressed women

Physiological doses treat women with climacteric depression

Pharmacological doses treat major depressive illness

Evidence for physiological doses benefiting subset of women with chronic fatigue syndrome

Chronic fatigue syndrome

During the past 6 months we have seen 28 premenopausal patients with chronic fatigue syndrome (CFS) diagnosed by consultant physicians of various disciplines. The patients all complained of lethargy, headaches, depression, weakness and loss of concentration, which were often worse in the premenstrual phase. There was a high incidence of severe PMS with 22 (79%) reporting this. There was also a high incidence of postnatal depression, in five out of 11 (45%). Also, nine out of 11 (81%) claimed to have been very well during pregnancy. Seven patients (25%) had estradiol levels below the normal 75 pmol/l with normal

follicle-stimulating hormone (FSH) levels. Four of these had a low bone density at the spine and hip. This is suggestive of a chronic estrogen-deficiency state in a subpopulation of these CFS sufferers, which improves in pregnancy when estrogen levels are high.

We believe that patients who have been diagnosed as having CFS represent a heterogeneous group, with a significant proportion suffering from a hypoestrogenic state and/or severe PMS. The fact that 22 of the 28 (79%) patients (seven of nine (78%) hypoestrogenic patients) improved using 200 μg-estradiol patches and cyclical progestogens supports this view. However, further comment on the efficacy of this therapy must await randomized controlled trials[35].

Conclusions

Therapeutic estrogens can produce significant improvement in the triad of estrogen-responsive psychological disorders: postnatal depression, premenstrual depression and climacteric depression. There is also preliminary evidence for a beneficial effect of estrogens in a subset of women suffering from chronic fatigue syndrome (Table 1). Future research should be directed at confirming the psychotherapeutic role of estrogen, as a treatment for the triad of depressive disorders and also as a therapeutic option for women with chronic fatigue syndrome, so that inappropriate treatment with antidepressant medication and electroconvulsive therapy can be avoided.

References

1. Maggi, A. and Perez, J. (1985). Role of female gonadal hormones in the CNS: clinical and experimental aspects. *Life Sci.*, **37**, 893–906
2. Sherwin, B. B. (1996). Hormones, mood and cognitive functioning in postmenopausal women. *Obstet. Gynecol.*, **87** (Suppl.2), 20–6
3. Crowley, W. R. (1982). Effects of ovarian hormones on norepinephrine and dopamine turnover in individual hypothalamic and extrahypothalamic nuclei. *Neuroendocrinology*, **34**, 381–6
4. Luine, V. N. and McEwen, B. S. (1977). Effect of estradiol on turnover of type A monoamine oxidase in brain. *J. Neurochem.*, **28**, 1221–7
5. Aylward, M. (1973). Plasma tryptophan levels and mental depression in postmenopausal subjects. Effects of oral piperazine oestrone sulphate. *IRCS Med. Sci.*, **1**, 30–4

6. Montgomery, J. C., Brincat, M., Studd, J. W. W., *et al.* (1987). Effect of oestrogen and testosterone implants on psychological disorders in the climacteric. *Lancet*, **1**, 297–9

7. Daly, E., Gray, A., Barlow, D., *et al.* (1993). Measuring the impact of menopausal symptoms on quality of life. *Br. Med. J.*, **307**, 836–40

8. Limouzin-Lamothe, M., Mairon, N., LeGal, J. *et al.* (1991). Quality of life after the menopause: influence of hormone replacement therapy. *Am. J. Obstet. Gynecol.*, **78**, 991–5

9. Ditkoff, E. C., Crary, W. G., Cristo, M. and Lobo, R. A. (1991). Estrogen improves psychological functioning in asymptomatic postmenopausal women. *Obstet. Gynecol.*, **78**, 991–5

10. Best, N., Rees, M., Barlow, D., *et al.* (1992). Effect of estradiol implant on noradrenergic function and mood in menopausal patients. *Psychoneurendocrinology*, **17**, 87–93

11. Klaiber, E. L., Broverman, D. M., Vogel, W., *et al.* (1979). Estrogen replacement therapy for severe persistent depression in women. *Arch. Gen. Psychiatr.*, **36**, 550–4

12. Magos, A. L. and Studd, J. W. W. (1984). The premenstrual syndrome. In Studd, J. W. W. (ed.) *Progress in Obstetrics and Gynaecology*, Vol. 4, pp. 334–50. (London: Churchill Livingstone)

13. Reid, R. L. (1991). Premenstrual syndrome. *N. Engl. J. Med.*, **324**, 1208–10

14. Studd, J. W. W. (1979). Premenstrual tension syndrome. *Br. Med., J.* **1**, 410

15. Watts, J. F., Butt, W. R. and Logan Edwards, R. (1987). A clinical trial using danazol for the treatment of premenstrual tension. *Br. J. Obstet. Gynaecol.*, **94**, 30–4

16. Leather, A. T., Studd, J. W. W., Watson, N. R. and Holland, E. F. N. (1993). The prevention of bone loss in young women treated with GnRH analogues with 'add-back' estrogen therapy. *Obstet. Gynecol.*, **81**, 104–7

17. Magos, A. L., Brincat, M. and Studd, J. W. W. (1986). Treatment of the premenstrual syndrome by subcutaneous oestradiol implants and cyclical oral norethisterone: placebo controlled study. *Br. Med. J.*, **292**, 1629–33

18. Watson, N. R., Studd, J. W. W., Riddle, A. F., *et al.* (1988). Suppression of ovulation by transdermal oestradiol patches. *Br. Med. J.*, **297**, 900–1

19. Watson, N. R., Studd, J. W. W., Savvas, M., *et al.* (1989). Treatment of severe premenstrual syndrome with oestradiol patches and cyclical oral norethisterone. *Lancet*, **1**, 730–4

20. Smith, R. N. J., Studd, J. W. W., Zamblera, D., *et al.* (1995). A randomised comparison over 8 months of 100 µg and 200 µg twice weekly doses of transdermal oestradiol in the treatment of severe premenstrual syndrome. *Br. J. Obstet. Gynaecol.*, **102**, 475–84

21. Smith, R. N. J. and Studd, J. W. W. (1994). Oestrogen and depression in women. In Lobo, R. A., (ed.) *Treatment of the Postmenopausal Woman*, pp. 129–36. (New York: Raven Press)

22. Pitt, B. (1968). Atypical depression following childbirth. *Br. J. Psychol.*, **114**, 1325–35

23. Henderson, A. and Studd, J. W. W. (1995). Oestrogens and postnatal depression. *Contemp. Rev. Obstet. Gynaecol.*, **7**, 90–6

24. Wagner, H. R. and Davis, J. N. (1980). Decreased beta-adrenoceptor responses in female rat are eliminated by ovariectomy: correlation of 3H-dihydroalprenolol binding and catecholamine stimulated cAMP levels. *Brain Res.*, **201**, 235–9

25. Harris, B., Johns, S., Fung, H., *et al.* (1989). The hormonal environment of postnatal depression. *Br. J. Psychol.*, **154**, 660–7

26. Harris, B., Lovett, L., Newcombe, R., *et al.* (1994). Maternity blues and major endocrine changes: Cardiff puerperal mood and hormone study II. *Br. Med. J.*, **308**, 49–53

27. Alder, E. M. and Cox, J. L. (1983). Breast feeding and postnatal depression. *J. Psychosom. Res.*, **27**, 139–44

28. Henderson, A., Gregoire, A. J. P., Kumar, R. and Studd, J. W. W. (1991). The treatment of severe postnatal depression with oestradiol skin patches. *Lancet*, **1**, 816

29. Gregoire, A. J. P., Kumar, R., Everitt, B., Henderson, A. F. and Studd J. W. W. (1996). Transdermal oestrogen is an effective treatment for severe postnatal depression. *Lancet*, **347**, 930–3

30. Magos, A. L., Brewster, E., Studd, J. W. W. *et al.* (1986). The effects of norethisterone in postmenopausal women on oestrogen replacement therapy: a model for premenstrual syndrome. *Br. J. Obstet. Gynaecol.*, **93**, 1290–6

31. Studd, J. W. W. (1992). Complications of hormone replacement therapy in postmenopausal women. *J. R. Soc. Med.*, **85**, 376–8

32. Raudaskoski, T. H., Tomas, E. I., Paakkari, I. A., Kauppila, A. J. and Laatikainen, T. J. (1995). Serum lipids and lipoproteins in postmenopausal women receiving transdermal oestrogen in combination with a levonorgestrel intrauterine device. *Maturitas*, **22**, 47–53

33. Suhonen, S. P., Holmstrom, T., Allonen, H. O. *et al.* (1995). Intrauterine and sub-dermal progestin administration in postmenopausal hormone replacement therapy. *Fertil. Steril.*, **63**, 336–42

34. Panay, N., Studd, J. W. W., Thomas, A., *et al.* (1996). The levonorgestrel intrauterine system as progestogenic opposition for oestrogen replacement therapy. Presented at *Annual Meeting of the British Menopause Society*, Exeter, UK, July

35. Studd, J. W. W. and Panay, N. (1996). Chronic fatigue syndrome. *Lancet*, **348**, 1384

Hormones and libido

56

A. Graziottin

Introduction

Human sexuality depends on a complex interaction among cognitive processes, neurophysiological and biochemical mechanisms, and mood[1]. Difficulties in evaluating the relative weight of these different factors are rooted both in the complexity of the human sexual experience and in the fogginess of words and concepts that refer to it.

Sexual appetite, desire and drive, sexual impulse and interest: many psychosexual and behavioral terms are used to describe basic human mental states, and their biological counterparts, involved in the beginning of sexual behavior[2].

'Libido', a comprehensive yet elusive term, is a Latin word that means 'desire'. It was first used by Sigmund Freud[3] to indicate the energy corresponding to the psychic side of the sex drive. Carl Jung[4] defined libido in a wider sense, as the psychic energy present in all that is 'appetitus', a kind of 'desire towards', not necessarily sexual. In recent literature, libido is again considered in its main sexual appetitive meaning that motivates a person to obtain sex and focuses his/her attention on that goal. This subjective experience is accompanied by and partly consists of various physiological changes, many of which are in preparation for sexual behavior[1]. From the biologist's point of view, this sexual appetite can be further divided into 'proceptivity' and 'receptivity'. The former refers to the willingness to initiate and invite sexual contact or sexual stimulation; the latter describes the preparedness of an individual (usually the female) to accept the sexual advances of another[5–7]. 'I never initiate sex but I respond when my husband approaches me' could be considered as a disorder of proceptivity, with receptivity being intact. Conversely, 'I feel the need for sex but lose interest when my husband approaches me' could be seen as a disorder of receptivity but not of proceptivity[7]. How much of this difference is secondary to biological or psychosexual and relational dynamics is far from being understood. Psychological processes play an important role in human libido: we learn to feel sexual drive at certain times and in certain situations, and for some this learning component dominates their sexual behavior, as it happens in the weekend sex of many stable couples. In recent years, the realm of libido has grown to include a deeper understanding of its biological roots[5–7] both endocrine and neurochemical, of the motivational and relational components[8–11] and of its vulnerability to personal factors and external agents.

Human beings undertake sexual activity for two primary reasons: to procreate – 'reproductive sex', and to give themselves pleasure – 'recreational sex'[2]. An old study in Sweden showed that only about 2% of sexual activity was performed with the conscious purpose of procreation[12]. A third reason, that widely runs through our sexual behavior, includes a host of motives[13] with a common denominator: 'instrumental sex', as a means to obtain advantages and express motivations different from pleasure and/or procreation. This happens when coitus is used to confirm one's identity, to achieve sexual competence, to rebel against authority, to control and dominate, to degrade and hurt, to overcome loneliness or boredom, to show that sexual access was possible, to obtain favors such as a better position or role in life, to satisfy masochistic needs or even for livelihood[2]. It is therefore evident that, in our species, libido has several roots, with a complex interplay among biological, motivational and relational factors, that may all have both an inhibiting or enhancing role[1,2,5-15].

Libido and sexual arousal

Libido – or sexual desire – is considered different from sexual arousal. Sexual desire is an attitude toward an object, while sexual arousal is a state with specific feelings, usually attached to the genitals. There can be sexual arousal without sexual desire, and sexual desire without arousal. Human sexual arousal can be characterized by three components: a central arousal, a non-genital peripheral arousal and a genital arousal[2]. Sexual desire and sexual arousal should therefore be kept distinguished.

A useful working definition is that 'sexual desire is normally an activated, unsatisfied mental state of variable intensity, created by external – via the sensory modalities – or internal stimuli – fantasy, memory, cognition . . . – that induces a feeling of a need or want to partake of sexual activity (usually with the object of desire) to satisfy the need'[2]. This sexually activated mental state may be set against and influenced by the mood of the moment. In a depressed mood we are less likely to interpret experiences in pleasant sexual terms[1,8]. A mood of inertia, typical of depression, reduces the likelihood of initiating overt sexual action, in spite of favorable external conditions, i.e. the availability of a willing partner. The relationship between hormones and libido may therefore be studied through the effects sexual hormones have on this peculiarly activated mental state and on the different stimuli that enhance or inhibit it.

Biological roots of libido

Hormones and the brain sexualization

In men, consistent evidence shows that androgens are necessary though not sufficient

factors to maintain a satisfying human libido, the best data coming from placebo-controlled studies of androgen replacement in hypogonadal men[16,17]. Androgen replacement affects mood in men, but in a less striking and less predictable fashion than is the case with sexual desire[17]. Erections during sleep are androgen dependent. They are manifestations of the neurophysiological substrate of sexual desire[1]. They are impaired in androgen-deficient men and are improved with androgen replacement[18]. Responses to fantasy may be androgen dependent, at least in some individuals[1]. The close relationship between level of androgens and sexual interest was well demonstrated in a study of boys around the age of puberty, where Udry and colleagues found that level of testosterone was the best predictor of the intensity of the boys' sexual interest and sexual activity, more so than stage of pubertal development or other social variables[19].

In women, the evidence for hormone–behavior relationships is much less consistent and often contradictory[1,7-11]. Estrogens prime the central nervous system, acting as neurotrophic and psychotrophic factors during the female life[14,15]. They contribute to neuro- and psychoplasticity that can be considered the neuroscientific translation of the Jungian 'psychic energy' involved in libido. They also prime the sensory organs – including skin – that are the key receptors for external sexual stimuli. Sensory organs transmit the basic information that, mixed with emotional and affective messages, contributes to the structuring of core sex identity and self-image, so relevant to the personal perception of being an 'object of desire' and to the direction (homo- or heterosexual) of the libido itself[8,20].

The interplay between estrogens and the dopaminergic system is the key process in determining the appetitive side of sexual behavior[6,7,15], which can be further thrilled by the peak of androgens at ovulation. This link is supported by the correlation between testosterone levels and frequency of masturbation[21] or vaginal response to erotic stimuli in the laboratory[22], that is with aspects of autoeroticism rather than partner sex. This latter has many more relational variables that may explain the contradictory findings in research trying to correlate the human female cycle with variations in libido[1,8,15]. Some consensus is found in the peak just before or after menstruation[23], and it is not clear how such a pattern could be hormonally determined, as it is opposite to the mid-cycle peak of androgens that are assumed to be the 'libido' hormone in men as well as in women. The improvement of mood in the post-menstrual phase could partly account for this favorable increase[1]. Progesterone seems to have an inhibitory effect: its premenstrual fall could contribute to the perimenstrual increase in sexual desire, at least in those women not suffering from premenstrual syndrome (PMS). Bancroft[1] suggests that these seemingly discrepant findings may be explained by a different brain effect of androgens during early female development, either because of different target-organ sensitivities or different timing of hormonal effects (in contrast with males who are relatively overdetermined by androgens during early development). This difference could lead to two types of androgen effect on female behavior that conflict partly with one another, i.e. an increase in 'sexiness' and an increase in 'assertiveness' which might make it more difficult for a person to conform comfortably with the stereotyped role of the conventional woman. Money and Ehrhard[20] had similar findings suggesting that the sensitivity of female sexual behavior to hormonal variations may depend not only on the actual fluctuations and/or levels, but also on the quality of central and peripheral estrogenic and androgenic priming. These early differences could also contribute to the biological basis of the following huge variations: in libido profile in women; in female sexuality after the menopausal hormonal fall; in the different responsiveness to hormonal treatment as far as libido is concerned. In the conflict between nature and culture, psychosocial factors seem to be more important in women than in men. Udry and co-workers[24], in their parallel study

of girls around the age of puberty, found that whereas testosterone levels in the blood predicted their levels of sexual interest or libido, their sexual activity, particularly coitus, was much more dependent on other psychosocial factors, such as peer group influences. Currently, androgens look nevertheless the most interesting hormones for the sexuality of women[1,6,7,15,25]. They could have a three-fold action: increase susceptibility to psychosexual stimulation, contributing to the 'sexually activated mental state', typical of a good libido; increase sensitivity of the external genitalia; increase the intensity of sexual gratification[26].

A recent review of Rubinow and Schmidt[27] suggests that in men androgen dependence takes the form of a threshold level, below which libido and sexual function are impaired, and above which they are not, with no correlation between either the ideational or erectile components of sexual function and testosterone levels in the normal range. In women, both a positive correlation[28], and the absence of it[29], between testosterone levels and sexual interest and behavior have been observed. Similarly, androgen replacement therapy increases libido in women who are androgen deficient (e.g. after surgical menopause[30,31]), but it does not affect sexual arousal and behavior in naturally menopausal women[32]. In humans, then, androgens play an important role in sexual function but are not its sole determinant as their action is 'context dependent'[27]. Prolactin has an inhibiting effect on libido and on the sexual cascade of neurovegetative and vascular responses, via the same dopaminergic system, though it is difficult to distinguish between the direct effects of prolactin itself on behavior and the effects of the underlying dopaminergic activity[1,6,15].

Hypothyroidism may inhibit libido, whilst hyperthyroidism seems to increase most of the biopsychological rhythms, without a specific positive effect on sexual desire[8].

Oxytocin is a nonapeptide secreted by the posterior pituitary and in neurons located in the supraoptic and paraventricular hypothalamus. Estrogen and testosterone stimulate the synthesis of oxytocin-binding sites, and recent evidence links oxytocin with the facilitation of sexual desire in both men and women[15]. In human females, masturbation to orgasm increases plasma oxytocin levels. Oxytocin may form part of a neurochemical axis that participates in the desire to affiliate with a sexual partner, to engage in sexual contact, and to achieve sexual satiety after extended matings. It could therefore be a modulating factor in the interplay between affective and erotic components of sexual behavior[6,15].

Hormones, in their complex interplay, seem to control the intensity of libido and sexual behavior, rather than its direction[5].

The brain is therefore the very first sex organ, as it is the biological and emotional realm of libido. It is the brain that: associates sensory stimuli and emotions (just think how important the olfactory and touch memory for love, affection, emotions, nostalgia is); anticipates the pleasures of love; colours our erotic and emotional life with fantasies, dreams, erotic fantasms, sexual day-dreams; maintains the internal coherence of ego that is the basis of sex identity, self-image and self-esteem[15,20,33,34].

Sex hormones are potent neurotrophic and psychoplastic factors in general[14], and specifically for the 'sexually activated mental state', thrilled and maintained by fantasies, memories and lively imaginations produced within the brain. Gynecologists should therefore pay more attention to the subtle functional (and morphological!) modifications of the brain and of psychosexual behaviour, during long-lasting hypoestrogenic states, in girls with persistent functional amenorrhea[35,36] as well as in postmenopausal women[8,25,26,37]. They should provide optimal hormone replacement therapy (HRT) to minimize this subtle damage that may contribute to a deterioration of the libido, the 'vital energy' in the Jungian sense, that is the most exciting fuel for the joy of living and the quality of life.

Therefore, as far as libido is concerned, estrogens contribute to the central and peripheral scenario of femininity that can be thrilled and lit up by appropriate levels of androgens, whilst oxytocin may mediate the affective quality of bonding involved in libido itself.

Hormones and the sensory organs

Sensory organs are well-known windows for the environmental sexual stimuli. Less attention is paid to the effect of hormones on the function and morphology of sensory organs themselves, both as sexual targets and sexual determinants of libido. A growing body of evidence shows that sexual hormones have a specific effect on:

Smell Chemoreception is the ability to receive chemical messages from the environment. In complex pluricellular organisms, specialized structures are devoted to receiving chemical stimuli and transmitting them as nervous impulses to the central nervous system (CNS). Olfaction is the most refined sense based on chemoreception. The receptor organ, the olfactory epithelium, is made of specialized neurons localized in an exceptionally peripheral position. The olfactory epithelium is a perfect example of hormone-dependent neuro-plasticity. It is made up of three cell types: the olfactory neurons, whose axons form the 'fila olfactoria'; the supporting cells; the basal cells [38]. Castration elicits structural alterations of the olfactory epithelium, that can improve after administration of sexual hormones[38,39]. Moreover, in female rhesus monkeys, the olfactory epithelium presents some changes during the preovulatory phase of the ovarian cycle, that could explain the increased olfactory sensitivity occuring at the time of ovulation. In animals and in humans, the olfactory epithelium shows a different appearance and different behavior of the olfactory, supporting and basal cells in pre- and postpuberty[38]. A close relationship between olfaction and gonadal activity is clinically confirmed by the Kalman syndrome[40], characterized by anosmia, eunuchoidism and hypogonadotropic hypogonadism due to a functional deficiency of the gonadotropic hypothalamic centers. The luteinizing hormone releasing hormone

(LHRH) cells arise in the olfactory placode and migrate via the nervus terminalis, preoptic septal area, to the hypothalamus. The hypogonadism of the Kalman syndrome could therefore be due to a defective migration of the LHRH cells to the hypothalamus. These data can explain the close relationship between olfaction and endocrine and sexual activity[38].

The involutional morphologic changes of the olfactory epithelium in hypoestrogenic states (long lasting functional amenorrhea and menopause) could also contribute to the biologically determined reduction of libido, so often reported in these conditions.

These changes could also reduce the responsivity to pheromones, chemical messages emitted by animals and able to influence behavior and physiology of other animals of the same species[15,38,39]. The invisible cloud of pheromones that envelops humans as a second dress is a potent factor in subliminal attraction, that enhances libido and activates sexual arousal. In women, reduction in the production of chemically attractive substances that contribute to the 'scent of woman', typical of the fertile age, could be responsible both for the reduced self-perception as an object of sexual desire and for the reduced attractivity for the partner. Therefore, even in a microsomatic animal as the human being is, hormone-dependent olfactory modifications may be important biological and functional contributors to the variation of libido in different phases of female life. Moreover, the functional model of cyclical neuroplasticity in the olfactory epithelium may add further information to the role of estrogens as central neurotrophic factors.

Taste Gustative receptors can also perceive pheromones[38]. Taste is another key biological and emotional factor in the thrilling of sex drive, especially in women. Increase of salivary secretion during sexual desire and arousal, and the pleasure for the taste of skin and of kisses, is a strong predictive factor of the quality of the sexual liking. Functional mouth dryness, more frequent in hypoestrogenic states, could be another understudied and underevaluated

factor in the biological modulation of libido.

Touch A highly sexually communicative skin depends on a happy mixture of good genes, optimal endocrine impregnation and good pheromone production and reception, plus excellent brain activity in the processing of peripheral information from the sensory organ enhanced with internal sexual and emotional stimuli: love, beyond libido, is the strongest attachment factor in the couple bonding through the skin touch[33,41]. Oxytocin seems to be a key neurochemical factor, enhanced in response to a desired skin touch, and a potent brain mediator of attachment needs and dynamics[15]. Touch, taste and smell contribute to the 'cenesthetic channel', that is considered the most important sensory contributor of libido in women. The sensory and emotional side of libido is deeply rooted in the quality of cenesthetic and loving bonding between mother and child, since early infancy[33].

Hearing This is a variable, usually strong attractive sense for women, mostly for the emotional vibration of the voice (the so-called 'feeling tone'), beyond the emotional, loving or sexual content of the message. Hormonal variations of hearing function are far from being clear, even if some interesting new findings begin to appear in the literature[42].

Vision This is the most potent sexual sense in men, but less in women. Estrogenic responsivity of ophthalmic structures is now well recognized for the anterior part of the eye (conjunctiva, lacrimal glands). According to Metka and colleagues[43], 35% of postmenopausal women complain of ophthalmic disturbances secondary to the lack of estrogens. Most of them improve with HRT. Whether variations of eye well-being contribute or not to modulation of libido is far from being defined. It is possible that all these subtle changes in sensory organ function and morphology could contribute to the deterioration of libido with age, and to the accelerated reduction it shows in many women in early postmenopausal years.

Hormones and genital responsivity

Physical pleasure enhances libido. Disappointment and frustration for a poor genital response inhibits it. Quality of peripheral, as well as central estrogenic and androgenic priming may be important in conditioning the quality of sexual response. Bailey[44] suggests an almost linear correlation between clitoral sensitivity, the ability to be 'turned on' and the orgasmic capacity. Riley and co-workers[26] found a correlation between low libido and poorly developed external genitalia, particularly the clitoris, which is often hypoplastic. These women can experience sexual arousal and can attain orgasm only with difficulty: this repeated failure may lead to a persistent block in sexual desire. Treatment with androgens is helpful in such patients, probably because of its effects on the androgenic receptivity of the clitoris.

Moreover, estrogens are important as 'permitting' factors that 'translate' libido and the neurovegetative pathway of neurotransmitters in the lubrication of the vagina[34].

Menopausal changes in libido

Lack of estrogens deprives the brain and all the female body of the natural lymph that contributes to the perception of female sex identity, of a satisfying sexual function and to the sensuality and seductivity that improve the quality of sexual relationships, causing a progressive loss of libido and a crisis of the self-perception as an object of desire[8,25,45].

Moreover, as previously mentioned, the lack of estrogens deprives sweat and sebaceous glands of the stimulus to produce the peculiar chemical secretion (pheromones) responsible for the 'scent of woman', so critical in sexual attraction[38,39]. Estrogens are the permitting factors for the action of vasoactive intestinal peptide (VIP), the key neurotransmitter for the endothelial and vasal changes that lead to vaginal lubrication[34]. That is why the absence of estrogens causes vaginal dryness and pain (dyspareunia) that can further inhibit libido through a negative feedback mechanism. Obviously, enhancing and inhibiting factors (medicines, drugs, alcohol[6,8,45]), plus other health problems can modify the biological impact of menopause on libido.

Motivational–affective and relational factors, implications and quality of couple relationship, and partner's attitude and problems, may further modulate the intensity and direction of libido[34,45] and contribute to the contradictory findings in the variability of libido in perimenopausal years[46].

Conclusion

Problems of libido are increasingly reported during the gynecological consultation, more frequently if the clinician is willing to listen and to look at the patient as a person who is emotionally suffering. A basic sexological training should become part of routine gynecological training, to enable physicians properly to diagnose the biological conditions they could adequately treat, and to encourage the patient to consult a psychosexologist if the problem reported during the consultation seems to be more rooted upon intrapsychic, motivational or relational bases.

Basic research is urgently needed to understand better and more the biological basis of human libido.

References

1. Bancroft, J. (1988). Sexual desire and the brain. *Sex. Marital Ther.*, **3**, 11–27
2. Levin, R. J. (1994). Human male sexuality: appetite and arousal, desire and drive. In Legg, C. and Boott, D. (eds.) Human Appetite: Neural and Behavioural Bases, pp. 127–64. (New York and London: Oxford University Press)
3. Freud, S. (1877). On sexuality. In Richards, A.

(ed.) *Three essays on the Theory of Sexuality and Other Works*. (London: The Pelican Freud Library, Vol. 7, Penguin Books, 1977)

4. Jung, C. G. (1938). In McGuire, W. and Hull, R. F. C. (eds.) *C. G. Jung Speaking*. (Princeton, NJ: Princeton University Press, 1977)

5. Levine, S. B. (1984). An essay on the nature of sexual desire. *J. Sex. Marital Ther.*, **10**, 83–96

6. Bloom, F. E. and Kupfer, D. (1995). *Psychopharmacology*. (New York: Raven Press)

7. Kaplan, H. S. (1979). *Disorders of Sexual Desire*. (New York: Simon and Schuster)

8. Graziottin, A. and Defilippi, A. (1995). Disfunzioni del desiderio sessuale. In Marandola P. (ed.) *Andrologia e Sessuologia Clinica*, pp. 229–37. (Pavia: La Goliardica)

9. Macphee, D. C., Johnson, S. M. and Van der Veer, M. M. (1995). Low sexual desire in women: the effect of marital therapy. *J. Sex. Marital Ther.*, **21**, 159–82

10. Talmadge, L. D. and Talmadge, W. C. (1986). Relational sexuality: an understanding of low sexual desire. *J. Sex. Marital Ther.*, **12**, 1–8

11. Beck Gayle, J., Bozman, A. W. and Qualtrough, T. (1991). The experience of sexual desire: psychological correlates in a college sample. *J. Sex. Res.*, **28**, 443–56

12. Linner, B. (1972). *Sex and Society in Sweden*. (New York: Harper and Row)

13. Neubeck, G. (1974). The myriad of motives for sex. In Gross, L. (ed.) *Sexual Behaviour Current Issues*, pp. 89–97. (Flushing: Spectrum)

14. Birge, S. J. (1994). The role of estrogen deficiency in the aging of the central nervous system. In Lobo, R. A. (ed.) *Treatment of Postmenopausal Women: Basic and Clinical Aspects*, pp. 153–7. (New York: Raven Press)

15. Pfaus, J. G. and Everitt, B. J. (1995). The psychopharmacology of sexual behaviour. In Bloom, F. E. and Kupfer, D. (eds.) *Psychopharmacology*, chap. 65, pp. 743–58. (New York: Raven Press)

16. Davidson, J. M., Camargo, C. A. and Smith, E. R. (1979). Effects of androgens on sexual behaviour of hypogonadal men. *J. Clin. Endocrinol. Metab.*, **48**, 955–8

17. Stakkebaek, N. E., Bancroft, J., Davidson, D. W. and Warner, P. (1981). Androgen replacement with oral testosterone undecanoate in hypogonadal men: a double blind controlled study. *Clin. Endocrinol.*, **14**, 49–67

18. O'Carroll, R., Shapiro, C. and Bancroft, J. (1985). Androgens, behaviour and nocturnal erections in hypogonadal men: the effect of varying the replacement dose. *Clin. Endocrinol.*, **23**, 527–38

19. Udry, J. R., Billy, J. O. G., Morris, N. M., Groff, T. R. and Raj M. H. (1985). Serum androgenic hormones motivate sexual behaviour in adolescent boys. *Fertil. Steril.*, **43**, 90–4

20. Money, J. and Ehrhardt, A. (1972). *Man and Woman, Boy and Girl*. (Baltimore: The John Hopkins University Press)

21. Bancroft, J., Sanders, D., Davidson, D. W. and Warner, P. (1983). Mood, sexuality, hormones and the menstrual cycle. III: Sexuality and the role of androgens. *Psychosom. Med.*, **45**, 509–16

22. Schreiner-Engel, P., Schiavi, R.C., Smith, H. and White, D. (1982). Plasma testosterone and female sexual behaviour. In Hoch, Z. and Lief, H. H. (eds.) *Proceedings of the 5th World Congress of Sexology*, pp. 80–3. (Amsterdam: Excerpta Medica)

23. Bancroft, J. (1988). *Human Sexuality and its Problems*, 2nd edn. (Edinburgh: Churchill Livingstone)

24. Udry, J. R., Talbert, L. M. and Morris, N. M. (1986). Biosocial foundations for adolescent female sexuality. *Demography*, **23**, 217–29

25. Sands, R. and Studd, J. (1995). Exogenous androgens in postmenopausal women. *Am. J. Med.*, **98**, 76–9

26. Riley, A., Riley, E. J. and Brown, P. (1986). Biological aspects of sexual desire in women. *Sex. Marital Ther.*, **1**, 35–42

27. Rubinow, D. R. and Schmidt, P. J. (1996). Androgens, brain and behaviour. *Am. J. Psychiatry*, **153**, 974–84

28. Alexander, G. M. and Sherwin, B. B. (1993). Sex steroids, sexual behaviour and selection attention for erotic stimuli in women using oral contraceptives. *Psychoneuroendocrinology*, **18**, 91–102

29. Morris, N. J., Udry, J. R., Kahn Dawood, F. and Dawood, M. Y. (1987). Marital sex frequency and midcycle female testosterone. *Arch. Sex. Behav.*, **16**, 27–37

30. Sherwin, B. B. and Gelfand, M. M. (1987). The role of androgen in the maintenance of sexual functioning in oophorectomized women. *Psychosom. Med.*, **49**, 397–409

31. Sherwin, B. B., Gelfand, M. M. and Brender, W. (1985). Androgens enhance sexual motivation in females: a prospective, crossover study of sex steroid administration in surgical menopause. *Psychosom. Med.*, **47**, 339–51

32. Myers, L. S., Dixen, J., Morrissette, D., Carmichael, M. and Davidson, J. M. (1990). Effects of estrogen, androgen and progestin on sexual psychophysiology and behaviour in postmenopausal women. *J. Clin. Endocrinol. Metab.*, **70**, 1124–31

33. Bowlby, J. (1988). *A Secure Base*. (London: Rutledge)

34. Levin, R. J. (1992). The mechanisms of human female sexual arousal. *Ann. Rev. Sex. Res.*, **3**, 1–48

35. Schmidt, H. (1995). Anorexia nervosa and psychosexual development. *Psychol. Med.*, **25**, 112–24

36. Treasure, J. L. (1995). Eating disorders. In Studd, J. (ed.) *Handbook of the Royal College of Obstetricians and Gynaecologists.* (London: Royal College)

37. Pearlstein, T. B. (1995). Hormones and depression: what are the facts about premenstrual syndrome, menopause and hormone replacement therapy? *Am. J. Obstet. Gynecol.*, **173**, 646–53

38. Balboni, G. C., Gheri, G., Gheri Bryk, S., Barni, T., Arimondi, C. and Vannelli, G. B. (1991). New trends in olfaction. In *Proceedings of the 45th Congress of the Italian Society of Anatomy*, pp. 14–46. (Florence: Mozzon)

39. Arimondi, C., Vannelli, G. B. and Balboni, G. C. (1993). Importance of olfaction in sexual life: morpho-functional and psychological studies in man. *Biomed. Res. (India)*, **4**, 43–52

40. Kalman, F., Schoenfeld, W. A. and Barrera, S. E. (1944). The genetic aspects of primary eunuchoidism. *Am. J. Ment. Defic.*, **48**, 203–36

41. Shaver, P. R. and Hazan, C. (1995). Adult romantic attachment process: theory and evidence. In Perlman, D. and Jones, W. (eds.) *Advances in Personal Relationship Outcomes*, Vol. IV, pp. 29–70. (London: J. Kingsey Publishing)

42. Leibenluft, E. (1996). Sex is complex. *Am. J. Psychiatry*, **153**, 969–76

43. Metka, M., Enzelsberger, H., Knogler, W., Schurz, B. and Aichmair, H. (1991). Ophthalmic complaint as a climacteric symptom. *Maturitas*, **14**, 3–8

44. Bailey, H. R., (1973). Studies in depression. II. Treatment of the depressed frigid woman. *Med. J. Aust.*, **1**, 834–7

45. Graziottin, A. (1996). Libido. In Studd, J. J. W. (ed.) *Progress in Obstetrics and Gynecology*, in press

46. Myers, L. S. (1995). Methodological review and meta-analysis of sexuality and menopause research. *Neurosci. Biobehav. Rev.*, **19**, 331–41

14

Hormones and the cardiovascular system

Mechanisms of action for estrogen in cardioprotection

57

G. I. Gorodeski

Introduction

Cardiovascular disease, and in particular cardiac ischemia, is the leading cause of morbidity and mortality in women[1]. Estrogen deficiency after the menopause is the single most important risk factor for cardiovascular disease in women[2]. Estrogen replacement therapy to postmenopausal women, on the other hand, significantly decreases the relative risks of cardiovascular disease and coronary artery heart disease, suggesting that estrogens directly affect the heart and confer a certain degree of protection[3]. Recent epidemiological studies have supported this hypothesis, and as a result, research has been focused on cellular and molecular mechanisms related to estrogen action on target organs including the heart and its vasculature. The objective of this review is to outline the existing data, and to emphasize their importance for the understanding of cardiac function *vis-à-vis* estrogen deficiency, and the role of estrogen replacement in cardio-protection.

Cellular and molecular mechanisms of action of estrogen

Estrogens regulate target cells directly and indirectly (Table 1). Direct effects include gene regulation, modulation of protein expression, modulation of ion-transport mechanisms and regulation of plasma membrane-related signal transduction mechanisms. Estrogens can also regulate cell homeostasis by affecting oxidation reactions extra- and intracellularly. The latter reactions are considered indirect by virtue of the nature of interaction of the hydroxy-phenolic ring of estrogen with free radicals, thus modulating exposure of the plasma membrane and membranes of intracellular structures to potential oxidative reactions.

The classical model of estrogen action is described by binding and activating a nuclear receptor[4]. Binding of estradiol in the nuclei of rat atrial myocytes has already been described two decades ago[5], and estrogen receptors were assayed in coronary arteries and cardiac tissues of various species, including women[6–15]. A detailed review of the physiology of coronary and cardiac estrogen receptors is beyond the scope of this paper, but these data are similar to those described for other estrogen-responsive tissues. Activation of the nuclear estrogen receptor triggers transcriptional regulation of protein synthesis within 10–60 min[4]. In most estrogen-responsive tissues, estrogen up-regulates its own receptors as well as receptors

Table 1 Estrogen action on target cells: cellular and molecular mechanisms

Modulation of protein synthesis – gene regulation via the nuclear receptor
Modulation of protein synthesis – post-transcriptional regulation
Modulation of ion-transport mechanisms – direct interaction with membrane transporters
Activation of (putative) plasma membrane receptors
Extra/intracellular effects dependent on the OH-phenolic ring

for progestins, and the effect is regulated by progesterone[12,17-19]. Similar effects were previously described in cardiovascular tissues of monkeys[20].

Another mechanism of regulation of protein expression is by modulation of post-transcriptional events[21]. While data in the heart are lacking, a number of investigators proposed such a mechanism of action for estrogen in the cardiovascular system, in view of the rapid effects of estrogen on the heart[22].

An important mode of regulation of cell activity is by activating membrane mechanisms which affect signal transduction. Estrogen has been shown by a number of investigators to interact with calcium influx mechanisms and to inhibit calcium entry into the cells[23-26]. These effects are most important for regulating excitable membranes in muscle cells and neurons, since acute modulation of electrical (and contractile) phenomena depends on rapid changes in intracellular calcium. However, other cell types can also be regulated by similar mechanisms, e.g. endothelial cells, which participate in the regulation of contraction of adjacent smooth muscle cells[26].

In contrast to transcription regulation, estrogen regulation of calcium influx occurs at estrogen concentrations which are 10^2–10^4-fold larger than the plasma levels of free estradiol in women *in vivo*, and a concern was raised that the findings *in vitro* as described by a number of investigators may not have physiological significance. It is possible, however, that estrogens, which are lipophilic molecules, accumulate in cytoplasmic domains of the plasma membrane at high concentrations that are sufficient to inhibit calcium entry mechanisms.

As a result of acute stimulation by estrogens, cytosolic calcium increases were reported in granulosa cells[27]. Effects were described at estrogen nanomolar concentrations, which are in the physiological range. The effects on cytosolic calcium resembled those produced by secretagogues which act on surface receptors and activate calcium release from intracellular stores, followed usually by augmented calcium influx via calcium channels. The significance of this mode of cell-function regulation by estrogen is at present unclear, because no membrane receptors for estrogen have been described.

All hydroxyphenolic compounds, including estrogens, have antioxidant properties *in vitro*[28]. Since free radicals are continually generated by living cells, it was suggested that estrogens indirectly may affect cells *in vivo* by interacting with free radicals. The antioxidant effects of estrogens depend on the type of estrogen, and on its concentrations. Based on a number of studies[28-35], the order of potency is diethyl-stilbestrol (DES) > 17α-ethinylestradiol > 2-hydroxyestradiol (catecholestrogens) > 17β-estradiol mestranol, equillins, estrone. Interestingly, 17α-estradiol, commonly regarded as a non-active estrogen, also has antioxidant properties by virtue of the hydroxyphenolic ring. Also of importance are the findings that estrogens exert antioxidant effects *in vitro* only at micromolar concentrations. However, *in vivo* 17β-estradiol may be an antioxidant at physiological (nanomolar) concentrations[36].

In conclusion, estrogens may affect cardiac cells via a number of potential mechanisms. Depending on the type of interaction between estrogens and the cell, effects can be immediate or delayed, and may involve acute activation of signal transduction mechanisms versus the more delayed protein synthesis. This spectrum of mechanisms may explain the diverse effects which are related to the heart. In addition, the antioxidant effects of estrogens may have a role in protecting the heart of women from repeated ischemia (see below).

Cardiac effects of estrogen in females

The effects of estrogen can be classified into those related to the coronary vasculature, and those related to cardiac myocytes (Table 2).

Effects on the coronary vasculature

These effects can be subclassified into effects on angiogenesis, inhibition of atherogenesis,

Table 2 Cardiac effects of estrogen in females

Effects on coronary vasculature
    angiogenesis
    inhibition of atherogenesis
    vasorelaxation
    modulation of endothelial tight junctions

Effects on cardiac myocytes
    metabolism
    contractility
    rate

---

vasodilator effects and modulation of endothelial tight junctions. Most of these effects are not specific to the coronary arteries, and have been also described in other vascular beds. However, due to the fact that coronary artery heart disease contributes significantly to morbidity and mortality in women, attention has been focused on the effects of sex hormones on female coronary vasculature.

Estrogens promote angiogenesis In a recent study, Schnaper and colleagues[37] found that endothelial cells invaded into matrigel implants placed under the skin of 9-week-old mice. Ovariectomy reduced invasion of the implants by endothelial cells by about 30% compared with controls. Estrogen promoted endothelial cell invasion to control levels, but the effect was blocked by the specific inhibitor of the estrogen receptor ICI 182,780. In contrast to endothelial cells, estrogen inhibits vascular smooth muscle growth. Kolodgic and co-workers[8] found that vascular smooth muscle cells' migration *in vitro* is inhibited by estrogen, and the effect does not depend on the active smooth muscle cell activator, e.g. fibronectine, platelet derived growth factor (PDGF)-BB, or insulin-like growth factor (IGF)-I. Estrogens also suppress collagen secretion and assembly[39,40]. Stimulation of endothelial cell growth coupled with controlled growth of smooth muscle cells and deposition of extracellular matrix are essential for coordinated angiogenesis.

Estrogens attenuate coronary atherosclerosis In addition to the systemic effects of estrogens which favorably affect the risk of atherosclerosis (for a review see references 1 and 2), estrogens mediate vasculoprotective mechanisms at the level of the coronary artery, e.g. attenuation of low-density lipoprotein (LDL) oxidation and influx of esterified cholesterol into the vessel wall, and enhancement of efflux of cholesterol from the vessel wall[41-46]. The net result of these effects is preservation of the endothelium, and attenuation of atherogenesis and coronary stenosis. Interesting evidence for the vasculo-preservative effects of estrogen were presented by a series of studies by Foegh and associates in relation to inhibition of neointimal hyperplasia[47,48]. It was shown that estrogen attenuates vascular stenosis by about 60%. The molecular mechanisms by which estrogens prevent coronary stenosis are not entirely understood. It was suggested that estrogens modulate expression of adhesion molecules[49-51] but more studies are needed to clarify these mechanisms.

Estrogens are vasodilators, and modulate reactivity of coronary arteries The vasodilator effects of estrogen occur at all levels of the coronary arterial tree and involve large proximal epicardial vessels[52-54] as well as the microscopic arterioles which determine the coronary vascular resistance[55,56]. Treatment of females (including women) with estrogens produces relaxation of the coronary arteries, increases the diameter of the vessels and therefore decreases the vascular resistance: the net effect is an increase in coronary flow.

Estrogens induce coronary vasodilation by up-regulating endothelium-dependent vasodilator mechanisms, e.g. nitric oxide synthase(s), prostacycline production and possibly potassium-related hyperpolarizing mechanisms[56,58-63]. All have been shown to promote coronary vasodilatation either directly (prostacyclines) or indirectly, by acting as distal messengers (nitric oxide) to stimuli originating from the endothelium (acetylcholine)[64-66]. In the normal heart of the female rabbit, 17β-estradiol reduces coronary vascular resistance by about 50% via a direct effect on the resistance vessels[56]. The decrease in coronary vascular resistance is mainly due to up-regulation of nitric oxide synthase mechanism(s), and it can be blocked by inhibiting nitric oxide production with specific nitric oxide synthase inhibitors.

Of clinical importance are the findings in animal models and in women that estrogens can promote vasorelaxation of atherosclerotic coronary vessels. Hypercholesterolemia and arteriosclerosis have a deleterious effect on the endothelium. As a result, normal vasodilator regulatory mechanisms are impaired. An example is the responsiveness to acetylcholine: under normal conditions, acetylcholine causes coronary vasorelaxation, in a process which is mediated via muscarinic endothelial receptors. In tissues with damaged endothelium (e.g. arteriosclerosis), acetylcholine is believed to bypass the endothelium and gain direct access to the underlying smooth muscle cells, and cause contraction and vasoconstriction[66-72]. In animals with various degrees of diet-induced coronary arteriosclerosis, or in women with abnormal coronary arteries, short pretreatment with estrogen (e.g. direct infusion into the coronary artery) reverses the vasoconstrictive effect of acetylcholine[73]. suggesting that estrogens protect endothelium-dependent coronary vasodilator mechanisms.

Recently, we have found that the effect is not entirely mediated by the endothelium, since direct administration of trypsin to the coronary vasculature (to damage the endothelium) did not abolish the beneficial effects of estrogen on coronary flow[74]. Our results support previous studies carried out on isolated coronary arteries[75]. Based on these results we have proposed that in the rabbit, the estrogen-sparing effect of coronary vasodilatation in females with damaged endothelium is up-regulation of nitric oxide synthase mechanism(s) in extraendothelial tissues. Nitric oxide is a critical step in the signal transduction leading to coronary vasorelaxation. Increased release of nitric oxide from extraendothelial sites may therefore amplify a signal which

originates even from a damaged endothelium, and result in net vasodilation.

An additional mechanism by which estrogens induce coronary vasodilatation is by down-regulating endothelium-dependent vasoconstrictive mechanisms, notably the endothelins and their receptors[76].

Estrogens also modulate autonomic regulation of the coronary vasculature, by sensitizing coronary arteries to the effects of β-adrenergic stimuli. Despite species differences, most (though not all) authors agree that estrogens promote release of β-adrenergic transmitters from nerve endings in the heart, and up-regulate β-adrenergic receptors in the coronary vasculature, resulting in vasodilatation[77,78].

A fourth mechanism by which estrogens produce coronary vasorelaxation is indirect modulation of the coronary microcirculation by affecting platelet activity. Coronary hemodynamics depend on the interaction between intraluminal factors and the vessel wall. Important for coronary vascular physiology are the effects of platelets on vascular reactivity. Platelets secrete potent vasoconstrictors, e.g. serotonin and thromboxane, as well as other endothelial secretagogues and mediators of inflammatory reaction. Under normal conditions, the effect of platelets on the microvasculature is small. However, when flow in the vascular tree is impaired, or in the presence of arteriosclerosis, platelets may aggregate and adhere to loci of injury or stenosis, secrete vasoconstrictors and aggravate the vasospasms. Bar and colleagues[79] have recently reported that estrogen replacement therapy exerts beneficial effects on platelet function as related to their vascular effects. Estrogen treatment to postmenopausal women confers decreased aggregability of platelets *in vitro*, and decreased adenosine triphosphate (ATP) release. These conditions are usually associated with decreased production of platelet-derived vasoconstrictors.

A fifth mechanism by which estrogens may promote coronary vasodilation is direct inhibition of smooth muscle cell contraction.

Such a mechanism is proposed by recent studies which demonstrate inhibition of calcium influx in vascular smooth muscle cells which are exposed to estrogen *in vitro*[23-26,80]. Since increases in cytosolic calcium mediate smooth muscle cell contractions, these results suggest that estrogens may directly relax the vessel. As was previously mentioned, one of the difficulties in the interpretation of these data is due to the fact that the concentrations *in vitro* required to elicit the response were significantly higher than the physiological levels of estrogens. More studies are necessary to clarify our understanding of this mechanism of estrogen action.

From the above, it is evident that estrogens play an important role in conferring vasorelaxation of the coronary vasculature in females. These data also suggest that estrogen deficiency such as that occurring after the menopause may promote coronary vasoconstriction, and that the effect may occur even in normal (i.e. atherosclerosis-free) vessels. Support for this hypothesis are clinical observations in estrogen-deficient post-menopausal women who have a higher incidence than men of non-stenotic angina. This syndrome, referred to as Syndrome-X[81,82] is believed to be the result of impaired coronary vasodilatation caused by estrogen deficiency. Replacement of estrogen alleviated some of the ensuing cardiac ischemia.

An interesting insight into the effects of estrogen deficiency or non-stenotic cardiac ischemia was provided by our results in female rabbits. We showed that *in vivo*, the amount of estrogen necessary to confer coronary vasodilatation is low, and that maximal effects of estrogen occur already at concentrations which are at the lower range of normalcy[56]. Based on these observations we concluded that estrogen deficiency after the menopause may be an aggravating factor for increased coronary vascular resistance even in women with normal (atherosclerosis free) arteries.

Previous studies in extracardiac tissues, e.g. the uterine artery vascular bed, revealed important kinetic information regarding the effects of estrogen on vascular resistance.

Studies by Killam and colleagues[83], and by Van Buren and co-workers[84] indicated that estrogen decreases vascular resistance within 30–60 min after direct administration of the hormone into the vascular bed, and it can be blocked by protein-synthesis inhibitors, or by blocking synthesis of nitric oxide. Similar results were obtained by Reis and associates[73] in women. Lack of an immediate effect of estrogen (10–20 min) suggests that the effect of estrogen on coronary vasodilatation is not only the result of acute modulation of signal transduction, but rather involves protein synthesis/modification by estrogens. This conclusion is also supported by our findings[85] and those of other investigators[83], that upon estrogen withdrawal the estrogen-induced increase in vascular (and coronary) flow dissipates slowly, rather than abruptly.

Estrogens stabilize endothelial tight junctions A novel mechanism of estrogen regulation of vascular function in females is the effect of estrogen on endothelial tight junctions. Movement of fluids and solutes across the vessel from the intraluminal compartment into the tissue is limited by the tight junctions. Tight junctions are intercellular communications between neighboring epithelial cells or endothelial cells which engulf the cells, thus creating a complex pattern of belt-like formation around the cells. The tight junctions are composed of a complex array of intercommunicating proteins, and the extracellular chains of these proteins are negatively charged[86,87]. In a recent study, Cho and colleagues reported that estrogen does not significantly modulate the transendothelial electrical resistance (an indicator of the intercellular permeability) across HUVEC cultures. In contrast, estrogen significantly attenuated the dilution potential across the cultures, generated by lowering NaCl concentrations in the luminal side from 130 mmol/l to 10 mmol/l. When expressed in terms of the relative mobilities of Cl^- versus Na^+, estrogen treatment reduced the ratio of uCl/uNa significantly from 1.34 to 1.31. Since cation selectivity is a property conferred by the tight

Table 3 Estrogen regulation of cardiac myocytes in females

Metabolism
  biochemistry (lysosomal enzymes)
  energy (glycogen)
  respiration (creatine kinase)
  signal transduction (nitric oxide mechanisms)

Contractility: enhanced inotropy
  myosin- and actin-activated (adenosine triphosphatase) activity
  myosin isoforms

Rate: estrogens induce bradycardia
  up-regulation of β-adrenergic and cholinergic receptors/activity in cardiac tissues
  inhibition of calcium influx

junctions[89], the results indicated for the first time that estrogen increases cation selectivity of endothelial tight junctions without significantly affecting baseline permeability. The conclusion was that estrogens increase stability of endothelial tight junctions, and therefore may protect tissues (e.g. cardiac myocytes) from sudden osmolar changes, such as those occurring during reperfusion (see below).

Estrogen regulation of cardiac myocytes in females

In addition to the regulation of coronary vasculature, estrogens also directly regulate cardiac myocytes in females (Table 3). The effects of estrogen can be classified into those on metabolism and signal transduction, contractility and heart rate. Most of these data were obtained via experiments done on animal models or on cells in culture. For obvious reasons our understanding of these mechanisms in women are limited.

Effects on metabolism and signal transduction Gallagher and Sloan[90] have shown in female rats that ovariectomy, as well as estrogen replacement, modulates activities of lysosomal enzymes in cardiac cells. For instance, ovariectomy increased the activities of Cathepsin B and acid phosphatase, and decreased the activity of Cathepsin D. Estrogen treatment decreased the activity of Cathepsin

B and restored activities of Cathepsin D and acid phosphatase. Lysosomes are membranous bags of hydrolytic enzymes used for controlled intracellular digestion of macromolecules. Since lysosomal enzymes are important for cell homeostasis, such changes may alter metabolic activity of cardiac cells. At present the significance of the specific changes in cardiac-cell lysosomal enzymes activities is unclear.

Estrogens increase glucagon content in hearts of female mice[91]. Glucagon is an intracellular source for glucose, which is an important energy source for cardiac myocytes. Estrogens may therefore affect the bioenergetic condition of cardiac cells by regulating intracellular carbohydrate storage.

Relatively little is known about the effects of estrogen on respiration. Indirect evidence suggests that estrogens may regulate cardiac myocyte respiration via effects on creatine kinase. The creatine kinases catalyze transfer of high-energy phosphates from ATP to creatine, and shuttle energy-rich molecules across the mitochondria in a very well-regulated manner. The B-type cytosolic creatine kinase isoenzyme, as well as the mitochondrial creatine kinase (MtCK), both expressed in heart tissues, are estrogen-regulated proteins[92].

The nitric oxide pathway is an important signal transduction mechanism in excitable cells. Cardiac cells express an abundance of nitric oxide synthase(s), which stimulate the formation of nitric oxide from L-arginine and oxygen[65]. In the heart, estrogens are potent modulators of nitric-oxide synthase mechanisms. In hearts of guinea-pigs, Weiner and associates[93] found that estrogens increase the expression of calcium-dependent nitric oxide synthase (eNOS) two-fold. Previous studies in other tissues revealed that other agents e.g. cytokines, and conditions e.g. infection or ischemia, may increase expression of calcium-independent nitric oxide synthase (iNOS) significantly[65,66,94]. Although nitric oxide is important for normal cardiovascular function, abnormal release of nitric oxide may lead to coronary and cardiac cell dysfunction (see below).

Estrogens enhance inotropy A number of investigations have previously reported augmented cardiac function in pregnancy, and in postmenopausal women treated with estrogens[95–99]. These data were difficult to interpret in terms of the direct effects of estrogens on cardiac cells, because estrogens also modulate other cardiovascular functions such as heart rate, blood pressure and systemic vascular resistance, and affect preload and afterload[96].

Scheuer and co-workers[100] studied the effects of estrogen on heart function in female rats and confirmed that ovariectomy decreased stroke work by 20% while estrogen replacement restored the effect. Interestingly, similar trends were found related to the activity of Ca-myosin ATPase, and actin-activated Mg-myosin ATPase. Biochemical analysis of cardiac myosin isoenzymes showed that ovariectomy reduces myosin isoenzyme type V_1, and increases types V_2 and V_3. In contrast, estrogen had opposite effects and tended to restore the biochemical profile of V_1, V_2 and V_3 myosin isoenzymes to control values. Since V_1 is associated with enhanced cardiac contractility, the estrogen-related changes in cardiac contractility in guinea-pigs may be the result of direct modulation by estrogen of the cardiac myocyte myosin apparatus.

A less well-understood phenomenon is the regulation of cardiac cell contractility by nitric oxide. Michel and Smith[101] have shown in isolated rat contracting ventricular myocytes that the inotropic effect of isoproterenol (β-adrenergic agent) was augmented by the inhibition of nitric oxide synthase, suggesting that nitric oxide has a role as mediator of negative inotropy. This effect may be similar to the effect of nitric oxide in the vascular system. Whether the effect of nitric oxide in cardiac cells is also mediated by cyclic guanylate monophosphate (cGMP) (as in vascular beds) remains to be determined.

Estrogens induce bradycardia Previous studies suggested that autonomic regulation of the cardiovascular system in females is different from that in men[102,103]. Johansson and Hjalmarson[104] reported that women are more sensitive than men to β-adrenergic stimulation of tachycardia. Other investigators reported that estrogens can modulate the responsiveness of the cardiovascular system in females. Williams and associates[105] found that estrogen sensitizes female monkeys to the effects of α- and β-adrenergic drugs, as was evident by alternation of increases in systemic vascular resistance and augmentation of increases in cardiac index. These and other studies[106,107] indicate that the gender-related differences in cardiovascular reactivity may be regulated by the sex hormones and mediated by changes in nitric oxide activity. The mechanisms of the gender-related differences are complex, and not entirely clear. A number of experiments showed that sex hormones modulate autonomic regulation of the peripheral vasculature. However, in addition to the autonomic regulation at peripheral sites, sex hormones also have direct effects on the coronary vasculature and cardiac cells.

Earlier studies in women and in animal models treated with estrogens reported that in addition to increased cardiac contractility, there was slowing of the heart rate. A more recent, well-controlled study in unanesthetized female rats showed significant estrogen-related decrease in heart rate which was unrelated to activity or sleep[108]. For methodological reasons these studies could not discern between direct effects of estrogen on the heart and secondary effects due to increased cardiac performance. In our studies in isolated perfused beating hearts of female rabbits, prior treatment with estrogen did not have a significant effect on the heart rate[56]. In contrast, Eckstein and colleagues[109] reported that direct exposure of isolated atria of male rats to 17β-estradiol decreased contraction rates in a dose-related manner. A similar effect was also noted in isolated spontaneous beating hearts. The authors concluded that estrogen directly affects chronotropy in rats. Since these effects required micromolar concentrations of estradiol, a possible explanation is direct inhibition of calcium entry, resulting in slowing of the cardiac cycle. Because the *in vitro* results correspond with those of Takezawa and co-workers in rats *in vivo*[108], it is possible that estrogens exert a direct and negative chronotropic effect *in vivo*.

In their study, Michel and Smith[101] also determined the role of nitric oxide in affecting rate of contraction of isolated rat ventricular myocytes. Carbachol (muscarinic agonist) produced slowing of contractions in a dose-related manner. This effect correlates well with cholinergic-induced bradycardia *in vivo*. Addition of L-NMMA (an inhibitor of nitric oxide synthase) abolished the effect of carbachol, suggesting that nitric oxide may be an important mediator of muscarinic stimulation of cardiac bradycardia. If a similar mechanism operates *in vivo*, it is possible that the estrogen-induced bradycardia is mediated by up-regulation of nitric oxide mechanisms in cardiac myocytes.

Another mode of regulation of estrogen-related changes in heart rate is modulation of cardiac autonomic mechanisms. A number of studies described that estrogens modulate the effects of adrenergic and cholinergic agents on coronary vascular reactivity[106,107] However, only a few studies looked into effects in cardiac cells. Klangkalya and Chan[110] studied regulation by sex hormones of expression and binding affinities of β-adrenergic and cholinergic receptors in hearts of female rats *in vivo*. Estrogen or progesterone alone had no

significant effect on the binding affinities of [³H]dihydroalprenolol (β-adrenergic agonist) and [³H]quinuclidinyl (muscarinic agonist). Treatment with estrogen increased the density of β-adrenergic receptors in the heart while progesterone had no effect. Combined estrogen plus progesterone treatment increased β-adrenergic receptors by two-fold. Treatment with estrogen or with progesterone alone decreased the density of muscarinic receptors mildly, while combined estrogen plus progesterone treatment increased the density of muscarinic receptors significantly. These results suggest a complex mode of regulation of autonomic receptors in cardiac cells by the sex hormones in the rat.

Cardioprotective effects of estrogens in females

The specific causes of cardiovascular disease in postmenopausal women are cardiac ischemia, arrhythmia, hypertension, stroke and degenerative changes related to aging[1,2]. The effects of estrogen on arrhythmia, hypertension and stroke are beyond the scope of this review.

Cardiac ischemia in postmenopausal women can be the result of three main mechanisms: stenosis of proximal coronary arteries, non-stenotic impaired coronary vasoreactivity, and ischemia-reperfusion syndrome. Estrogen deficiency after the menopause is a major risk factor for all three mechanisms (for details see references 1 and 2). Estrogen replacement therapy to postmenopausal women attenuates development of atherosclerosis of proximal coronary arteries, coronary stenosis, coronary thrombosis and impaired vasoreactivity due to estrogen-deficiency. Thus, estrogens are important for prevention and for risk reduction of cardiac ischemia in postmenopausal women (Table 4).

Estrogens may also affect the ischemic heart in women. Of clinical importance is the recently described ischemia-reperfusion syndrome. This syndrome is characterized by repeated insults to the myocardium following reperfusion of ischemic cardiac segments[111,112]. During

Table 4 Cardioprotective effects of estrogens in females

Effects on coronary vascular resistance
    coronary vasodilatation and increased coronary flow

Effects on stenosis of proximal vessels
    attenuation of atherosclerosis
    modulation of impaired angiogenesis
        stimulate endothelial growth
        inhibit smooth muscle hypertrophy
        modulate collagen production
    attenuation of thombosis
    modulation of vasoreactivity of diseased vessels (and attenuation of vasospasm)

Effects on cardiac hypoxia
    modulation of consequences of ischemia-reperfusion insults
    modulation of oxidation by free radicals

---

ischemia, vital organelles become damaged, particularly those which operate at a high energy level, or those which undergo rapid turnover. Examples are ion transporters (e.g. calcium efflux mechanisms which have to extrude calcium in order to maintain a 10^4 gradient of extracellular/intracellular concentration), enzymes involved in respiration and maintenance of transmembranal electrochemical gradients, scavenger mechanisms (e.g. antioxidants) and more. Following blood reperfusion to a previously ischemic area, there is a sudden flow of fresh blood to the partially damaged tissues. These cells are limited in their capacity to withstand the influx of blood-born chemicals. As a result, the affected cells are subject to further injury and accelerated death.

Pathophysiological mechanisms known to be associated with cardiac ischemia-reperfusion syndrome are impaired production of nitric oxide with a decrease in the production of eNOS-related nitric oxide, and an increase in the production of iNOS-related nitric oxide[113–122] It is believed that the former is a more regulated process while the latter results in excess release of the product. Nitric oxide is an oxidant, and when released in large quantities it can cause irreversible cardiac damage. Other mechanisms of cardiac ischemia-reperfusion syndrome involve impaired prostaglandin production, rapid overproduction and release of free radicals (oxidants), enhanced polymorphonuclear activation, and enhanced platelet adhesion and aggregation[123–130]. All may lead to impaired blood flow in the coronary microvasculature, recurrent thrombosis, increased vascular resistance, invasion of the myocardia with polymorphonuclear leukocytes, accelerated necrosis and increased injury to the affected cardiac segment[131].

With the progress in diagnostic and surgical techniques, more patients are now exposed to procedures, e.g. coronary bypasses, balloon angioplasty, coronary atherectomy, thrombolysis and elective cardioplegia (during open heart surgery), which increase the incidence and prevalence of the syndrome among men and women[132].

Previous epidemiological studies[3] indicated that current users of estrogen-replacement therapy have a higher degree of protection from coronary artery heart disease than previous users by a factor of 3:1[3]. This suggests, among other things, an effect of estrogen which depends on the presence of the hormone at target tissues at the time of the insult to the heart. At present, only a few studies have been conducted to test this hypothesis. Martin and associates[133] examined the effects of hormonal treatment on myocardial anoxia in female rats. In estrogen-treated animals, 10 min of anoxia lowered the contractility of right ventricular strips *in vitro* to 22% of pre-anoxic value, compared to 8% in vehicle-treated animals. Pretreatment with testosterone, or estrogen plus testosterone, lowered the contractility to 12% of pre-anoxic value. These results indicate that estrogens confer a certain degree of protection on the heart from anoxic insults.

We have studied the effects of estrogen on cardiac stunning in female rabbits, and preliminary data indicate that estrogen shortens the recovery of cardiac contractility from ischemia and facilitates preconditioning. Interestingly, stunning also led to decreased coronary vascular resistance (i.e. post-ischemic hyperemia), but the changes in flow were independent of the increases in flow that were induced by estrogen (Gorodeski and coworkers, unpublished results). These results therefore rule out estrogen-related increases in coronary flow as a mechanism of the estrogen protection of cardiac tissues from repeat ischemia.

The mechanisms of estrogen-related cardioprotection are unclear. A possible mechanism of the cardioprotective effects of estrogen is modulation of recurrent tissue damage by free radicals *in situ*, notably antioxidation. Oxidative damage to macromolecules e.g. lipo- and glycoproteins, and nucleic acids, is the main effector of tissue degeneration and aging[134–137]. *In vivo*, the main oxidants are free radicals which are by-products of normal metabolism, including aerobic respiration, phagocytosis, leakage from peroxisomes, and reactions catalyzed by cytochrome P_{450} enzymes[134]. Known defense mechanisms against oxidation are reductive enzymes (e.g. catalase and superoxidedismutase), DNA and protein repair enzymes, peroxisomes, plasma proteins (e.g. transferrin, ferritin, ceruloplasmin), and dietary antioxidants (vitamins C, E, and β-carotens)[134–137]. Estrogens may have an important antioxidant effect *in vivo*, due to their chemical structure which contains a hydroxyphenolic ring, but little is known about the effects on the cardiovascular system. Recently, Behl and

colleagues reported that estrogen protects neurons from oxidative stress-induced cell death *in vitro*. While their data were convincing from an experimental point of view, the concentrations of estrogen required to elicit the protective response were high, at micromolar levels. In rabbits, estradiol does not influence myocardial superoxidedismutase activity[139], but little is known of the effects of estrogen on cardiac antioxidant mechanisms in the human. More studies are needed to understand the antioxidant, cardioprotective role of estrogens *in vivo*.

Another possible mechanism for the estrogen-related cardioprotection is changes in cardiac nitric oxide system(s). Most, although not all authors suggest that endogenous nitric oxide protects against ischemia-reperfusion injury in the rabbit and in other species, including in the human[140–152].

Summary and conclusions

Data from experimental studies suggest that estrogens are important regulators of cardiac tissues in females *in vivo*. Hypoestrogenism invariably leads to changes which may be considered non-advantageous to women. These effects can be reversed, to a degree, by estrogen replacement therapy. From a clinical point of view, two types of conclusions can be drawn from these studies: first, that estrogen replacement therapy reduces the occurrence and impact of risk factors of cardiac ischemia in women; second, that estrogens can protect the ischemic heart in women. Understanding the cellular and molecular mechanisms by which estrogens regulate cardiovascular functions in females is important for instituting appropriate treatment modalities to postmenopausal women.

Acknowledgements

Mrs Ellie McBride and Mrs Marci Rothstein are acknowledged for technical support. Funding for some of the experiments in the author's lab was obtained by grants from Noven Pharmaceuticals and from Bristol-Myers Squibb.

References

1. Gorodeski, G. I. and Utian, W. H.(1994). Epidemiology and risk factors of cardiovascular disease in postmenopausal women. In Lobo, R. A. (ed.) *Treatment of the Postmenopausal Woman, Basic and Clinical Aspects*, pp.199–221. (New York: Raven Press)

2. Gorodeski, G. I. (1994). Impact of the menopause on the epidemiology and risk factors of coronary artery heart disease in women. *Exp. Gerontol.*, **29**, 75

3. Stampfer, M.J. and Colditz G. A. (1991). Estrogen replacement therapy and coronary heart disease: a quantitative assessment of the epidemiologic evidence. *Prevent. Med.*, **20**, 47–63

4. Elderman, I. S. (1975). Mechanism of action of steroid hormones. *J. Steroid Biochem.*, **6**,145–59

5. Stumpf, W. E., Sar, M. and Aumuller, G. (1977). The heart: a target organ for estradiol. *Science*, **196**, 319–21

6. McGill, H. C. and Sheridan, P. J. (1981). Nuclear uptake of sex steroid hormones in the cardiovascular system of the baboon. *Circ. Res.*, **48**, 238–44

7. Horwitz, K. B. and Horwitz, L. D. (1982). Canine vascular tissues are targets for androgens, estrogens, progestins and glucocorticoids. *J. Clin. Invest.*, **69**, 750–8

8. Lin, A. L., McGill, H. C. and Shain, S. A. (1982). Hormone receptors of the baboon cardiovascular system. Biochemical characterization of aortic and myocardial cytoplasmic progesterone receptors. *Circ. Res.*, **50**, 610–16

9. Sheridan, P. J. and McGill, H. C. Jr (1984). The nuclear uptake and retention of a synthetic progestin in the cardiovascular system of the baboon. *Endocrinology*, **114**, 2015

10. Hochner-Celnikier, D., Marandici, A., Iohan, F. and Monder, C. (1986). Estrogen and progesterone receptors in the organs of prenatal cynomolgus monkey and laboratory mouse. *Biol. Reprod.*, **35**, 633–40

11. Stumpf, W. E. (1990). Steroid hormones and the cardiovascular system: direct action of estradiol, progesterone, testosterone, gluco and mineralocorticoids and soltriol (Vitamin D) on central nervous regulatory and peripheral tissues. *Experiential*, **46**,13–25

12. White, M. M., Zamudio, S., Stevens, T., Tyler, R., Lindenfeld, J., Leslie, K. and Moore, L. G.(1995). Estrogen, progesterone, and vascular reactivity: potential cellular mechanisms. *Endocr. Rev.*, **16**, 739–51

13. Baysal, K. and Losordo, D. W. (1996). Oestrogen receptors and cardiovascular disease. *Clin. Exp. Pharmacol. Physiol.*, **23**, 537–48

14. Kim-Schulze, S., McGowan, K. A., Hubchak, S. C., Cid, M. C., Martin, B., Kleinman, H. K., Greene, G. L. and Schnaper, H. W. (1996). Expression of an estrogen receptor by human coronary artery and umbilical vein endothelial cells. *Circulation*, **94**, 1402–7

15. Venkov, C. D., Rankin, A. B. and Vaughan, D. E. (1996). Identification of authentic estrogen receptor in cultured endothelial cells. *Circulation*, **94**, 727–33

16. Muldoon, T. G.(1980). Regulation of steroid hormone receptor activity. *Endocrinol. Rev.*, **1**, 339–64

17. Eckert, R. L. and Katzenellenbogen, B. A. (1982). Effects of estrogens and antiestrogens on estrogen receptor dynamics and the induction of progesterone receptor in MCF-7 human breast cancer cells. *Cancer Res.*, **42**, 139–48

18. Gorodeski, I. G., Bahary, C. M., Beery, R., Lunenfeld, B. and Geier, A. (1986). Characterization and assay of the nuclear and cytosolic progesterone receptors in premarin primed human endometrium and myometrium after single dose progesterone administration. *Fertil. Steril.*, **45**, 788–93

19. Ingegno, M. D., Money, S. R., Thelmo, W., Greene, G. L., Davidian, M., Jaffe, B. M. and Pertschuk, L .P. (1988). Progesterone receptors in the human heart and great vessels. *Lab. Invest.*, **59**, 353–6

20. Lin, A. L., Gonzalez, R., Carey, K. D. and Shain, S. A. (1986). Estradiol-17β affects estrogen receptor distribution and elevates progesterone receptor content in baboon aorta. *Arteriosclerosis*, **6**, 495–504

21. Chilton, B. S., Kaplan, H. A. and Lennarz, W. J. (1988). Estrogen regulation of the central enzymes involved in O- and N-linked glycoprotein assembly in the developing and the adult rabbit endocervix. *Endocrinology*, **123**, 1237–44

22. Weiner, C. P. (1996). Sex hormonal regulation of nitric oxide during ovulation and pregnancy. Presented at ASPET Colloquium: *Effects of Gonadal Steroids on Vascular Function*, Washington, DC, April

23. Ishi, K., Kano, T. and Ando J. (1986). Calcium channel, Ca^{++} mobilization and mechanical reactivity of estrogen- and progesterone-treated rat uterus. *J. J. Pharmacol.*, **41**, 47–54

24. Collins, P., Rosano, G. M., Jiang, C., Lindsay, D., Sarrel, P. M. and Poole-Wilson, P. A. (1993). Cardiovascular protection by oestrogen – a calcium antagonist effect? *Lancet*, **341**, 1264–5

25. Yamamoto, T. (1995). Effects of estrogens on Ca channels in myometrial cells isolated from pregnant rats. *Am. J. Physiol.*, **268**, C64–9

26. Lippert, T. H., Seeger, H., Mueck, A. O., Hanke, H. and Haasis, R. (1996). Effect of estradiol, progesterone and progestogens on calcium influx in cell cultures of human vessels. *Menopause*, **3**, 33–7

27. Morley, P., Whitfield, J. F., Vanderhyden, B. C., Tsang, B. K. and Schwartz, J. L. (1992). A new, nongenomic estrogen action: the rapid release of intracellular calcium. Endocrinology, **131**, 1305–12

28. Subbiah, M. T. R., Kessel, B., Agrawal, M., Rajan, R., Abplanalp, W. and Rymaszewski, Z. (1993). Antioxidant potential of specific estrogens on lipid peroxidation. *J. Clin. Endocrilol. Metab.*, **77**, 1095–7

29. Yagi, K. and Komura, S. (1986). Inhibitory effect of female hormones on lipid peroxidation. *Biochem. Int.*, **13**, 1051–5

30. Schwartz, J., Freeman, R. and Frishman, W. (1994). Clinical pharmacology of estrogens: cardiovascular actions and cardioprotective benefits of replacement therapy in postmenopausal women. *J. Clin. Pharmacol.*, **35**, 1–16

31. Taniguchi, S., Yanase, T., Kobayashi, K., Takayanagi, R., Haji, M., Umeda, F. and Nawata, H. (1994). Catechol estrogens are more potent antioxidants than estrogens for the Cu^{2+}-catalyzed oxidation of low or high density lipoprotein: antioxidative effects of steroids on lipoproteins. *Endocr. J.*, **41**, 605–11

32. Lacort, M., Leal, A. M., Liza, M., Martin, C., Martinez, R. and Ruiz-Larrea, M. B. (1995). Protective effect of estrogens and catecholestrogens against peroxidative membrane damage *in vitro*. *Lipids*, **30**, 141–6

33. Tang, M., Abplanalp, W., Ayres, S., and Subbiah, M. T. R. (1996). Superior and distinct antioxidant effects of selected estrogen metabolites on lipid peroxidation. *Metab. Clin. Exp.*, **45**, 411–14

34. Tranquilli, A. L., Mazzanti, L., Cugini, A. M., Cester, N., Garzetti, G. G. and Romanini, C. (1995). Transdermal estradiol and medroxy-progesterone acetate in hormone replacement therapy are both antioxidants. *Gynecol. Endocrinol.*, **9**,137–41

35. Takanashi, K., Watanabe, K. and Yoshizawa, I. (1995). On the inhibitory effect of E_{17}-sulfoconjugated catechol estrogens upon lipid peroxidation of rat liver microsomes. *Biol. Pharm. Bull.*, **18**, 1120–5

36. Keany, J. (1996). Antioxidant effects of estrogen. Presented at ASPET Colloquium: *Effects of Gonadal Steroids on Vascular Function*, Washington, DC, April

37. Schnaper, H. W., McGowan, K. A., Kim-Schulze, S. and Cid, M. C. (1996) Oestrogen and endothelial cell angiogenic activity. *Clin. & Exper. Pharmacol. & Physiol.*, **23**, 247–50

38. Kolodgic, F. D., Jacob, A., Wilson, P. S., Carlson, G. C., Farb, A., Verma, A. and Virmani, R. (1996). Estradiol attenuates directed migration of vascular smooth muscle cells *in vitro*. *Am. J. Pathol.*, **148**, 969–76

39. Fischer, G. M., Cherian, K. and Swain, M. L. (1981). Increased synthesis of aortic collagen and elastin in experimental atherosclerosis: inhibition by contraceptive steroids. *Atherosclerosis*, **39**, 463–76

40. Fischer, G. M. and Swain, M. L. (1985). Effects of estradiol and progesterone on the increased synthesis of collagen in atherosclerotic rabbit aortas. *Atherosclerosis*, **54**, 177–85

41. Wagner, J. D., Clarkson, T. B., St Clair, R. W., Schwenke, D. C., Shively, C. A. and Adams, M. R. (1991). Estrogen and progesterone replacement therapy reduces low density lipoprotein accumulation in the coronary arteries of surgically postmenopausal cyno-molgus monkeys. *J. Clin. Invest.*, **88**, 1995-2002

42. Rifici, V.A. and Khachadurian, A. K. (1992). The inhibition of low-density lipoprotein oxidation by 17-beta estradiol. *Metab. Clin. Exp.*, **41**, 1110–4

43. Sack, M. N., Rader, D. J. and Cannon, R. O. III (1994). Estrogen and inhibition of oxidation of low density lipoproteins in postmenopausal women. *Lancet*, **343**, 269–70

44. Fitzpatrick, L. A. (1996). Gender-related differences in the development of atherosclerosis: studies at the cellular level. *Clin. Exp. Pharmacol.*, **23**, 267–9

45. Hough, J. L. and Zilversmith, D. B. (1986). Effect of 17-beta estradiol on aortic cholesterol content and metabolism in cholesterol-fed rabbits. *Arteriosclerosis*, **6**, 57–63

46. Adams, M. R., Kaplan J. R., Manuck, S. B., *et al.* (1990). Inhibition of coronary artery atherosclerosis by 17-beta estradiol in ovariectomized monkeys. *Arteriosclerosis*, **10**, 1051–7

47. Cheng, L. P., Kuwahara, M., Jacobsson, J. and Foegh, M. L. (1991). Inhibition of myointimal hyperplasia and macrophage infiltration by estradiol in aorta allografts. *Transplantation*, **52**, 967–72

48. Foegh, M. L., Asotra, S., Howell, M. H. and Ramwell, P. W. (1994). Estradiol inhibition of arterial neointimal hyperplasia after balloon injury. *J. Vasc. Surg.*, **19**, 722–6

49. Dejana, E., Corada, M. and Lampugnani, M. G. (1995). Endothelial cell-to-cell junctions. *FASEB J.*, **9**, 910–18

50. Caulin-Glaser, T., Watson, C. A. and Bender, J. R. (1996). Effects of 17β-estradiol on cytokine-induced endothelial cell adhesion molecule expression. *J. Clin. Invest.*, **98**, 36–42

51. Farhat, M. Y., Lavigne, M. C. and Ramwell, P. W. (1996). The vascular protective effects of estrogen. *FASEB J.*, **10**, 615–24

52. Gisclard, V., Miller, V. M. and Vanhoutte, P. M. (1988). Effect of 17β-estradiol on endothelium-dependent responses in the rabbit. *J. Pharmacol. Exp. Ther.*, **244**, 19–22

53. Lieberman, E. H., Gerhard, M. D., Uchata, A. , *et al.* (1994). Estrogen improves endothelium-dependent flow-mediated vasodilation in postmenopausal women. *Ann. Intern. Med.*, **121**, 936–41

54. Gorodeski, G. I., Sheean, L. A. and Utian, W. H. (1995). Sex hormone modulation of flow velocity in the parametrial artery of the pregnant rat. *Am. J. Physiol.*, **268**, R614–24

55. Gilligan, D. M., Badar, D. M., Panza, J. A., Quyyumi, A. A. and Cannon, R. O. (1995). Effects of estrogen replacement therapy on peripheral vasomotor function in post-menopausal women. *Am. J. Cardiol.*, **75**, 264–8

56. Gorodeski, G. I., Yang, T., Levy, M. N., Goldfarb, J. and Utian, W. H. (1995). Effects of estrogen *in vivo* on coronary vascular resistance in perfused rabbit hearts. *Am. J. Physiol.*, **269**, R1333–8

57. Gilligan, D. M., Quyyumi, A. A. and Cannon, R. O. (1994). Effects of physiological levels of estrogen on coronary vasomotor function in postmenopausal women. *Circulation*, **89**, 2545–51

58. Ignarro, L. J., Buga, G. M., Wood, K. S., Byrns, R. E. and Chaudhuri, G. (1987). Endothelium-derived relaxing factor produced and released from artery and vein is nitric oxide. *Proc. Natl. Acad. Sci. USA*, **84**, 9265–9

59. Hayashi, T., Fukuto, J. M., Ignarro, L. J. and Chaudhuri, G. (1992). Basal release of nitric oxide from aortic rings is greater in female rabbits than in male rabbits: implication for atherosclerosis. *Proc. Natl. Acad. Sci. USA*, **89**, 11259–63

60. Zeiher, A. M., Drexler, H., Saurbier, B. and Just, H. (1993). Endothelium-mediated coronary blood flow modulation in humans. *J. Clin. Invest.*, **92**, 652–62

61. Harrison, D. G., Sayegh, H., Ohara, Y., Inoue, N and Venema, R. C.(1996). Regulation of expression of the endothelial cell nitric oxide synthase. *Clin. Exp. Pharmacol. Physiol.*, **23**, 251–5

62. Wellman, G. C., Brayden, J. E. and Nelson, M. T. (1996). A proposed mechanism for the cardioprotective effect of oestrogen in women: enhanced endothelial nitric oxide release decreases coronary artery reactivity. *Clin. Exp. Pharmacol. Physiol.*, **23**, 260–6

63. Lamontagne, D., Konig, A., Bassenge, E. and Busse, R. (1992). Prostacyclin and nitric oxide contribute to the vasodilator action of acetylcholine and bradykinin in the intact rabbit coronary bed. *J. Cardiovasc. Pharmacol.*, **20**, 652–7

64. Ludmer, P. L., Selwyn, A. P., Shook, T. L., Wayne, R. R., Mudge, G. H., Alexander, W. and Ganz, P. (1986). Paradoxical vasoconstriction induced by acetylcholine in atherosclerotic coronary arteries. *N. Engl. J. Med.*, **315**, 1046–51

65. Moncada, S. and Higgs, A. (1993). The L-arginine-nitric oxide pathway. *N. Eng. J. Med.*, **329**, 2002–12

66. Furchgott, R. F. and Vanhoutte, P. M. (1989). Endothelium-derived relaxing and contracting factors. *FASEB J.*, **3**, 2007–18

67. Osborne, J. A., Siegman, M. J., Sedar, A. W., Moores, A. U. and Lefer, A. M. (1989). Lack of endothelium dependent relaxation in coronary resistance arteries of cholesterol-fed rabbits. *Am. J. Physiol.*, **256**, 6591–7

68. Williams, J. K., Adams, M. R. and Klopfenstein, H. S. (1990). Estrogen modulates responses of atherosclerotic coronary arteries. *Circulation*, **81**, 1680–7

69. Galle, J., Busse, R. R. and Bassenge, E. (1991). Hypercholesterolemia and atherosclerosis change vascular reactivity in rabbits by different mechanisms. *Arterioscl. Thromb.*, **11**, 1712–18

70. Williams, J. K., Adams, M. R., Herrington, D. M. and Clarkson, T. B. (1992). Short-term administration of estrogen and vascular responses of atherosclerotic coronary arteries. *J. Am. Coll. Cardiol.*, **20**, 452–7

71. Egashira, K., Inou, T., Hirooka, Y., Yamada, A., Maruoka, Y., Kai, H., Sugimachi, M., Suzuki, S. and Takeshita, A. (1993). Impaired coronary blood flow response to acetylcholin in patients with coronary risk factors and proximal atherosclerotic lesions. *J. Clin. Invest.*, **91**, 29–37

72. Luscher, T. F., Tanner, F. C., Tschudi, M. R. and Noll, G. (1993). Endothelial dysfunction in coronary artery disease. *Annu. Rev. Med.*, **44**, 395–418

73. Reis, S. E., Gloth, S. T., Blumenthal, R. S., Resar, J. R., Zacur, H. A., Gerstenblith, G., *et al.* (1994). Ethinyl estradiol acutely attenuates abnormal coronary vasomotor responses to acetylcholine in postmenopausal women. *Circulation*, **89**, 52–60

74. Gorodeski, G. I., Yang, T., Matsuda, M., Levy, M. N., Goldfarb, J., and Utian, W.H. (1996). Modulation of coronary vascular resistance in female rabbits by estrogen and progesterone. Submitted for publication

75. Mugge, A., Riedel, M., Barton, M., Kuhn, M. and Lichtlen, P. R. (1993). Endothelium independent relaxation of human coronary arteries by 17β-oestradiol *in vitro. Cardiovasc. Res.*, **27**, 1939–42

76. Miller, V. M., Barber, D. A., Fenton, A. M., Wang, X. and Sieck, G. C. (1996). Gender differences in response to endothelin-1 in coronary arteries: transcription, receptors and calcium regulation. *Clin. Exp. Pharmacol. Physiol.*, **23**, 256–9

77. Colucci, W. S., Gimbrone, M. A., McLaughlin, M. K., Halpern, W. and Alexander, R. W. (1982). Increased vascular catecholamine sensitivity and α-adrenergic receptor affinity in female and estrogen-treated male rats. *Circ. Res.*, **50**, 805–11

78. Fregly, M. J and Thrasher, T. N. (1977). Response of heart rate to acute administration of isoproterenol in rats treated chronically with norethynodrel, ethinyl estradiol, and both combined. *Endocrinology*, **100**, 148–54

79. Bar, J., Tepper, R., Fuchs, J., Pardo, Y., Goldberger, S. and Ovadia, J. (1993). The effect of estrogen replacement therapy on platelet aggregation and adenosine triphosphate release in postmenopausal women. *Obstet. Gynecol.*, **81**, 261–4

80. Han, S. Z., Karaki, H., Ouchi, Y., Akishita, M. and Orimo, H. (1995). 17β-estradiol inhibits Ca^{2+} influx and Ca^{2+} release induced by thromboxane A_2 in porcine coronary artery. *Circulation*, **91**, 2619–26

81. Kessler, K. M. (1992). Syndrome X: the epicardial view. *J. Am. Coll. Cardiol.*, **19**, 32–3

82. Sarrel, P. M., Lindsay, D., Rosano, G. M. C. and Poole-Wilson, P. A. (1992). Angina and normal coronary arteries in women: gynecologic findings. *Am. J. Obstet. Gynecol.*, **167**, 467–72

83. Killam, A. O., Rosefeld, C. R., Battaglia, F. C., Makowski, E. L. and Meschia, G. (1973). Effect of estrogens on the uterine blood flow of oophorectomized ewes. *Am. J. Obstet. Gynecol.*, **115**, 1045–52

84. Van Buren, G. A., Yang, D. S. and Clark, K. E. (1992). Estrogen-induced uterine vasodilatation is antagonized by L-nitroarginine methyl ester, an inhibitor of nitric oxide synthesis. *Am. J. Obstet. Gynecol.*, **167**, 828–33

85. Gorodeski, G. I., Utian, W. H. and Levy, M. N. (1994). Estrogen increases coronary flow by a nitric oxide related mechanism. Presented at 5th Annual Meeting of the North American Menopause Society, Washington DC, September

86. Furie, M. B., Cramer, E. B., Naprstek, B. L. and Silverstein, S. C. (1984). Cultured endothelial cell monolayers that restrict the transendothelial passage of macromolecules and electrical current. *J. Cell Biol.*, **98**, 1033–41

87. Schneeberger, E. E. and Lynch, R. D. (1992). Structure, function, and regulation of cellular tight junctions. *Am. J. Physiol.*, **262**, L647–61

88. Cho, M., Ziats, N., Goldfarb, J., Utian, W. H. and Gorodeski, G. I. (1996). Estrogen increases transendothelial cation selectivity: a novel vasculoprotective mechanism. Presented at *7th Annual Meeting of the North American Menopause Society*, Chicago, Il, September

89. Reuss, L. (1991). Tight junction permeability to ions and water. In Cereijido, M. (ed.) *Tight Junctions*, pp. 49–66. (Boca Raton, Ann Arbor, London: CRC Press)

90. Gallagher, L. J and Sloane, B. F. (1984). Effect of estrogen on lysosomal enzyme activities in rat heart. *Proc. Soc. Exp. Bio. Med.*, **177**, 428–33

91. Carrington, L. J. and Bailey, C. J. (1985). Effects of natural and synthetic estrogens and progestins on glycogen deposition in female mice. *Horm. Res.*, **21**, 199–203

92. Payne, R. M., Friedman, D. L., Grant, J. W., Perryman, M. B. and Strauss, A. W. (1993). Creatine kinase isoenzymes are highly regulated during pregnancy in rat uterus and placenta. *Am. J. Physiol.*, **265**, E624–35

93. Weiner, C. P., Lizasoain, I., Baylis, S. A., Knowles, R. G., Charles, I. G. and Moncada, S. (1994). Induction of calcium-dependent nitric oxide synthases by sex hormones. *Proc. Natl. Acad. Sci. USA*, **91**, 5212–16

94. Busse, R. and Mulsch, A. (1990). Induction of nitric oxide synthase by cytokines in vascular smooth muscle cells. *FEBS lett.*, **275**, 87–90

95. Shiverick, K. T., Hutchins, K., Kikta, D. C., Squires, N. and Fregly, M. J. (1983). Effects of chronic administration of mestranol on alpha and beta adrenergic responsiveness in female rats. *J. Pharm. Exp. Ther.*, **226**, 362–7

96. Magness, R. R. and Rosenfeld, C. R. (1989). Local and systemic estradiol 17β: Effects on uterine and systemic vasodilation. *Am. J. Physiol.*, **256**, E536–42

97. Pines, A., Fisman, E. Z., Levo, Y., Averbuch, D., Lidor, A., Drory, Y., *et al.* (1991). The effects of hormone replacement therapy in normal postmenopausal women: measurements of Doppler-derived parameters of aortic flow. *Am. J. Obstet. Gynecol.*, **164**, 806–12

98. Davis, L. E., Magness, R. R. and Rosenfeld, C. R. (1992). Role of angiotensin II and α-adrenergic receptors during estrogen-induced vasodilation in ewes. *Am. Physiol. Soc.*, E837–43

99. Pines, A., Fisman, E. Z., Shemesh, J., Levo, Y., Ayalon, D., Kellermann, J. J., *et al.* (1992). Menopause-related changes in left ventricular function in healthy women. *Cardiology*, **80**, 413-16

100. Scheuer, J., Malhotra, A., Schaible, T. F., and Capasso, J. (1987). Effects of gonadectomy and hormonal replacement on rat hearts. *Circ. Res.*, **61**, 12–19

101. Michel, T. and Smith, T. W. (1993). Nitric oxide synthases and cardiovascular signaling. *Am. J. Cardiol.*, **72**, 33C–8C

102. Barone, S., Panek, D., Bennett, L., Stitzel, R. E. and Head, R. J. (1987). The influence of oestrogen and oestrogen metabolites on the sensitivity of the isolated rabbit aorta to catecholamines. *Arch. Pharmacol.*, **335**, 518–20

103. Gisclard, V., Flavahan, N. A. and Vanhoutte, P. M. (1987). Alpha adrenergic responses of blood vessels of rabbits after ovariectomy and administration of 17β estradiol. *J. Pharmacol. Exp. Ther.*, **240**, 466–70

104. Johansson, S. R. and Hjalmarson, A. (1988). Age and sex differences in cardiovascular reactivity to adrenergic agonists, mental stress and isometric excercise in normal subjects. *Scand. J. Clin. Lab. Invest.*, **48**, 183–91

105. Williams, J. K., Kim, Y. D., Adams, M. R., Chen, M.-F., Myers, A. K. and Ramwell, P. W. (1994). Effects of estrogen on cardiovascular responses of premenopausal monkeys. *J. Pharmacol. Exp. Ther.*, **271**, 671–6

106. Colucci, W. S., Gimbrone, M. A. and Alexander, R. W. (1984). Regulation of myocardial and vascular α-adrenergic receptor affinity. *Circ. Res.*, **55**, 78-88

107. Schwarz, P., Diem, R., Dun, N. J. and Forstermann, U. (1995). Endogenous and exogenous nitric oxide inhibits norepinephrine release from rat heart sympathetic nerves. *Circ. Res.*, **77**, 841–8

108. Takesawa, H., Hayashi, H., Sano, H., Saito, H. and Ebihara, S. (1994). Circadian and estrous cycle-dependent variations in blood pressure and heart rate in female rats. *Am. J. Physiol.*, **267**, R1250–6

109. Eckstein, N., Nadler, E., Barnea, O., Shavit, G. and Ayalon, D. (1994). Acute effects of 17β-estradiol on the rat heart. *Am. J. Obstet. Gynecol.*, **171**, 844–8

110. Klangkalya, B. and Chan, A. (1988). The effects of ovarian hormones on beta-adrenergic and muscarinic receptors in rat heart. *Life Sci.*, **42**, 2307–14

111. Hasan, A. and McDonough, K. H. (1995). Effects of short term ischemia and reperfusion on coronary vascular reactivity and myocardial function. *Life Sci.*, **57**, 2171–85

112. Vinten-Johansen, J., Sato, H. and Zhao, Z. Q. (1995). The role of nitric oxide and NO-donor agents in myocardial protection from surgical ischemic-reperfusion injury. *Int. J. Cardiol.*, **50**, 273–81

113. Nakanishi, K., Vinten-Johansen, J., Lefer, D. J., Zhao, Z., Fowler, W. C. III, McGee, D. S. and Johnston, W. E. (1992). Intracoronary L-arginine during reperfusion improves endothelial function and reduces infarct size. *Am. J. Physiol.*, **263**, H1650–8

114. Lefer, D. J., Nakanishi, K. and Vinten-Johansen, J. (1993). Endothelial and myocardial cell protection by a cysteine-containing nitric oxide donor after myocardial ischemia and reperfusion. *J. Cardiovasc. Pharmacol.*, **22** (Suppl.7), S34–43

115. Fung, K. P., Wu, T. W., Zeng, L. H and Wu. J. (1994). The opposing effects of an inhibitor of nitric oxide synthesis and of a donor of nitric oxide in rabbits undergoing myocardial ischemia reperfusion. *Life Sci.*, **54**, PL491–6

116. Hattler, B. G., Gorcsan, J. III, Shah, N., Oddis, C. V., Billiar, T. R., Simmons, R. L. and Finkel, M. S. (1994). A potential role for nitric oxide in myocardial stunning. *J. Cardiac Surg.*, May; **9**, 425–9

117. Seccombe, J. F., Pearson, P. J. and Schaff, H. V. (1994). Oxygen radical-mediated vascular injury selectively inhibits receptor-dependent release of nitric oxide from canine coronary arteries. *J. Thoracic Cardiovasc. Surg.*, **107**, 505–9

118. Engelman, D. T., Watanabe, M., Engelman, R. M., Rousou, J. A., Flack, J. E. III, Deaton, D. W. and Das, D. K. (1995). Constitutive nitric oxide release is impaired after ischemia and reperfusion. *J. Thoracic Cardiovasc Surg.*, **110**, 1047–53

119. Hammon, J. W. Jr and Vinten-Johansen, J. (1995). Augmentation of microvascular nitric oxide improves myocardial performance following global ischemia. *J. Cardiac Surg.*, **10**, 423–7

120. Hiramatsu, T., Forbess, J. M., Miura, T. and Mayer, J. E. Jr (1995). Effects of L-arginine and L-nitro-arginine methyl ester on recovery of neonatal lamb hearts after cold ischemia. Evidence for an important role of endothelial production of nitric oxide. *J. Thoracic Cardiovasc. Surg.*, **109**, 81–6, discussion 87

121. Maulik, N., Engelman, D. T., Watanabe, M., Engelman, R. M., Maulik, G., Cordis, G. A. and Das, D. K. (1995). Nitric oxide signaling in ischemic heart. *Cardiovasc. Res.*, **30**, 593–601

122. Seccombe, J. F. and Schaff, H. V. (1995). Coronary artery endothelial function after myocardial ischemia and reperfusion. *Ann. Thoracic Surg.*, **60**, 778–88

123. Pearson, P. J., Lin, P. J. and Schaff, H. V. (1992). Global myocardial ischemia and reperfusion impair endothelium-dependent relaxations to aggregating platelets in the canine coronary artery. A possible cause of vasospasm after cardiopulmonary bypass. *J. Thoracic Cardiovasc. Surg.*, **103**, 1147–54

124. Schror, K. and Woditsch, I. (1992). Endogenous prostacyclin preserves myocardial function and endothelium-derived nitric oxide formation in myocardial ischemia. *Agents Actions*, **37** (Suppl.), 312–19

125. Vegh, A., Szekeres, L. and Parratt, J. (1992). Preconditioning of the ischaemic myocardium; involvement of the L-arginine nitric oxide pathway. *Br. J. Pharmacol.*, **107**, 648–52

126. Woditsch, I. and Schror, K. (1992). Prostacyclin rather than endogenous nitric oxide is a tissue protective factor in myocardial ischemia. *Am. J. Physiol.*, **263**, H1390–6

127. Hiramatsu, T., Forbess, J., Miura, T., Roth, S. J., Cioffi, M. A. and Mayer, J. E. Jr (1995). Effects of endothelin-l and endothelin-A receptor antagonist on recovery after hypothermic cardioplegic ischemia in neonatal lamb hearts. *Circulation*, **92**, 400–4

128. Wang, Q. D., Uriuda, Y., Pernow, J., Hemsen, A., Sjoquist, P. O. and Ryden L. (1995). Myocardial release of endothelin (ET) and enhanced ET(A) receptor-mediated coronary vasoconstriction after coronary thrombosis and thrombolysis in pigs. *J. Cardiovasc. Pharmacol.*, **26**, 770–6

129. Wanna, F. S., Obayashi, D. Y., Young, J. N., and DeCampli, W. M. (1995). Simultaneous manipulation of the nitric oxide and prostanoid pathways reduces myocardial reperfusion injury. *J. Thoracic Cardiovasc. Surg.*, **110**, 1054–62

130. Pabla, R., Buda, A. J., Flynn, D. M., Blesse, S. A., Shin, A. M., Curtis, M. J. and Lefer, D. J. (1996). Nitric oxide attenuates neutrophil-mediated myocardial contractile dysfunction after ischemia and reperfusion. *Circ. Res.*, **78**, 65–72

131. Lefer, D. J. (1995). Myocardial protective actions of nitric oxide donors after myocardial ischemia and reperfusion. *New Horizons*, **3**, 105–12

132. Vinten-Johansen, J., Zhao, Z. Q. and Sato, H. (1995). Reduction in surgical ischemic-gynecological endocrinology reperfusion injury with adenosine and nitric oxide therapy. *Ann. Thoracic Surg.*, **60**, 852–7

133. Martin, L. G., Brenner, G. M., Jarolim, K. L., Banschbach, M. W., Coons, D. L. and Wolfe, A. K. (1993). Effects of sex steroids on myocardial anoxic resistance. *Pro. Soc. Exp. Biol. Med.*, **202**, 288–94

134. Ames, B. N., Shigenaga, M. K. and Hagen, T. M. (1995). Oxidants, antioxidants, and the degenerative diseases of aging. *Proc. Natl. Acad. Sci. USA*, **90**, 7915–22

135. Kendall, M. J., Rajman, I. and Maxwell, S. R. J. (1994). Cardioprotective therapeutics – drugs used in hypertension, hyperlipidaemia, thromboembolism, arrhythmias, the post-menopausal state and as anti-oxidants. *Postgrad. Med. J.*, **70**, 329–43

136. Sato, I., Morita, I., Kaji, K., Ikeda, M., Nagao, M. and Murota, S.-I. (1993). Reduction of nitric oxide producing activity associated with *in vitro* aging in cultured human umbilical vein. *Biochem. Biophys. Res. Comm.*, **195**, 1070–6

137. Brunet, J., Boily, M. J., Cordeau, S. and Des Rosiers, C. (1995). Effects of N-acetylcysteine in the rat heart reperfused after low-flow ischemia: evidence for a direct scavenging of hydroxyl radicals and a nitric oxide-dependent increase in coronary flow. *Free Radical Biol. Med.*, **19**, 627–38

138. Behl, C., Widmann, M., Trapp, T. and Holsboer, F. (1995). 17-beta estradiol protects neurons from oxidative stress-induced cell death *in vitro*. *Biochem. Biophys. Res. Comm.*, **216**, 473–82

139. Furuya, K. and Chaudhuri, G. (1993). Estradiol does not influence myocardial superoxide dismutase activity in rabbits. *J. Cardiovasc. Pharmacol.*, **68**, 65–8

140. Coughlan, M. G., Kenny, D., Kampine, J. P., Bosnjak, Z. J. and Warltier, D. C. (1993). Differential sensitivity of proximal and distal coronary arteries to a nitric oxide donor following reperfusion injury or inhibition of nitric oxide synthesis. *Cardiovasc. Res.*, **27**, 1444–8

141. Patel, V. C., Yellon, D. M., Singh, K. J., Neild, G. H. and Woolfson, R. G. (1993). Inhibition of nitric oxide limits infarct size in the *in situ* rabbit heart. *Biochem. Biophys. Res. Comm.*, **194**, 234–8

142. Pernow, J., Uriuda, Y., Wang, Q. D., Li, X. S., Nordlander, R. and Rydeen, L. (1994). The protective effect of L-arginine on myocardial injury and endothelial function following ischaemia and reperfusion in the pig. *Eur. Heart J.*, **15**, 1712–19

143. Amrani, M., Chester, A. H., Jayakumar, J., Schyns, C. J. and Yacoub, M. H. (1995). L-arginine reverses low coronary reflow and enhances postischaemic recovery of cardiac mechanical function. *Cardiovasc. Res.*, **30**, 200–4

144. Depre, C., Vanoverschelde, J. L., Goudemant, J. F., Mottet, I. and Hue, L. (1995). Protection against ischemic injury by nonvasoactive concentrations of nitric oxide synthase inhibitors in the perfused rabbit heart. *Circulation*, **92**, 1911–18

145. Engelman, D. T., Watanabe, M., Maulik, N., Cordis, G. A., Engelman, R. M., Rousou, J. A., Flack, J. E. III, Deaton, D. W. and Das, D. K. (1995). L-arginine reduces endothelial inflammation and myocardial stunning during ischemia/reperfusion. *Ann. Thoracic Surg.*, **60**, 1275-81

146. Naseem, S. A., Kontos, M. C., Rao, P. S., Jesse, R. L., Hess, M. L. and Kukreja, R. C. (1995). Sustained inhibition of nitric oxide by NG-nitro-L-arginine improves myocardial function following ischemia/reperfusion in isolated perfused rat heart. *J. Mol. Cell Cardiol.*, **27**, 419–26

147. Hoshida, S., Yamashita, N., Igarashi, J., Nishida, M., Hori, M., Kamada, T., Kuzuya, T. and Tada, M. (1995). Nitric oxide synthase protects the heart against ischemia-reperfusion injury in rabbits. *J. Pharmacol. Exp. Ther.*, **274**, 413–18

148. Sato, H., Zhao, Z. Q., McGee, D. S., Williams, M. W., Hammon, J. W. Jr and Vinten-Johansen, J. (1995). Supplemental L-arginine during cardioplegic arrest and reperfusion avoids regional postischemic injury. *J. Thoracic Cardiovasc. Surg.*, **110**, 302–14

149. Schulz, R. and Wambolt, R. (1995). Inhibition of nitric oxide synthesis protects the isolated working rabbit heart from ischaemia-reperfusion injury. *Cardiovasc. Res.*, **30**, 432–9

150. Takeuchi, K., McGowan, F. X., Danh, H. C., Glynn, P., Simplaceanu, E. and del Nido, P. J. (1995). Direct detrimental effects of L-arginine upon ischemia-reperfusion injury to myocardium. *J. Mol. Cell Cardiol.*, **27**, 1405–14

151. Weselcouch, E. O., Baird, A. J., Sleph, P. and Grover, G. J. (1995). Inhibition of nitric oxide synthesis does not affect ischemic preconditioning in isolated perfused rat hearts. *Am. J. Physiol.*, **268**, H242–9

152. Williams, M. W., Taft, C. S., Ramnauth, S., Zhao, Z. Q. and Vinten-Johansen, J. (1995). Endogenous nitric oxide (NO) protects against ischaemia-reperfusion injury in the rabbit. *Cardiovasc. Res.*, **30**, 79–86

Progestogens do not attenuate cardiovascular benefits by estrogens

58

G. Samsioe

Introduction

A growing body of evidence supports the notion that cardiovascular disease, especially myocardial infarction, may be substantially reduced following estrogen therapy. In the general population the risk of myocardial infarction may be halved during estrogen replacement therapy. Although few have been carried out, secondary prevention trials suggest an even greater benefit (a relative risk of 0.2) in women with a sustained myocardial infarction. In addition, studies have also indicated that women carrying risk factors for cardiovascular disease like smoking or hypertension may also benefit to a greater extent than those without risk factors[1,2].

Cardiovascular disease is the main killer both in men and women in modern western society. Reductions of its incidence and prevalence have a vast influence on the health care sectors of any given country. Theoretically, deaths prevented by estrogen replacement therapy outnumber its potential risks in use as indicated by Ross and colleagues[3,4]. One of several problems in preventive medicine is the lag time preceding the majority of events. Myocardial infarction in women is of little importance before the age of 55 years and not until two to three decades later do cardiovascular diseases become a significant burden to the health care system.

Treating women with estrogen monotherapy for periods of a decade or more greatly increases the risk of endometrial cancer and other endometrial pathology. In addition, endometrial hyperplasia and/or irregular vaginal bleeds often follow estrogen monotherapy.

Clinical realities, as well as fear of cancer, provide serious obstacles to the long-term use of estrogen monotherapy and impede compliance substantially. It has been repeatedly shown that progestogen comedication prevents the development of hyperplasia as well as endometrial cancer. In the majority of cases, a socially acceptable bleeding pattern can also be obtained.

In several biochemical as well as physiological processes progestogens seem to counteract the effects of estrogens. This concept seems to be true also for some metabolic markers of cardiovascular disease.

Cardioprotection by estrogens: mechanisms of action

Angiographic studies (Table 1) demonstrate a reduction in coronary stenosis by estrogen monotherapy. This reduction seems to be more marked in those with the more severe stenosis[4].

Two major explanatory mechanisms contribute to this. First, an effect via arterial function, i.e. leading to vasodilatation, and second, a reduction of atherosclerosis. Vasodilatation results either from an increase in factors promoting vasodilatation or a decrease of factors responsible for vaso-constriction. Estrogens and progestogens may well affect several factors belonging to each category.

Atherosclerosis is of multifactorial origin. Hemostasis, blood pressure, lipid and carbohydrate metabolism are of importance for the long-term development and may also

419

Table 1 Effects of estrogens on coronary atherosclerosis as verified by angiographic studies. From reference 4, with permission

Reference	Study design	Study size	Endpoints	Risk estimates
Hong	cross-sectional	18 users	coronary stenosis	0.13
		72 non-users		
Sullivan	case–control	cases = 1178	> 70% stenosis	0.44*
Gruchow	cross-sectional	users = 154	severe occlusion	0.37*
		non-users = 779	moderate occlusion	0.59*
McFarland	case–control	cases = 137	> 70% stenosis	0.50*

*$p < 0.05$

contribute to the physicochemical properties of the atherosclerotic plaque. Newly formed instable plaques seem to be more deleterious than older chronic atherosclerotic lesions. It is well known that estrogens as well as progestogens may influence several of the parameters belonging to hemostasis as well as carbohydrate and lipid metabolism.

Atherosclerotic process: effects of estrogens and progestogens

Even if hemostasis, lipid and carbohydrate metabolisms are often discussed separately, it should be remembered that different metabolic disturbances are extraordinarily interconnected. Hence changes in one system can knock on to another aspect and actually generate self-sustaining systems of metabolic disturbance which all converge on atherogenesis (Figure 1). In other words, independent tips of apparently different icebergs are really part of the same system. Insulin resistance may well be a common characteristic.

Blood pressure

In most studies blood pressure changes have been small. Several studies fail to demonstrate any major effect of blood pressure, although the general impression is that there is a small reduction of between 3 and 6 mmHg; reductions of diastolic blood pressure have been more uniformly found than those of systolic blood pressure. The introduction of progestogens does not seem to alter this picture and the overall conclusion is that progestogen addition irrespective of type does not have an adverse effect on blood pressure. It should be remembered, however, that 2–3% of women in

Metabolism		Vessel wall	
HDL cholesterol	↑	Endothelin(s)	↓
LDL cholesterol	↓	EDRF (NO)	↑
Oxidized LDL	↓	Thromboxane A$_2$	↓
Triglycerides	↓	Prostacyclin	(↑)
Insulin	↓	Calcium channel blocking	↑
Coagulation factors	↓		
Fibrinolysis	(↑)		
Anticoagulation factors	↑		

Blood pressure	↓
Blood flow	↑
Vascular resistance	↓

Figure 1 Estrogen cardioprotection is conceivably mediated via known risk factors for cardiovascular disease. Estrogens have been described to influence a variety of markers for metabolism as well as vessel-wall physiology. Only qualitative changes are marked. Importance of each change in quantitative terms vis-á-vis cardioprotection remains to be clarified. Figure represents only recognized activities of estrogens and additional mechanisms of importance may well exist. HDL, high-density lipoprotein; LDL, low-density lipoprotein; EDRF, endothelium-derived relaxing factor; NO, nitric oxide

the general population may have an idiosyncratic response to estrogens and display a marked increase in blood pressure. Overall, there is consensus to state that blood pressure changes seem to be of little, if any, importance for the cardioprotective effects of estrogens or estrogen–progestogen combinations[5].

Hemostasis

Estrogen replacement therapy induces profound changes within parameters belonging to the hemostasis system. This is true for factors promoting clotting as well as for those of importance for fibrinolysis and anticoagulation. Following menopause, the loss of ovarian function results in a time-since-menopause-dependent course of events of factors belonging to the hemostatic systems[6]. Antithrombin III and protein C activity increase as well as plasminogen and plasminogen activator inhibitor (PAI)-1. In addition factor VII and fibrinogen are commonly increased. By estrogen monotreatment, plasminogen activity increases further. Oral estrogens also increase factor VII and fibrinogen[7].

Fibrinogen, factor VII and PAI-1 all decrease following a combined therapy of transdermal estradiol with medroxyprogesterone acetate[8]. As a whole, progestogens have little effect on factors promoting clotting whereas they might further augment fibrinolysis. In other words, the addition of a progestogen to estrogen replacement therapy seems to have no adverse effects, rather the contrary seems to be true[9].

Observational studies on venous thromboembolism and hormone replacement therapy (HRT) are few, the number of cases small and the methodology sometimes questionable in studies published up to 1995. Recent studies[10–12] provided evidence of a two- to four-fold increase of venous thrombo-embolism by estrogen replacement therapy as well as combined HRT. Both oral and transdermal estrogen were used in these studies. These findings are somewhat surprising in view of results obtained on intermittent markers of hemostatis. However, the risk of venous complications by the combined therapy is not greater than for estrogen alone, which again emphasizes the fact that progestogens are inert with respect to venous events.

Carbohydrate metabolism

The effect of estrogens on parameters of importance for carbohydrate metabolism is variable and possibly also dependent on the type of estrogen as well as route of administration. It would seem that estradiol performs better than conjugated equine estrogens although the database is not very large. In addition, transdermal estradiol may have an even more favorable effect.

Levonorgestrel and medroxyprogesterone induce insulin resistance whereas natural progesterone and possibly also dydrogesterone appear to have relatively minute effects. Norethisterone alone also seems to be relatively inert[13]. The postmenopausal estrogen/progestin interventions (PEPI) study[14] showed, during the oral glucose tolerance test, changes in the 2-h insulin response or 2-h glucose response. There was a significant deterioration in glucose tolerance associated with the Premarin plus medroxyprogesterone acetate (MPA) combi-nations. No overall changes in insulin were seen which is not too surprising considering the precision of the assay used in the study.

In a combination with estradiol plus dydrogesterone there were no changes in glucose reduction by insulin but some increase in C peptide, i.e. very similar to the pattern seen by estradiol alone. A comparative study with Premarin plus levonorgestrel and estradiol plus norethisterone acetate[15] found no difference between the two groups in the insulin sensitivity index. There was however, a significant deterioration with the Premarin plus levonorgestrel group in the intravenous glucose tolerance test, with no change in the reference of the norethisterone plus estradiol group. There was also a marked reduction in the initial plasma insulin response to glucose with the Premarin plus levonorgestrel combination,

421

which could well be responsible for the deterioration in glucose tolerance that was encountered in that group.

Lipid and lipoprotein metabolism

The bulk of data on metabolic effects by sex hormones is confined to lipids. In the routine serum lipid profile all estrogens reduce total and low-density lipoprotein (LDL) cholesterol but elevate high-density lipoprotein (HDL) cholesterol as well as triglycerides. Conjugated equine estrogens and particularly ethinyl-estradiol increase triglycerides more than does oral 17β-estradiol. Transdermal estradiol has little or no effect on HDL cholesterol, a similar effect on LDL cholesterol and tends to reduce triglycerides.

The effects of the addition of a progestogen vary depending on type and dose of the substance and conceivably by route of administration. The PEPI study[14] is a placebo-controlled study in which continuous and cyclical MPA plus Premarin were compared with Premarin alone and Premarin plus cyclical micronized progesterone. Again the typical changes were found in the MPA group with less of an increase in HDL than in the other treatment arms. The least impact on the lipid metabolic effects was seen in the group receiving natural progesterone. However, oral progesterone has a poor and variable bioavailability, but as data were also related to the effect on the endometrium, it is conceivable that the oral progesterone was absorbed in sufficient amounts. These data also support the view that progestogenic compounds derived from natural progesterone have the least impact on lipid metabolism. This is true to some extent for medroxyprogesterone but also for dydrogesterone. Other progesterones belonging to the 19-norethisterone derivatives have a lipid metabolic profile more closely related to their androgen properties.

The changes in HDL have also been studied in more detail; most of the reduction seems to be confined to the HDL-2 component in short-term studies. However, prolonged treatment with combined preparations also reduces HDL-3. Long-term studies on lipid metabolism are few, but in one 5-year study with estradiol and continuous norethisterone acetate the initially-observed reduction of HDL was not significant after 5 years[16]. However, the reduction in LDL cholesterol and total cholesterol persisted with time.

There are ample data to suggest that estrogen favorably affects certain aspects of the postmenopausal metabolic syndrome. The effect of the addition of progestogens is difficult to interpret especially in general terms, and each combination must be assessed on its own as the metabolic effect cannot be predicted from results of other combinations in any great detail. The clinical significance of these changes remains unclear.

Using the Cox proportional hazards model, Manolio and co-workers[17] determined that in an observational study the cardioprotective effect varied with HDL cholesterol and that roughly one-third of the protective mechanisms could be explained by increased HDL cholesterol. However, estrogen and progestogens affect so many of the parameters, and serum HDL cholesterol could simply be a marker of metabolic estrogenicity comprising several hundreds of variables.

An increasing number of reports have also emphasized the role of estradiol as an antioxidant. Albeit limited, existing data on the combined preparations and on progestogens imply that the antioxidant effect exerted by estrogens is not disturbed by the presence of a progestogen, at least not in doses of clinical significance in hormone replacement therapy[18,19].

Lipoprotein(a) is another substance that has recently come into focus. Both progestogens[20] and estrogens[21] on their own reduce levels of lipoprotein(a). Also combinations of estrogen and progestogen seem to have the same effect[22]. The clinical significance of this is under debate and it has recently been stated that the androgenicity of lipoprotein(a) is largely dependent on the prevailing LDL cholesterol concentration[23].

Low-density lipoprotein reduction seen after oral as well as transdermal estradiol is probably dependent on an increase in LDL receptors and thereby augmentation of the excretion of cholesterol into the bile. However, transdermal estradiol seems to lower LDL cholesterol as efficiently as the oral compound, despite the fact that the liver concentration of estrogen is much lower. Transdermal estradiol also seems to lower triglycerides. Lipoprotein lipase, after hydrolysing triglycerides in the periphery, attaches to lipoprotein remnants[24] which make existing hepatic LDL receptors more efficient. This may be at least part of the explanation as to why transdermal estradiol is as efficient an LDL cholesterol-lowering agent as is the oral compound.

Vessel wall physiology

Administration of 17β-estradiol to women with coronary artery disease seems to increase the time to ST-segment depression on exercise electrocardiogram (ECG). In hypertensive women (Pines and colleagues, personal communication) 6-month oral HRT induced a number of changes; however, there were no acute effects by the estrogen. After 6 months peak flow velocity increased and the mean acceleration time increased.

Acute effects on the vessel wall by estrogens may be different from more long-term effects. For the acute effects it would seem that estradiol can reverse and block the coronary constriction induced by acetylcholine in women with coronary artery disease. Gilligan and co-workers[25,26] have shown that women with hypertension or coronary artery disease respond to estrogens by vasodilatation both of large coronary conductance arteries and also the microvascular resistance arteries. In contrast to these profound effects in women they cannot be repeated in men[27]. These results with a gender difference also question the relevance of several animal experiments. Some arteries may respond differently when adding progestogens. Arteries belonging to the uterus or the vagina may be more sensitive to sex steroids than others. At least in short-term studies the addition of various progestogens diminishes the estrogenic vasodilatation and decreases blood flow in the genitalia. However, the relevance to the coronary artery of these studies is questionable. In cynomolgus monkeys the addition of MPA to estrogen-primed animals reduced blood flow in the coronary arteries. However, when the extent of atherosclerosis was considered along with the alterations of the arterial lumen, these changes were less abundant[28]. In humans data are still lacking on specific progestogen effects on the coronary arteries.

Vessel wall biochemistry

The reasons for effects on arteries by sex steroids are still obscure. It has been demonstrated that estrogens reduce endothelins and also impair the function of one of the endothelin receptors, and thereby impede endothelin-induced vasoconstriction. Estrogens have also been shown to have a calcium-blocking effect which again promotes vasodilatation. In addition, estrogens seem to influence nitric oxide metabolism again yielding vasodilatation[26].

Estrogen and possibly also progesterone receptors have been demonstrated within the heart itself and also in the coronary arteries. However, vasodilatation of coronary arteries is immediate rendering unlikely a classic genomic effect via the classical receptors. Much more research is needed to address these issues in greater detail.

Data on progestogens and progestogen addition are even less abundant than those of estrogens. Mechanisms, influenced by progestogens, in the vessel wall physiology and biochemistry are largely unknown.

Observational studies

An accumulating body of evidence also suggests that intermediate markers and metabolic endpoints are difficult to interpret in terms of importance for future cardiovascular disease. This is particularly prudent for various

Table 2 Cardiovascular disease and combined estrogen–progestogen replacement therapy. Swedish study by Falkeborn *et al.* used largely levonorgestrel, and in study by Hunt *et al.* norethisterone was also used. Medroxyprogesterone was predominating progestogen in other two studies

Reference (year)	Study design	Study size	Endpoints	Risk estimates
Nabulsi (1993)	cross-sectional	173 users	CHD	< 0.58
Nachtigall (1979)	clinical trial	84 pairs	MI	no increase
Thompson (1989) E alone, RR = 1.1	case–control	603 cases 1.206 controls	MI + CVD stroke	RR = 0.9
Hunt (1990)	cohort	4544	IHD	RR = 0.3
Falkeborn (1992)	cohort	23 000	MI, stroke	RR = 0.5
Psaty (1994) E alone, RR = 0.69	case–control	502 cases	MI	RR = 0.68

E, estrogen; CHD, coronary heart disease; MI, myocardial infarction; CVD, cardiovascular disease; IHD, ischemic heart disease; RR, relative risk

Table 3 Relative risk of cadiovascular disease among current users of conjugated estrogens alone or with progestogens as compared with non-users. Data from the Nurse Health Cohort Study. Reproduced from references 29 with permission

Hormone use	Person years	Major coronary disease			Stroke (all types)		
		No. of cases	Relative risk (95% CI)		No. of cases	Relative risk (95% CI)	
			Age adjusted	Multivariate adjusted*		Age adjusted	Multivariate adjusted*
Never used	304 744	431	1.0		270	1.0	
Currently used							
Estrogen alone	82 626	47	0.45 (0.34–0.60)	0.60 (0.43–0.83)	74	1.13 (0.88–1.46)	1.27 (0.95–1.69)
Estrogen with progestin	27 161	8	0.22 (0.12–0.41)	0.39 (0.19–0.78)	17	0.74 (0.45–1.20)	1.09 (0.66–1.80)

*The analysis was adjusted for age (in 5-year categories), time (in 2-year categories), age at menopause (in 2-year categories), body mass index (in quintiles), diabetes (yes or no), high blood pressure (yes or no), high cholesterol level (yes or no), cigarette smoking (never, formerly, or currently [1–14, 15–24, or 25 or more cigarettes per day]), past oral contraceptive use (yes or no), parental history of myocardial infarction before the age of 60 years (yes or no), and type of menopause (natural or surgical); CI, confidence interval

combinations of estrogens and progestogens where little data with hard endpoints are available. Unfortunately, few observational studies on combined therapy have been published, and Table 2 summarizes the published data. As can be inferred from this table it would seem that estrogen plus progestogen combinations have virtually the same cardioprotective effect as estrogen given alone. It seems to be true for levonorgestrel and MPA which are the two dominating progestogens that have been used. In the study by Hunt and associates some women also used norethisterone.

In addition, data from the Nurse Health Cohort Study indicate that there is at least the same degree of cardioprotection in women receiving conjugated equine estrogens alone as in those receiving estrogen plus MPA (Table 3)[29].

Acknowledgement

We are grateful to Marie Elmér for her assistance in the preparation of this report.

References

1. Bush, T. L., Barrett-Connor, E., Cowan, L. D., *et al.* (1987). Cardiovascular mortality and non-contraceptive estrogen use in women: results from the Lipid Research Clinic's Program Follow-Up Study. *Circulation*, **75**, 1002–9

2. Sullivan, J. M. (1994). Atherosclerosis and estrogen replacement therapy. *Int. J. Fertil.*, **39**, 28–35

3. Henderson, B. E., Ross, R. K., Lobo, R. A., Pike, M. C. and Mack, T. M. (1988). Re-evaluating the role of progestogen therapy after the menopause. *Fertil. Steril.*, **49**, 9S–15S

4. Ross, R. K., Pike, M. C., Henderson, B. E., Mack, T. M. and Lobo, R. A. (1989). Stroke prevention and oestrogen replacement therapy. *Lancet*, **1**, 505–7

5. Wren, B. (1994). Effects of estrogen and management of hypertension in women. In Lobo, R. (ed.) *Treatment of the Postmenopausal Woman. Basic and Clinical Effects*, pp. 283–7 (New York: Raven Press)

6. Lindoff, C., Peterson, F., Lecander, I., Martinsson, G. and Åstedt, B. (1993). Passage of the menopause is followed by haemostatic changes. *Maturitas*, **17**, 17–22

7. Winkler, U. H. (1992). Menopause, hormone replacement therapy and cardiovascular disease: a review of haemostaseological findings. *Fibrinolysis*, **6**, 5–10

8. Lindoff, C., Peterson, F., Lecander, I., Martinsson, G. and Åstedt, B. (1996). Transdermal oestrogen replacement therapy: beneficial effects on haemostatic risk factors for cardiovascular disease. *Maturitas*, **24**, 43–50

9. Notelovitz, M., Kitchens, C., Ware, M. *et al.* (1985). Combination estrogen and progestogen replacement therapy does not adversely affect coagulation. *Obstet. Gynecol. Surv.*, **44**, 425–36

10. Daly, E., Vessey, M. P., Hawkins, M. M. *et al.* (1996). Risk of venous thromboembolism in users of hormone replacement therapy. *Lancet*, **348**, 977–80

11. Jick, H., Derby, L. E., Wald Myers, M. *et al.* (1996). Risk of hospital admission for idiopathic venous thromboembolism among users of post-menopausal oestrogens. *Lancet*, **348**, 981–3

12. Grodstein, F., Stumpfer, M. J., Goldhaber, S. Z., *et al.* (1996). Prospective study of exogenous hormones and risk of pulmonary embolism in women. *Lancet*, **348**, 983–7

13. Stevenson, J. C., Proudler, A. J., Walton, C. and Godsland, I. F. (1994). HRT mechanism of action: carbohydrates. *Int. J. Fertil.*, **39**, 50–5

14. The Writing Group for the PEPI Trial. (1995). Effects of estrogen and estrogen/progestin regimens on heart disease: risk factors in postmenopausal women. The postmenopausal estrogen/progestin interventions (PEPI) trial. *J. Am. Med. Assoc.*, **273**, 199–207

15. Godsland, I. F., Gangar, K.F., Walton, C., *et al.* (1993). Insulin resistance, secretion and elimination in postmenopausal women receiving oral or transdermal hormone replacement therapy. *Metabolism*, **42**, 846–53

16. Christiansen, C. and Juel-Riis, B. (1990). Five years with continuous combined oestrogen/progestogen therapy. Effects on calcium metabolism, lipoproteins and bleeding pattern. *Br. J. Obstet. Gynaecol.*, **97**, 1087–92

17. Manolio, T. A., Furberg, C. D., Schemanski, L., Psaty, B. M., O'Leary, D. H., Tracy, R. P. and Bush, T. L. (1993). Associations of postmenopausal estrogen use with cardiovascular disease and its risk factors in older women. *Circulation*, **88**, 2163–71

18. Samsioe, G., Andersson, K. and Mattsson, L. Å. Relative fatty acid composition of serum lethitin in postmenopausal women receiving oral oestradiol combined with levonorgestrel in an intrauterine device or as tablets. Submitted for publication

19. Wiegratz, I., Hertwig, B., Jung-Hoffman, C. and Kuhl, H. (1996). Inhibition of low-density lipoprotein oxidation *in vitro* and *ex vivo* by several estrogens and oral contraceptives. *Gynecol. Endocrinol.*, **10** (Suppl. 2), 149–52

20. Farish, E., Rolton, H. A., Barnes, J. F. and Hart, D. M. (1991). Lipoprotein (a) concentrations in

postmenopausal women taking norethisterone. *Br. Med. J.,* **303**, 694–5

21. Kim, C. J., Jang, H. C., Cho, D. H., *et al.* (1994). Effects of hormone replacement therapy in lipoprotein(a) and lipids in postmenopausal women. *Arterioscler. Thromb.,* **14**, 275–81

22. Nabulsi, A. A., Aaron, B., Folsom, R., *et al.* (1993). Association of hormone replacement therapy with various cardiovascular risk factors in postmenopausal women. *N. Engl. J. Med.,* **328**, 1070–5

23. Maher, V. M. G. and Brown, G. (1995). Lipoprotein(a) and coronary heart disease. *Curr. Opin. Lipidol.,* **6**, 229–35

24. Beisiegel, U. (1995). Receptors for triglyceride-rich lipoproteins and their role in lipoprotein metabolism. *Curr. Opin. Lipidol.,* **6**, 117–22

25. Gilligan, D. M., Badar, D. M., Panza, J. A., Quyyumi, A. A. and Cannon, R. O. (1994). Acute vascular effects of estrogen in postmenopausal women. *Circulation,* **90**, 786–91

26. Gilligan, D. M., Badar, D. M., Panza, J. A., Quyyumi, A. A. and Cannon, R. O. (1995). Effects of estrogen replacement therapy on peripheral vasomotor function in post-menopausal women. *Am. J. Cardiol.,* **75**, 264–8

27. Collins, P., Rosano, G. M. C., Sarrel, P. M., *et al.* (1995). Estradiol-17β attenuates acetylcholine-induced coronary arterial constriction in women but not men with coronary heart disease. *Circulation,* **92**, 24–30

28. Clarkson, T. B., Adams, M. R., Williams, J. K., *et al.* (1993). Clinical implications of animal models of gender difference in heart disease. In Douglas, P. S. (ed.) *Cardiovascular Health and Disease in Women,* pp. 283–302. (Philadelphia, PA: W. B. Saunders)

29. Grodstein, F., Stampfer, M. J., Manson, J. E., *et al.* (1996). Postmenopausal estrogen and progestin use and the risk of cardiovascular disease. *N. Engl. J. Med.,* **335**, 453–61

In vitro and *in vivo* effects of estrogens on prostacyclin and thromboxane and on other vasoactive compounds

59

A. O. Mueck, H. Seeger and T. H. Lippert

Introduction

Estrogens may influence vasomotor tone by endothelium-dependent and endothelium-independent mechanism(s). Effects of estrogens on the synthesis of vasoactive agents like nitric oxide (NO) and the eicosanoids prostacyclin and thromboxane, as well as on alteration of intracellular calcium concentrations in vascular cells may be responsible for their vasodilatory properties.

In the following our *in vitro* investigations regarding the influence of estrogens on the synthesis of vasoactive substances and on calcium homeostasis in human vascular cell cultures will be summarized and discussed. In addition, we report on our *in vivo* studies, measuring the urinary excretion of vasoactive substances or their stable metabolites as surrogate markers, for the effect of treatment with transdermal and oral estradiol in postmenopausal women.

In vitro investigations

The prostacyclin/thromboxane ratio is important for the regulation of vasomotor tone, since prostacyclin is a vasodilatory, and thromboxane a vasoconstrictory agent. Prostacyclin is mainly synthesized in endothelial cells, whereas thromboxane is mainly produced in platelets but also can be generated in endothelial cells. We evaluated prostacyclin and thromboxane synthesis in cell cultures of human endothelial veins after addition of 17β-estradiol, by measuring the stable metabolites 6-keto-prostaglandin $F_{1\alpha}$ (6-keto-PGF$_{1\alpha}$) and

thromboxane B_2 (TXB$_2$), respectively. After incubation for 24, 48 and 72 h no significant changes in the concentrations of 6-keto-PGF$_{1\alpha}$ and TXB$_2$ could be observed[1]. An interesting result, however, could be obtained by the addition of endothelin-1, a vasoconstrictory endothelium-derived agent, to estradiol. Endothelin alone only slightly increased the production of 6-keto-PGF$_{1\alpha}$ which can be interpreted as an endothelium counteraction. In combination with estradiol, however, the 6-keto-PGF$_{1\alpha}$ production was enhanced by a factor of nearly 10 compared with the effect of endothelin alone (Figure 1). This result alludes to a potent estradiol-mediated compensatory vasodilating reaction of the vasoconstrictory-stimulated endothelium.

Nitric oxide (NO) is a potent vasodilatory and anti-thrombogenic substance, which is produced in the vascular endothelium. Since methods for its determination in biological fluids are difficult to perform, we measured cyclic guanylate monophosphate (cGMP) which closely reflects the NO production. We have evaluated the effect of 17β-estradiol in homogenates of human leg veins obtained at bypass operations[2]. Estradiol was not able to increase cGMP concentrations after addition of L-arginine, the natural substrate for NO-synthase, although a tendency to higher values compared with the control values was observed. Statistical significance is lacking probably due to the short incubation time of 1 h. Estradiol seems to affect the activity of NO-synthase thereby elevating cGMP concentrations *in vitro*

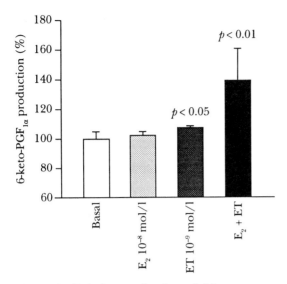

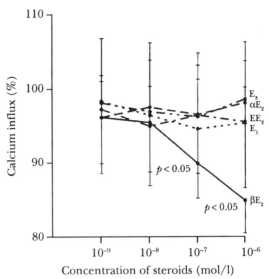

Figure 1 Relative production of 6-keto-prostaglandin $F_{1\alpha}$ (6-keto-$PGF_{1\alpha}$), expressed as percentages of basal values, in endothelial cell cultures from human umbilical cord veins after addition of endothelin-1 (ET) and 17β-estradiol (E_2) alone or in combination (mean + SD, $n = 5$). Significant differences compared with basal value

Figure 2 Changes in intracellular ^{45}Ca-uptake in depolarized human vascular smooth muscle cell cultures after addition of 17β-estradiol (βE_2), estrone (E_1), estriol (E_3), 17α-estradiol (αE_2) and 17α-ethinylestradiol (EE_2). Ordinate, percentage of ^{45}Ca-uptake in relation to basal value = 100%; abscissa, molar concentrations of steroids (mean ± SD, $n = 8$). Significant differences compared with basal value

only after long-term incubation. Measuring urinary excretion of cGMP in postmenopausal women after 4 weeks' treatment with estradiol likewise revealed only a tendency of cGMP levels to increase[2]. This result may indicate that only intracellularly measured cGMP concentrations can reflect NO production correctly.

Recently evidence emerged in animal experiments of a vasodilatory estradiol effect by influencing voltage-dependent calcium channels directly. In cell cultures of human aortic smooth muscle cells we have examined the effect of the estrogens 17β-estradiol, 17α-estradiol, estrone, estriol and 17α-ethinyl-estradiol on calcium influx, by investigating the intracellular uptake of radio-labelled calcium after depolarization of the cells with KCl solution. Only 17β-estradiol had an inhibitory effect on calcium influx at the concentrations of 10^{-6} and 10^{-7} mol/l, the greatest reduction being about 20% (Figure 2). However, the other estrogens also may exhibit a calcium-antagonistic effect which might be measurable

only with more sensitive methods like the patch-clamp technique.

We also compared 17β-estradiol with the well-known antagonist nifedipine, and found that the inhibition of calcium influx by estradiol was only one-third that of nifedipine[3]. Further experiments were conducted in polarized, i.e. resting cell cultures. Under these conditions, 17β-estradiol inhibited calcium influx to the same degree as observed under depolarized conditions. This may hint at an effect of estradiol on so-called leak calcium channels.

In vivo investigations

In our *in vivo* investigations we measured urinary excretion of vasoactive substances or their stable metabolites as surrogate markers for the effect of estradiol on the vascular endothelium.

Table 1 Ratios of prostacyclin to thromboxane (TX) metabolites in urine of postmenopausal women, before and after 14 and 28 days of estrogen treatment (mean ± SD). PG, prostaglandin

	$6\text{-keto-PGF}_{1\alpha}/TXB_2$	$Dinor\text{-}6\text{-keto-PGF}_{1\alpha}/Dinor\text{-}TXB_2$
Transdermal estrogen ($n = 19$)		
Before treatment	3.9 ± 4.1	3.6 ± 1.8
14 days' treatment	4.6 ± 3.5	4.9 ± 3.8
28 days' treatment	6.1 ± 4.4**	7.5 ± 5.4
Oral estrogen ($n = 18$)		
Before treatment	4.9 ± 7.0	5.8 ± 4.5
14 days' treatment	5.8 ± 4.5**	8.2 ± 8.8**
28 days' treatment	5.8 ± 4.1**	10.9 ± 11.3**

**$p < 0.01$

The urinary excretion of the following stable metabolites of prostacyclin and thromboxane were determined during treatment with transdermal and oral estradiol for 4 weeks in 40 postmenopausal women: 6-keto-PGF$_{1\alpha}$, 2,3-dinor-6-keto-PGF$_{1\alpha}$, TXB$_2$ and 2,3-dinor-TXB$_2$. In addition, the urinary concentrations of the stable serotonin metabolite, 5-hydroxindole acetic acid, the stable melatonin metabolite, 6-sulfatoxy-melatonin and the urinary excretion of relaxin were measured. Urine, excreted between 22.00 and 6.00, was collected before and after 2 and 4 weeks' estradiol treatment. The collection of urine during the night provided a convenient and reliable way of sampling as well as a concise comparable time period, well defined by the resting condition during sleep.

The prostacyclin metabolites were enhanced after oral estradiol treatment, and the thromboxane metabolites were decreased after transdermal treatment compared with the pretreatment value. Thus both administration routes positively influenced the prostacyclin/thromboxane ratio as shown in Table 1[4].

The indoleamine serotonin has been shown to elicit vasodilatation in human coronary arteries with an intact endothelium, whereas it provokes vasoconstriction in coronary arteries with a damaged endothelium. We found a significant urinary increase of the serotonin-metabolite after transdermal estradiol treatment (Figure 3). This hints at a possible participation of serotonin in mediating the vasodilatory action of estradiol[5].

The pineal hormone melatonin is believed to influence vascular tonus. However, neither transdermal nor oral estradiol treatment for 4 weeks exhibited significant effects on melatonin production. It was remarkable that although the response of different patients was not predictable, individual profiles consistently show either stimulation or inhibition after estradiol treatment. Currently, this is under further investigation.

Another vasoactive substance is relaxin, a polypeptide hormone mainly known for its uterus relaxing activity in pregnant women. Evidence is emerging that relaxin influences the cardiovascular system by developing inotropic and chronotropic effects as well as vasodilatation and lowering of blood pressure[6]. Figure 4 shows the results of our investigation. Urinary relaxin concentrations were significantly elevated after 4 weeks of transdermal estradiol treatment. Thus relaxin may also play a role as mediator of estradiol-elicited vasodilatation. However, the source of relaxin in women with atrophic ovaries and uteri is still unclear.

Administration of transdermal or oral estradiol treatment apparently leads to different urinary excretion profiles of the surrogate

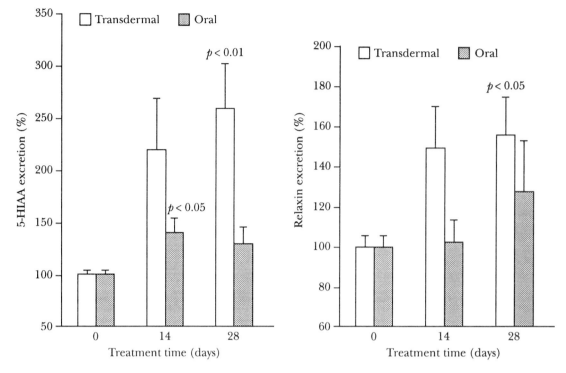

Figure 3 Urinary excretion of 5-hydroxyindole acetic acid (5-HIAA) as percentage of pretreatment value (100%) after transdermal ($n = 18$) and oral ($n = 17$) estradiol treatment (mean ± SEM). Significant differences compared with basal value

Figure 4 Urinary excretion of relaxin as percentage of pretreatment value (100%) after transdermal ($n = 13$) and oral ($n = 12$) estradiol treatment (mean ± SEM). Significant difference compared with basal value

markers measured. The reason for this phenomenon may be the different pharmacokinetic profiles of the two treatment routes. Continuous steady-state plasma levels of estradiol, as achieved by transdermal application, perhaps affect peripheral vasculature to a greater extent than oral administration with its high peak levels which are reached only for a short time after

administration. This issue has to be elucidated by further studies.

Conclusion

In summary, our *in vitro* and *in vivo* investigations of the mechanisms of vasodilatation elicited by estrogens indicate an involvement of a complex array of mediators.

References

1. Mueck, A. O., Seeger, H., Korte, K., Dartsch, P. C. and Lippert, T. H. (1993). Natural and synthetic estrogens on prostacyclin production in human endothelial cells from umbilical cord and leg veins. *Prostaglandins*, **45**, 517–25
2. Mueck, A. O., Seeger, H., Korte, K., Haasis, R. and Lippert, T. H. (1994). Is there any effect of estradiol on the vasodilating NO/cGMP-system? Investigations of the mechanism of cardiovascular protection by estrogen substitution in postmenopausal women. *Zentralbl. Gynäkol.*, **116**, 507–11

3. Seeger, H., Mueck, A. O. and Lippert, T. H. (1995). Comparison of the effect of estradiol with calcium channel blockers – *in vitro* investigations of calcium influx in human aortic smooth muscle cells. *Pharm. Pharmacol. Lett.*, **5**, 132–4

4. Mueck, A. O., Seeger, H., Wiesner, J., Korte, K. and Lippert, T. H. (1994). Urinary prostanoids in postmenopausal women after transdermal and oral oestrogen. *J. Obstet. Gynaecol.*, **14**, 341–5

5. Lippert, T. H., Filshie, G. M., Mueck, A. O., Seeger, H. and Zwirner, M. (1996). Serotonin metabolite excretion after postmenopausal estradiol therapy. *Maturitas*, **24**, 37–41

6. Lippert, T. H., Armbruster, F. P., Seeger, H., Mueck, A. O., Zwirner, M. and Voelter, W. (1996). Urinary excretion of relaxin after estradiol treatment of postmenopausal women. *Clin. Exp. Obstet. Gynecol.*, **23**, 65–9

Long-term effects of cyclic combined conjugated estrogens and dydrogesterone in postmenopausal women

60

M. Gambacciani, M. Ciaponi, B. Cappagli, L. Piaggesi, C. Benussi,
S. Picchetti and A. R. Genazzani

Introduction

Hormonal replacement therapy is currently used for the control of climacteric symptoms, and for the prevention of long-term consequences of menopause. Chronic hypoestrogenism in postmenopausal years causes a critical decrease in bone mineral density (BMD) that is an important determinant of fracture risk[1-3]. Estrogen replacement therapy prevents the lowering of BMD related to peri- and postmenopausal hypoestrogenism[4-7]. In addition, postmenopausal estrogen supplementation can exert cardioprotective effects with substantial reduction of morbidity and mortality for cardiovascular disease[8-16]. During estrogen therapy, progestin supplementation is mandatory to prevent endometrial hyperstimulation[17-23]. However, the administration of progestogens can jeopardize the beneficial effects of estrogens on cardiovascular protection[24,25]. The metabolic effects depend on the type and dose of progestogens. Dydrogesterone (DD) is a potent orally active progestogen, similar to endogenous progesterone in its molecular structure and biological actions, and devoid of any androgenic, anabolic or estrogenic effect[26-31]. Sequential DD administration was reported to antagonize the estrogenic effect on endometrial proliferation[26-31]. In the present paper we report clinical and metabolic effects of the long-term administration of DD in combination with conjugated estrogens (CE) in early postmenopausal women.

Materials and methods

We report the data concerning postmenopausal women recruited from the Climacteric Clinic of our department. The women had amenorrhea for at least 6 months before treatment, and plasma gonadotropin and estradiol levels in the postmenopausal range according to our laboratory (follicle-stimulating hormone (FSH) > 40 U/l; estradiol < 25 pg/ml). All patients were free of disease known to influence calcium metabolism, and none had a history of glucocorticoid treatment. They all had normal thyroid, adrenal and renal function, as assessed by clinical, biochemical and hormonal evaluations. None had been treated with hormones in the 6 months before the study. Of these postmenopausal women, 20 subjects (group 1) received a single calcium supplement (calcium carbonate and lactogluconate at the dose of 500 mg/day) with the evening meal; 20 postmenopausal women were treated with cyclic combined CE (0.625 mg/day) and DD (5 mg/day) for 21 days with a 7-day free interval (group 2). The groups were well matched with no difference in age, menopausal state, or hormonal levels. The subjects in the CE + DD group underwent either an outpatient's hysteroscopy or endometrial biopsy before and after 36 months of treatment. No other medication was allowed during the study. At the end of the study period we were able to evaluate 10 subjects in the control group; the others were lost to follow-up or required treatment for their climacteric symptoms. The 10 control subjects also presented mild to moderate menopausal symptoms, and no abnormal uterine bleeding. In the CE + DD group data were available for 18 patients; two patients were lost to follow-up. The lipid profile, as well as fasting urinary hydroxyproline/creatinine (FU Hpr/Cr) and lumbar spine (L2–L4) bone mineral density (BMD) were measured as previously reported[32]. The results are reported as the mean ± SD. Factorial analysis of variance was used to compare baseline values, and two-way analysis of variance for repeated measures was used to analyze the longitudinal data, as appropriate. The *post-hoc* comparison was made using Scheffe's F-test.

Results

No significant differences in the basal values of lipid parameters, FU Hpr/Cr and lumbar spine BMD were evidenced between the two groups before the study (data not shown). The administration of CE + DD was highly effective in reducing hot flushes and other clinical symptoms related to the estrogen deficiency (data not shown). In Group 1 constant levels of urinary excretion of FU Hpr/Cr were observed (Figure 1). In this group vertebral BMD showed a significant ($p < 0.05$) decrease after 12, 18, 24 and 36 months (Figure 2). In group 2 urinary excretion of FU Hpr/Cr significantly ($p < 0.05$) decreased after 6, 12, 18, 24 and 36 months (Figure 1). In this group vertebral BMD showed a significant ($p < 0.05$) increase after 12, 18, 24 and 36 months (Figure 2). The two-way analysis of variance showed that the patterns of bone biochemical marker and BMD were significantly ($p < 0.001$) different in the two groups. In group 1 a slight but significant ($p < 0.05$) increase in serum low-density lipoprotein (LDL) cholesterol levels was detected after 12 months of observation (Figure 3), whereas no significant modification in total cholesterol, high-density lipoprotein (HDL) cholesterol and triglycerides was observed (Figures 4, 5 and 6). In CE + DD-treated subjects, total cholesterol significantly ($p < 0.05$) decreased after 6, 12, 18, 24 and 36 months (Figure 4). Plasma LDL

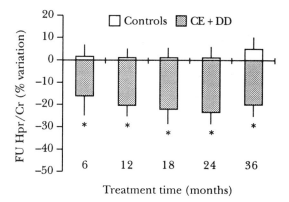

Figure 1 Fasting urinary hydroxyproline/creatinine (FU Hpr/Cr) excretion in control and conjugated estrogens plus dydrogesterone (CE + DD)-treated group during 3-year follow-up study. Results are reported as percentage variation over corresponding basal values. *$p < 0.05$ vs. corresponding basal values

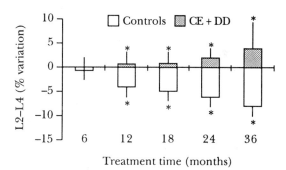

Figure 2 Lumbar spine (L2–L4) bone mineral density (BMD) in control and conjugated estrogens plus dydrogesterone (CE + DD)-treated group during 3-year follow-up study. Results are reported as percentage variation over corresponding basal values. *$p < 0.05$ vs. corresponding basal values

cholesterol significantly ($p < 0.05$) decreased after 6, 18, 24 and 36 months (Figure 3), while triglyceride levels showed a slight but not significant increase throughout the study (Figure 6). In this group HDL cholesterol levels showed a significant ($p < 0.05$) increase after 6, 18, 24 and 36 months (Figure 5). The two-way analysis of variance showed that total cholesterol, HDL and LDL cholesterol profiles were significantly ($p < 0.01$) different in the two

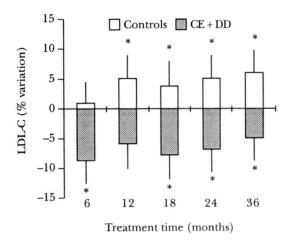

Figure 3 Low-density lipoprotein cholesterol (LDL-C) in control and conjugated estrogens plus dydrogesterone (CE + DD)-treated group during 3-year follow-up study. Results are reported as percentage variation over corresponding basal values. *$p < 0.05$ vs. corresponding basal values

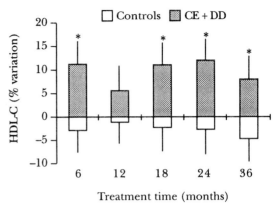

Figure 5 Serum high-density lipoprotein cholesterol (HDL-C) levels in control and conjugated estrogens plus dydrogesterone (CE + DD)-treated group during 3-year follow-up study. Results are reported as percentage variation over corresponding basal values. *$p < 0.05$ vs. corresponding basal values

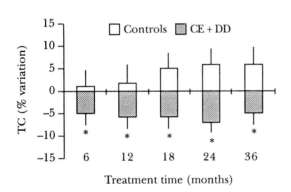

Figure 4 Serum total cholesterol (TC) levels in control and conjugated estrogens plus dydrogesterone (CE + DD)-treated group during 3-year follow-up study. Results are reported as percentage variation over corresponding basal values. *$p < 0.05$ vs. corresponding basal values

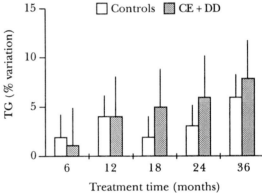

Figure 6 Serum triglycerides (TG) levels in control and conjugated estrogens plus dydrogesterone (CE + DD)-treated group during 3-year follow-up study. Results are reported as percentage variation over corresponding basal values. *$p < 0.05$ vs. corresponding basal values

groups, whereas no difference was observed in triglyceride profiles. Dydrogesterone did not induce premenstrual syndrome (PMS)-like symptoms. Only a mild breast tenderness was experienced during the first 3 months of treatment in five subjects. To analyze the effects of CE + DD on bleeding pattern, we reviewed

the patients' diaries and calculated and recorded the days with bleeding during each study month. Of 24 patients, eight postmenopausal women were amenorrheic after 1 month, five after 3 and three after 6 months throughout the study. The other women reported a regular, short-lasting bleeding

(Figure 7). Withdrawal bleeds were regular, starting 1–2 days after the last treatment day and defined as light or mild. After 36 months of treatment, no sign of endometrial hyperstimulation was evident at the hysteroscopic and bioptic evaluation (Figure 8).

Conclusion

This study extends a previous report[32], showing that the DD low dose in combination with CE provides effective protection against postmenopausal osteopenia, and can antagonize the endometrial proliferation, but does not negate the effects of estrogens on lipid profile. The potentially negative metabolic effects of added progestogen are related to the dose and the androgenic potency of the hormone preparation, and the concomitant dose of estrogens[8–16]. It is often stated that the pregnane derivatives exert no adverse effects on lipid profile. However, we also have to take into account that pregnane derivatives may negate or even reverse the beneficial estrogen effects, depending on the dose and the type (cyclic vs. continuous) of regimen[33–35]. A dose of 10 mg/day of DD can be as effective as 5 mg of medroxyprogesterone acetate (MPA) on postmenopausal estrogen-primed endometrium[22]. In addition, MPA in doses as low as 2.5 mg/day on a sequential basis can be sufficient to reverse the estrogenic endometrial stimuli in terms of the number of estrogen receptors[23], and thus virtually eliminate the risk of endometrial hyperplasia. In a large prospective study[36], endometrial hyperplasia was present in less than 1% of 279 patients taking 0.625 mg CE plus 2.5 mg/day of MPA. In the present study, we have used a dose of DD that could be seen as equivalent to a 2.5 mg dose of MPA. The hysteroscopic and histological results seem to demonstrate that the dose of 5 mg/day DD is able to induce a safe endo-metrial transformation and well-controlled endometrial shedding. No evidence of endometrial hyperplasia was found after 36 months of treatment in the hysteroscopic–bioptic evaluation. In the present study most women

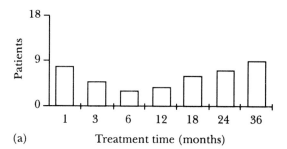

(a)

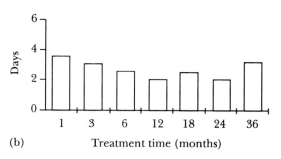

(b)

Figure 7 Number of subjects presenting with amenorrhea (a) and mean days of bleeding (b) in patients treated with cyclic combined conjugated estrogens plus dydrogesterone

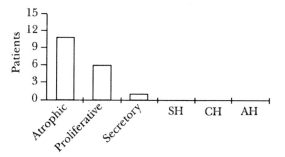

Figure 8 Histological results from endometrial specimens obtained after 36 months of treatment with cyclic combined conjugated estrogens plus dydrogesterone. SH, simple hyperplasia; CH, cystic hyperplasia; AH, atypical hyperplasia

had regular bleeding that was moderate in the early treatment period. After a few months bleedings were further reduced. Sequential progestogens are widely used in addition to continuous estrogens, but most postmenopausal women treated for 10 or more days on a monthly basis will experience withdrawal bleeding which can be copious and long-lasting. Bleeding can be a cause of a high drop-out rate. Different studies have reported that continuous combined estrogen–progestin formulations offer several benefits in com-parison to the standard sequential admini-stration of hormones[35–37]. However, the daily continuous combined hormone replacement therapy can induce annoying breakthrough bleeding and spotting that can result in a drop-out rate as high as 38% during the first few months of treatment[35]. The formula for cyclic combined estrogen–progestogen therapy reduces bleeding disturbances and results in a high continuation rate. Further studies are required to confirm the long-term beneficial effects of this formula on cardiovascular protection and fracture rate.

References

1. Riggs, B. L., Wahner, H. W., Dunn, W. L., Mazess, R. B., Offord, K. P. and Melton, L. J. III. (1981). Differential changes in bone mineral density of the appendicular and axial skeleton with ageing. *J. Clin. Invest.*, **67**, 328–35
2. Gambacciani, M., Spinetti, A., De Simone, L., Cappagli, B., Maffei, S., Taponeco, F. and Fioretti, P. (1993). The relative contribution of menopause and aging to postmenopausal vertebral osteopenia. *J. Clin. Endocrinol. Metab.*, **77**, 1148–52
3. Nilas, L. and Christiansen, C. (1989). The pathophysiology of peri- and postmenopausal bone loss. *Br. J. Obstet. Gynaecol.*, **96**, 580–7
4. Wallach, S. and Henneman, P. (1959). Prolonged estrogen therapy in postmenopausal women. *J. Am. Med. Assoc.*, **171**, 1637–40
5. Lindsay, R. (1987). Estrogen therapy in the prevention and management of osteoporosis. *Am. J. Obstet. Gynecol.*, **156**, 1347–51
6. Gambacciani, M., Spinetti, A., Taponeco, F., Cappagli, B., Manetti, P., Piaggesi, L. and Fioretti, P. (1994). Longitudinal evaluation of pre-menopausal vertebral bone loss: effects of a low dose oral contraceptive preparation on bone mincral density and metabolism. *Obstet. Gynecol.*, **8**, 392–4
7. Noteloviz, M. (1993). Osteoporosis: screening, prevention, and management. *Fertil. Steril.*, **59**, 707–25
8. Bush, T. L. and Barrett-Connor, E. (1985). Noncontraceptive estrogen use and cardiovascular disease. *Epidemiol. Rev.*, **7**, 80–104
9. Rosenberg, L., Armstrong, B. and Jick, H. (1976). Myocardial infarction and estrogen therapy in postmenopausal women. *N. Engl. J. Med.*, **294**, 1256–9
10. Ross, R. K., Paganini-Hill, A., Mack, T. M., *et al.*, (1981). Menopausal oestrogen therapy and protection from death from ischaemic heart disease. *Lancet*, **18**, 858–62
11. Henderson, B. E., Ross, R. K., Paganini-Hill, A. and Mach, T. M. (1986). Estrogen use and cardiovascular disease. *Am. J. Obstet. Gynecol.*, **154**, 1181–6
12. Henderson, B. E., Paganini-Hill, A. and Ross, R. K. (1988). Estrogen replacement therapy and protection from acute myocardial infarction. *Am. J. Obstet. Gynecol.*, **159**, 312–17
13. Stampfer, M. J., Colditz, G. A., Willet, W. C., *et al.* (1991). Postmenopausal estrogen therapy and cardiovascular disease: ten-year follow-up from the Nurses' Health Study. *N. Engl. J. Med.*, **325**, 756–62
14. Session, D. R., Kelly, A. C. and Jewelewicz, R. (1993). Current concepts in estrogen replace-ment therapy in the menopause. *Fertil. Steril.*, **2**, 277–84
15. Mason, C. A. (1994). Primary care for postreproductive women: further thoughts concerning steroid replacement. *Am. J. Obstet. Gynecol.*, **170**, 936–66
16. Lobo, R. A. and Speroff, L. (1994). International consensus conference on postmenopausal hormone therapy and the cardiovascular system. *Fertil. Steril.*, **61**, 592–5
17. Whitehead, M. I., Townsend, P. T., Pryse-Davies, J., *et al.* (1982). Effects of various types and dosages of progestogens on the postmenopausal endometrium. *J. Reprod. Med.*, **27**, 539
18. Campbell, S., Minardi, J., McQueen, J., *et al.* (1978). Endometrial factors: the modifying effect of progestogen on the response of the postmenopausal endometrium to exogenous estrogens. *Postgrad. Med. J.*, **54**, 59–61
19. Gambrell, R. D., Massey, F. M., Castanedo, T. A., Ugenas, A. Y., Ricci, C. A. and Wright, Y. M. (1980). Use of the progestogen challenge test to reduce the risk of endometrial cancer. *Obstet. Gynecol.*, **55**, 732–8
20. Sturdel, D. W., Wade-Evans, T., Paterson, M. E. L., Thom, M. and Studd, J. W. W. (1978). Re-

lations between bleeding pattern, endometrial histology, and estrogen treatment in menopausal women. *Br. Med. J.*, **1**, 1575–7

21. Paterson, M. E. L., Wade-Evans, T., Sturdee, D. W., Thom, M. H. and Studd, J. W. W. (1980). Endometrial disease with oestrogens and progestogens in the climacteric. *Br. Med. J.*, **280**, 822–4

22. King, R. Y. B. and Whitehead, M. I. (1986). Assessment of the potency of orally administered progestins in women. *Fertil. Steril.*, **46**, 1062–5

23. Gibbson, W. E., Moyer, D. L., Lobo, R. A., Roy, S. and Mishell, D. R. (1986). Biochemical and histologic effects of sequential estrogen/progestin therapy on the endometrium of postmenopausal women. *Am. J. Obstet. Gynecol.*, **154**, 456–61

24. Ottson, U. B. (1984). Oral progesterone and estrogen–progesterone therapy. Effects of natural and synthetic hormones on subfractions of HDL cholesterol and liver proteins. *Acta Obstet. Gynecol. Scand.*, **127**, 1–37

25. Fahraeus, L., Larsson-Cohn, U. and Wallentin, L. (1983). L-norgestrel and progesterone have different influences on plasma lipoproteins. *Eur. J. Clin. Invest.*, **13**, 447–53

26. Campagnoli, C., Belforte, P., Maraschiello, T., *et al.* (1986). Oral estradiol valerate for treatment of the climacteric syndrome and prevention of bone loss in women in spontaneous menopause. In Genazzani, A. R., Volpe, A., Facchinetti, F., (eds.) *Research on Gynecological Endocrinology*, pp. 495–9. (Carnforth, UK: Parthenon Publishing)

27. Candron, Y. and Hendrickx, B. (1988). Comparison of two equine estrogen–dydrogesterone regimens in the climacteric. *Maturitas*, **10**, 133–41

28. Fletcher, C. D., Farish, E., Dagen, M. M., *et al.* (1988). The effects of conjugated equine estrogens plus cyclical dydrogesterone on serum lipoproteins and apoproteins in postmenopausal women. *Acta Endocrinol.*, **117**, 339–42

29. Henderson, B. E., Ross, R. K., Lobo, R. A., Pike, M. C. and Mack, T. M. (1988). Re-evaluating the role of progestogen therapy after the menopause. *Fertil. Steril.*, **49**(Suppl.), 9–15

30. De Cleyn, K., Buytaert, P., Delbeke, L. and Gerris, J. (1986). Equine estrogen–dydrogesterone therapy in the management of postmenopausal women. *Eur. J. Obstet. Gynecol. Reprod. Biol.*, **23**, 201–9

31. Whitehead, M. I., Hillard, T. C. and Crook, D. (1990). The role and use of progestogens. *Obstet. Gynecol.*, **4**(Suppl.), 59–76

32. Gambacciani, M., Spinetti, A., *et al.* (1995). Cyclic-combined conjugated estrogens and dydrogesterone in the treatment of post-menopausal syndrome. *Menopause*, **2**, 19–25

33. Miller, V. T., Muesing, R. A., LaRosa, J. C., Stoy, D., Fowler, S. E. and Robert, J. S. (1994). Quantitative and qualitative changes in lipids, lipoproteins, apolipoprotein A-I, and sex hormone-binding globulin due to two doses of conjugated equine estrogen with and without a progestin. *Obstet. Gynecol.*, **83**, 173–9

34. Hirvonen, E., Malkonen, M. and Mannien, V. (1981). Effects of different progestogens on lipoproteins during postmenopausal replacement therapy. *N. Eng. J. Med.*, **304**, 560–3

35. Weinstein, L., Bewtra, C. and Gallagher, C. (1990). Evaluation of a continuous combined low-dose regimen of estrogen–progestin for treatment of the menopausal patient. *Am. J. Obstet. Gynecol.*, **162**, 1534–9

36. Woodruff, D. J. and Pickar, J. H. (1994). Incidence of endometrial hyperplasia in postmenopausal women taking conjugated estrogens (Premarin) with medroxyprogesterone acetate or conjugated estrogens alone. *Am. J. Obstet. Gynecol.*, **170**, 1213–23

37. Magos, A. L., Brincat, M., Studd, J. W. W., *et al.* (1985). Amenorrhea and endometrial atrophy with continuous oral estrogen and progestogen therapy in postmenopausal women. *Obstet. Gynecol.*, **65**, 496–8

15

Compliance with hormonal therapy

How can compliance be improved in a general practice setting?   61

P.-J. Roberts

Compliance

Compliance has been defined as 'the extent to which a patient's behavior coincides with the medical or health advice given'[1]. Hormone replacement therapy (HRT) needs to be taken long-term to prevent osteoporosis and cardiovascular disease[2] with poor long-term compliance reducing the effectiveness of HRT. The problem of non-compliance was recognized by Hippocrates in 200 BC. Non-compliance with HRT encompasses a spectrum of activities and behaviors ranging from failure to redeem prescriptions[3,4] and intermittent use of therapy[5], to discontinuation of therapy once it has been commenced[6].

Current use of hormone replacement therapy

The majority of perimenopausal and postmenopausal women internationally do not use HRT and of those who commence HRT, a high proportion discontinue it within a year.

Women's use of HRT varies between countries and ranges from 3% of women in Italy to 12% of women in France and 25% of women in Germany[7]. Less than 20% of American women[8] and less than 10% of British women use HRT[7,9–12]. Compliance has been found to be low amongst women in the UK[13], Belgium[14], The Netherlands[15], Australia[16] and the USA[17].

Factors affecting compliance

Patient-related factors

Low use of HRT results from poor uptake and discontinuation of therapy. The poor uptake of HRT is due to a lack of awareness amongst women about HRT[18], incomplete and often inaccurate knowledge about both the menopause and HRT[11,13,19], women not consulting their health advisors about menopausal problems and HRT[11,18,20], and reluctance to take HRT[21]. Women may not wish to take HRT for a number of reasons including the fear of breast cancer, concerns about side-effects and viewing the menopause as a natural transition[22]. Uptake of HRT appears to be the main constraining factor on the use of HRT for osteoporosis prevention in the UK[23].

Women discontinue HRT because of bleeding[13,16] and other side-effects[24,25] and because HRT does not meet their expectations[26]. Other reasons for discontinuing HRT include concerns about long-term side-effects[23] and fear of weight gain[27]. Women who develop problems with HRT tend to discontinue therapy rather than request modification of the regime[28] and many stop HRT without telling their general practitioner[13]. The majority of women use HRT to treat menopausal symptoms[13,19,23], some women completing a 'course' but forgetting to get a renewal of their HRT[13,16].

The media are a powerful source of information about HRT for many women[7,19,20]. However, although women's images of the media are mostly positive, some women find the media to be unhelpful or incorrect[29]. General practitioners felt that media interest had led to increased patient anxiety, expectations, requests for HRT and consulting rates[30].

Doctor-related factors and primary health care

The medical profession is the third commonest source of information on the menopause and HRT amongst European women after the media, friends and relatives[7]. Nevertheless, the advice of a doctor is a major influence on women's decisions whether or not to use HRT[11,31,32]. In Germany and France gynecologists are an important source of information about the menopause and HRT. In contrast, in the UK women have access to a gynecologist only via their general practitioners, and general practitioners and practice nurses are the most important people in helping women to decide about therapy[29].

In the UK both general practitioners' attitudes to prescribing HRT and prescribing rates for HRT have varied widely[9,10]. There has been confusion about the reported effects of HRT on the risks of endometrial carcinoma and on ischemic heart disease[33], and there is considerable variation of opinion amongst general practitioners about the long-term use of HRT[12,33,34]. General practitioners were found to need more information about HRT and more evidence about long-term benefits before they offered this therapy to more women[33]. Concerns have been expressed about the long-term side-effects such as breast cancer and the time required for supervision and monitoring, financial costs and likely poor patient compliance[33]. In the past women have had to apply pressure to their general practitioner to obtain HRT[20] although more recent studies have suggested that general practitioners are no longer a major obstacle to women receiving HRT[29].

Methods of improving compliance

Increasing women's awareness of HRT

The association between women's poor knowledge about the menopause and HRT and poor uptake of HRT has led to suggestions for specific health education campaigns, using consumer-friendly educational materials to highlight the benefits of HRT[11]. In one general practice the use of personalized letters containing information leaflets about HRT increased the uptake of HRT from 46 to 68 hysterectomized women over 3 months[35] although no information was available on long-term use. The uptake of HRT could be increased by targeting specific groups of women, e.g. younger women before they reach menopausal age and women at increased risk of cardiovascular disease[36] and osteoporosis[37-39].

The presentation of accurate and balanced information about HRT by the media could be facilitated by co-operation between the medical profession and those responsible for the presentation of media material[19]. The use of HRT might be increased by dissemination of information about osteoporosis to women[40], particularly women found to be at increased risk of fracture following bone scanning[39].

Education of health care professionals

To increase the prescribing rate of HRT doctors should be made aware of their role in advising women about HRT, and need to be informed about the true benefits and risks of HRT[41]. It is important that accurate and up-to-date information and guidance are effectively disseminated to general practitioners.

Within primary care in the UK, the establishing of a general practitioner with interest and expertise in the menopause and HRT in each practice might improve compliance. Better compliance has been achieved in other clinical fields by both UK general practitioners[42] and US physicians[43] with a special interest in their particular fields.

Education and counseling

Assessing patient beliefs, dispelling unrealistic expectations[44] and explaining about the problem and its treatment increase patient compliance in general practice[45]. Addressing women's fears about side-effects, specifically weight gain, when commencing HRT may improve uptake and long-term compliance with HRT[27].

Formal and informal counseling by menopause counselors has been found to be a much needed form of therapy complementing HRT at specialist clinics[46] which could be adapted for primary care. A need has been identified for involvement of a woman's partner in menopause care[47,48] and enlisting the aid of the patient's family or friends can improve compliance[45].

Booklets about the menopause, HRT and osteoporosis may help in the education process[28] together with a telephone question line[48].

Structured care

Compliance is increased by structured care incorporating planned follow-up visits[43], in-depth discussion[49] and explicit review of compliance[45]. Formal follow-up, e.g. 3 months after therapy has been commenced, helps identify problems and provides the opportunity to answer questions and alter therapy as appropriate[28]. In addition, encouraging patients to attend with problems following reading of literature or following media reports enables concerns to be discussed further[28].

The introduction of a formal protocol in the management of HRT users in one general practice resulted in HRT use by 28.7% of 40–80-year-olds and a long-term compliance rate of 60% for 5 years and 19% for 10 years[50]. Attendance of women at a general practice-based clinic following postal invitation led to increased uptake of HRT from 15 to 45% and a long-term compliance with HRT of 84%[51]. HRT users attending another general practice-based clinic expressed a high degree of satisfaction with care[52] although this did not improve short-term compliance with HRT[53].

Complementary to general practice-based care are community-based menopause clinics, one of which resulted in a compliance rate of 79.1% after 9 months or longer after discharge[54]. After initial assessment, counseling, prescription of HRT and a review appointment most women were discharged back to the care of their general practitioners. The recognition

that specialist hospital menopausal clinics are unable to cope with demand[55] together with the very high levels of satisfaction with community menopause services[56] have confirmed the need for these specialist menopause clinics within the community[57].

The practice nurse

The practice nurse already has an important role in counseling perimenopausal women about HRT[58], although the present activity of practice nurses in this area varies between practices[59]. The practice nurse is regarded by women as influencing their decision to take HRT[29] and can be an important source of information about lifestyle and facilities such as clinics[52].

Counseling and education are vital to improve compliance with HRT. As the time of the general practitioner is limited, the practice nurse is in an ideal situation to be trained as a specialist menopause nurse to take on some of the teaching, training and counseling within the primary health care team[60]. However, general practitioners have recently expressed reservations about delegation of this role owing to concerns about breast-cancer risk and HRT[61].

Choice of hormonal preparations

Discussion of treatment options[13] and individualizing treatment result in greater compliance[41,44]. When problems occur it is often possible to modify the type of estrogen, progestogen, pattern of administration and route of administration[28]. The development of new preparations such as continuous combined HRT and inclusion of alternative progestogens in opposed therapy should lead to fewer problems with bleeding and side-effects, and so to improved compliance[41]. Use of easy-to-take medication with calendar devices or reminders may facilitate long-term use of medication[14].

Resource allocation

There is likely to be increased use of HRT in the future[62,63]. The vast majority of British women who seek help for their menopausal problems consult their general practitioner[9] and only a minority of general practitioners and consultant gynecologists in the UK consider that HRT should be initiated by consultants[64]. Personalized care by an informed general practitioner over three to four visits to allow for titration of therapy and adequate counseling can result in a high rate of compliance[48], and compliance with HRT in general practice appears to be improving[23].

Primary care, at least in the UK, is therefore likely to be the main provider of HRT in coming years. The substantial resources required to meet the potential demand have been recognized[18] and resource problems related to HRT prescribing within general practice have been highlighted[65]. General practitioners have expressed concerns about the ability of the National Health Service (NHS) to afford HRT[30], and limitation of prescribing budgets may deter general practitioners from prescribing HRT as a preventive measure[55].

As the increased use of HRT will have major implications for primary care staff and drug budgets, targeting care to those most at risk and increasing primary care staff and drug budgets will be required[61].

Conclusions

HRT is underused internationally despite its many benefits. In the UK, the bulk of menopausal care is undertaken within general practice. Within this primary care setting a number of strategies can he employed to improve women's uptake of and compliance with HRT, ranging from structuring of care within general practice to education of women and health care professionals (Table 1).

Table 1 Summary of methods to improve compliance with hormone replacement therapy (HRT)

Increasing women's awareness of HRT through health education and media information

Education of health care professionals about HRT and their roles in advising women

Education and counseling of women

Structuring care and development of the practice nurse's role

Choice of hormonal preparations and individualization of treatment

Resource allocation particularly to primary care

References

1. Griffith, S. (1990). A review of the factors associated with patient compliance and the taking of prescribed medicines. *Br. J. Gen. Pract.*, **40**, 114–16
2. Belchetz, P. E. (1994). Hormonal treatment of postmenopausal women. *N. Engl. J. Med.*, **330**, 1062–71
3. Ravnikar, V. A. (1987). Compliance with hormone therapy. *Am. J. Obstet. Gynecol.*, **156**, 1332–4
4. Beardon, P. H. G., McGilchrist, M. M., McKendrick, A. D., McDevitt, D. G. and MacDonald, T. M. (1993). Primary non-compliance with prescribed medication in primary care. *Br. Med. J.*, **307**, 846–8
5. Cano, A. (1995). Compliance to hormone replacement therapy in menopausal women controlled in a third level academic centre. *Maturitas*, **20**, 91–9
6. Coope, J. and Marsh J. (1992). Can we improve compliance with long-term HRT? *Maturitas*, **15**, 151–8
7. Oddens, B. J., Boulet, M. J., Lehert, P. and Visser, A. P. (1992). Has the climacteric been medicalized? A study on the use of medication for climacteric complaints in four countries. *Maturitas*, **15**, 171–81
8. Cauley, J. A., Cummings, S. R., Black, D. M., Mascioli, S. R. and Seeley, D. G. (1990). Prevalence and determinants of estrogen replacement therapy in elderly women. *Am. J. Obstet. Gynecol.*, **163**, 1438–44
9. Barlow, D. H., Grosset, K. A., Hart, H. and Hart, D. M. (1989). A study of the experience of Glasgow women in the climacteric years. *Br. J. Obstet. Gynaecol.*, **96**, 1192–7
10. Barlow, D. H., Brockie, J. A. and Rees, C. M. P.

(1991). Study of general practice consultations and menopausal problems. *Br. Med. J.*, **302**, 274–6

11. Sinclair, H. K., Bond, C. M. and Taylor, R. J. (1993). Hormone replacement therapy: a study of women's knowledge and attitudes. *Br. J. Gen. Pract.*, **43**, 365–70

12. Wilkes, H. C. and Meade, T. W. (1991). Hormone replacement therapy in general practice: a survey of doctors in the MRC's general practice research framework. *Br. Med. J.*, **302**, 1317–20

13. Hope S. and Rees, M. C. P. (1995). Why do British women start and stop hormone replacement therapy? *J. Br. Menopause Soc.*, **1**(2), 26–8

14. Rozenberg, S., Vandromme, J., Kroll, M., Twagirayezu, P. and Vyankandondera, J. (1995). Compliance with hormone replacement therapy. *Rev. Med. Bruxelles*, **16**, 295–8

15. Groenveld, F. P., Bareman, F. P., Barentsen, R., Dokter, H. J., Drogendijk, A. C. and Hoes, A. W. (1994). Determinants of first prescription of hormone replacement therapy. A follow-up study among 1689 women aged 45–60 years. *Maturitas*, **20**, 81–9

16. Wren, B. G. and Brown, L. (1991). Compliance with hormonal replacement therapy. *Maturitas*, **13**, 17–21

17. Hammond, C. B. (1994). Women's concerns with hormone replacement therapy – compliance issues. *Fertil. Steril.*, **62** (Suppl. 2), 157S–60S

18. Draper, J. and Roland, M. (1990). Perimenopausal women's views on taking hormone replacement therapy to prevent osteoporosis. *Br. Med. J.*, **300**, 786–8

19. Roberts, P.-J. (1991). The menopause and hormone replacement therapy: views of women in general practice receiving hormone replacement therapy. *Br. J. Gen. Pract.*, **41**, 421–4

20. Kadri, A. Z. (1991). Hormone replacement therapy – a survey of perimenopausal women in a community setting. *Br. J. Gen. Pract.*, **41**, 109–12

21. Wallace, W. A., Price, V. H., Elliot, C. A., MacPherson, M. B. A. and Scott, B. W. (1990). Hormone replacement therapy acceptability to Nottingham post-menopausal women with a risk factor for osteoporosis. *J. R. Soc. Med.*, **83**, 699–701

22. O'Leary Cobb, J. (1993). Why women choose not to take hormone therapy. In Berg, G. and Hammer, M. (eds.) *The Modern Management of the Menopause*, pp. 525–32. (New York and London: Parthenon Publishing)

23. Griffiths, F. and Convery, B. (1995). Women's use of hormone replacement therapy for relief of menopausal symptoms, for prevention of osteoporosis, and after hysterectomy. *Br. J. Gen. Pract.*, **45**, 355–8

24. Hahn, R. G. (1989). Compliance considerations with estrogen replacement: withdrawal bleeding and other factors. *Am. J. Obstet. Gynecol.*, **161**, 1854–8

25. Marsh, M. S. and Whitehead, M. I. (1993). The practicalities of hormone replacement therapy (review). *Bail. Clin. Endocrinol. Metab.*, **7**, 183–202

26. Liao, K. L. M, Hunter, M. S. and White, P. (1994). Beliefs about menopause of general practitioners and mid-aged women. *Fam. Pract.*, **11**, 408–12

27. O'Connor, R., McCaffery, M. and Pitkin J. (1993). Weight gain at the menopause: a real fear. Presented at the *7th International Congress on the Menopause*, Stockholm, June

28. Stumpf, P. G. and Trolice, M. P. (1994). Compliance problems with hormone replacement therapy. *Obstet. Gynecol. Clin. N. Am.*, **21**, 219–29

29. Griffiths, F. (1995). Women's decisions about whether or not to take hormone replacement therapy: influence of social and medical factors. *Br. J. Gen. Pract.*, **45**, 477–80

30. Kadri, A. Z. (1990). Attitudes to HRT. *Practitioner*, **234**, 880–4

31. Ferguson, K. J., Hoegh, C. and Johnson, M. D. (1989). Estrogen replacement therapy. A survey of women's knowledge and attitudes. *Arch. Intern. Med.*, **149**, 133–6

32. Hunskaar, S. and Backe, B. (1992). Attitudes towards and level of information on perimenopausal and postmenopausal hormone replacement therapy among Norwegian women. *Maturitas*, **15**, 183–94

33. Bryce, F. C. and Lilford, R. J. (1990). General practitioners' use of hormone replacement therapy in Yorkshire. *Eur. J. Obstet. Gynaecol.*, **37**, 55–61

34. Shears, M. R. (1989). Brighton practitioners' attitudes to HRT. *Practitioner*, **233**, 146–9

35. Salt, S. (1995). Personal letter and use of hormone replacement therapy (letter). *Br. J. Gen. Pract.*, **45**, 216

36. Griffiths, F. (1995). Women's health concerns: is the promotion of hormone replacement therapy for prevention important to women? *Fam. Pract.*, **12**, 54–9

37. Spector, T. M. (1989). Use of oestrogen replacement therapy in high risk groups in the United Kingdom. *Br. Med. J.*, **299**, 1434

38. Seeley, T. (1992). Oestrogen replacement therapy after hysterectomy. *Br. Med. J.*, **305**, 811–12

39. Garton, M., Reid, D. and Rennie, E. (1995). The climacteric, osteoporosis and hormone replacement therapy; views of women aged 45–49. *Maturitas*, **21**, 7–15

40. Ringa, V., Ledesert, B. and Breart, G. (1994). Determinants of hormone replacement therapy

among postmenopausal women enroled in the French GAZEL cohort. *Osteoporosis Int.*, **4**, 16–20

41. (1991). More than hot flushes (editorial). *Lancet*, **338**, 917–18

42. Pringle, M., Stewart-Evans, C., Coupland, C., Williams, I., Allison, S. and Sterland, J. (1993). Influences on control in diabetes mellitus: patient, doctor, practice or delivery of care? *Br. Med. J.*, **306**, 630–4

43. DiMatteo, M. R., Sherbourne, C. D., Hays, R. D., Ordway, L., Kravitz, R. L., McGlynn, E. A., Kaplan, S. and Rogers, W. H. (1993). Physicians' characteristics influence patients' adherence to medical treatment: results from the Medical Outcomes Study. *Health Psychol.*, **12**, 93–102

44. Gangar, E. (1992). Appropriate use of HRT post-menopause. *Nurs. Stand.*, **7**, 28–30

45. Carr, A. (1990). Compliance with medical advice (editorial). *Br. J. Gen. Pract.*, **338**, 358–60

46. Lilley, C. and Pitkin, J. (1993). Counselling as additional therapy in the menopause. Presented at the *7th International Congress on the Menopause*, Stockholm, June

47. O'Connor, R., Stafford, M. and Pitkin, J. (1993). Partners should share the menopause. Presented at the *7th International Congress on the Menopause*, Stockholm, June

48. MacLennan, A. H. (1993). Running a menopause clinic. *Bail. Clin. Endocrinol. Metab.*, **7**, 243–53

49. Sarrel, L. and Sarrel, P. M. (1994). Helping women decide about hormone replacement therapy: approaches to counselling and medical practices. In Berg, G. and Hammer, M. (eds.) *The Modern Management of the Menopause*, pp. 499–509. (New York and London: Parthenon Publishing)

50. Sethi, K. and Pitkin, J. (1995). HRT uptake and compliance. Menopause Society communications. *Eur. Menopause J.*, **2**, 33–4

51. Coope, J. and Roberts, D. (1990). A clinic for the prevention of osteoporosis in general practice. *Br. J. Gen. Pract.*, **40**, 295–9

52. Roberts, P.-J. (1995). Reported satisfaction among women receiving hormone replacement therapy in a dedicated general practice clinic and in a normal consultation. *Br. J. Gen. Pract.*, **45**, 79–81

53. Roberts, P.-J. (1995). Hormone replacement therapy (letter). *Br. J. Gen. Pract.*, **45**, 562–3

54. McCleery, J. M. and Gebbie, A. E. (1994). Compliance with hormone replacement therapy at a menopause clinic in a community setting. *Br. J. Fam. Plann.*, **20**, 73–5

55. Garnett, T., Mitchell, A. and Studd, J. (1991). Patterns of referral to a menopause clinic. *J. R. Soc. Med.*, **84**, 128–30

56. Hanlon, L., Welsh, S., Rajoriya, V. and Clarke, A. (1996). A survey of women aged 44–54 years to determine their perceptions of menopause services in primary care and community clinics. *Br. J. Fam. Plann.*, **22**, 97–100

57. Gebbie, A. E., Caird, L. and Glasier, A. (1996). A community menopause clinic in Edinburgh – five years' experience. *Br. J. Fam. Plann.*, **22**, 46–8

58. Brockie, J. (1996). Role of the nurse in patient compliance with HRT. *J. Br. Menopause Soc.*, **29**, 19–21

59. Jeffreys, L. A., Clerk, A. L. and Koperski, M. (1995). Practice nurses' workload and consultation patterns. *Br. J. Gen. Pract.*, **45**, 415–18

60. Pitkin, J. (1995). HRT: are we achieving compliance? *Eur. Menopause J.*, **2** (Suppl. 4), 36–40

61. Pereira Gray, D., Evans, P., Sweeney, K. and Steele, R. (1996). HRT prescribing – a paradigm for the complexity of prescribing in general practice. In Brown, J.S., Pereira Gray, D., Mathie, A. G and Reith, W. (eds.) *RCGP Members' Reference Book 1996*, pp. 245–50. (London: Sterling Publications)

62. Griffiths, F. and Jones, K. (1995). The use of hormone replacement therapy; results of a community survey. *Fam. Pract.*, **12**, 163–5

63. Isaacs, A. J., Britton, A. R. and McPhearson, K. (1995). Utilisation of hormone replacement therapy by women doctors. *Br. Med. J.*, **311**, 1399–401

64. Norman, S. G. and Studd, J. W. (1994). A survey of views on hormone replacement therapy. *Br. J. Obstet. Gynaecol.*, **101**, 879–87

65. Roberts, P.-J. (1996). Comparison of care between a general practice clinic and general surgeries: the views of women using HRT. *J. Br. Menopause Soc.*, **29**, 15–18

What measures should we adopt to improve hormone replacement therapy compliance during the next decade?

62

A. H. MacLennan

Introduction

Compliance or adherence to therapy presumes knowledge by the patient and the prescriber of an optimum length of time for therapy. This knowledge only comes from an understanding of the best scientific evidence available to date and an individualization of this evidence to the particular woman's risk factors, needs and wishes. Clearly it also requires informed consent. Thus, on the basis of the available long-term observational studies and the short-term randomized controlled trials conducted to date, compliance to therapy may currently be generalized as being appropriate for the control of menopausal symptoms for 5–10 years, for the management of low bone density over 15–20 years, and for those with cardiovascular risk factors perhaps for 25 years or more. The debate about breast cancer risk continues but current overviews are reassuring, with any increased risk with long-term therapy likely to be relatively small if any at all[1,2]. Indeed, the largest cohort study published to date shows a significant 16% reduction (relative risk 0.84, 95% confidence interval 0.75–0.94) in breast cancer fatalities among postmenopausal women who had ever used estrogen replacement therapy compared to non-users[3]. This study of 422 373 women over 9 years will do much to improve compliance. A family history of dementia may also prove in the future to be an indication for longer compliance. However, without long-term randomized trials it will not be possible to clearly define the optimal length of therapy

for any individual, and all governments should be encouraged to fund and conduct such trials.

Previous speakers and papers in this session of the proceedings will have emphasized the need for extensive medical and public education and access to adequate information, if high usage and compliance rates for the above indications and time limits suggested above are to be achieved. This paper first presents evidence from a large population survey that high usage and compliance rates can be achieved, and then suggests how this occurred and can be achieved elsewhere.

HRT compliance rates in South Australia

It has been possible to accurately assess the use of hormone replacement therapy (HRT) for non-contraceptive reasons in South Australia (population 1.4 million) using the South Australian Health Omnibus Survey which obtains a yearly random and representative sample of over 4500 metropolitan and country households. In each household women over the age of 40 are questioned personally by trained interviewers about multiple health issues. Details of HRT usage and non-usage were obtained in 1991[4], 1993[5] and 1995 (submitted). In 1987 industry figures estimated HRT use in South Australia at 2–3% of the female population. For women between the ages of 45 and 59 years the Omnibus surveys recorded current use (% ever use) of HRT at 26.6% (39.0) in 1991, 35.3% (46.9) in 1993

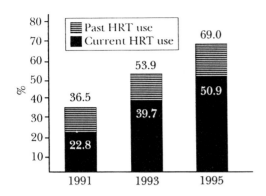

Figure 1 Percentage ever use (current plus past use) of hormone replacement therapy (HRT) in South Australian population in 1991, 1993 and 1995 in the age group 55–59 years

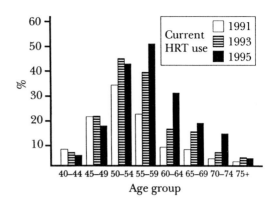

Figure 2 Percentage of current hormone replacement therapy (HRT) use by 5-year age groups in South Australian population surveyed in 1991, 1993 and 1995

and 38.3% (49.8) in 1995. In 1991 and 1993 highest use was in the 5-year age bracket 50–54 years but in 1995 the highest prevalence was in the age group 55–59 years where current HRT use was 50.9% and ever use was 69.0% (Figure 1). This reflects a continuance rate in this presumably early postmenopausal group of 74%. Such compliance rates compare very favorably with other long-term preventive therapies in this country such as lipid-lowering drugs where compliance rates are only 40% after 12 months[6].

Figure 2 shows the trends of current use by 5-year age groups in the three surveys. Although prevalence rates have increased overall in 1995, it is interesting to note in 1995 a small drop in current use in all age groups under 55 years and a significant increase in use in all age groups over 55 years. The 1995 survey was conducted a few months after the publication of the Nurses Health Study[7] which highlighted a possible increase in breast cancer rates with long-term HRT use. This precipitated much media attention in Australia and often the findings were taken out of context and exaggerated. It is interesting to speculate if and why this adverse publicity may have influenced the younger users of HRT and not older women.

The length of use of HRT has continued to increase in the surveys with mean current use

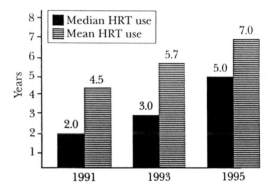

Figure 3 Median and mean current length of use of hormone replacement therapy (HRT) by all women over 50 years surveyed in South Australia in 1991, 1993 and 1995

in 1991, 1993 and 1995 in all women over 50 being 4.5, 5.7 and 7.0 years respectively (Figure 3). The earlier surveys suggested that HRT users were more likely to be upper social class, higher-income earners, metropolitan dwelling, smokers, UK or Ireland born and have had a hysterectomy. Later surveys when HRT use was higher suggested a wider use of HRT in middle class, middle-income, country dwelling, Australian born and non-smoking women. In each survey, hysterectomized women had a high usage and compliance with HRT.

447

Table 1 Main reason why postmenopausal women had stopped or never started hormone replacement therapy (HRT) in 1995

	%
Side-effects	21.5
No further need	17.5
Not natural	16.5
Fear of breast cancer	6.0
Fear of weight gain	2.5
Dissuaded by others/media	1.5
Other reasons	34.5

Excluding women who were not yet perimenopausal, the earliest survey suggested non-users had a greater ignorance of HRT and its possible benefits than was seen in the most recent survey. In 1991 49% of those who had stopped HRT did so because of side-effects and most of these women had stopped after only 1 to 6 months of therapy without returning to the prescriber. Table 1 shows the reasons given in 1995 as to why they had stopped or never started HRT. Only 21% stopped HRT in 1995 owing to side-effects. This may reflect greater experience in the prescribers and their greater ability to tailor the therapies.

How have such high prevalence and compliance rates been obtained?

The South Australian population is relatively compact with 1.1 of the 1.4 million residents living in the city of Adelaide. Most of the medical professionals are metropolitan based and this facilitates postgraduate medical education. Thus it has perhaps been easier than in other more widespread populations to run multiple medical and lay education courses. However, the lay media and the medical press have been actively cultivated through educational messages and articles. The Australian Menopause Society has been active with many meetings together with other educational meetings run by professional colleges and medical groups. Video education of both the lay and medical professions may also have contributed greatly as a very large number of menopause education videos[8,9] have been distributed in this state allowing information to reach those who cannot attend educational meetings. There is a great opportunity for similar information to be distributed world-wide on the Internet. Currently there is a variety of menopause information on the Internet and it would be important in the future to clearly identify independent, evidence-based advice. Computer-assisted learning programs are another recent option and are being demonstrated at this congress.

Future goals for the next decade to facilitate compliance

Menopause societies

As other speakers have clearly emphasized, medical and lay education must be a priority using verbal, written, video and electronic communication. The media must not be avoided or feared, and independent evidence-based consensus messages should be clearly provided to the media by appropriate spokespersons for bodies such as the national or international menopause societies. Indeed, we need to be proactive and not just slowly respond to scare-headlines, misinformation or potentially bad news that can be easily misinterpreted.

It is important that our menopause and professional societies and spokespersons are (and are seen to be) independent of the pharmaceutical industry, the alternative medicine industry and any other pressure groups. Opinions should be founded on evidence-based medicine, and patient compliance is likely to be greater if such opinions are seen to be clearly independent with only their interests at heart.

The Cochrane Collaboration and its systematic reviews should be supported by all societies as it brings together carefully assessed comprehensive scientific data on the menopause. This will be a corner-stone of our future advice to patients on menopause management.

Goals for industry

Production information   More accurate product information is required for most estrogen and progestogen preparations on the market. Some of the product information for patients is out of date, creates unnecessary anxiety and includes inappropriate contraindications or unsubstantiated warnings such as an increased thrombosis risk with hormone replacement therapy[10]. Pharmaceutical companies need to negotiate with the registering authorities, perhaps with the help of the local national menopause society, for accurate, balanced and sensible patient information to accompany their products.

Packaging of some products could also be improved. As most menopausal women need glasses to read the details on a calendar pack, small print and colors such as red on a reflective background should not be used.

Policing and restriction of negative advertising   Two recent examples of inaccurate and destructive advertising by companies with products in competition with HRT have been dealt with by the Code of Conduct Sub-Committee of the Australian Pharmaceutical Manufacturers Association. The first purported to warn doctors of the risks of breast cancer for women on HRT by selectively quoting parts of the Nurses Health Study[7] without balancing references to the main literature, while suggesting a switch to their product for the treatment of osteoporosis. This generated much concern and misinformation amongst general practitioners who did not have access at first to the original article, or an overview of the literature. Some practitioners are purported to have stopped prescribing or re-prescribing HRT following this letter in 1995.

A second more subtle negative campaign was conducted by the manufacturer of an alternative product for the treatment of hot flushes, where a female cartoon character exclaimed without qualification that she could not take HRT because of a history of thrombosis, migraine or a family history of breast cancer. All of these are not, in practice, contraindications. Without qualifying 'family history' the high prevalence of breast cancer means that almost everyone would have a family history of breast cancer if they knew the medical history of their extended family and ancestors. These advertisements were belatedly stopped, but not before much misinformation and unnecessary concern about HRT had been spread.

Increased product efficacy and decreased cost   Industry must continue to support long-term trials of efficacy, to seek products that are specific to the action that is required, and to minimize the cost of long-term HRT which is an important factor for those with low incomes. Industry must also be encouraged to fund and conduct product comparison trials.

Side-effects   Up to one-half of all women commencing HRT experience mild side-effects[11]. Side-effects are a common reason for women ceasing HRT early in therapy[4]. Efforts are being made by manufacturers to reduce side-effects. Postmenopausal bleeding can be avoided by the use of a progestogen-containing intrauterine device, Tibilone, new estrogen analogs and continuous combined estrogen and progestogen regimens. Oral agents are currently less effective where bowel disorders such as irritable bowel syndrome are present, or agents that may inhibit estrogen absorption are being used such as H_2 antagonists or proton-pump inhibitors for gastric reflux or gastric ulcers. Oral preparations that avoid such problems would enhance compliance. Similarly, transdermal therapies that do not cause irritation and adhere well will increase compliance with this route. Finally, better slow- and constant-release estrogen implants may reduce the significant problem of tachyphylaxis associated with this route of administration.

Health professionals

Counseling time   Time for counseling should be made available and rewarded by the national public or private remuneration systems. In many health systems surgical procedures are financially rewarded but taking time to listen, counsel, explain options and tailor therapeutic regimens to the individual is often greatly undervalued.

Counseling skills Students and professionals in this area should be taught counseling skills. Compliance is greatly helped by supplementing verbal counseling with written information (counseling booklets[12] are freely available in this country) and video education[8]. This may overcome memory problems and adds authority to the verbal counseling.

Investigations and compliance A study by Ahmed and colleagues[13] has suggested that long-term compliance may be increased when bone density measurements predict an increased risk of osteoporosis. This does not necessarily support a policy of universal screening of bone density in all perimenopausal women, but rather supports a policy of the option of bone density measurements before women cease therapy or in women who would not commence HRT unless they were at risk of osteoporosis.

Identification of risk factors for coronary heart disease may also increase compliance if these are adequately explained together with the probable protective effect of estrogen. Thus, a lipid profile or a random cholesterol test may help decision making when HRT is being considered, together with ascertaining other risk factors such as high blood pressure, excess weight, personal and family history of cardiovascular disease, diabetes and smoking.

Tailoring HRT Like wearing a suit, compliance depends on a good fit and up to 50% of women require a readjustment of their therapy in the first year. Thus early follow-up is important and 3 months is a practical time to assess the therapy. Easy telephone access for advice is important to tide users through early minor start-up side-effects, frequent misinformation from 'friends', apprehension

and side-effects that require adjustment of dosage. Yearly medical checks also help compliance and allow a general review of health and time for questions.

Alternative medicines and practitioners Doctors should be aware that approximately 50% of perimenopausal women use over the counter non-registered alternative medicines such as Chinese herbal medicines, ginseng, evening primrose oil etc., and that about 20% of women visit alternative practitioners such as naturopaths, iridologists etc.[14]. The cost of alternative medicines and practitioners in Australia is estimated at one billion dollars per year and equates with similar estimates in other first world countries, e.g. 13.7 billion US dollars in the USA[13]. The Australian public spends almost twice as much on alternative medicines as it contributes to all types of pharmaceutical drugs. The efficacy and safety of many of these costly medicines are unproven and some may interact with, enhance or detract from the effect of HRT, indirectly affecting compliance. The alternative medicine industry could potentially see HRT as an undermining factor in their market as perimenopausal women are the greatest users of their products and services[12]. Although respect must be given to the beliefs and wishes of patients to use other remedies, it is helpful to know of their use and understand any interaction together with any misinformation about HRT that might have derived from their experiences with alternative medicine.

Conclusion

Compliance starts with our beliefs and evidence for the value of complying. We still need more evidence from randomized prospective trials to be sure that our current advice on compliance is appropriate. Also we need to define appropriate times to review therapy and advise cessation rather than continuance! High HRT compliance rates in menopausal women (74%) with a mean of 7 years' therapy have already been achieved in the general population of South Australia. Such rates depend on education of the health professional, the media and the lay public. Professional societies such as the International Menopause Society should lead the way with independent evidence-based advice, the pharmaceutical industry should try to provide what women need and want, and individual health professionals should take time to individualize the therapeutic options for each woman to ensure that she understands these options and can adhere to her chosen course.

Acknowledgements

The South Australian Health Omnibus data have been analyzed in collaboration with Dr David Wilson and Mrs Anne Taylor of the Behavioural Epidemiology Unit, Public and Environmental Health Service, South Australian Health Commission: my thanks to them both.

References

1. Speroff, L. (1996). Postmenopausal hormone therapy and breast cancer. *Obstet. Gynecol.*, **87**, 44S–54S
2. MacLennan, A. H. (1995). Hormone replacement therapy and breast cancer: what are the facts? *Med. J. Aust.*, **163**, 483–5
3. Willis, D. B., Calle, E. E., Miracle-McMahill, H. L. and Heath C. W. Jr (1996). Estrogen replacement therapy and risk of fatal breast cancer in a prospective cohort of post-menopausal women in the United States. *Cancer Causes Control*, **7**, 449–57
4. MacLennan, A. H., MacLennan, A. and Wilson, D. H. (1993). The prevalence of oestrogen replacement therapy in South Australia. *Maturitas*, **16**, 175–83
5. MacLennan, A. H., Taylor, A. W. and Wilson, D. H. (1995). Changes in the use of hormone replacement therapy in South Australia. *Med. J. Aust.*, **162**, 175–83
6. Simons, L. A., Levis, G. and Simons, J. (1996). Apparent discontinuation rates in patients prescribed lipid-lowering drugs. *Med. J. Aust.*, **164**, 208–11
7. Colditz, G. A., Hankinson, S. E., Hunter D. J., Willet, W. C., Manson, J. E., Stampfer, M. J., Hennekens, C., Rosner, B. and Speizer, F. E. (1995). The use of estrogens and progestins and the risk of breast cancer in postmenopausal women. *N. Engl. J. Med.*, **332**, 1589–93
8. Foundation Studios (1991). *Understanding the Menopause.* A video for the lay public. (North Adelaide, South Australia: Foundation Studios, Women's & Children's Hospital)
9. Foundation Studios (1993). *Modern Management of the Menopause.* A video for health professionals. (North Adelaide, South Australia: Foundation Studios, Women's & Children's Hospital)
10. Young, R. L., Goepfert, A. R. and Goldzieher, H. W. (1991). Estrogen replacement therapy is not conducive of venous thromboembolism. *Maturitas*, **13**, 189–92
11. MacLennan, A. H., MacLennan, A., O'Neill, S., Kirkgard, Y., Wenzel, S. and Chambers, H. M. (1992). Oestrogen and cyclical progestogen in postmenopausal hormone replacement therapy. *Med. J. Aust.*, **157**, 167–70
12. Wyeth-Ayerst (1996). *Presenting a Positive Outlook on the Menopause. Answers to Some Commonly Asked Questions About the Menopause and HRT*, 5th edn. (Parramatta, NSW: Wyeth-Ayerst)
13. Ahmed, A. I. H., Ryan, P. J., Snelling, T., Blake, G. M., Rymer, J. and Fogelman, I. (1996). Long term compliance with hormone replacement treatment following screening for post-menopausal osteoporosis by bone density measurements. *J. Obstet. Gynaecol.*, **16**, 41–4
14. MacLennan, A. H., Wilson, D. H. and Taylor, A. W. (1996). Prevalence and cost of alternative medicine in Australia. *Lancet*, **347**, 569–73

A general practitioner's outlook on long-term hormone replacement therapy and the general practitioner/specialist relationship

63

S. V. Drew

Introduction

In many countries the primary care physician (general practitioner, GP) is the confidante of the family; this is no more so than in the UK where individual patients register with a specific doctor. In recent years primary health-care teams have been developed where partnerships of GPs pool their expertise and share the management of patients with practice nurses and other health-care professionals such as district nurses and health visitors. Good liaison within this group should help to improve the standards of health promotion generally, and chronic-disease management and prevention in particular. Those patients at potential risk of long-term morbidity such as cardiovascular disease and osteoporosis can be identified and monitored.

In the UK it is not usual for patients to have direct access to a specialist. Patients are normally seen first by their GP who may initiate treatment before an appropriate specialist referral is made, if deemed necessary. After consultation with the specialist, specific treatment may be started, but the patient is usually returned to the care of the GP for further management and long-term care. Good liaison between GP and specialist is therefore vital.

Role of the general practitioner

The prime role of the GP in the UK has been modified in recent years. We are now encouraged to promote and provide a disease-prevention approach. Women make up 50% of our average list, and account for at least two-thirds of our usual number of consultations. The average GP has just under 2000 registered patients, of whom currently around 300 are women over the age of 50 years. This number is predicted to rise to around 400 over the next 10 years. The majority of these women will reach 80 years of age, having spent 30 years in a post-menopausal state, achieving a high risk for osteoporosis and cardiovascular disease. These risks are significant for all women to varying degrees. The GP, with special knowledge of the woman and her family, is ideally placed to identify her individual risks and provide sound advice, treatment and support.

Many menopausal women will have received contraceptive and maternity services from their GP, and will probably have attended the surgery regularly with their children over the years. Hopefully they will have developed a trusting relationship, and will value the opinion and advice of their GP. They should be familiar with the services offered at the practice. It is therefore very important that women feel welcome to seek advice, and that advice is readily available. This of course requires time, which is invariably at a premium.

Today's women want and need to be properly informed so that they can be involved in decisions surrounding their menopause and the long-term implications of estrogen deficiency and its prevention. They need to be reassured about the relative risks of cancer compared with the benefits from hormone replacement therapy (HRT), to balance the simplistic and frequently distorted and alarmist messages they receive from the media and their well-meaning but ill informed 'friends'. GPs and their team have a vital and valuable role to play. They can help women understand the menopause and the potential benefits of HRT, and put their personal benefits/risks in context. Importantly, they can present HRT not just as an alleviator of menopausal symptoms if taken for a few months or years, but in terms of the long-term benefits to the skeletal, cardiovascular and other systems if continued for 5, 10 or more years. Good GP management guidelines are necessary to achieve long-term compliance.

GP/specialist relationship

Collaboration between GPs and specialists is essential. Primary care physicians are an important link between women and their specialist care. Those at particular risk should be identified, whoever eventually initiates therapy. Hospital doctors may have special skills to choose the most appropriate therapy, but the primary care team is best placed to offer education and support around the menopause and in the long term. There is strong evidence that women are more likely to comply with HRT if they understand the menopause and its treatment.

In many areas of the UK, joint protocols of care management between GPs and specialist hospital departments are proving very effective. These particularly involve departments of obstetrics/gynecology, geriatrics and rheumatology, who are able to identify women most at risk from osteoporosis. Cardiologists, chest physicians and orthopedic surgeons are also beginning to co-operate. Many women present at casualty departments and fracture clinics with low impact fractures, often suspiciously early, in their 50s and early 60s. Those with chronic and debilitating diseases, especially those on long-term steroids, are regular attenders at hospital clinics. A

premature menopause may be associated with an early presentation of heart disease, as well as early fracture. Identification of these women and a joint management approach between specialist and GP will significantly improve both their quality of life and life expectancy. Shared management also allows for the sharing of expertise and facilities. Perimenopausal women often present at well-women clinics with an unclear relative risk for osteoporosis. Some are only prepared to consider HRT if their risk can be proved. Sadly the majority of GPs do not have direct access to bone densitometry; liaison with a specialist department to provide densitometry would be very beneficial.

Outlook on long-term HRT

The GP is most frequently involved with the needs of perimenopausal and recently postmenopausal women. The later post-menopausal women have often 'weathered the storm' of vasomotor symptoms, and are under the mistaken impression that it is too late for them to benefit from HRT. They are also put off the thought of HRT because of perceived side-effects and the need for the return of periods. Some may have been on HRT in the past and have stopped because of bleeding and side-effects, particularly if they had received little or no information. We know that many women, even those at known risk, give up treatment within 6 months of starting and some never resume[1].

Long-term compliance with treatment is one of the major challenges facing the GP. A recent survey of women doctors in the UK[2] showed that 55% of postmenopausal doctors aged between 45 and 65 years had at some time used HRT, with 41% being current users, most had been taking HRT for more than 5 years (Figure 1). Hopefully these figures may be achieved by the population as a whole if better levels of information and support are accomplished. A recent study of HRT usage in the UK, as compared to other European countries[3] shows only 7% ongoing usage amongst post-menopausal women (Figure 2). This and other

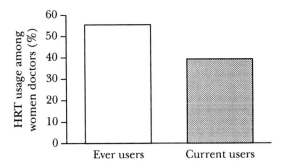

Figure 1 Utilization of hormone replacement therapy (HRT) by postmenopausal women doctors aged 45–65 years in the UK. Data from reference 2

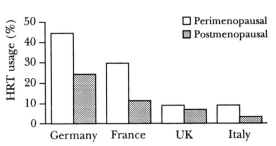

Figure 2 Country variation in the uptake of hormone replacement therapy (HRT). Data from reference 3

surveys suggest that HRT use in the UK is one of the lowest in the Western world. I am convinced that the lack of time generally given to information and support is a critical factor, as is poor communication between GP and specialist. Hopefully, increasing information to all health-care professionals will reduce this handicap.

HRT fears

The fear of breast cancer and the return of periods are two of the most quoted reasons for not starting HRT, or discontinuing. The former fear is universal throughout the age ranges, and only sound unbiased information can put this in perspective. Reputable studies have not shown a link between breast cancer and up to 5 years of treatment, and only a small increase in incidence with longer-term treatment. This information alone should encourage women to start HRT and continue for a significant time. The resistance to the return and prolongation of periods is definitely related to menopausal status. Pre- and perimenopausal women are significantly less resistant to the continuation or return of withdrawal bleeding than postmenopausal women[4], but even perimenopausal women are not happy with the thought that they might go on bleeding indefinitely (Figure 3). GPs must counsel perimenopausal women that sequential estrogen/progestogen therapy is still the most

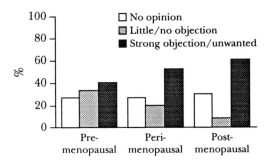

Figure 3 Opinion of women regarding continuation or reintroduction of monthly withdrawal bleeds after menopause. Data from reference 4

appropriate HRT for women with a uterus until they can be considered to be at least 1 year postmenopausal. After this time they can be offered continuous combined estrogen/progestogen therapy with the opportunity for long-term period-free HRT.

HRT regimen

A continuous combined regimen, such as Kliogest® (2 mg 17β-estradiol, 1 mg norethisterone acetate), may offer a number of advantages over sequential therapies. Data from the UK Multicentre Kliofem® (Kliogest) Study show that Kliogest has been developed to induce/maintain an atrophic endometrium, and may well offer better long-term endometrial protection than other HRT regimens. This offers the potential for safe, long-term, period-free HRT for postmenopausal women. Some women do bleed initially, but the majority cease any regular bleeding or spotting within 6–9 months. Good initial patient selection and counseling by the GP should minimize the withdrawal of women from treatment and encourage women to continue until amenorrhea is achieved. In my experience, women are more concerned about the persistence and irregularity of bleeding than they are about the amount at any one time. A good supportive protocol is therefore essential over the early stages of therapy. It is important to note that significant early bleeding is more common in those women who fail to achieve amenorrhea. Furthermore, as Kliogest avoids the cyclical hormonal changes that can be associated with sequential regimens, women who are used to experiencing the 'premenstrual syndrome-like' peaks and troughs of interrupted progestogen therapy report a feeling of calmness on continuous combined therapy, which is another aid to compliance. In recent trials in the UK, over 80% of women on Kliogest expressed a wish to stay on treatment in preference to returning to sequential therapy. It would therefore seem logical to suppose that, if long-term compliance can be improved, benefits can be gained in terms of the prevention of osteoporosis, cardiovascular disease and other aging diseases now associated with long-term estrogen deficiency.

Summary

The primary care physician is best placed to educate, treat and support the peri- and postmenopausal woman. The support of specialist colleagues is vital in helping the woman to balance the risks and benefits of a proposed course of HRT. It is through the holistic, 'whole woman' approach that the GP can be most effective. Cardiologists, rheumatologists, or gynecologists may be constrained by their particular specialty. The GP is in a privileged position to evaluate a woman's overall need for HRT, and to encourage and monitor compliance with any such treatment she may choose to use in the long term.

References

1. Ryan, P. J., Harrison, R., Blake, G. M. and Fogelman, I. (1992). Compliance with HRT after screening for postmenopausal osteoporosis. *Br. J. Obstet. Gynaecol.*, **99**(4), 325–8
2. Isaacs, A. J., Britton, A. R. and McPherson, K. (1995). Utilisation of hormone replacement therapy by women doctors. *Br. Med. J.*, **311**, 1399–401
3. Oddens, B. J., Boulet, M. J., Lehert, P. and Visser, A. P. (1992). Has the climacteric been medicalized? A study on the use of medication for climacteric complaints in four countries. *Maturitas*, **15**, 171–81
4. Barentsen, R., Groeneveld, F. P., Bareman, F. P., Hoes, A. W., Dokter, H. J. and Drogendijk, A. C. (1993). Women's opinion on withdrawal bleeding with hormone replacement therapy. *Eur. J. Obstet. Gynecol. Reprod. Biol.*, **51**, 203–7

16

Hormone replacement therapy in women over 60

Hormone replacement therapy in women over 60: management of osteoporosis prevention

64

S. Palacios

Introduction

Numerous studies have shown that estrogen deficiency results in accelerated loss of bone mineral density (BMD)[1,2]. The average decrease in BMD during a 10-year period among untreated postmenopausal women corresponds to a doubling of fracture risk[3]. By age 60–70 years, only one in nine women in the United States has normal BMD, almost one in three has osteoporosis and the rest have osteopenia. Beyond 80 years, about 70% of women have osteoporosis[4,5].

In early postmenopausal women, numerous studies have demonstrated that estrogen and estrogen/progestogen regimens stop bone loss and even reverse the loss of bone that normally occurs during these years[6,7]. However, there are few data about whether the effects of hormone replacement therapy (HRT) persist, or whether 'catch-up' bone loss occurs[8–10]. This is an important issue since HRT is most often received by women soon after the menopause and is commonly recommended for up to 10 years, and the prevalence of use declines as women reach their sixties; but the incidence of fractures related to bone fragility increases with age[11].

This article reviews the existing literature about HRT and osteoporosis prevention in women over 60 years.

Role of HRT in women over 60

Does HRT prevent bone loss in women over 60?

After menopause there is rapid bone loss of about 2–4% per year on average, which seems to subside gradually within 5–10 years in the absence of treatment[12,13]. Women who are more than 5 years postmenopausal lose BMD at a rate of about 1–2% per year. Recent studies, however, have shown that this rate of bone loss persists or accelerates after the age of 70 years[14,15].

Several studies of women over the age of 60 have shown that HRT stops and prevents bone loss[16,17]. In a study of 64-year-old postmenopausal women[16], it was found that, after 2 years of treatment, the group receiving HRT had 7–10% higher cortical bone mass than the control group. In another 2-year longitudinal study[15], it was demonstrated that administration of 1.5 mg of 17β-estradiol (one dose of 2.5 g of gel on to the skin), even more than 10 years after menopause, is capable of arresting bone loss and even of causing a significant gain in BMD at the level of the vertebrae.

The literature contains clear evidence that HRT prevents bone loss at all stages of the postmenopause[16–19].

Does HRT decrease fracture risk in women over 60?

Lufkin and colleagues[20] conducted a 1-year prospective, randomized, double-blind placebo-controlled trial of transdermal estradiol therapy in postmenopausal women with vertebral fractures due to established osteoporosis, and their results showed that, in the lumbar spine, bone mineral density increased after 1 year. Recently, it has also been found that transdermal treatment for 1 year significantly decreases the incidence of fracture[19].

Recent evidence implies that detectable serum estradiol levels in women over the age of 65 years correspond to a decrease in the risk of vertebral fracture[21].

Thus, there are sufficient studies suggesting that HRT administration after the age of 60 years does decrease fracture risk.

What dose and for how long?

The estrogenic effect on bone is dose-dependent[22], indicating that, if a sufficient serum concentration of estrogen is not obtained, bone loss will not be arrested completely.

Studies of oral estrogen/progestogen therapy have demonstrated that doses of 0.3–0.6 mg conjugated estrogens daily with a calcium supplement of 1000 mg[23], or 1–2 mg of 17β-estradiol[24], are optimum in the prevention of late postmenopausal bone loss. In the case of transdermally applied estrogen a dose of 50 μg per day[25], and 1.5 mg per day of percutaneous estrogen gel[2], appear to be sufficient (Table 1).

Conversely, the adverse effects of estrogen therapy are also dose-dependent. It is, therefore, of major importance to reduce the dose of estrogen required to prevent bone loss and osteoporosis, if possible. It is logical to start with a low dose and then to wait for the outcome.

The required duration of HRT is not clear, but if started at the age of 60 years in a patient with low bone mass, therapy should continue for at least 10 years. Perhaps the optimal solution would be to give therapy throughout her remaining lifetime (Figure 1).

Should we start HRT with women in their fifties or in their sixties?

With increasing menopausal age, there may be a tendency towards a slowing down in bone turnover, and thereby in the rate of bone loss. The greatest benefit from HRT is, therefore,

Table 1 Estrogen dose for prevention of late post-menopausal bone loss

Administration routes	Daily dose (mg)
Oral	0.3–0.6, conjugated estrogens 1–2, estradiol
Percutaneous	1.5, estradiol
Transdermal	0.05, estradiol

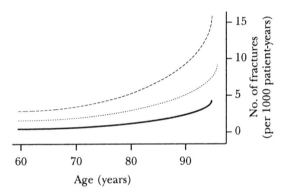

Figure 1 Duration of hormone replacement therapy and relationship with femoral neck fracture incidence. Broken line shows age-specific fracture incidence without HRT; dotted line shows fracture incidence after 10 years' HRT; unbroken line shows fracture incidence after lifetime HRT

obtained if it is instituted shortly after the menopause.

However, the effect of estrogen does not seem to persist long after the discontinuation of therapy according to some studies. Felson and colleagues[26] suggested that even 10 years of early postmenopausal estrogen therapy would have a trivial residual effect on bone mineral density at age 75. Epidemiological studies[27-29] have conversely reported that estrogen therapy protects women against later hip fracture, suggesting that there may be a residual effect of estrogen on bone density.

Perhaps it would be logical to start HRT in the early postmenopause, with administration of a low-dose estrogen regimen for more than 10 years.

Management of osteoporosis prevention in women over 60

Before initiation of HRT, the woman's state of health must be evaluated. For the purpose of prevention of osteoporosis it is useful to obtain an estimate of bone mass, and repeat the measurement after 1 year to determine if the treatment is effective. There is some site-specificity as might be expected, and measurement of the hip is a better predictor of the risk of hip fracture than results from other sites in the skeleton. For patients over 60 years with above average BMD, measurements at 5-year intervals are probably sufficient. In contrast, measurements at 1–2-year intervals are recommended if there are potent risk factors for bone loss. Women with below average BMD may benefit from measurements at 2–3-year intervals (Figure 2). In addition to a complete history, other useful pre-treatment evaluations may include a mammogram, and if any postmenopausal bleeding has occurred prior to therapy, evaluation of endometrial status is necessary.

In the management of osteoporosis prevention in women over 60 years with HRT, other factors should be taken into account, such as: the coprescription of other medications (e.g. hypnotics); low calcium intake and reduced intestinal calcium resorption; and decreasing physical activity.

For patients who have undergone a natural menopause, estrogens are normally given along with a progestin to protect the endometrium. In women over 60 years, we would initially recommend a low daily dose of estrogens and progestogens concomitant with 1000 mg of calcium.

Especial care must be taken to avoid secondary effects and the treatment should be tailored according to the individual patient, increasing the dose as required to achieve the desired goal with minimum side-effects.

Figure 3 summarizes the different mechanisms leading to an osteoporotic fracture. The most important preventive measure would be to stop increased bone resorption in women

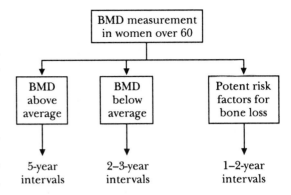

Figure 2 Management of osteoporosis prevention. BMD, bone mineral density

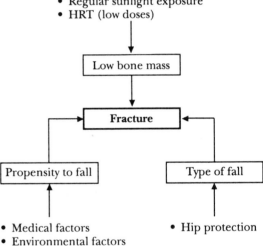

Figure 3 Prevention of fractures in women over 60 years. HRT, hormone replacement therapy

over 60 years. A positive calcium balance, a daily exercise program, regular exposure to sunlight and low-dose HRT will be the first choices for avoiding rapid bone loss in management of fracture prevention.

In general hip fracture is a combination of bone fragility and trauma. A large number of potential risk factors for falling in the elderly have been identified; avoidance of such risk factors could reduce the incidence of fracture.

It is possible to distinguish medical factors, e.g. cataracts, dementia; environmental factors, e.g. carpet folds, darkness ; and influence of medication, e.g. hypnotics, sedatives. Finally, it is important to ascertain the type of falling; there are specific hip protectors available that can reduce hip fractures by 56% in comparison with controls[30].

Conclusion

The literature contains clear evidence that HRT prevents bone loss and decreases the incidence of fractures at all stages of postmenopausal life. Most direct evidence suggests that bone that has been preserved is not rapidly lost when estrogen treatment is stopped.

Indirect evidence also suggests that the estrogen effect may persist for as long as 20–25 years. However, several epidemiological case–control studies have shown that, although the protective effect of estrogen persists into extreme old age, the effects are less than those in younger individuals more recently exposed to estrogen. This is an important area for further research.

References

1. Prior, J. C., Vigna, J. M., Schechter, M. T. and Burgess, A. G. (1990). Spinal bone loss and ovulatory disturbances. *N. Engl. J. Med.*, **323**, 1221–7
2. Palacios, S., Menendez, C., Jurado, A. R. and Vargas, J. C. (1995). Effects of percutaneous oestradiol versus oral oestrogens on bone density. *Maturitas*, **20**, 209–13
3. Davis, J. W., Ross, P. D., Waswich, R. D., Maclean, C. J. and Vogel, J. M. (1991). The long-term precision of bone loss rate measurements among postmenopausal women. *Ann. Intern. Med.*, **117**, 1–9
4. Melton, J. L. III (1995). How many women have osteoporosis now? *J. Bone Miner. Res.*, **10**, 175–7
5. Ross, P. (1996). Osteoporosis: frequency, consequences and risk factors. *Arch. Intern. Med.*, **156**, 1399–411
6. Barzel, U. S. (1988). Estrogens in the prevention and treatment of postmenopausal osteoporosis: a review. *Am. J. Med.*, **85**, 847–50
7. Lindsay, R. (1991). Why do oestrogens prevent bone loss? *Baill. Clin. Obstet. Gynaecol.*, **5**, 837–52
8. World Health Organization (1991). Consensus development conference: diagnosis, prophylaxis and treatment of osteoporosis. *Am. J. Med.*, **90**, 107–10
9. Law, M. R., Wald, N. J. and Meade, T. W. (1991). Strategies for prevention of osteoporosis and hip fracture. *Br. Med. J.*, **303**, 453–9
10. Pitt, E. A. (1990). The costs and benefits of screening and preventing postmenopausal osteoporosis in the Trent Region. *Report of the Trent Osteoporosis Working Group.* (Sheffield: Trent Regional Health Authority)
11. Melton, L. J. III, O'Fallon, W. M. and Riggs, B. L. (1987). Secular trends in the incidence of hip fractures. *Calcif. Tissue Int.*, **41**, 57–64
12. Hansen, M. A., Overgaard, K. and Christiansen, C. (1995). Spontaneous postmenopause bone loss in different skeletal areas: followed up for 15 years. *J. Bone Miner. Res.*, **10**, 205–10
13. Palacios, S., Menendez, C. and Jurado, A. R. (1994). Prevention and treatment of postmenopausal osteoporosis. In Palacios, S. (ed.) *Menopause Present and Future*, pp. 27–35. (Madrid: Mirpal)
14. Greenspan, S. L., Maitland, L. A., Myers, E. R., Krasnow, M. B. and Kido, T. H. (1994). Femoral bone loss progresses with age: a longitudinal study in women age 65. *J. Bone Miner. Res.*, **9** (Suppl. 1), 153
15. Hannan, M. T., Kiel, D. P., Mercier, C. E., Anderson, J. J. and Felson, D. T. (1994). Longitudinal bone mineral density (BMD) change in elderly men and women; the Framingham Osteoporosis Study. *J. Bone Miner. Res.*, **9** (Suppl. 1), 153
16. Christiansen, C. and Riis, B. J. (1990). 17β estradiol and continuous norethisterone: a unique treatment for established osteoporosis in elderly women. *J. Clin. Endocrinol. Metab.*, **71**, 836–41
17. Tremollieres, F., Pouilles, J. M., Louvet, J. P. and Ribot, C. (1990). Preventive effects on postmenopausal bone loss of percutaneous 17β estradiol in early and late menopause. In Christiansen, C. and Overgaard, K. (eds.) *Osteoporosis 1990. Proceedings of the Third International Symposium on Osteoporosis*, pp. 1910–15. (Denmark: Osteopress)

18. Quigley, M. E. T., Martin, P. L., Burnier, A. M. and Brooks, P. (1987). Estrogen therapy arrests bone loss in elderly women. *Am. J. Obstet. Gynecol.*, **156**, 1516–23

19. Lufkin, E. G., Hodeson, S. F., Kotowicz, M. A., O'Fallon, W. M., Wahner, H. W. and Riggs, B. L. (1990). The use of transdermal estrogen treatment in osteoporosis. In Christiansen, C. and Overgaard, K. (eds.) *Osteoporosis 1990. Proceedings of the Third International Symposium on Osteoporosis*, pp. 1995–8. (Denmark: Osteopress)

20. Lufkin, E., Wahner, H. W., O'Fallon, W. M. O., Hodson, S. F., Kotowicz, M. A., Lane, A. W., Juss, H. L., Caplan, R. H. and Riggs, B. L. (1992). Treatment of postmenopausal osteoporosis with transdermal estrogen. *Ann. Intern. Med.*, **117**, 1–9

21. Bauer, D. C., Cauley, J. A., Ensrud, K. G., Neviit, M. C., Stone, N. and Cummings, S. R. (1996). Women with low serum estradiol have an increased risk of vertebral fracture: a prospective study. *Osteoporosis Intern.*, **6**, 92

22. Horsman, A., Jones, M., Francis, R. and Nordin, B. B. C. (1983). The effect of estrogen dose on postmenopausal bone loss. *N. Engl. J. Med.*, **309**, 1405–7

23. Ettinger, B., Genant, H. K. and Cann, C. E. (1987). Postmenopausal bone loss is prevented by treatment with low-dosage estrogen with calcium. *Ann. Intern. Med.*, **104**, 40–4

24. Lindsay, R., Hart, C. M. and Clark, D. M. (1983). The minimum effective dose of estrogen for prevention of postmenopausal bone loss. *Obstet. Gynecol.*, **63**, 759–63

25. Ribbot, C., Tremollieres, F. and Oilles, J. M. (1990). Cyclic Estraderm TTS plus oral progestogen in the prevention of post-menopausal bone loss over 24 months. In Christiansen, C. and Overgaard, K. (eds.) *Osteoporosis 1990. Proceedings of the Third International Symposium on Osteoporosis*, pp. 1979–84. (Denmark: Osteopress)

26. Felson, D., Zhang, Y., Hannan, M., Kiel, D., Wilson, P. and Anderson, J. (1993). The effect of postmenopausal estrogen therapy on bone density in elderly women. *N. Engl. J. Med.*, **329**, 1141–6

27. Kiel, D. P., Felson, D. T., Anderson, J. J., Wilson, P. N. F. and Moskowirz, M. A. (1987). Hip fracture and the use of estrogens in postmenopausal women; the Framingham Study. *N. Engl. J. Med.*, **317**, 1169–74

28. Weiss, N. S., Ure, C. L., Ballard, J. H., Williams, A. R. and Daling, Y. R. (1980). Decreased risk of fractures of the hip and lower forearm with postmenopausal use of estrogen. *N. Engl. J. Med.*, **303**, 1195–8

29. Paganini-Hill, A., Ross, R. K., Gerkins, U. R., Henderson, B. E., Arthur, M. and Mak, T. M. (1981). Menopausal estrogen therapy and hip fractures. *Ann. Intern. Med.*, **95**, 28–31

30. Lauritzen, J. B. and Askegaard, V. (1992). Protection against hip fracture by energy absorption. *Dan. Med. Bull.*, **39**, 91

Hormone replacement therapy in women over 60: management of cancer risks   65

J. M. Foidart, J. Desreux, A. Beliard, A. C. Delvigne, X. Denoo, C. Colin, S. Fournier and B. de Lignières

Introduction

Long-term hormone replacement therapy is necessary since most cardiovascular benefits and osteoporosis prevention wane soon after discontinuation.

The risk of breast, endometrial and cervical cancer increases with age (Figure 1) and the risk of estrogen-induced endometrial cancer has been substantially reduced by the addition of progestins[1]. However, concern about whether or not exogenous steroids increase the risk of breast cancer remains. Over 40 epidemiological studies of breast cancer in relation to estrogen replacement therapy (ERT) or combined therapy have been conducted, with inconsistent results[2]. Efforts to analyze these investigations are hampered by differences in design and inclusion criteria (menopausal status, age and *in situ* breast cancer). Most studies find that the incidence of breast cancer in women who have previously used ERT or combined therapy is not different from that of untreated postmenopausal women (Figure 2). Discrepancies are, however, observed with respect to recency and long-term use[3,4].

It is uncertain whether the modest increase in the risk of breast cancer with hormone use found in some epidemiological studies reflects a causal association or rather the influence of one or several forms of bias (for a discussion see reference 2).

Even more conflicting data are produced with respect to ever, recent and long-term use of combined therapy[3,4]. A limited randomized trial found no cases of breast cancer among women who used combined therapy for 10

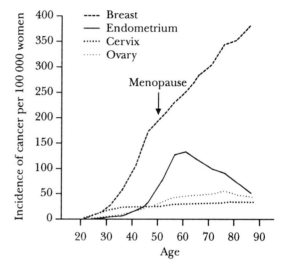

Figure 1 Incidences of breast, endometrial, cervical and ovarian cancer as a function of age. (Adapted from Gambrell, R. D. Breast disease in the postmenopausal years. *Semin. Reprod. Endocrinol.*, 1983, **1**, 27)

years, whereas 4.8% of those who did not use hormone therapy developed breast cancer over the 10 years' duration of the trial[5]. No cases occurred in the women receiving combined hormone replacement therapy (HRT) during 12 additional years of follow-up[5]. Two other non-randomized trials also concluded that women who used combined HRT were at lower risk of breast cancer[1,6]. Six studies found no association of breast cancer with ever use of combined therapy[7-12]. Two others found an increased risk of 30–40%[13,14].

Altogether these studies indicate that, if recent or long-term use of HRT truly does increase the risk of breast cancer, this increase

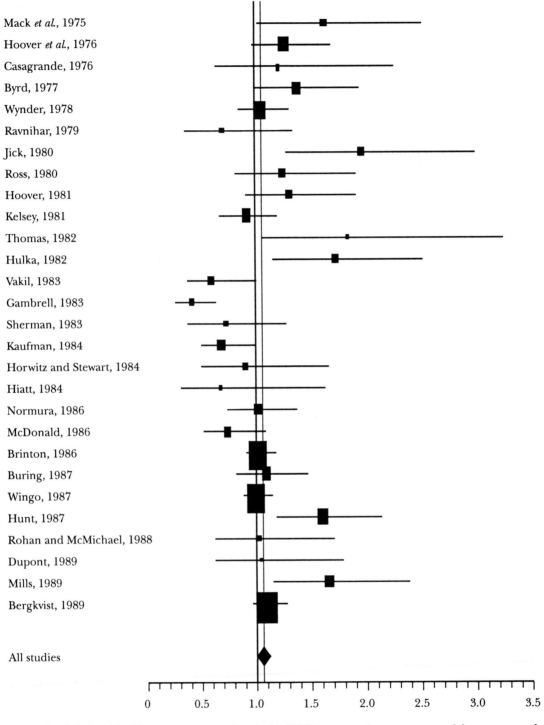

Figure 2 Relative risk of breast cancer associated with HRT in comparison to women of the same age who did not use HRT. The horizontal lines represent 95% confidence intervals. (Adapted from Dupont, W. D. and Page, D. L. (1991). *Arch. Intern. Med.*, **151**, 67–72)

seems to be modest. However, small relative increases in risk may have great public health importance. A 30% increase in relative risk of breast cancer would result in approximately 5000 additional cases in the USA[15]. Attempts are being made to determine whether the possible small relative increase in risk of breast cancer does or does not reflect a causal relation. Randomized trials of ERT and combined therapy are under way[16]. Pending the results of these trials, benefit–risk rates can only be estimated.

Similarly, the endocrine regulation of normal breast cell proliferation remains a matter of debate. 17β-Estradiol, in physiological concentrations, stimulates the proliferation of normal breast epithelial cells while the influence of progesterone and progestins has been controversial for two decades.

Depending upon the models used (animal or human, *in vitro* or *in vivo* studies), the timing of progesterone administration and the method of evaluation (mitotic index, proliferation cell nuclear antigen (PCNA) immunostaining, K_i 67 or [³H]thymidine labelling) progesterone is reported to stimulate, reduce or be neutral on mitotic activity and proliferation of breast epithelial cells[17–19]. Therefore, the therapeutical suggestions of progesterone treatment or avoidance are based on insufficient and controversial epidemiological evidence and on a lack of adequately controlled data about the influence of progesterone on normal breast epithelium.

In this study, we evaluated the effect of 17β-estradiol and progesterone on the epithelial cell cycle of normal human breast *in vivo* in 40 postmenopausal women undergoing breast surgery for the removal of a benign lesion.

Study design

Forty postmenopausal women were blindly and randomly allocated to four treatment groups and treated for 14 days prior to surgery. Only women with levels of plasma follicle stimulating hormone (FSH) > 30 mIU/ml and plasma 17β-estradiol < 20 pg/ml were enrolled. A gel containing either a placebo, 17β-estradiol (1.5 mg/day), progesterone (25 mg/day) or a combination of 17β-estradiol and progesterone (1.5 mg 17β-estradiol + 25 mg progesterone/day) was daily applied on both breasts for 14 days.

Plasma and breast tissue concentrations of 17β-estradiol and progesterone were determined as previously documented[20]. Proliferation of epithelial breast cells was evaluated by the PCNA labelling index[20].

Results

The hormone plasma and tissue levels corresponded to the expected figures. The progesterone concentration was elevated in the group treated with the progesterone gel (plasma progesterone, 1266 ± 280 pg/ml; tissue progesterone, 18 ± 20 ng/g) and the gel containing 17β-estradiol + progesterone (plasma progesterone, 950 ± 300 pg/ml; tissue progesterone, 12 ± 8 ng/g) in comparison with the placebo-controlled group (plasma progesterone, 280 ± 220 pg/ml; tissue progesterone, 3 ± 2.5 ng/g). These differences were statistically significant ($p < 0.05$, Kruskal–Wallis non-parametric test of variance and Student's t test).

Similarly the mean 17β-estradiol tissue and plasma concentrations were significantly higher in the 17β-estradiol group (659 ± 462 pg/g and 74 ± 20 pg/ml, respectively) and in the 17β-estradiol + progesterone group (566 ± 355 pg/g and 75 ± 68 pg/ml, respectively) than in the placebo group (278 ± 104 pg/g and 30 ± 11 pg/ml).

The PCNA labelling index confirmed the absence of proliferation in the untreated women. The women receiving 17β-estradiol displayed an intense proliferative response of their breast epithelial cells ($11.5 \pm 2.3\%$) (Figure 3). The progesterone group also showed low levels ($1.5 \pm 0.6\%$) of proliferation which were significantly higher than the placebo group ($0.1 \pm 0.1\%$) ($p < 0.01$). Finally, the PCNA labelling index was reduced significantly in the 17β-estradiol + progesterone group ($1.3 \pm 1.1\%$) in comparison with the 17β-estradiol group

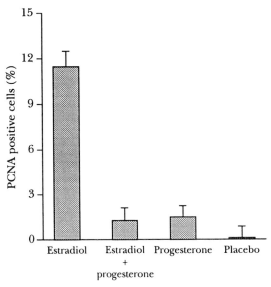

Figure 3 Proliferation of normal breast epithelial cells in postmenopausal women as a function of various percutaneous treatments

($p < 0.001$), to reach levels identical to that of the progesterone group ($1.5 \pm 0.6\%$).

Discussion

This study was designed as a double-blind randomized trial on 40 postmenopausal women undergoing breast surgery for plastic reasons or for benign breast mammary lesions. The daily percutaneous administration of progesterone, 17β-estradiol, progesterone + 17β-estradiol or placebo for 14 days resulted in the expected changes in plasma and tissue concentrations of steroids.

As expected from previous *in vitro* studies by others, 17β-estradiol considerably stimulated the proliferation of normal human breast epithelial cells in comparison with the placebo group ($11.5 \pm 2.3\%$ versus $0.1 \pm 0.1\%$). This proliferation index was also considerably higher in comparison with the progesterone group ($1.5 \pm 0.6\%$) or the progesterone + 17β-estradiol group ($1.3 \pm 1.1\%$). Progesterone administration thus dramatically reduced the 17β-estradiol-induced proliferation of normal human breast epithelial cells.

The progesterone and progesterone + 17β-estradiol treatment induced low levels of proliferation of galactophoric cells. This growth rate was significantly higher than in the placebo group. This low level of PCNA-positive cells could, in fact, reflect the capacity of progesterone to engage breast epithelial cells in the G_1 phase of the cell cycle. PCNA immunostaining identifies all cycling cells from G_1 to the G_2–M phases. In contrast to the [³H]thymidine labelling index, it does not only measure those cells in the S phase but also detects cells in the G_1, G_2 and M phases[21,22]. The PCNA-positive cells in these two groups could, therefore, represent cells in the G_1 phase. Such cells are not necessarily committed to becoming mitotic since they may also undergo apoptosis.

Our data strongly support the observations by Barrat and colleagues[23] and by Chang and colleagues[20] that progesterone participates in the control of human breast epithelial cell proliferation. They also suggest that progesterone may have a therapeutic value to prevent breast epithelial hyperplasia when used for 14 days per month at substitutive doses.

Our results clearly differ from observations by others which indicate that optimal proliferation occurs during the luteal (progestogenic) phase of the menstrual cycle[24–29] or in women receiving an oral contraceptive estrogen and progestin combination or a progestin-only oral contraception[27]. These data were interpreted as the demonstration of a positive influence of progesterone and progestins on breast epithelial proliferation. These data were obtained directly with histologically normal breast terminal duct-lobular units (TDLU) adjacent to benign fibroadenoma. If such tissue is excised and grown in hormonally treated, immunodeficient mice, a different picture emerges. 17β-Estradiol stimulates growth of the TDLU and progesterone or progestins have no effect[30].

Epithelial cells cultured from normal human breast are also stimulated by 17β-estradiol and not by progestin[31]. These conflicting data obtained by different techniques do not allow clear confirmation as to whether progestins either alone, or in combination with estrogen, are breast mitogens. It must finally be remembered that progesterone and synthetic progestins may induce different responses. It is indeed well-known that progestins of the 19 nortestosterone family, present in second- and third-generation oral contraceptives, display an estrogenic potential *in vitro* and *in vivo*, bind to the 17β-estradiol receptor and stimulate in this way human breast and endometrial cancer cell proliferation[32–34]. The intrinsic estrogenicity of some progestogenic drugs could, therefore, at least in part, elucidate these apparent controversies[35].

Altogether, our *in vivo* data indicate that, in contrast to indirect evidence from correlative studies between [³H]thymidine incorporation and day of the menstrual cycle, the direct administration of progesterone to post-menopausal women does not result in a mitogenic activity of breast epithelium. On the contrary, progesterone administration is able to counteract the estrogen-induced proliferation of human mammary epithelial cells and, in this way, may be protective against hyperplasia.

Acknowledgements

This work was supported by grants from the Communauté Française de Belgique (Actions de Recherche Concertées 93/98-171 and 95/00-191), the CGER-Assurances and asbl VIVA 1993/1996 in Belgium, the Association contre le Cancer in Belgium, the Association Sportive contre le Cancer in Belgium, the Fonds de la Recherche Scientifique Médicale in Belgium (n° 3.4573.95), the Fonds National de la Recherche Scientifique – Televie in Belgium (n° 7.4568.95), the Centre Anticancéreux près l'Université de Liège in Belgium, the Fondation Léon Frédéricq, University of Liège, Belgium and a grant from Industry (Boehringer Mannheim GmbH, Penzberg, Germany).

References

1. Don Gambrell, R. (1987). Use of progestogen therapy. *Am. J. Obstet. Gynecol.*, **156**, 1304–13
2. Voigt, L. F., Weiss, N. S. and Stanford, J. L. (1996). Review of the epidemiologic data on hormone replacement therapy in relation to the risk of breast cancer. In Calvo, F., Crepin, M. and Magdelenat, H. (eds.) *Breast Cancer, Advances in Biology and Therapeutics*, pp. 321–7. (Montrouge: John Libbey Eurotext Ltd.)
3. Dupont, W. D. and Page, D. L. (1991) Menopausal estrogen replacement therapy and breast cancer. *Arch. Intern. Med.*, **151**, 67–72
4. Colditz, G. A., Hankinson, S. E., Hunter, D. J., Willett, W. C., Manson, J. E., Stampfer, M. J., Hennekens, C., Rosner, B. and Speizer, F. E. (1995). The use of estrogens and progestins and the risk of breast cancer in postmenopausal women. *N. Engl. J. Med.*, **332**, 1589–93
5. Nachtigall, M. J., Smilen, S. W., Nachtigall, R. D., Nachtigall, R. H. and Nachtigall, L. E. (1992). Incidence of breast cancer in a 22-year study of women receiving estrogen–progestin replacement therapy. *Obstet. Gynecol.*, **80**, 827–30
6. Palmer, J. R., Rosenberg, L., Clarke, E. A., Miller, D. R. and Shapiro, S. (1991). Breast cancer risk after estrogen replacement therapy: results from the Toronto Breast Cancer Study. *Am. J. Epidemiol.*, **134**, 1386–95
7. Yang, C. P., Daling, J. R., Band, P. R., Gallagher, R. P., White, E. and Weiss, N. S. (1992). Non contraceptive hormone use and risk of breast cancer. *Cancer Causes Control*, **3**, 475–9
8. Schuurman, A. G., van den Brandt, P. A. and Goldbohm, R. A. (1995). Exogenous hormone use and the risk of postmenopausal breast cancer: results from The Netherlands Cohort Study. *Cancer Causes Control*, **6**, 416–24
9. Newcomb, P. A., Longnecker, M. P., Storer, B. E., Mittendorf, R., Baron, J., Clapp, R. W., Bogdan, G. and Willett, W. C. (1995). Long term hormone replacement therapy and risk of breast cancer in postmenopausal women. *Am. J. Epidemiol.*, **142**, 788–95
10. Stanford, J. L., Weiss, N. S., Voigt, L. F., Daling, J. R., Habel, L. A. and Rossing, M. A. (1995). Combined estrogen and progestin hormone replacement therapy in relation to risk of breast cancer in middle-aged women. *J. Am. Med. Assoc.*, **274**, 137–42
11. Bergkvist, L., Adami, H. O., Persson, I., Hoover,

R. and Schairer, C. (1989). The risk of breast cancer after estrogen and estrogen–progestin treatment replacement. *N. Engl. J. Med.*, **321**, 293–7

12. Risch, H. A. and Howe, G. R. (1994). Menopausal hormone usage and breast cancer in Saskatchewan: a second record-linkage and cohort study. *Am. J. Epidemiol.*, **139**, 670–83

13. Persson, I., Yuen, J., Bergkvist, L., Adami, H. O., Hoover, R. and Schairer, C. (1992). Combined estrogen–progestogen replacement and breast cancer risk. *Lancet*, **340**, 1044

14. Ewertz, M. (1988) Influence of non contraceptive exogenous and endogenous sex hormones on breast cancer risks in Denmark. *Int. J. Cancer*, **42**, 832–8

15. Steinberg, K. K., Smith, S. J., Thacker, S. B. and Stroup, D. F. (1994). Breast cancer risk and duration of estrogen use: the role of study design in meta-analysis. *Epidemiology*, **5**, 415–21

16. Barrett-Connor, E. (1996). Hormones and heart disease and women. Presented at the 8th *International Congress on the Menopause*, Sydney, November, Abstract S57

17. Key, D. L. and Pike, M. (1988). The role of estrogens and progestogens in the epidemiology and prevention of breast cancer. *Eur. J. Cancer Clin. Oncol.*, **24**, 29–43

18. Going, J., Anderson, T. and Battersby, S. (1988). Proliferative and secretory activity in human breast during natural and artificial menstrual cycle. *Am. J. Pathol.*, **130**, 193–204

19. Vorherr, H. (1986). Fibrocystic breast disease: pathophysiology, pathomorphology, clinical picture, and management. *Am. J. Obstet. Gynecol.*, **154**, 161–79

20. Chang, K. J., Lee, T. T. Y., Linares-Cruz, G., Fournier, S. and de Lignières, B. (1995). Influences of percutaneous administration of estradiol and progesterone on human breast epithelial cell cycle *in vivo. Fertil. Steril.*, **663**, 785–91

21. Dietrich, D. R. (1993). Toxicological and pathological applications of proliferating cell nuclear antigen (PCNA), a novel endogenous marker for cell proliferation. *Crit. Rev. Toxicol.*, **23**, 77–109

22. Bravo, R., Frank, R., Bundell, P. A. and MacDonald-Bravo, H. (1987). Cyclin/PCNA is the auxillary protein of DNA polymerase-d. *Nature (London)*, **326**, 515–17

23. Barrat, J., de Lignières, B., Marpeau, L., Larue, L., Fournier, S., Nahoul, K., Linares, G., Giorgi, H. and Contesso, G. (1990). Effet *in vivo* de l'administration locale de progestérone sur l'activité mitotique des galactophores humains. *J. Gynécol. Obstét. Biol. Reprod.*, **19**, 269–74

24. King, R. J. B. (1991). A discussion of the roles of estrogen and progestin in human mammary carcinogenesis. *J. Steroid Biochem. Mol. Biol.*, **39**, 811–18

25. Going, J. J., Anderson, T. J., Battersby, S. and MacIntyre, C. C. A. (1988). Proliferative and secretory activity in human breast during natural and artificial menstrual cycles. *Am. J. Pathol.*, **130**, 193–203

26. Anderson, T. J., Battersby, S., King, R. J. B., McPherson, K. and Going, J. J. (1989). Oral contraceptive use influences resting breast proliferation. *Hum. Pathol.*, **20**, 1139–44

27. Meyer, J. S. (1977). Cell proliferation in normal human breast ducts, fibroadenomas, and other duct hyperplasias measured by nuclear labelling with tritiated thymidine: effects of menstrual phase, age, and oral contraceptive hormones. *Hum. Pathol.*, **8**, 67–81

28. Longacre, T. A. and Bartow, S. A. (1986). A correlation morphologic study of human breast and endometrium in the menstrual cycle. *Am. J. Surg. Pathol.*, **10**, 382–93

29. Potten, C. S., Watson, R. J., Williams, G. T., Tickle, S., Roberts, S. A., Harris, M. and Howell, A. (1988). The effect of age and menstrual cycle upon proliferative activity of the normal human breast. *Br. J. Cancer*, **58**, 163–70

30. McManus, M. J. and Welsch, C. W. (1984). The effect of estrogen, progesterone, thyroxine and human placental lactogen on DNA synthesis of human breast ductal epithelium maintained in athymic nude mice. *Cancer*, **54**, 1920–7

31. Mauvais-Jarvis, P., Kuttenn, F. and Gompel, A. (1986). Anti-estrogen action of progesterone in breast cancer. *Breast Cancer Res. Treat.*, **8**, 179–88

32. Botella, J., Duc, I., Delansorne, R., Paris, J. and Lahlou, B. (1989). Regulation of rat uterine steroid receptors by nomegestriol acetate, a new 19-nor-progesterone derivative *J. Pharmacol. Exp. Ther.*, **248**, 758–61

33. Jeng, M. H., Parker, C. J. and Jordan, V. C. (1992). Estrogenic potential of progestins in oral contraceptives to stimulate human breast cancer cell proliferation. *Cancer Res.*, **52**, 6539–46

34. Markiewicz, L., Hochberg, R. B. and Gurpide, E. (1992). Intrinsic estrogenicity of some progestagenic drugs. *J. Steroid Biochem. Mol. Biol.*, **41**, 53–8

35. Botella, J., Duranti, E., Viader, V., Duc, I., Delansorne, R. and Paris, J. (1994). Lack of estrogenic potential of progesterone or 19-nor-progesterone derived progestins as opposed to testosterone or 19-nor-testosterone derivatives on endometrial Ishikawa cells. *J. Steroid Biochem. Mol. Biol.*, **50**, 41–7

Hormone replacement therapy in women over 60: management of compliance

B. de Lignières

Introduction

Since the promised decrease in risk of fracture and vascular disease is observed exclusively in current estrogen users, compliance to hormone replacement therapy (HRT) must be improved primarily in women aged 60 years and more. In today's average situation only a very small selected group of women, likely to be the healthiest part of the population, remain compliant to HRT long enough to secure preventive benefits, while most women never use HRT or stop taking it after only a short time. Without striking improvements in the management of compliance in elderly women, therefore, the type of HRT currently prescribed today is not likely to be effective in preventive medicine.

Consistency of medical message

Recent epidemiological surveys show that at least 50% of postmenopausal women still never use HRT, even when they are nurses who have volunteered to participate in a menopause survey and likely to be better informed about the consequences of osteoporosis and vascular disease than the average population[1]. This suggests that the medical message about the benefits and risks of long-term HRT is far from being convincingly positive for many educated women. Some major inconsistencies prevent many potential users from sharing in the enthusiasm of the prescribers.

Epidemiological studies conducted in similar North American populations using the same kind of HRT, at the same doses and apparently using the same schedule, come to quite different conclusions regarding the relative risk of breast cancer[2–4]. This is the opportunity for women to discover that doctors have prescribed different doses and schedules of progesterone and synthetic progestins for decades without a precise knowledge of the consequences for breast or even for normal tissue in the short term[5], which is not exactly reassuring.

A 50% decrease in relative risk of almost all vascular events is enthusiastically promised to all HRT users, especially to those at high risk. However, more experts today conclude that no study is powerful enough to support this claim[7–9]. The largest observational surveys, comparing the small self-selected group of users to the large group of past or never users, find only a non-significant decrease in the risk of coronary events in women over 60 years[1] or even an increase[10,11], but a significant increase in idiopathic deep venous thromboembolism[12,13], pulmonary embolism[14] and also in ischemic strokes[1] or all strokes[10]. Then an increasing number of investigators come to the conclusion that the most popular oral route for estrogen administration may not be optimal because the pharmacological liver first-pass effect creates more side-effects (specifically on coagulation factors, triglycerides and low-density lipoprotein (LDL) particle size) than benefits, since the increase of high-density lipoprotein (HDL) cholesterol is far lower than expected[15–18]. The rising debate on the relative safety of oral and non-oral routes of administration for estrogen substitution is also not reassuring for the potential users of today.

Moreover, the use of the most popular formulation of synthetic progestin has recently been shown to consistently annihilate all the vascular benefits of estrogens in experimental and human studies[19-21]. So the usual recommendation, to improve the education of women in order to improve HRT compliance, seems difficult to follow until the major discrepancies in the education program are solved.

Clinical side-effects

Most studies show a large rate of drop-out during the first months of HRT even in volunteers having signed an informed consent to participate in a clinical trial, and therefore unlikely to have serious safety concerns *a priori*.

In one recent multicenter study[22] 1724 non-hysterectomized postmenopausal volunteers were randomized within five treatment groups all using conjugated equine estrogens 0.625 mg/day every day for 12 months, combined with various schedules and doses of medroxyprogesterone acetate (MPA). Only 972 (56%) completed the study while 44% discontinued. Several other studies show a similar rate of drop-out in volunteers, around 25% after 6 months and 40–60% after 12 months[23,24]. Occurrence of irregular bleeding seems to be the major reason to discontinue HRT in approximately 25% of the cases. A cyclic regimen of progestin is claimed to induce bleeding at time of withdrawal of the progestin. However, several studies conducted with MPA or norethisterone at various doses show that almost 50% of women actually bleed before the cylic withdrawal of the progestin[22-24]. A continuous combined regimen is claimed to induce amenorrhea in almost all users. However, around 50% of women experience some unpredicted bleeding episodes during the first 12 months of continuous combined regimens[22]. Some studies suggest that the incidence of 'irregular' bleeding decreases with time. One explanation for this may be related to the high rate of drop-out during the first year, likely to leave HRT users free of clinical side-effects available for study[25]. A second explanation is related to the possibility for patients involved in some studies to customize their HRT during the first months of treatment

in selecting their own individual optimal dosages[26,27]. Mainly because of large interindividual variability in bioavailability of both estrogens and progestins, no fixed dose and schedule is optimal for all individuals, and HRT must be customized instead of standardized to improve compliance[28].

Obviously the major influence on bleeding pattern comes from the progestin/estrogen combination method. The highest rate of cyclic bleeding (> 80% of cycles) is obtained with cyclic addition of a progestin to estrogen leaving an unopposed estrogen phase of more than 7 days per cycle. On the contrary, reducing or suppressing the unopposed estrogen phase reduces the incidence of cyclic bleeding and increases the incidence of amenorrhea to 60–95% of the cycles. However, the highest incidence of unscheduled (and unacceptable) bleeding is observed with a non-stop continuous combined regimen (25–40% of cycles)[22] while interruption of the progestin treatment for a few days each month is associated with a lower incidence (5–16% of cycles)[27]. These results may be explained by the regulation of vascular growth factors and progesterone receptors in endometrial stroma, but do not support the simplistic, exclusive 'withdrawal' explanation of bleeding[29].

Occurrence of irregular bleeding is not the only the reason to discontinue HRT and in hysterectomized volunteers a 30–40% rate of drop-out has been observed during a 24-month study[30]. Many clinical side-effects are related to an estrogen or estrogen/progestin combination unadapted to a single individual[31]. One of the most frequent and poorly tolerated is mastodynia, which is an unpleasant symptom raising anxiety about potential harmful effects of HRT on the breast. Its incidence increases with estrogen daily dose[32]. The incidence of other common symptoms such as asthenia, depressive mood, headache and back pain tend to increase with progestin daily dose[31]. Thus individual dose titration should be based first on clinical symptoms when they are clear enough, but this is not often the case in older women, who especially remain poorly symptomatic in a hypoestrogenic state.

Periodic evaluation

Since climacteric symptoms, bone loss and vascular risks are dissociated in a large number of individuals over the age of 60, it is not possible to assume that the lack of hot flushes, for example, indicates that the hormonal situation is optimal for the bone and vascular protection of one individual. A standardized dose of estrogen determined to induce a sufficient bone response in approximately 90% of users is likely to be excessive and to induce clinical side-effects in a large number of them[32]. On the contrary, a small dose determined to avoid clinical side-effects in 90% of users is likely to be ineffective for bone loss prevention in a large number of them. With the current estrogen dosages recommended by consensus conferences on osteoporosis, the percentage of users with suboptimal responses in bone is likely to reach 20–25%, but the percentage of patients with suboptimal clinical responses, likely to lead to drop-out, may reach 30–60%[32,33]. Obviously these number can only be decreased by an adequate flexibility in dose level based on some individual periodic evaluation.

Changes in urinary bone resorption markers are poorly correlated to bone protection in a single individual. Bone density measurements are more predictive but expensive, and do not deliver information fast enough. Regarding vascular risks, the predictive value of parallel increases in HDL cholesterol and triglycerides, decreases in LDL cholesterol and LDL particle size and increases in coagulation and fibrinolysis observed during oral estrogen regimens seems unreliable in animal studies and human surveys[16]. Therefore it seems desirable to try to follow estrogen replacement, as is done for thyroid replacement, with an easy and relatively cheap hormonal blood test. The reliability of periodic estradiol and estrone dosages can be greatly improved by careful selection of the appropriate assays and the use of flexible non-oral formulations, slowly releasing estradiol. According to available animal and human studies, estradiol and estrone levels around 80 pg/ml, similar to mid-follicular phase levels, are associated with optimal efficacy on bone and vessels, while inducing the lowest rate of clinical side-effects, even in women over 60[31]. The daily dose of estradiol required to reach these levels is quite variable in different individuals, and periodic serum controls may help to customize the dose. These controls also deliver to the patient objective evidence of the physiological level of the substitution, and improve long-term compliance.

Conclusion

To attain the promised benefits for bone and vascular diseases, compliance to HRT must be strikingly improved in women over 60. The worrying inconsistencies in evaluating the relative safety of various HRT formulations must be solved instead of denied. Doses should be customized instead of standardized, and identification of simple, cheap and reliable tools to periodically evaluate individual safety and efficacy is mandatory.

References

1. Grodstein, F., Stampfer, M. J., Manson, J. E. *et al.* (1996). Postmenopausal estrogen and progestin use and the risk of cardiovascular disease. *N. Engl. J. Med.*, **335**, 453–61
2. Colditz, G. A., Hankinson, S. E., Hunter, D. J. *et al.* (1995). The use of estrogens and progestins and the risk of breast cancer in postmenopausal women. *N. Engl. J. Med.*, **332**, 1589–93
3. Stanford, J. L., Weiss, N. S., Voigt, L. F. *et al.* (1995). Combined estrogen and progestin hormone replacement therapy in relation to risk of breast cancer in middle-aged women. *J. Am. Med. Assoc.*, **274**, 137–42
4. Risch, H. A. and Howe, G. R. (1994). Menopausal hormone usage and breast cancer in Saskatchewan: a record-linkage cohort study. *Am. J. Epidemiol.*, **139**, 670–83
5. Chang, K. J., Fournier, S., Lee, T. T. Y. *et al.* (1995).

Influences of percutaneous administration of estradiol and progesterone on human breast epithelial cell cycle *in vivo. Fertil. Steril.*, **63**, 785–91

6. Rossouw, J. E. (1996). Estrogens for prevention of coronary heart disease. *Circulation*, **94**, 2982–5

7. Sturgeon, S. R., Schairer, C., Brinton, L. A. *et al.* (1995). Evidence of a healthy estrogen user survivor effect. *Epidemiology*, **6**, 227–31

8. Matthews, K. A., Kuller, L. H., Wing, R. R. *et al.* (1996). Prior to use of estrogen replacement therapy, are users healthier than nonusers? *Am. J. Epidemiol.*, **143**, 971–8

9. Barrett-Connor, E. (1996). The menopause, hormone replacement, and cardiovascular disease: the epidemiologic evidence. *Maturitas*, **23**, 227–34

10. Wilson, P. W., Garrison, R. J. and Castelli, W. P. (1985). Postmenopausal estrogen use, cigarette smoking and cardiovascular morbidity in women over 50: the Framingham study. *N. Engl. J. Med.*, **313**, 1038–43

11. Psaty, B. M., Heckbert, S. R., Atkins, D. *et al.* (1993). A review of the association of estrogens and progestins with cardiovascular disease in postmenopausal women. *Arch. Intern. Med.*, **153**, 1421–7

12. Daly, E., Vessey, M. P., Hawkins, M. M. *et al.* (1996). Risk of venous thromboembolism in users of hormone replacement therapy. *Lancet*, **348**, 977–80

13. Jick, H., Derby, L. E., Myers, M. W. *et al.* (1996). Risk of hospital admission for idiopathic venous thromboembolism among users of post-menopausal oestrogens. *Lancet*, **348**, 981–3

14. Grodstein, F., Stampfer, M. J., Goldhaber, S. Z. *et al.* (1996). Prospective study of exogenous hormones and risk of pulmonary embolism in women. *Lancet*, **348**, 983–7

15. Moorjani, S., Dupont, A., Labrie, F. *et al.* (1991). Changes in plasma lipoprotein and apolipoprotein composition in relation to oral versus percutaneous administration of estrogen alone or in cyclic association with Utrogestan in menopausal women. *J. Clin. Endocrinol. Metab.*, **73**, 373–9

16. de Lignières, B. (1993). The case for a non plasma lipoprotein etiology of reduced vascular risk in estrogen replacement therapy. *Curr. Opin. Obstet. Gynecol.*, **5**, 389–95

17. Tikkanen, M. J. (1996). The menopause and hormone replacement therapy: lipids, lipoproteins, coagulation and fibrinolytic factors. *Maturitas*, **23**, 209–16

18. Writing Group for the PEPI Trial. (1995). Effects of estrogen or estrogen/progestin regimens on heart disease risk factors in postmenopausal women. *J. Am. Med. Assoc.*, **273**, 199–208

19. Clarkson, T. B., Anthony, M. S. and Klein, K. P. (1996). Hormone replacement therapy and coronary artery atherosclerosis: the monkey model. *Br. J. Obstet. Gynaecol.*, **103**, 53–8

20. Sullivan, J. M., Shala, B. A., Miller, L. A. *et al.* (1995). Progestin enhances vasoconstrictor responses in postmenopausal women receiving estrogen replacement therapy. *J. N. Am. Menopause Soc.*, **2**, 193–9

21. Giraud, G. D., Morton, M. J., Wilson, R. A. *et al.* (1996). Effects of estrogen and progestin on aortic size and compliance in postmenopausal women. *Am. J. Obstet. Gynecol.*, **174**, 1708–18

22. Archer, D. F., Pickar, J. H. and Bottiglioni, F. (1994). Bleeding patterns in postmenopausal women taking continuous combined or sequential regimens of conjugated estrogens with medroxyprogesterone acetate. *Obstet. Gynecol.*, **83**, 686–92

23. Habiba, M. A., Bell, S. C., Abrams, K. and Al-Azzawi, F. (1996). Endometrial responses to hormone replacement therapy: the bleeding pattern. *Hum. Reprod.*, **11**, 503–8

24. Saure, A., Hirvonen, E., Milsom, I. *et al.* (1996). A randomized, double-blind, multicentre study comparing the clinical effects of two sequential estradiol–progestin combinations containing either desogestrel or norethisterone acetate in climacteric women with estrogen deficiency symptoms. *Maturitas*, **24**, 111–18

25. Hillard, T. C., Siddle, N. C., Whitehead, M. I. *et al.* (1992). Continuous combined conjugated equine estrogen–progestogen therapy: effects of medroxyprogesterone acetate and norethindrone acetate on bleeding patterns and endometrial histologic diagnosis. *Am. J. Obstet. Gynecol.*, **167**, 1–7

26. Moyer, D. I., de Lignières, B., Driguez, P. and Pez, J. P. (1993). Prevention of endometrial hyperplasia by progesterone during long-term estradiol replacement: influence of bleeding pattern and secretory changes. *Fertil. Steril.*, **59**, 992–7

27. Gillet, J. Y., Andre, G., Faguer, B. *et al.* (1994). Induction of amenorrhea during hormone replacement therapy: optimal micronized progesterone dose. A multicenter study. *Maturitas*, **19**, 103–15

28. de Lignières, B. (1996). Estrogen replacement therapy must be customized. *Eur. Menopause J.*, **3**, 21–5

29. de Lignières, B. and Moyer, D. L. (1994). Influence of sex hormones on hyperplasia/carcinoma risks. In Lobo, R. A. (ed.) *Treatment of the Postmenopausal Woman: Basic and Clinical Aspects*, pp. 373–83. (New York: Raven Press)

30. Meade, T. W. (1996). Randomized comparison of oestrogen versus oestrogen plus progestogen

hormone replacement therapy in women with hysterectomy. *Br. Med. J.*, **312**, 473–8

31. de Lignières, B. (1996). Hormone replacement therapy: clinical benefits and side-effects. *Maturitas*, **23**, S31–6

32. Ettinger, B., Genant, H. K., Steiger, P. and Madvig, P. (1992). Low-dosage micronized 17β-estradiol prevents bone loss in postmenopausal women. *Am. J. Obstet. Gynecol.*, **166**, 479–88

33. Dupont, A., Dupont, P., Cusan, L. *et al.* (1991). Comparative endocrinological and clinical effects of percutaneous estradiol and oral conjugated estrogens as replacement therapy in menopausal women. *Maturitas*, **13**, 297–311

17

Towards better recognition of urogenital aging

The female perspective: women's attitudes towards urogenital aging 67

H. J. Wright

The experience of menopause varies from woman to woman and, like menstruation, it is surrounded by myths and misinformation. It often carries a cultural taboo and many women feel unable to discuss the menopause and its symptoms with their doctors, family or friends.

However, in recent years, the subject of menopause has made the front covers of *Vanity Fair* (October 1991), *Good Housekeeping* (January 1992) and *Newsweek* (May 25, 1992). Gail Sheehy wrote in *Vanity Fair* (1992) that the silence and the apprehension surrounding the subject in North America were mainly due to the phobia about aging. In a culture where desirability and youth go hand-in-hand, it is not surprising that menopause is a subject that causes embarrassment and shame. Women are judged by their physical appearance more than anything else, and with so much emphasis on beauty, fashion, figure and youth it is difficult for women to value themselves when they see their exterior aging.

There are signs that, in North America at least, attitudes are changing. In the past, relatively few women lived for many years after the menopause. Now, the majority of women live approximately one-third of their lives post menopause – perhaps 30 years (Figure 1)[1]. Many are determined to make the best of those years, and, especially in North America, are becoming more vocal and more visible than before.

While there is now more public emphasis on the varied experiences of women as they live through the perimenopausal phase, there is less discussion about the period after the acute symptoms have subsided, when the symptoms of urogenital aging are likely to arise. This paper will address some of the issues surrounding that

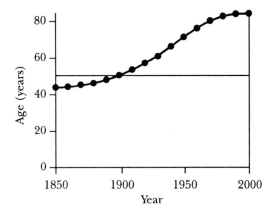

Figure 1 Age at menopause and life expectancy. Adapted from reference 1

postmenopausal phase, and in particular look at the attitudes of women in a number of European countries towards their symptoms. Mankowitz, a psychologist based in Canada who has studied the menopause, said[2],

'If the beginning of reproductive life is recognised as crucial, and if the fruits of reproductive life are celebrated, how can the ending of it not have deep meaning? There is a great need for the understanding and support of a life change as crucial as puberty or the first childbirth . . . Each woman's menopause, when she comes to it, is a deadly secret, can not be told, must be hidden away – got through as well as possible with nobody knowing.'

This feeling that women must hide their problems, not just during but after the menopause, is confirmed by research in Europe.

During consultation work for Pharmacia & Upjohn, Burson-Marsteller set up two focus groups in Denmark in 1995 to look at qualitative issues surrounding urogenital aging. One group consisted of women aged between 55 and 67; the second consisted of women aged 67–80. The focus groups lasted 3 h and consisted of a series of questionnaires and interviews. Half the participants were chosen at random and half were chosen because they recognized symptoms of, or were undergoing treatment for, postmenopausal hormone deficiency. Approximately one-half of the women were married or had a partner.

Responses in both groups were characterized by beliefs that were either handed down or traditional, to the effect that postmenopausal gynecological problems were either 'private matters' or 'something you have to sort out for yourself'. Other comments made included:

Women have always had problems, that's how it is.
Women have to make sure they keep going. Men don't understand what it's all about.
Problems related to and after the menopause are a woman's own problem.
You have to just get on with your work and forget about your problems.

Denmark is a country thought of as very 'open', with a relaxed attitude towards discussing matters such as sexuality. It was quite surprising, therefore, that modesty in both groups was so dominant and activated defence mechanisms to such an extent that the women tried to divert the conversation by all possible means, especially when discussing vaginal matters.

In both groups it was obvious that it was difficult to describe vaginal problems. Phrases such as 'down there', 'the womb', 'dryness' and 'when I'm with my husband' were commonly used. However, as the interview progressed and words like 'vagina' and 'sexual intercourse' were used by the interviewers, the participants themselves began to use the correct terminology and agreed that it was better to do so.

The women in the focus groups wanted to solve their problems, but in accordance with tradition, wanted to solve them by themselves. They felt intimidated and embarrassed when

too much attention was paid in relation to the menopause and were particularly reticent to questions about their sex lives.

The older age group took 30 min before taking an active part in the discussion, but once they started talking they were more open about their problems than the younger group. This may be because fewer of the older group were still sexually active and were therefore able to distance themselves from the problem, whereas the younger age group clearly found the problem closer to their daily life.

The conclusion from these focus groups was that dialog about gynecological problems was hard to establish. However, it is possible to establish dialog if the right amount of time is allowed in an atmosphere of mutual trust. Considering the brief amount of time a woman spends in consultation with her doctor and that many doctors, male or female, may be much younger than the patient, it is not surprising that many women do not feel able to talk to their doctors about their symptoms.

Another focus group set up by Burson-Marsteller in Sweden, also a country thought of as 'open', interviewed women between the ages of 60 and 70 years living in Stockholm. The study found urogenital problems among the women were considered personal, private and embarrassing, and affected self-confidence.

The women in this study were disappointed in their doctors and felt that they had received no information regarding the menopause. There was clearly a communication problem and the women felt unable to talk to their doctor, husband or friends. They were very aware of their doctor's lack of time, and tended to take a passive role during the consultation, trusting their doctor to make all the decisions.

The Farmland study[3], carried out in a small country settlement of Norway by the Norwegian Menopause Project, consisted of personal interviews with over 60 women of different ages, exploring beliefs and attitudes towards the menopause. The study showed that the women in the Farmland valley rarely talked to each other about the menopause; their knowledge about the menopause came only to a small extent from personal relationships with other women such as their mothers and female friends. Their main sources of information were women's magazines, books, radio and TV, reflecting a medical view based on experiences with patients.

Similar results were found by the Project group in Drammen and Oslo. These studies again highlight the unwillingness of women to discuss problems associated with the menopause, even with family and friends.

Unwillingness to discuss menopausal or postmenopausal symptoms is not confined to Scandinavian countries. In 1994 a study[4] was carried out on behalf of Pharmacia in six European countries to examine the perceived impact of symptoms of urogenital aging on quality of life. Data were collected from 3000 women between the ages of 55 and 75. The response rate from the study was 65% and results showed that the average proportion of women over 55 years of age who report symptoms of urogenital aging is 29%, with Italian women suffering the most problems (40%). Forty-eight per cent of affected women considered urogenital aging as only a minor problem, 22% found the problems irritating and 30% perceived their urogenital aging symptoms as strongly affecting their daily lives (Figure 2).

Although most of the women who reported an irritating urogenital aging problem which impacted on their daily life went to see their physician, 21% did not seek any help for it. French women were the most likely to regard their urogenital aging problems as embarrassing (44%): however, they discussed their problems most frequently and were the most active at seeking help. In comparison, only 7% of women in The Netherlands described their urogenital aging symptoms as embarrassing, and this figure was even lower in Denmark (2%). It is difficult to relate this to the findings from the Danish focus groups, but it suggests that even though a woman may not admit to being embarrassed by her symptoms, she may still regard them as private and personal – her own problem.

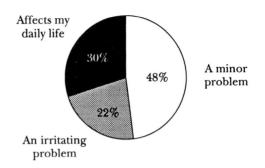

Figure 2 European study on prevalence of urogenital aging and its perceived impact on quality of life[4]

Approximately 67% of all the women in this study who had a partner did not believe that there was an age when they should stop having sex. It is difficult to persuade older people to talk about their sexuality, particularly women. There is a general belief in society that older people are, or should be, asexual and a false assumption exists that sexual desire and activity cease – or should cease – to exist at the onset of old age.

The pan-European urogenital aging study showed that 50% of women subjects had been in a sexual relationship in the year preceding the study, and of those that were sexually inactive, 63% were so because of the loss of their partner. In comparison, sexual inactivity due to the woman's loss of interest was reported by only 23% of women subjects. Male partners may also experience altered sexual responsiveness and diminished sexual desire, but it is easy to blame the postmenopausal woman for dysfunction and miss the problem in the male partner. Sarrel[5] found that in 25% of sexually dysfunctional postmenopausal couples the problems existed in the male.

A questionnaire-based study in The Netherlands of nearly 5000 women aged between 39 and 60, all of whom had a partner, compared women with a regular menstrual pattern to women with an irregular menstrual cycle in the preceding year[6]. Most of the women in both groups were sexually active and 84% of women who had not menstruated for at least 10 years still engaged in sex, with 34% enjoying sex most of the time and 60% reporting an absence of vaginal dryness or pain. However, there was a large decrease in the percentage of women reporting pleasure in sex most of the time, from over 70% of the regularly menstruating women to around 35% of women who had not menstruated for at least 10 years (Figure 3). This study did not look at the number of women who sought treatment, but there can be little doubt that in societies that regard sexuality as the prerogative of youth, many postmenopausal women will hesitate to ask their physicians about diminishing pleasure in sex.

The comments above have all related to Western attitudes and ideas. In Japan, there appears to be a similar reticence to discuss symptoms of urogenital aging, although menopause as the end of menstruation does not exist as such a clear-cut concept. *Konenki*, which is the closest equivalent to our use of the term menopause, is perhaps better translated as the rather outdated term 'change of life'. Some people in Japan believe it is a long gradual change lasting from the mid-30s to about 60 years, others that it lasts from about 45 to 55 or that it coincides with the end of menstruation and lasts 1 or 2 years at most. Japanese women rarely complain of the symptoms usually associated with menopause in the West, such as hot flushes and night sweats. Symptoms such as stiffness in the shoulders, headache, lumbago and constipation were the most common complaints in a survey of Japanese women between the ages of 45 and 55[7].

However, some Japanese doctors, at least[8], report that many of the women that present have sexual problems which they do not want to discuss directly:

> Since people in Japan traditionally haven't talked about sex, certainly not older people, they come and talk about other symptoms and no matter how many tests we do, we can't find anything wrong, but sometimes we can guess the problem is related to sex and give the women some counselling.

Another Japanese doctor quoted in the same work said that until recently, it was not possible

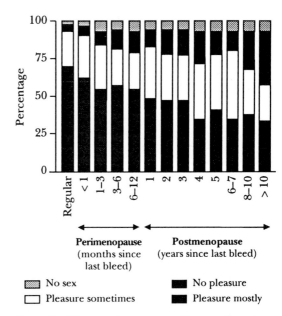

Figure 3 Pleasure in sex according to climacteric status in women with partner ($n = 4788$)[6]

for Japanese women to discuss the menopause at all and middle-aged women found it very hard to talk about it with a doctor:

> People who're in their fifties now are the ones who got their education during the war, they're in a sort of valley, cut off both from the people who are older and the younger ones. They're a very special generation, and they don't have anywhere to go with their problems.

Anthropologist Margaret Mead referred to the 'postmenopausal zest' many women feel once the acute changes of the menopause are over. It is tragic that many women may be prevented from realizing their potential and achieving the quality of life that could be theirs, through unwillingness to share their problems. Future generations of women may find it easier to discuss their symptoms. But in the meantime, there is a vast number of women who could be helped, if they could overcome the emotional and cultural barriers which presently inhibit them from seeking that help.

In Europe, certainly, but in other countries as well, doctors need to be better equipped to improve communication between themselves and their postmenopausal patients, recognizing that this is unlikely to happen in a short consultation. In particular, physicians need to 'ask the question', as many women will simply not raise the subject of urogenital symptoms without prompting, and indeed may need to be encouraged to talk about the subject at all.

In addition, there is a great need for women to be 'given permission' to discuss their problems, which, as it may conflict with deep-seated traditions and beliefs, is no easy task.

References

1. Cope (1976). Physical changes associated with the post-menopausal years. In Campbell, S. (ed.) *The Management of the Menopause and Postmenopausal Years*, p. 33. (Baltimore: University Park Press)
2. Mankowitz, A. (1984). *Change of Life: a Psychological Study of Dreams and the Menopause*, pp. 104–7. (Toronto: Inner City Books)
3. Holte, A. and Mikkelsen, A. (1981). Cultural myths and climacteric reaction: a small scale Norwegian study. Presented at *III International Congress on Menopause*, Ostende
4. Linde, M. (1995). A European survey of the perceived impact of urogenital ageing on quality of life. In Barlow, D. H. (ed.) *Towards Better Recognition of Urogenital Ageing*, pp. 15–20. (London: RSM Press)
5. Sarrel, P. (1987). Sexuality in the middle years. *Obstet. Gynecol. Clin. North Am.*, **14** (1), 49–62
6. Oldenhave, A. (1993). Some aspects of sexuality during the normal climacteric. In von Schoultz, B. (ed.) *Urogenital Aging*, pp. 15–26. (Carnforth, UK: Parthenon Publishing)
7. Lock, M. (1993). *Encounters with Ageing: Mythologies of Menopause in Japan and North America*, Ch. 1, p. 24. (University of California Press)
8. Lock, M. (1993). *Encounters with Ageing: Mythologies of Menopause in Japan and North America*, Ch. 10, pp. 268–72. (California: University of California Press)

Index